Gateway to Crack

GPAT

&

PHARMACY

Competitive Entrance Exams

25000+ Solved MCQs and Model Practice Paper

Gateway to Crack

GPAT

&

PHARMACY

Competitive Entrance Exams

25000+ Solved MCQs and Model Practice Paper

SERIES OF MCQS OF COMPLETE PHARMACY SYLLABUS USEFUL TO PREPARE FOR GPAT AND OTHER PHARMACY COMPETITION EXAMINATIONS PHARMACY COMPETITIONS & ENTRANCE EXAMINATIONS

Authors

DR. NEELESH MALVIYA

Dr. Rajiv Saxena, Mrs. Arti Majumdar, Dr. Kushagra Dubey, Dr. Tahir Nizami

Mrs. Ruchi Gupta, Mr. Anindya Goswami, Dr. Neelima Naneriya, Mr. Ankit Mangal

Ms. Priya Mourya, Mrs. Himani Singh, Ms. Vishakha Chauhan, Ms. Namrata Rathore

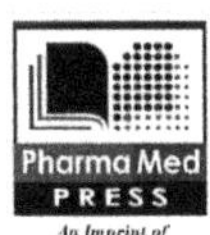

PharmaMed Press

An imprint of BSP Books pvt. Ltd

4-4-309/316, Giriraj Lane,

Sultan Bazar, Hyderabad - 500 095.

Gateway to Crack GPAT & PHARMACY Competitive Entrance Exams by ***Dr. Neelesh Malviya***

Disclaimer: The authors and the publishers have taken due care to provide the authentic, reliable and up to date information related to the subject. However, neither the authors nor the publisher shall be responsible for any liability for any damage caused as a result of use of this book. The respective user must check the accuracy from other sources too.

Published by:

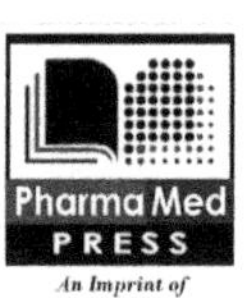

PharmaMed Press

An imprint of BSP Books Pvt. Ltd.

4-4-309/316, Giriraj Lane, Sultan Bazar, Hyderabad - 500 095.
Phone: 040-23445688; Fax: 91+40-23445611
e-mail: info@pharmamedpress.com
www.pharmamedpress.com/pharmamedpress.net

ISBN: 978-93-95039-15-4 (Hardback)

Contents

CHAPTER 1

Pharmaceutics

1. **How does the addition of magnesia and alumina affect soda lime glass?**
   A. Enhances mechanical strength
   B. Increases softening temperature
   C. Reduces porosity
   D. Improves chemical durability

2. **What are lead glasses used for?**
   A. Kitchenware
   B. Electronic tubes
   C. Optical components
   D. Temperature thermometers

3. **Which type of glass is regarded as the most heat resistant?**
   A. Fused silica B. 96% silica
   C. Alumino silicate D. Borosilicate

4. **What is 96% silica glass used for?**
   A. Heat shield
   B. Temperature thermometers
   C. Combustion tubes
   D. Electronic tubes

5. **Which of the following packaging material is protect the drug content against light ?**
   A. Plastic containers
   B. Amber coloured glass container
   C. Both
   D. None of the above

6. **Major Disadvantage of glass as a packaging material is:**
   A. Fragility B. Weight
   C. Both D. None of the above

7. **To produce molten glass, which of the following method is used**
   A. Blowing B. Pressing
   C. Drawing D. Casting

8. **Which of the following one is a broken glass & acts as fusion agent**
   A. Cullet B. Lime stone
   C. Soda Ash D. Sand

9. **Type I glass is also known as**
   A. Borosilicate glass
   B. Regular soda lime glass
   C. Treated soda lime glass
   D. None

10. **Which of the following test is performed on crushed grains, to evaluate the chemical resistance of glass?**
    A. Powder glass test
    B. Water attack test
    C. Both
    D. None

11. **The advantages of plastic containers over glass containers are**
    A. Easy formation
    B. Resistance to breakage
    C. Freedom of design
    D. All of the above

12. **To protect the contents of a bottle from the effects of sunlight by UV rays, which glass is used?**
    A. Amber glass B. Red glass
    C. Both D. None

13. **Soda ash also known as**
    A. Pure silica
    B. Lime stone
    C. Sodium carbonate
    D. Calcium carbonate

14. **Type NP glass is also known as**
    A. Borosilicate glass
    B. General purpose glass
    C. Soda lime glass
    D. Treated soda lime glass

15. Type III glass is also known as
A. Borosilicate glass
B. General purpose glass
C. Regular soda lime glass
D. Treated soda lime glass

16. Process of use of compressed air to form molten glass in the cavity of a metal mold is called
A. Drawing B. Casting
C. Blowing D. Pressing

17. The process in which molten glass is pulled through dies which shape the soft glass is called
A. Drawing B. Casting
C. Blowing D. Pressing

18. The process of production of glass containers which makes use of centrifugal force is called
A. Casting B. Drawing
C. Pressing D. Blowing

19. The process of production of glass containers which makes use of mechanical force is called
A. Casting B. Drawing
C. Pressing D. Blowing

20. The USP specifications for light resistance containers require the glass to provide protection against ....wavelength of light.
A. 7800-8000 angstroms
B. Below 1000 angstroms
C. 2900-4500 angstroms
D. None of the above

21. Test for evaluating chemical resistance described in NF
A. Powdered glass test
B. Water attack test
C. Both A and B
D. None

22. Water attack test is used only to evaluate
A. Borosilicate glass
B. General purpose glass
C. Regular soda lime glass
D. Treated soda lime glass

23. Powdered glass test is used only to evaluate
A. Borosilicate glass
B. Regular soda lime glass
C. Treated soda lime glass
D. All of above

24. Distilled water stored for one year in regular soda lime glass picks up to .... sodium hydroxide.
A. 10 to 15 ppm B. 40 to 50 ppm
C. 100 ppm D. None

25. Percentage of Boron in Type I borosilicate glass is approximately
A. 6% B. 10%
C. 17% D. 25%

26. Distilled water stored for one year in treated soda lime glass picks up to .... sodium hydroxide.
A. 0.5 ppm B. 5 ppm
C. 10 to 15ppm D. None

27. Weathering can be prevented by the use of
A. Commercial soda lime glass
B. De-alkalized soda lime glass
C. Regular soda lime glass
D. None

28. Sulphate bloom appears on treated soda lime glass due to deposition of
A. Alkali B. Acid
C. Sulphur D. None

29. The density of polyethylene is in the range
A. 0.91-0.96 B. 0.89-0.90
C. 1.09-1.14 D. None

30. Water absorption property is comparatively higher in case of which plastic
A. Low density polyethylene
B. High density polyethylene
C. Polypropylene
D. Polystyrene

31. **Permeability to water vapour is comparatively higher in case of which plastic**
A. Low density polyethylene
B. High density polyethylene
C. Polypropylene
D. Polystyrene

32. **Oxygen permeability to is comparatively lower in case of which plastic**
A. PVC
B. High density polyethylene
C. Polypropylene
D. Polystyrene

33. **Which of the following packaging material have very good resistance to acids?**
A. Nitrile polymers B. PVC
C. Polystyrene D. None of the above

34. **Which of the following packaging material have a good heat resistance?**
A. Low density polyethylene
B. High density polyethylene
C. Polypropylene
D. Polystyrene

35. **Which of the following plastic material cannot be stored at low temperature?**
A. PVC
B. Low density polyethylene
C. High density polyethylene
D. Polypropylene

36. **Which of the following packaging material has an excellent resistance to impact?**
A. Low density polyethylene
B. High density polyethylene
C. Styrene acrylonitrile
D. Polystyrene

37. **Which of the following plastic material has the highest unit cost**
A. Nitrile polymers
B. Low density polyethylene
C. High density polyethylene
D. Styrene acrylonitrile

38. **Density of polyethylene directly determines which property of the polymer**
A. Stiffness B. Stress cracking
C. Clarity D. All the above

39. **Dilauryl thiopropionate is used as**
A. Antioxidant B. Antistatic agent
C. Plasticizer D. Impact modifiers

40. **Polyethylene glycols in concentration range of 0.1% to 0.2% is used as**
A. Antistatic agent B. Antioxidant
C. Impact modifiers D. Plasticizer

41. **One of the drawback of polypropylene is**
A. Lack of clarity
B. Lack of acid resistance
C. Low melting point
D. It stress crack easily

42. **Dioctyl-tin mercaptoacetate is added to PVC with the purpose to prevent**
A. Yellowing when exposed to heat
B. Stress cracking
C. Water vapour permeation
D. None

43. **Tin compounds are added to PVC for the purpose of**
A. Antistatic agent B. Plasticizer
C. Impact modifiers D. Stabilizer

44. **Angiosarcoma is observed in some patient exposed to**
A. Vinyl chloride monomers
B. PVC
C. Polyethylene
D. None

45. **Impact resistance in PVC containers is found to be**
A. Increased on storage at low temperature
B. Not effected
C. Decreased on storage at low temperature
D. None of above

46. **The properties of polystyrene is**
A. High water vapour tranmission
B. Low resistance to impact
C. Low melting point
D. All the above

47. **To improve impact resistance and brittleness polystyrene is combine with**
A. Sulphur
B. Rubber and acrylic compounds
C. Tin
D. None of the above

48. High impact, super impact and inter-mediate impact are the classification of

A. Glass B. Polystyrene
C. Rubber D. None of the above

49. The properties of polyamide is

A. High oxygen impermeability
B. Low resistance to impact
C. High water vapour impermeability
D. All the above

50. Water vapor permeability of polyamide can be reduced by laminating it with

A. Polyethylene B. Polystyrene
C. Acrylic polymer D. None

51. Highest impact resistance is observed in which plastic

A. Polycarbonate B. Polystyrene
C. Polypropylene D. None

52. Which of the following plastics is set by FDA for food along with pharmaceutical packaging?

A. Acrylic Multipolymers
B. Polyvinyl Chloride
C. Polystyrene
D. None

53. Limit of acrylic monomer in Acrylic polymers is

A. Less than 0.3 ppm
B. Less than 15 ppm
C. Less than 20 ppm
D. Less than 11ppm

54. Allowable limits for migration of acylic monomer in food products is

A. Less than 10 ppm
B. Less than 20 ppm
C. Less than 0.3 ppm
D. Less than 0.5 ppm

55. Which of the following is an exampl of condensation polymer

A. Polystyrene
B. Polypropylene
C. Polyethylene terephthalate
D. None of above

56. Coextrusion technology may be used to increase

A. Barrier to moisture
B. Barrier to gas
C. Impact resistance
D. All of above

57. Transmission of gases, vapours or liquids through plastic packaging materials is called

A. Sorption B. Leaching
C. Chemical reaction D. Permeation

58. Permeation through plastic containers present problem to dosage forms which are sensitive to

A. Hydrolysis B. Oxidation
C. Both D. None

59. Migration of additives from plastic container to the formulation stored in it is termed as

A. Leaching B. Sorption
C. Permeation D. Chemical reaction

60. The process of removal of constituents from drug product by the packaging material is called as

A. Sorption
B. Leaching
C. Chemical reaction
D. Permeation

61. Factors influencing sorption from product are

A. Chemical structure
B. Temperature
C. Concentration of active ingredients
D. All the above

62. The physical and chemical alteration of the packaging material by the drug product is called

A. Chemical reactivity B. Leaching
C. Modification D. Sorption

63. Softening effect on polyethylene due to oils stored in it is an example of

A. Modification B. Leaching
C. Chemical reactivity D. Sorption

64. Main purpose of adding antimony to lead in the preparation of collapsible tubes is to
A. Enhances pliability
B. Increases malleability
C. Reduces porosity
D. Increase hardness

65. Main purpose of adding antimony to lead in the preparation of collapsible tubes is to
A. Enhances pliability
B. Increases malleability
C. Reduces porosity
D. Increase hardness

66. Which metal tube hardens on use and may develop leaks
A. Tin B. Lead
C. Aluminium D. None

67. Which is the most expensive metal used in the preparation of collapsible tubes?
A. Tin B. Lead
C. Aluminium D. Iron

68. Which material is used for linings in the preparation of metal collapsible tubes?
A. Wax
B. Phenolics
C. Epoxides and vinyls
D. All the above

69. Which of the following packaging material is used in the preparation of collapsible tubes?
A. Low density polyethylene
B. High density polyethylene
C. Polypropylene
D. All the above

70. Sideseamer is a machine which is used in the preparation of
A. Metal collapsible tube
B. Plastic collapsible tube
C. Laminated tube
D. None of the above

71. Press-on, roll-on, friction etc are the designs of:
A. Clo sures
B. Laminates
C. Metal collapsible tube
D. None of the above

72. The Owens-Illinois torque tester is used in the evaluation of:
A. Glass containers
B. Plastic containers
C. Metal containers
D. Plastic moulded closures

73. Facing material and backing are the part of:
A. Homogenous Liner
B. Rubber closure
C. Heterogenous Liner
D. None of the above

74. Cushioning and sealing properties of cap are provided by
A. Resilient backing
B. Facing material
C. Both the above
D. None of the above

75. The rubber polymers commonly used for rubber stoppers are:
A. Natural rubber B. Neoprene
C. Butyl rubber D. All the above

76. Sulphur is added in the manufacturing of rubber closures as
A. Vulcanizing agent B. Antioxidant
C. Accelerator D. Pigment

77. Zinc oxide is added in the manufacturing of rubber closures as
A. Vulcanizing agent B. Antioxidant
C. Accelerator D. Pigment

78. Phenolics are the example of
A. Thermosetting resins
B. Thermoplastics resins
C. Both the above
D. None of the above

79. Polystyrene is an example of
A. Thermosetting resins
B Thermoplastics resins
C. Both the above
D. None of the above

80. Which of the following is capable of meeting the requirements of tamper-resistance packaging as defined by FDA regulation 21 C.F.R. Parts 211, 314 and 700

A. Film wrappers B. Tape seals
C. Blister package D. All the above

81. End-folded and fin seal are the types of

A. Film wrappers B. Tape seals
C. Sealed cartons D. Blister package

82. Heat sealable acrylic coatings are applied to impart heat sealing characteristics to

A. Polypropylene B. Cellophane
C. Both D. None

83. Nitrocellulose is applied to cellophane to impart

A. Crystal clarity
B. Machinability
C. Heat sealable characteristic
D. None

84. Comparatively highest seal integrity is observed in

A. End-folded wrapper
B. Fin seal wrapper
C. Shrink wrapper
D. None

85. Which is an example of heat sealable material:

A. Polyethylene B. Surlyn
C. Nitrocellulose D. All the above

86. Polyvinylidene chloride laminations are available under the trade name of

A. Saran B. Aclar
C. Surlyn D. None of the above

87. Aclar is chemically

A. Poly vinyl chloride
B. Polyvinylidene
C. Polychlorotrifluroethylene
D. None of the above

88. Main purpose of applying saran and aclar laminates is to impart

A. Moisture resistance
B. Heat sealability
C. Tensile strength
D. None of the above

89. Ointment tubes are the example of:

A. Primary packaging system
B. secondary packaging system
C. tertiary packaging system
D. All the above

90. The container that protects the contents from extraneous solids and from loss of the article under ordinary or customary conditions of handling, shipment, storage and distribution, according to USP XXVII is called

A. Well closed container
B. Tight container
C. Hermatic container
D. Light resistant container

91. The container that is impervious to air or any other gas under ordinary or customary conditions of handling, shipment, storage and distribution, according to USP XXVII is called

A. Well closed container
B. Tight container
C. Hermetic container
D. Light resistant container

92. The container that protects the contents from contamination by extraneous liquid, solids or vapors and from loss of the article, and from efflorescence, deliquescence or evaporation under ordinary or customary conditions of handling, shipment, storage and distribution, according to USP XXVII is called

A. Tight container
B. Well closed container
C. Light resistant container
D. Hermetic container

93. According to IP 1996, official test for rubber closures are:

A. Fragmentation test
B. Self sealability test
C. Sterilization test
D. All the above

94. As per IP 1996, for fragmentation test number of vials taken initially is

A. 5 B. 8
C. 10 D. 12

95. As per IP 1996, for fragmentation test closures are pierced with the hypodermic needle

A. 21 SWG B. 1 SWG
C. 11 SWG D. 31 SWG

96. As per IP 1996, for fragmentation test closures are pierced with the 21 SWG hypodermic needle

A. 2 times B. 4 times
C. 6 times D. 10 times

97. As per IP 1996, for fragmentation test closures are pierced with the 21 SWG hypodermic needle 4 times and the liquid is passed through the filter with pore size of:

A. 0.45 μm B. 0.05 μm
C. 0.5 μm D. None

98. As per IP 1996, for fragmentation test closures are pierced with the 21 SWG hypodermic needle 4 times and the liquid is passed through the filter with pore size of 0.5 μm. The total number of fragments visible to naked eye should not be more than:

A. 5 B. 10
C. 15 D. None

99. As per IP 1996, for fragmentation test closures are pierced with the 21 SWG hypodermic needle 4 times and the liquid is passed through the filter with pore size of 0.5 μm. The total number of fragments of butyl rubber, visible to naked eye should not be more than:

A. 5 B. 10
C. 15 D. None

100. As per IP 1996, self sealability test for rubber closure is applicable for

A. Single dose containers
B. Multi dose containers
C. Both
D. None of the above

101. As per IP 1996, for Self sealability test number

A. 5 B. 10
C. 15 D. 20

102. As per IP 1996, for Self sealability test closures are pierced with the 21 SWG hypodermic needle

A. 2 times B. 5 times
C. 10 times D. 15 times

103. As per IP 1996, for Self sealability test closures are pierced with the 21 SWG hypodermic needle for 10 times and immersed in

A. 0.1% Methyl red
B. 0.1% Methyl orange
C. 0.1% Methylene blue
D. None

104. As per IP 1996, for Self sealability test closures are pierced with the 21 SWG hypodermic needle for 10 times and immersed in 0.1% methylene blue at the pressure of

A. 27 KPa B. 27 Pa
C. 30 KPa D. 30 Pa

105. Main constituent of non-stick coating is

A. Polytetrafluoroethylene
B. Polyethylene terephthalate
C. Polystyrene
D. Polypropylene

106. Mylar, Arnite, Impet and Rynite are the trade names of which poltmers

A. Polyethylene terephthalate
B. Polytetrafluoroethylene
C. Polypropylene
D. Polystyrene

107. Presently, Tinfoil is made up of

A. Tin B. Aluminium
C. Silver D. All the above

108. Putting a foil lid over the tray section and sealing it to the blister is called

A. Cold form foil blisters
B. Thermoformed blister
C. Tropicalised blister
D. None of above

109. When an aluminium based laminate film is pressed into a mold by means of a stamp so that aluminium is elongated and maintains the formed shape, the blister thus formed is called as

A. Cold form foil blisters
B. Thermoformed blister
C. Tropicalised blister
D. None of above

110. Pinholes are the characteristics feature of

A. Aluminium foil B. Glass
C. plastics D. None of above

111. Package integrity test on blister packages can be of

A. Destructive type
B. Non destructive type
C. Both the above
D. None

112. As per USP, for powdered glass test prepared glass specimen should be autoclaved to

A. 121oC for 30 minutes
B. 121oC for 60 minutes
C. 121oC for 15 minutes
D. None

113. As per USP, for powdered glass test prepared glass specimen after autoclaving are titrated with

A. 0.05 N Sulphuric acid
B. 0.05 N Nitric acid
C. 0.02 N Sulphuric acid
D. 0.02 N Nitric acid

114. As per USP Water attack test is carried out at

A. 100 oC
B. 121 oC
C. 27 oC
D. At room temperature

115. As per IP 1996, Leakage test for plastic container is carried out on how many containers?

A. 5 B. 10
C. 15 D. 20

116. As per IP 1996, for Water vopour permeability test for plastic containers for injectable preparations, the condition are:

A. 50 ± 5% at 20 to 25 oC
B. 60 ± 10% at 20 to 25 oC
C. 60 ± 5% at 20 to 25 oC
D. 60 ± 10% at 20 to 25 oC

117. As per IP 1996, for collapsibility test for plastic containers, the container should squeeze at least

A. 50% of its nominal content
B. 70% of its nominal content
C. 90% of its nominal content
D. 100% of its nominal content

118. Missing liner in closure is an example of

A. Critical defect B. Major defect
C. Minor defect D. None of above

119. Which type of defect makes the container unacceptable for use:

A. Class A B. Class B
C. Class C D. None of above

120. Pulping is the process of manufacture of:

A. Paper B. Glass
C. Rubber D. Plastic

121. Fourdrinier System is used for the manufacture of:

A. Glass B. Paper
C. Plastic D. Rubber

122. The finishing process in the manufacture of paper is done by applying a solution of gelatin to the paper is called:

A. Finishing B. Glazing
C. Tub-sizing D. None of above

123. Which of the following is the process of surface treatment for paper:

A. Cloaking
B. Impregnations
C. Laminations
D. All of above

124. Cobb test is used for testing which of the following:

A. Paper and Board B. Glass
C. plastics D. Aluminium foil

125. Flute sizes A, B, C, D, E and F are in the manufacture of

A. Capsule B. Ampoule
C. Corrugated board D. None of the above

126. TAPPI and ASTM test methods are used for the evaluation of

A. Corrugated board B. Plastic containers
C. Rubber closures D. None of the above

127. Biochemical and physiological effects of the drug and its mechanism of action is studied in the

A. Pharmaceutical Phase
B. Pharmacokinetic Phase
C. Pharmacodynamic Phase
D. Therapeutic Phase

128. Designing of proper dosage regimen is very tedious process for

A. Drugs having low therapeutic index
B. All Drugs
C. Drugs having high therapeutic index
D. Less potent drugs

129. Rapid absorption of lipid-soluble drugs can be achieved by ....

A. Intravenous route
B. Subcutaneous route
C. Intramuscular route
D. Sublingual route

130. Molecular weight of drug is an important criteria for the drug delivery through

A. Intravenous route
B. Oral route
C. Subcutaneous route
D. Transdermal route

131. Lowest degree of variation in the rate of absorption has been observed in ...

A. Intravenous route
B. Inhalation
C. Oral route
D. Transdermal route

132. Aqueous filled pore are present in cell membrane structure allowing inorganic ions and some organic molecules have diameter of ...

A. 40-100 Å B. 40-100 μm
C. 40-100 nm D. None of above

133. Core of phospholipids in cell membrane is.

A. Hydrophilic B. Hydrophobic
C. Amphillic D. None of above

134. Active and passive processes are the major transport mechanism in case of

A. Transcellular absorption
B. Corpuscular absorption
C. Paracellular absorption
D. None of above

135. Compounds of high molecular weight even above 16,000 can be well absorbed by

A. Splanchnic Circulation
B. Lymphatic Circulation
C. First-pass effect
D. None of above

136. Pharmacokinetics can be defined as:

A. The study of biological and therapeutic effects of drugs
B. The study of absorption, distribution, metabolism and excretion of drugs
C. The study of mechanisms of drug action
D. The study of methods of new drug development

137. The preferable mechanism of absorption for most of drugs in GI tract is:

A. Active transport or carrier-mediated diffusion
B. Filtration or aqueous diffusion
C. Passive diffusion or lipid diffusion
D. Endocytosis and exocytosis

138. Which of the following substances cannot permeate cell membranes by passive diffusion?

A. Unionized substances
B. Lipid-soluble
C. Hydrophobic substances
D. Hydrophilic substances

139. Drugs with lower value of partition coefficient (Ko/w) has the following property:

A. Lower rate of permeation through the lipidic cell membrane
B. Permeation through cell membrane by means of endocytosis
C. Easy permeation through the blood-brain barrier
D. High reabsorption in renal tubules

140. Which is the characteristic of active transport:

A. transport of drug particle by a cell membrane with a new vesicle formation

B. Transport against the concentration gradient

C. Transport of drugs through a membrane by means of diffusion

D. Transport without energy consumption

141. "Bioavailability" may be define as?

A. Fraction of an uncharged drug reaching the systemic circulation following any route of administration

B. Amount of a substance in urine relative to the initial dose

C. Permeability through the brain-blood barrier

D. Degree of plasma protein binding of drug substance

142. The main objective for the determination of bioavailability is to study:

A. Extent of absorption and hepatic first-pass effect

B. Rheological parameters of blood

C. Amount of a substance obtained orally and quantity of intakes

D. Glomerular filtration rate

143. Minimum first pass metabolism is observed in which of the following alimentary routes of administration:

A. Oral B. Transdermal

C. Rectal D. Intraduodenal

144. Highest first-pass effect is observed in which route of drug administration:

A. Intravenous route B. Sublingual

C. Oral D. Intramuscular

145. Characteristic feature of the oral route is:

A. Fast onset of effect

B. The sterilization of medicinal forms is obligatory

C. Absorption depends on GI tract secretion

D. A drug reaches the blood bypassing the liver

146. Characteristic feature of the sublingual route:

A. A drug is exposed to gastric secretion

B. Fast absorption

C. A drug is exposed more prominent liver metabolism

D. A drug can be administered in a variety of doses

147. Which of the following is the parenteral route of medicinal agent administration:

A. Rectal B. Sublingual

C Oral D. Inhalation

148. Characteristic feature of parenteral administration is that:

A. It cannot be used with unconsciousness patients

B. It usually produces a more rapid response than oral administration

C. It generally results in a less accurate dosage than oral administration

D. It is too slow for emergency use

149. Characteristic feature of the intramuscular route of drug administration:

A. Only water solutions can be injected

B. Opportunity of hypertonic solution injections

C. Oily solutions can be injected

D. The action develops slower, than at oral administration

150. Drugs poses difficulty in crossing brain-blood barrier due to:

A. Absence of pores in the brain capillary endothelium

B. High octanol- water partition coefficient of a drug

C. Prominent endocytotic nature of the brain capillaries

D. Meningitis and other inflamed conditions of brain

151. Urinary flow rate often affects the excretion of compounds

A. Whose tubular reabsorption is pH sensitive

B. Whose tubular reabsorption is not affected by pH

C. Whose tubular reabsorption is absent

D. Like strong acids and strong bases

152. Which of the following substances cannot permeate cell membranes by passive diffusion?

A. Unionized substances
B. Lipid-soluble
C. Hydrophobic substances
D. Hydrophilic substances

153. Drugs having pKa values 4-6 are:

A. Weak bases B. Strong bases
C. Weak acids D. Strong acids

154. Reabsorption of acidic drugs having pKa values more than 8

A. Does not occurs
B. Occurs at all urinary pH values
C. Occurs at low urinary pH values
D. Occurs at high urinary pH values

155. Reabsorption of acidic drugs having pKa values less than 2

A. Does not occurs
B. Occurs at all urinary pH values
C. Occurs at low urinary pH values
D. Occurs at high urinary pH values

156. Reabsorption of weakly basic drugs having pKa values 6 or below

A. Does not occurs
B. Occurs at all urinary pH values
C. Occurs at low urinary pH values
D. Occurs at high urinary pH values

157. Susceptibility to interference by metabolic or competitive inhibitors is the characteristic feature of

A. Active transport
B. Filtration
C. Passive diffusion
D. Endocytosis and exocytosis

158. Permeability constant is independent of:

A. Diffusion coefficient of the drug through the membrane
B. Membrane thickness
C. Partition coefficient of the drug between membrane and donor medium
D. Surface area of membrane

159. Under Biopharmaceutics Classification System drugs are classified on the basis of:

A. Intestinal permeability of drugs
B. Solubility of drugs
C. Both the parameters
D. None of the above

160. A drug with high solubility and high permeability is classified as

A. BCS Class I drug
B. BCS Class II drug
C. BCS Class III drug
D. BCS Class IV drug

161. A drug with low solubility and low permeability is classified as

A. BCS Class I drug
B. B CS Class II drug
C. BCS Class III drug
D. BCS Class IV drug

162. A drug with high solubility and low permeability is classified as

A. BCS Class I drug
B. BCS Class II drug
C. BCS Class III drug
D. BCS Class IV drug

163. A drug with low solubility and high permeability is classified as

A. BCS Class I drug B. BCS Class II drug
C. BCS Class III drug D. BCS Class IV drug

164. Which statement is correct in context to Absolute solubility and Dissolution rate:

A. Both are static process
B. Both are dynamic process
C. Absolute solubility is a static process while Dissolution rate is a dynamic process
D. None of above

165. In vivo dissolution rate is always .... than in vitro dissolution rate

A. Lesser B. Greater
C. Similar D. None of above

166. Which of the following equations accounts for change in surface area accompanying dissolution

A. Noyes – Whitney's Equation
B. Fick's law
C. Hixson Crowell cube root law of dissolution
D. None of above

167. In case of carrier mediated transport, the area in which the carrier system is most dense is called

A. Absorption window
B. Carrier window
C. Diffusion window
D. None of above

168. The oesophageal transit of most of the dosage forms is of order of

A. 10-15 minutes B. 4-5 minutes
C. 1-2 minutes D. 10-15 seconds

169. Pepsin is denatured at pH

A. 1-2 B. 3-4
C. 4-5 D. 6-7

170. The controlling factor in the onset of drug absorption from the small intestine is

A. Rate of drug dissolution
B. Rate of gastric emptying
C. Rate of chewing
D. None of above

171. Small intestine is an excellent site of absorption due to the presence of

A. Folds of Kerckring B. Villi
C. Microvilli D. All of above

172. Which of the phase of gastric emptying process is called housekeeper wave

A. Phase I B. Phase II
C. Phase III D. Phase IV

173. Blood flow to gastrointestinal tract is and liver is

A. Increased after meals
B. Decreased after meals
C. Not affected by the meals
D. None of above

174. In which transport mechanism, no further increase in rate of absorption is observed at higher concentrations

A. Passive process
B. Active process
C. First-pass effect
D. None of above

175. Vitamin A, D, E and K are mainly absorbed by

A. Endocytosis B. Pinocytosis
C. Facilitated diffusion D. Phagocytosis

176. Polio and other vaccines administered orally are mainly absorbed through the process of

A. Pinocytosis B. Endocytosis
C. Phagocytosis D. Facilitated diffusion

177. The process by which the material is internalised by the membrane is transported through the cell and is secreted on the other side is called

A. Pinocytosis B. Endocytosis
C. Phagocytosis D. Transcytosis

178. The molecular weight cut off for paracellular route is

A. 200 Da B. 400 Da
C. 700 Da D. 50 Da

179. The most common example of counter transport efflux protein that is responsible for expelling specific drugs back into the lumen of gastrointestinal tract is

A. Albumin B. P- glycoprotein
C. Globulin D. None of the above

180. Bioavailability of drugs which are unstable in gastric fluids can be

A. Increased on reducing particle size
B. Decreased on reducing particle size
C. Remain uneffective on reducing particle size
D. None of the above

181. Some drugs particularly those that are of hydrophobic in nature dry particle size reduction techniques

A. Result in aggregation of particles
B. Result in enhanced bioavailability
C. No effect on bioavailability
D. Result in increase in effective surface area

182. A strongly basic salt of a weakly acidic drug is expected to give

A. More absorption from git than free acid form
B. Less absorption from git than free acid form
C. Similar absorption from git than free acid form
D. None of the above

183. A strongly acidic salt of a weakly basic drug is expected to give
A. More absorption from git than free acid form
B. Less absorption from git than free acid form
C. Similar absorption from git than free acid form
D. None of the above

184. Solubility of sulphate salt of a drug is
A. Equal to its hydrochloride salt in git
B. More than its hydrochloride salt in git
C. Less its hydrochloride salt in git
D. None of the above

185. The inclusion of basic excipients in the formulation of aspirin tablet can
A. Enhance dissolution and bioavailability
B. Reduce dissolution and bioavailability
C. Not alter dissolution and bioavailability
D. None of the above

186. Higher bioavailability is observed in case of
A. Stable polymorphs
B. Metastable polymorphs
C. Unstable polymorphs
D. All the above

187. In ancient time dried animal parts, herbs, plant parts, honey and minerals were used as:
A. Food source B. Dentifrices
C. Vehicles D. Non of above

188. Abrasives, Detergent, Flavours are the ingredients of:
A. Face wash B. Cream
C. Tooth pest D. Soap

189. Hardness of an abrasive used in tooth pest preparation is depends on
A. Partial size B. Chemical nature
C. Impurities D. Both A and C

190. The amount of an abrasive should be .... Of total weight of tooth pest.
A. 50% B. 70%
C. 30% D. 80%

191. Most commonly used abrasive is:
A. Aluminium sulphate
B. Calcium carbonate
C. Magnesium trisilicate
D. Dicalcium phosphate

192. Calcium carbonate imparts........... To the rooth pest preparation
A. Acidity B. Alkalinity
C. Both D. No one

193. .... Is the native form of raw calcium carbonate
A. Stone B. Sand
C. Chalk D. Clay

194. Dicalcium phosphate imparts........... PH in the tooth pest preparation.
A. Acidic B. Neutral
C. Basic D. All of above

195. Hydrated magnesium silicate is used as an abrasive and...........
A. Antacid B. Laxatiive
C. Purgative D. Anti emetic

196. Most commonly used detergent is:
A. Sodium lauryl sulfate
B. Magnesium lauryl sulfate
C. Diethyl sodium lauryl sulphosuccinate
D. All of above

197. The higher amount of humectant in a tooth paste formulation is:
A. 10% B. 20%
C. 30% D. 40%

198. The actual amount of humectant in a tooth paste formulation is decided by
A. Viscosity B. Density
C. Molecular weight D. All of above

199. In which concentration binding agents are used:
A. 1-2.5 B. 1-2
C. 1-3 D. 1-1.5

200. To prevent the formation of lumps in a tooth paste formulation what is added:
A. Glycerin B. Alcohol
C. Tragacanth D. Both A and B

201. Mucilages of chondrus and Irish moss is Incorporated in a tooth paste formulation as a:
A. Detergent B. Binding agent
C. Humectant D. Flavours

202. Sodium saccharine is used in .... In tooth paste

A. 0.05 to 0.1 B. 0.05 to 0.23
C. 0.05 to 0.31 D. 0.05 to 0.38

203. .... Is a sweetening agent which is band due to its toxicity.

A. Cyclamate B. Sucrose
C. Maltose D. None of above

204. Cinnamon oil, clove oil, peppermint oil, cassia oil are used in a tooth paste as :

A. Sweetening agent B. Flavours
C. Both A and B D. No one

205. Which is used as a bleaching agent in tooth paste

A. Sodium benzoate
B. Sodium perborate
C. Sodium selisylate
D. Sodium carbonate

206. What can be used in a tooth paste for halitosis:

A. Carbohydrates B. Chlorophyll
C. Starch D. Resins

207. Which part of a teeth does not contain living cells but is like bone

A. Enamel B. Dentine
C. Cementum D. All of above

208. The periodontal ligament is made up of:

A. Collagen fibers B. Elastic fibers
C. Lignin fiber D. None of above

209. The outer layer of teeth enemal is made up of

A. Calcium carbonate
B. Calcium citrate
C. Calcium phosphate
D. Calcium gluconate

210. The hardest biologically substance is

A. Bone B. Muscle
C. Dentine D. Nail

211. Which glycoprotein is responsible for the lubrication action of the saliva:

A. Albumin B. Casin
C. Mucin D. Muceins

212. 75% of saliva is secreted by

A. Submandibular gland
B. Parotid gland
C. Sublingual
D. All of above

213. Which immunoglobulin is present in saliva for control of bacteria:

A. Ig G B. Ig A
C. Ig E D. Ig B

214. The bacteria responsible for pulpits is

A. Acne vulgeris B. S. Mutans
C. B. Vulgeris D. E. Coli

215. Sodium lauryl sarcosinate is used as:

A. Anti - cariogenic
B. Anti - enzyme
C. Bacteriostatic
D. Bacteriostatic

216. Which one combines with tooth enamel and form insoluble tin oxide to prevent pith decay:

A. Stannous chloride
B. Strontium chloride
C. Stannous fluoride
D. All of above

217. In the manufacturing of tooth powder the mixer is used:

A. Ribbon type B. Agitator type
C. Sigma type D. Both A and B

218. What is the percentage of the soap in soap containing solid dental products:

A. 20-30% B. 20-40%
C. 20-50% D. 20-60%

219. Evaluation parameters for a tooth paste is:

A. Abrasiveness
B. Limit test of arsenic and lead
C. Consistency
D. All of above

220. A good mouthwash should have

A. Quick antiseptic action
B. Sweet taste
C. Non irritant
D. All of above

221. Mouthwashes are .... Solutions which are used in oral cavity.

A. Acidic B. Alcoholic
C. Basic D. None of above

222. In a mouthwash preparation, phenol is used as:
A. Antiseptic B. Flavour
C. Astringent D. All of above

223. In which concentration the chlorothymol is used in a mouth wash preparation
A. 0.1-1% B 0.3-0.5%
C 0.05-0.1% D 0.05-0.3%

224. The quaternary ammonium compounds are active at which pH
A. Acidic B. Basic
C. Neutral D. All of above

225. Tincture of cinchona, benzoin tincture are Incorporated in a mouthwash for:
A. Astringent B. Stimulant
C. Flavouring agent D. All of above

226. Which is used am a vehicle in mouthwash
A. Alcohol
B. Water
C. Alcohol and water in combination
D. None of above

227. Glycerin is Incorporated in a mouthwash preparation for
A. Sweetening agent B. Flavor
C. Demulcent D. All of above

228. Which instrument is used to detect the deodorizing effect of mouthwash:
A. Gas chromatograph
B. Fair-wells osmoscope
C. Both A and B
D. None of above

229. What is evaluation parameters fir mouthwash:
A. Spreadability B. Dilution test
C. Burning test D. None of above

230. Deodorizing effect of mouthwash is done by:
A. Chemical analysis B. Surface tension
C. Physical analysis D. All of above

231. The essential growth factor or component of nails are:
A. Amino acids
B. Vitamins
C. Essential fatty acids
D. All of above

232. Eponychium is formed by the extension of a portion of..............of the nail root.
A. Stratum corneum
B. Stratum granulosam
C. Stratum spinosam
D. Stratum germilative

233. The pale crescent produced by abscured blood vessels near the nail root is called:
A. Hyponychium B. Lunula
C. Eponychium D. None of above

234. In AIDS, Thyroid and Respiratory disease diagnosis which colour of nail is a indication:
A. Red B. Black
C. Yellow D. None of above

235. In .... the nail may become pitted and distorted.
A. Geridiasis B. Trichomoniasis
C. Vaginitis D. Psoriasis

236. The content of water water in nail is:
A. 10-15% B. 10-12%
C. 12-14% D. 14-18%

237. Leukonychia is disorder of:
A. Hair B. Nail
C. Skin D. Teeth

238. Brittleness of nail is caused by:
A. Anaemia B. Avitaminosis
C. Both A and B D. None of above

239. Which is not a characteristic of a good nail lacquer:
A. Good gloss B. Good adhesion
C. Good cleansing D. Quick drying

240. In an Nail preparation Nitrocellulose, ethyl cellulose, methacrylate and vinyl resin are used for the purpose of
A. Solvent
B. Resin
C. Film forming substance
D. Pigments

241. Nitrocellulose film is better in terms of:
A. Toughness
B. Hardness
C. Low solvent retention
D. All of above

242. **Modified resin is used along with nitrocellulose to overcome the:**
A. Poor adherence B. Poor gloss
C. None of obove D. Both A and B

243. **Presently used resin in an Nail preparation is:**
A. Gum damar
B. Sulphonamide - formaldehyde resin
C. Gum copal
D. Shellac

244. **Polyvinyl acetate, Epoxy ester, coumaron inden polymer is used as:**
A. Resin B. Solvent
C. Film former D. Colours

245. **Ether, Acetone, Benzen and toluene is used as ....n an Nail preparation.**
A. Solvent B. Diluent
C. Plasticizer D. Colours

246. **Diluents are Incorporated in an Nail preparation to**
A. Stabilize the viscosity
B. Solubilization of resin
C. Better effect on enamel
D. All of above

247. **Non solvent plasticizer act as .... In the Nail paint preparation.**
A. Softener B. Filmformer
C. Both D. None of above

248. **The total percentage of plasticizer in nail preparation is**
A. 2% B. 5%
C. 8% D. 10%

249. **Which is a plasticizer**
A. Urea derivative B. Resorcinol
C. Castor oil D. All of above

250. **.................% of titanium dioxide or lithopone is Incorporated in nail preparation to achieve opacity.**
A. 2% B. 4%
C. 5% D. 7%

251. **In an Nail preparation to obtain brown and tan shades what is used:**
A. Iron sulfate
B. Copper sulfate
C. Magnesium oxide
D. Iron oxide

252. **Nacreous pigment used to impart .... Appearance.**
A. Iridescent B. Gold
C. Silver D. Creamy

253. **Acetone, ethyl acetate, and toluene applied on nail as a**
A. Detergent B. Perfume
C. Lacquer remover D. All of above

254. **To overcome the unpleasant odour of lacquer what is added into it:**
A. Orang oil B. Terpenes
C. Terpienol D. All of above

255. **What is evaluation parameters for Nail lacquer:**
A. Drying rate B. Hardness
C. Viscosity D. All of above

256. **Which is not an auxiliary productor nails:**
A. Nail cream B. Nail bleach
C. Nail lacquer D. Nail whitener

257. **In cutical Softener the concentration of Quaternary ammonium compounds is**
A. 3-5% B. 3-10%
C. 3-15% D. 3-20%

258. **In cutical Softener for swelling of keratin and softening of cutical what is used:**
A. Quaternary ammonium compounds
B. Urea
C. Lanolin
D. None of above

259. **Potassium hydroxide is used as .... In Nail care preparation.**
A. Cutical Softener B. Cutical remover
C. Both D. None of above

260. **What is Incorporated in cutical remover to counteract the irritation coused by alkali.**
A. Humectant B. Disinfectant
C. Acidifier D. All of above

261. **What type of preparation is used to remove the nail strains and to discoloration of nail.**
A. Cutical remover B. Nail paint
C. Nail bleaches D. All of above

262. Oxidizing agents used for bleaching of nail is
A. Hydrogen peroxide
B. Sodium perborate
C. Both
D. None of above

263. Population density of normal adult scalp hair is:
A. 225 hair cm square
B. 335 hair cm square
C. 445 hair cm square
D. 555 hair cm square

264. which part of body hairs have highest rate of growth
A. Scalp B. Chin
C. Eyelashes D. Both A and B

265. The per day growth of hair on scalp is:
A. 0.25 - 0.42 mm per day
B. 0.27 - 0.40 mm per day
C. 0.32 - 0.51mm per day
D. 0.34 - 0.38 mm per day

266. Carbon, nitrogen, phosphorus, and sulfur are responsible for .... Of hair.
A. Red B. Brown
C. Grey D. white

267. What is present in more quantity in red hair
A. Iron B. Sulfur
C. Phosphorus D. Carbon

268. A good shampoo have characteristics like
A. Removal of wast substance
B. Produce sof, lustrous hair
C. Imparts fragrance
D. All of above

269. What is main component of shampoo:
A. Surfactant B. Sequestrant
C. Pearlscent agents D. All of above

270. Which type of surfactant are used in shampoo
A. Cationic B. Anionic
C. Ampholytic D. All of above

271. What is used as principal surfactant:
A. Anionic surfactant
B. Non ionic surfactant
C. Cationic surfactant
D. Ampholytic surfactant

272. What is widely used for anionic surfactant in shampoo
A. Alkyl sulphates
B. Alkyl glycol sulphates
C. Both
D. None of above

273. Alkyl sulphonate are formed of catalytic reduction of fatty acid of..............
A. Coconut B. Butter
C. Soya D. All of above

274. Which is not an example of anionic surfactant:
A. Sodium lauryl sulfate
B. Triethanol
C. Methyl taurides
D. Monoethanol

275. Which one is used in powder sampoos because of less hygroscopicity:
A. Sodium lauryl sulfate
B. Magnesium lauryl sulfate
C. Monoethanol lauryl sulfate
D. Ammonium lauryl sulfate

276. Methyl taurides is .... type of surfactant
A. Anionic B. Cationic
C. Non ionic D. Amphoteric

277. In sodium lauryl sulfate, monoethanolamides are added to increase:
A. Viscosity B. Solubility
C. Density D. All of above

278. Mono alkyl sulphosuccinates are non irritant to eyes thus may be used in:
A. Hair shampo B. Body shampo
C. Both D. None of above

279. Methyl taurides leave the gairon excellent condition because of the presence of:
A. Amide group B. Ether group
C. Ester group D. All of above

280. Acyl sarcosins contain CON group and have conditioning effect and used along with:
A. Alkyl nitrates B. Alkyl carbonates
C. Alkyl sulphates D. Alkyl acetates

281. Which one of this is used in oil shampoo to form a light coating:
A. Turkey red oils B. Turkey green oil
C. Turkey clean oil D. All of above

282. Benzalkonium chloride is Incorporated in a shampoo preparation as a:
A. Detergent
B. Anti-dandruff
C. Conditioning agent
D. Thickening agent

283. Which one is a phenol derivative used as Germicide in a shampoo preparation?
A. Benzalkonium chloride
B. Cadmium sulphide
C. Sodium sulphacitamide
D. Tetramethyl thiuram sulphide

284. Which one of this a Anti dandruff agent:
A. Selenium sulphide
B. Sulphonated caster oil
C. Methyl cellulose
D. All of above

285. Conditioning agents are fatty acid substance like:
A. Lanolin B. Oils
C. Amino acids D. All of above

286. What is the PH rang at which pearlscent agents show their better action:
A. 4-5 B. 4.5-5
C. 5-6 D. 5.5-6

287. What concentration of a pearlscent agent is used in a shampoo preparation.
A. 0.2-1% B. 0.5-1%
C. 0.5-2% D. 0.5-0.8

288. Sodium salt of EDTA is Incorporated in shampoo preparation as a
A. Thickening agent B. Detergent
C. Sequestrant D. Pearlscent agent

289. Example of thickening agent is:
A. Alginates B. Methyl cellulose
C. Colloidal silica D. All of above

290. Formaldehyde ans p-hydroxy benzoic acids added in shampoo preparation as
A. Perfume C. Colour
C. Preservatives D. All of above

291. Liquid cream shampoo are expected to be mild and ....in action.
A. Emollient B. Demulcent
C. Anti adherent D. None of above

292. what is the characteristic of a hair tonic:
A. Counter irritant B. Antiseptic
C. Conditioning D. All of above

293. For dry scalp which type of hair tonic is used
A. Oily tonic B. Alkaline tonic
C. Acidic tonic D. None of above

294. For oily scalp which type of tonic is used
A. Oily tonic B. Acidic tonic
C. Alkaline tonic D. All of above

295. The concentration range of alcohol for vehicle in hair tonic is
A. 10-90% B. 10-85%
C. 10-95% D. All of above

296. Which of the action is imparted by alcohol present in hair tonic.
A. Removal of acid-protein complex
B. Addition of fatty acid-protein complex
C. Removal of dust particals
D. None of above

297. What can also be used in place of alcohol to get emollient and lubricant action:
A. Isopropyl alcohol B. Glycerin
C. Cholesterol D. Resorcinol

298. What kind of drugs are Incorporated in hair tonic to stimulate hair growth:
A. Emollient B. Demulcent
C. Rubefacient D. All of above

299. Agents used in hair tonic to increase temperature and localized circulation are
A. Capsicum B. Sulphur
C. Mercuric chloride D. All of above

300. Which one of this have an effect on the activity of sebaceous gland and hair formation.
A. Mercuric chloride B. Pilocarpine
C. Ammonia D. Cholesterol

301. Polyxyethylene condensation product of wool wax alcohol is used as
A. Solubilizer
B. Permeation enhancer
C. Viscosity enhancer
D. Conditioner

302. What is used to treat skin irregularities
A. Vitamin E B. Vitamin F
C. Vitamin C D. Vitamin B

303. Resorcinol and it's mono acetate have powerful........... Action.
A. Antiseptic B. Antispasmodic
C. Anti arrhythmic D. None of above

304. What is responsible for the toxicity of resorcinol used in hair tonic:
A. Cetomacrogol B. Pantothenic acid
C. Resorcinol D. Mercuric chloride

305. Which one of these used to increase the solubility of beta napthol used in hair tonic.
A. Boric acid B. Tartaric acid
C. Sulfuric acid D. None of above

306. Which form of capsaicin is used in hair tonic?
A. Solution B. Tincture
C. Paste D. All of above

307. Conditioners are usually based on .... And fatty materials.
A. Anionic detergent
B. Cationic detergent
C. Non ionic detergent
D. Amphoteric detergent

308. Which country used natural occurring colouring agent Kohl as a hair colourant.
A. Egyptian B. Unani
C. American D. Russian

309. What is the constituent of Kohl used as hair color?
A. Lead acetate B. Lead chloride
C. Lead sulfate D. All of above

310. What is the characteristics of hair color.
A. Non toxic B. Dermititic sensitizer
C. Easy to apply D. All of above

311. What is the important factor while selecting a hair dye?
A. Molecular size B. PH
C. Solubility D. Both A and B

312. What is the color imparting duration of temporary colorants?
A. First shampoo B. Fourth shampoo
C. Sixth shampoo D. Both B and C

313. Vinegar or lemon oil is used in early time to neutralize the effect of
A. Detergent B. Alkali
C. Conditioner D. All of above

314. Simple powder dyestuff are used in a
A. Sachet B. Tablet
C. Capsule D. Both A and C

315. Temporary colorants penetrate which membrane of hair
A. Cutical B. Cortex
C. Medulla D. All of above

316. What is the PH of temporary colorants
A. 3 B. 5
C. 7 D. 8

317. The time duration of semi permanent colorants is:
A. First shampoo
B. Six to eight shampoo
C. More than eight shampoo
D. None of above

318. The semi permanent has
A. High risk to damage hair
B. Less risk to damage hair
C. No risk
D. None of above

319. What is basic dyestuff of semi permanent colorants
A. Nitro amino dye
B. P toluenediamine dye
C. Quaternary ammonium dye
D. All of above

320. Which color imparted by picramic acid in semipermanent colourant
A. Red B. Yellow
C. Both C. None of above

321. What color imparted by anthraquinone to make brown shade
A. Green B. Blue
C. Light brown D. Chocolaty

322. By which process color complex formed
A. Mixing of anionic surfactant with dyestuff solution
B. Mixing of cationic surfactant with Anionic dyestuff
C. Mixing of anionic surfactant with cationic surfactant
D. All of above

323. P-phenylene diamine is a .... dye
A. Oxidation dye
B. Vegetable dye
C. Salt of heavy material
D. None of above

324. P-tolulenediamine is a type of .... dye
A. Temporary B. Semi permanent
C. Permanent D. All of above

325. P-TOLULENEDIAMINE is also incorporate .... In hair
A. Conditioning effect
B. Cleaning effect
C. Toxicity
D. Surfactant

326. What is the example of vegetable dye
A. Lawsonia alba B. P-toluenediamine
C. Picramic acid D. None of above

327. What is the example of vegetable dye
A. Lawsonia alba B. P-toluenediamine
C. Picramic acid D. All of above

328. At what ph the henna works properly
A. 2.5 B. 4.5
C. 5.5 D. 6.5

329. What is responsible for production of color by metallic dyes
A. Formation of sulfides by sulfur
B. Formation of metallic oxides
C. Both
D. None of above

330. Which one affects the colouring property of lead dyes
A. Concentration of lead
B. Nature of dye
C. Air
D. Light

331. What can be added to modify the colour produced by the silver dyes
A. Copper B. Aluminium
C. Iron D. Arsenic

332. Bleaches imparts it's action by the mechanism:
A. Production of karatin
B. Destruction of karatin
C. Production of Melanin
D. Destruction of melanine

333. What is the percentage of hydrogen peroxide for the domestic use as the bleach:
A. 3-4% B. 5-6%
C. 7-8% D. 10%

334. In what percentage the alkaline hydrogen peroxide is used as a bleaching agent:-
A. 3-4% B. 5-6%
C. 7-8% D. 10%

335. Acetanilide, diluted acids, and ammonium bisulphate is used as .... In bleaching agent.
A. Solubility enhancer
B. Stabilizer
C. Permeation enhancer
D. None of above

336. Turkey red oil is used as ....
A. Bleaching agent B. Hair softener
C. Dye remover D. All of above

337. Which one used as a oxidation dye remover:-
A. Turkey red oil
B. Sodium dithionate
C. Hydrogen peroxide
D. None of above

338. What should be the iodine number for a vegetable oil used in brilliantine.
A. Less than 105 B. More than 105
C. 105 D. None of above

339. For what tocopherol is used in brilliantine preparation.
A. Antioxidant B. Bleaching agent
C. Reductant D. None of above

340. Which one is used to prevent rancidity
A. Propyl p-hydroxy benzoate
B. NDGA
C. Both
D. None of above

341. What is the strength of phenol derivatives used as Preservatives
A. 10% B. 20%
C. 30% D. 50%

342. Which is the non ionic surfactant used in hair cream
A. Span B. Wool alcohol
C. Lanolin D. All of above

343. What is the strength of calcium hydroxide in hair cream
A. 0.1% B. 0.14%
C. 0.12% D. 0.18%

344. Which can be used in a hair cream to impart higher concentration:-
A. Calcium adipate
B. Calcium oxalate
C. Calcium saccharate
D. All of above

345. What is the action of zinc stearate in a hair cream:-
A. Viscosity enhancer
B. Smoothness provider
C. Solublizer
D. Stabilizer

346. The concentration of fatty substance in shaving soap is:-
A. 30% B. 50%
C. 67% D. 80%

347. Which one of these is a widely used and advanced preparation used for shaving with razor blade:-
A. Shaving soap
B. Brush less shaving cream
C. Aerosol preparation
D. None of above

348. Determination of potash soap, foam formation and Determination of total fatty acid are the evaluation parameters of
A. For shaving preparation
B. For after shave preparation
C. Both D. None

349. Which one of these is a evaluation parameter for after shave preparation:-
A. Skin sensitization test
B. Determination of alcohol content
C. Determination of fatty materials
D. Stability of cream

350. Which layer of the skin is in direct contact of any cosmetic preparation
A. Stratum corneum
B. Stratum lucidium
C. Stratum granulosa
D. Stratum germilative

351. What is the characteristics of an ideal face powder
A. Adhere to skin
B. Must ne absorbant
C. Hide skin blemishes
D. All of above

352. Which one is not an ideal characteristics of good raw material used in power
A. Non irritating and non toxic
B. Chemically neutral
C. Should not hard
D. Nome of above

353. For what purpose titanium dioxide is Incorporated in powder
A. As a frosted look material
B. As a material imparting slip
C. Material imparting covering character
D. All of above

354. What should be tha particles size rang for song oxide to show good covering:-
A. Below 0.25 um B. 0.25um
C. Above 0.25um D. All of above

355. Which one of these used for face powder and talcum powder
A. Magnesium stearate for face powder and zinc stearate for talcum powder
B. Zinc stearate for face powder and magnesium stearate for talcum powder
C. Both
D. None of above

356. Which is the best quality talc for gave and body powder:-
A. Italian talk B. Russian talc
C. American talk D. Indian talc

357. What is the main use of colloidal kaolin in a face, body or baby powder
A. Absorbance characteristic
B. Imparts patch like finish
C. Imparts adhesion
D. Cover the face and body

358. Which one is not a material that impart absorbency in a face powder:-
A. Colloidal kaolin
B. Linolin
C. Calcium carbonate
D. Bentonite

359. What is the swelling power of bentonite of its own volume:-
A. 8 times B. 10 times
C. 12 times D. 15 times

360. What should be the maximum percentage of powdered silica used as material imparting peach like finish in face powder.
A. 20% B. 30%
C. 50% D. 80%

361. Which type of starch grade is used as the material imparting peach like finish.
A. Maize starch B. Starch 180
C. Starch 360 D. None of above

362. What is the alternative replacement of guanine which was used for frosted look material?
A. Bismuth subnitrate
B. Bismuth subcitrate
C. Bismuth oxychloride
D. All of above

363. Mica, aluminum and bronze are the substance used as..........
A. Colouring substance
B. Material imparting peach like finish
C. Slip and softners
D. Frosted look material

364. Which one is not uses the colouring agents in the preparation?
A. Face powder B. Compacts
C. Both D. None

365. Covering power of a face powder is
A. Mask alone shine B. Enlarged force
C. Minor blemishes D. All of above

366. What should we call the ability to impart velvety, peach like finish produced by face powder?
A. Slip B. Adhesivness
C. Bloom D. Absorbancy

367. What is Incorporated in the medium type of face powder to balance it's cohesiveness?
A. Zinc oxide B. Zinc stearate
C. Zinc Fluoride D. Zinc chloride

368. What is the introduction year of compact powder in america:-
A. 1920 B. 1930
C. 1940 D. 1950

369. What is the example of dry binder used in compact face powder?
A. Zinc stearate B. Isopropyl myristate
C. PVP D. None of above

370. What is required to impart firm compacting in compact face powder?
A. Increased temperature
B. Increased pressure
C. Increased density
D. None of above

371. Which is not an example of water soluble binder used in compact face powder
A. PVP
B. Methyl cellulose
C. Gum tragacanth
D. Glycerol mono stearate

372. To overcome the problem of nonuniformity, loss of moisture, which type or binder is used in compact powder:-
A. Emulsion binder
B. Water soluble binder
C. Oil binder
D. Dry binder

373. Which method is widely and commercially used for the production of compact powder:-
A. Dry mathod B. Wet mathod
C. Damp method D. None of above

374. Whach ingredient is used in highest quantity in powders
A. Talc B. Colouring agents
C. Binders D. Perfume

375. What is the other name of body powder:-
A. Talcum powder B. Dusting powder
C. Both D. None

376. What is the main use of body powder
A. To absorb moisture
B. Perspiration after bathing
C. Cover large surface area
D. All of above

377. What ingredient body powder have which become it different:-
A. Adhesive B. Slip
C. Antiseptic D. Covering material

378. For which purpose Boric acid and bithional are Incorporated in body powder:-
A. Slip B. Antiseptic
C. Covering material D. Adhesive

379. What is the evaluation parameter for powder
A. Pay off B. Flow property
C. Particle size D. All of above

380. What should be the height limit for the breakage test of powder evaluation:-
A. 10 inch B. 15 inch
C. 20 inch D. 25inch

381. What is beauty aids:-
A. Skin colorants B. Powders
C. Cream D. None of above

382. What is the psychological motives to use skin colourant:-
A. Decoration
B. Well groomed appearance
C. Attract opposite sex
D. All of above

383. What is absent in the lip skin
A. Sweat glands B. Salivary glands
C. Both D. None

384. Lips are almost entirely free from........
A. Muscle B. Fat
C. Hypodermis D. All of above

385. Which layer of lip tends to dry and cracks lip in cold or dry weather:-
A. Stratum germinative
B. Hypodermis
C. Corneal layer
D. None of above

386. What should not impart by the lipstick
A. Brittleness B. Tacky
C. Both D. None

387. Plasticity is the characteristics of ....
A. Powder B. Hair remover
C. Lipstick D. None of above

388. What is the characteristics of a lipstick:-
A. Good degree of indelibilit
B. Free from bloom
C. Retain plasticity
D. All of above

389. What should be the melting point of base used in lipstick to withstand weather
A. 60 B. 62
C. 65 D. 70

390. Which one is used in lipstick as raw material:-
A. Wax mixture B. Oil mixture
C. Bromo mixture D. All of above

391. What is responsible for the gloss and hardness property of lipstick:-
A. Waxes B. Oils
C. Bromo mixture D. Preservatives

392. What is the percentage of white beeswax of total formula
A. 3 to 10% B. 5 to 12 %
C. 4 to 8 % D. None of above

393. What is the additional property of beeswax
A. Shrinks on heating
B. Distribute on heating
C. Distribute on heating
D. Distribute on cooling

394. Which one is used in lipstick having melting point of 65-69 C and used in 5-10% :-
A. Bees wax B. Candelilla wax
C. Ceresin wax D. Carnauba wax

395. What is used in excess in lipstick to get smooth and glossy appearance:-
A. Ozokwrite wax B. Cetyl alcohol
C. Bees wax D. Candelilla wax

396. Cetostearyl alcohol is Incorporated to impart

A. Emollient action B. Demulcent action
C. Anti roughness D. None of above

397. What happens when lipstick have high concentration of cetyl alcohol:-

A. Leads to smooth appearance
B. Leads to crystal formation on the surface of lipstick
C. Crumble effect
D. All of above

398. Which one is good plasticizing agent used in lipstick

A. Castor oil B. Bees wax
C. Bromo acid D. All of above

399. Which one is not prone to rancidification:-

A. Olive oil B. Castor oil
C. Almond oil D. All of above

400. High ....of castore oil makes dispersion of pigments long stable.

A. High ....of castore oil makes dispersion of pigments long stable
B. Solubility
C. Viscosity
D. Stability

401. Which ester of Tetrahydrofurfuryl alcohol has very good solvent property for eosin dye:-

A. Acetate B. Stearate
C. Ricinolate D. Perborate

402. What property of solvent can lead to smudging of outline by evaporation in lipstick:-

A. Solubility B. Viscosity
C. Volatility D. Density

403. What should be the percentage of paraffin oil in the lipstick

A. Less than 2% B. Not more than 5%
C. More than 5% D. None of above

404. Isopropyl myristate have a good wetting effect on ....dyes used in lipstick

A. Soluble B. Insoluble
C. Partially soluble D. Slightly soluble

405. Why binder is used with isopropyl myristate used in lipstick

A. To remove separation
B. Because of its low surface tension
C. To increase bulk
D. Both A and B

406. What is Incorporated in lipstick to improve thixotropic properties of sticks.

A. Monoglycerides B. Triglycerides
C. Acetoglycerides D. None of above

407. The portion of the lipstick product which imparts an indelible stain is called

A. Bromo mixture B. Colouring agents
C. Pigments D. Dye's

408. What is composition of bromo acids

A. Floureceins
B. Halogenated fluorescein
C. Water insoluble dye
D. All of above

409. What is concentration of bromo acid in lipstick formulation

A. 2-3% B. 4-5%
C. 10% D. 15%

410. What can produced by the use of fluorescein and it's derivative

A. Sensitization B. Photosensitization
C. Cheilitis D. All of above

411. Which dye is used in transparent lipstick.

A. Fluorescein B. Calcium lakes
C. Barium lakes D. Aluminum lakes

412. What is the lake toner?

A. Azotype dyestuff of calcium
B. Azotype dyestuff of barium
C. Floureceins
D. Both A and B

413. What is the formulation problems associated with titanium dioxide:-

A. Oily exudation B. Streaking
C. Dullness D. All of above

414. What is the concentration of propyl parahydroxybenzoate used as Preservative in lipstick:-

A. 0.1% B. .02%
C. .01% D. 1.2%

415. In what proportion the perfume is added in lipstick formulation:-

A. 2-4% B. 2-6%
C. 4-5% D. None of above

416. BHA, propyl gallate and citric acid are .... Present in lipstick.
A. Antiseptic B. Antioxidant
C. Additives D. None of above

417. What is used as fixation in lipstick formulation?
A. Silicon fluid B. Silicon dyestuff
C. Both D. None of the above

418. For what purpose the polyvinyl pyrrolidine is esse in lipstick formulation?
A. Film former B. Film remover
C. Additive D. None of above

419. What is used for large quantities production of lipstick formulation.
A. Split moulds
B. Automatic ejection moulds
C. Normal moulds
D. All of above

420. Splits moulds are used for the ....
A. Small scale production
B. Large scale production
C. Intermediate production
D. All of the above

421. In rouge preparation what os used for colouration??
A. Iron oxide B. Iron sulfate
C. Iron trisilicate D. All of above

422. What problem can arise with the use of pigments in rouge preparation?
A. Bleeding B. Irritation
C. Colour fading D. None of above

423. In Ancient time the people used .... As rouge
A. Sandalwood B. Cinnabar
C. Brazilwood D. All of above

424. Liquid Rouge's, dry Rouge's, and grease rouge were used in.........
A. Early nineties B. Early twenties
C. Early eighties D. None of above

425. What is the oldest form of rouge preparation?
A. Powder roage B. Liquid Rouge
C. Cream rouge D. All of above

426. What should be the concentration of binder in compact rouge produced by dry process?
A. 1% B. 2%
C. 5% D. 8%

427. Which type of base is used in anhydrous cream rouge:-
A. Fat-wax base B. Oil- wax base
C. Fat-oil base D. Fat-oil-wax base

428. Which type of rouge required cleaning with cleaning cream after use?
A. Emulsion cream rouge
B. Anhydrous cream rouge
C. Liquid Rouge
D. None of above

429. Droop point test is done for......
A. Melting point B. Cracking point
C. Aging stability D. Oxidative ability

430. What is difference between the droop point
A. Time B. Temperature
C. Method D. Both B and C

431. For what purpose the breaking point test is done?
A. To check viscosity
B. To check strength
C. To check density
D. All of above

432. which apparatus is used to done thixotropic character?
A. Plethizmometer B. Penetrometer
C. Monometer D. Hydrometer

433. Dynamometer is used to measure...........
A. Thixotropic character
B. Breaking point
C. Force of application
D. None of above

434. By which one of these oxidative stability is determined:-
A. Peroxide value
B. Acid value
C. Saponification value
D. Detergent value

435. What is the particle size limit of colour dispersion in rouge:-

A. 20mue B. 50mue
C. 75mue D. None of above

436. Which one is not a type of skin cream:-

A. According to function
B. According to characteristics
C. According to type of emulsion
D. According to skin

437. Which one is a type of cream according to function:-

A. Cold cream B. Vanishing cream
C. Foundation D. O/w cream

438. Cold cream is a type of cream according to............

A. Function B. Characteristics
C. Nature D. All of above

439. What is preferred than soap to remove sebum and solidified skin oil :-

A. Commercial cleaning cream
B. Polyethylene glycol 400
C. Olive oil
D. All of above

440. Which one is not remove solid sebum but remove surface oil:-

A. Dioxane
B. Acetone
C. Chloroform
D. Polyethylene glycol 400

441. Jata is the characteristics of a good cream:-

A. Emollient action Should be remain on skin
B. Melt on skin
C. Should be able to remove oil and water soluble material
D. All of above

442. Beeswax borax type of cleaning cream is:-

A. Oil in water
B. Water in oil
C. Oil in water in oil
D. Water in oil in water

443. What is acts as emulsifier in cleansing cream

A. Borax
B. Free fatty acids
C. Borax with free fatty acid present in bees wax
D. None of above

444. Liquefying cleansing cream is .... type have thixotropic character.

A. Hydrous B. Anhydrous
C. Volatile D. All of above

445. What problem can arise by disproportion of oil and wax in liquefying cleansing cream?

A. Separation
B. Sweating
C. Granular appearance
D. All of above

446. In vanishing cream what should be the neutralization limit for fatty acid?

A. 10-15% B. 16-20%
C. 10-25% D. 16-25%

447. What factor is responsible for the consistency and texture of vanishing cream?

A. Amount of acid added
B. Amount of acid saponified
C. Amount of alkali added
D. Both B andC

448. Foundation is applied on skin .... because of good holding power.

A. Before B. After
C. With make up D. None of above

449. What is additional features of massage cream

A. Provide nutrition
B. Can be a supplement for hormones
C. Supplement for vitamins
D. All of above

450. What is the synonyms of night cream:-

A. Hormones cream
B. Vitamin cream
C. Massage cream
D. All of above

451. Which one is not a humectant used in massage cream:-

A. Glucose B. Sorbitol
C. Allatonin D. Methanol

452. Which vitamin is used in massage cream to provide nutrition

A. Vitamin A B. Vitamin C

C. Vitamin K D. All of above

453. Which hormone is added in night cream for hormone therapy?

A. Adrenaline B. Thyroid

C. Progestin D. All of above

454. What is Incorporated in body cream to prevent the loss of water:-

A. Humectant B. Demulcent

C. Emollient D. None of above

455. Which one is a humectant used in body cream to prevent loss of water:-

A. Sucrose B. Glucose

C. Sorbitol D. Manitol

456. What is the main basis to choose the humectant for the cream used on body or hands?

A. Nature B. Viscosity

C. Application D. Skin type

457. Which one in not a synthetic film former:-

A. Acacia

B. Agar agar

C. Carboxy cellulose

D. None of above

458. What result is shown by the Alkyl fatty acids Incorporated in body creams:-

A. Make thinner film on skin

B. Make thicker film on skin

C. Impart roughness

D. All of above

459. Which one is a healing agent to enhance granulation of the skin?

A. Iron oxide B. Benzoic acid

C. Allatonin D. None of above

460. Which type of solvent is used to dissolve Methyl ester and propyl ester respectively:-

A. Aqueous/oil phase

B. Oil/aqueous phase

C. Combination of Aqueous and oily phase

D. None of above

461. Which one is above mentioned is a essential oil based perfume:-

A. Geraniol

B. Cinnamon aldehyde

C. Rose de mai absolute

D. Light floral

462. By what the wool alcohol is obtained:-

A. Got fat B. Sheep wool

C. Cow wool D. All of above

463. Which method is used to obtained wool alcohol used in all purpose cream:-

A. Iodination B. Saponification

C. Rancidification D. Esterification

464. What should be concentration of cholesterol in wool alcohol use in all purpose cream:-

A. 20% B. 25%

C. 28% D. 30%

465. Which antioxidant is used to prevent oxidation in all purpose cream:-

A. Butylated hydroxyanisole

B. Propyl para hydroxybenzoate

C. Methyl para hydroxybenzoate

D. None of above

466. Which type of fluid is considered to the cream formulation:-

A. Newtonian B. Non- newtonian

C. Both of above D. None of above

467. Which one of equipment is used to check rheological property of creams:-

A. Sphygmomanometer

B. Hydrometer

C. Viscometer

D. RD bottle

468. What is use of zinc oxide in a power preparation:-

A. Reflect UV rays B. Absorb UV rays

C. Both D. None

469. Which substance form brown complex with keratin and cause tanning

A. Acetone B. Dioxy acetone

C. Trioxy acetone D. None of above

470. Which natural substance show good reflection to UV rays:-

A. Clay B. Sand
C. Snow D. Stone

471. Which one of these is a sun burn protective substance:-

A. PABA
B. Coumarine derivative
C. Selisylate
D. All of above

472. What is widely used to treat steam burn:-

A. Calamine B. Acacia
C. Agar D. Tregacanth

473. What is the use of phenol and camphor in steam burn preparation:-

A. Mild anaesthetic B. Analgesic
C. Hypertensive D. None of above

474. Which one is used as a vehicle for steam burn preparation;-

A. Alcohol B. Acetone
C. Rose water D. All of above

475. Which country used ammonium as the pigmentation enhancer:-

A. Egypt B. America
C. India D. Japan

476. What should be the PH of preparation contain dihydroxyacetone:-

A. 6-6.5 B. 7
C. 8 D. 9

477. What should be the concentration of dihydroxyacetone in preparation:-

A. 2% B. 4%
C. 6% D. 8%

478. What is used as sun tan agent with dihydroxyacetone:-

A. Juglon B. Lawson
C. Both A and B D. None of above

479. What is the equation for Erythemal dosage:-

A. E-vitons B. E-vitons/cm2
C. E-cm2 D. None of above

480. What is the time duration of a muskara :-

A. 2 month B. 4 month
C. 5 month D. 8 month

481. The word pigmentation means:-

A. Colour B. Powder
C. Tanning D. None of above

482. What is the concentration of calcium hydroxide in hair cream:-

A. 0.12% B. 0.14%
C. 0.15% D. 0.16%

483. In which year the heating method for hair wavers is developed in England:-

A. 1920 B. 1923
C. 1950 C. 1955

484. What is the time duration taken by the thioglycollate to remove the hair from scalp:-

A. 5-15 min B. 20 min
C. 25 min D. 25 min

485. For what purpose the cream are used after shaving:-

A. To remove hairs B. To heal cuts
C. Both A and B D. None of above

486. What is the main aim to use potassium, sodium and ammonium on nail

A. Nail whitener
B. Nail darkner
C. Nail preparation remover
D. All of above

487. Bioavailability can be elucidated as :

A. Extent and rate at which drug is absorbed in the body
B. extent and rate at which active ingredient is in systemic circulation
C. That is administered through sub-lingual route and are entirely bio-available
D. None of the above

488. FDx=CL/CLr Ux∞ = Ux∞/fr is a generalised mathematical representation for :

A. Non-intravenous dose
B. sub-cutaneous dose
C. Intravenous dose
D. Intramuscular dose

489. Instead of using intravenous route for bioavailability, what can be used as a reference standard ?

A. Non-intravenous B. Pellets
C. Oral solution D. Tablets

490. The bioavailability of drug is maximum of oral solution.

2. Ideally, intravenous and oral solution dose are both responded as solid dosage form.

3. The bioavailabilty of drug is maximum of non-intravenous route.

Which of the following options are correct?

A. a and c B. Only a
C. a and b D. all of the above

491. The drugs that are poorly absorbed and have poor bioavailability can:

A. Not improved by formulation
B. Improve first-pass metabolism
C. Improved by formulation
D. Achieve high rate absorption

492. Bioavailable doses are those doses which have:

A. Dose with high bioavailability
B. Dose that reaches to systemic circulation
C. Dose with high absorption rate
D. Dose available to patient

493. F= bioavailable dose / administered dose. In the above formula F confronts?

A. Systemic bioavailability
B. Bioavailable dose
C. Extent of absorption rate
D. Relative bioavailability

494. The availability of drug when in systemic circulation administered orally, is determined when compared to intravenous administration.

The above statement elaborates the concept of :

A. Comparative bioavailability
B. Systemic bioavailability
C. Absolute bioavailability
D. Relative bioavailability

495. The concept of absolute bioavailability is mainly based upon the criteria of:

A. To avoid absorption step
B. Poor water soluble drugs
C. Increase systemic availability
D. Bioavailable dose

496. Which of the following are limitations of absolute bioavailabilty :

a. Applicable to one compartment model.
b. Can be applied to two compartment model
c. Unabsorbed dose of drug calculated
d. Can't determine elimination rate if oral absorption rate is less

A. 1 and 2 B. 3 and 2
C. 2 and 4 D. 1 and 4

497. In solid dosage forms, dissolution rate limitation in drug absorption can be differentiated when :

A. Intramuscular dose is used as standard
B. Oral solution used in conjugation with intravenous route
C. Oral solution is used as standard
D. Intravenous route is used to interpret absorption properties

498. Comparative bioavailability is essential for:

A. Used to characterize drugs absorption properties from e.v. site
B. Used to characterize oral absorption rate
C. Orally administered drug compared with availability in circulation
D. Used to characterize absorption of drug from its formula

499. Single dose bioavailability can't offer :

A. Exposure to drugs
B. Prediction of peak
C. Half-life terminal
D. Steady-state characteristics of drug and inter-subject variability with such studies

500. Advantages for multiple dose study can be elicited as:

A. Predict terminal half-life
B. Blood levels can't be measured at same concentration
C. Predict peak and valley characteristics of drug
D. Non-linearity in pharmacokinetics can't be determined

501. The adverse drug reactions can be increased due to exposure of patient in test drug. This limitis conjured in:

A. Single dose study
B. Multiple dose study
C. Absolute bioavailabilty
D. Dose availability

502. In multiple dose study, when the steady state is reached it is ensured by:

A. Drug administered for 5-6 elimination half life

B. Drug administered 6 hours before sample collection

C. Sample taken immediately after administerd drug

D. Half-life attained, then sample is removed

503. Healthy volunteers used in bioavailabilty study should be:

A. 20-40 years male ; ± 10% body weight

B. 20-40 years male and female ; ± 10% body weight

C. 25-40 years male and female patients ; ± 5% body weight

D. 25-40 years male and female; ± 10% body weight

504. Volunteers as female can only be used for testing for:

A. Oral contraceptives

B. Uterus contraceptives

C. Any disease purpose

D. None of the above

505. Volunteers when ongoing tests, are instructed to restrain from :

A. No fasting

B. Only fluid in diet

C. Administered drug after few hours

D. Administered drug for at least a week and fast overnight

506. Indirect methods can further be categorised into:

A. Therapeutic response

B. pharmacodynamic

C. Plasma level time studies

D. Acute pharmacological response

507. A method where there is measurement of drug effect on patho physiological process as a function of time. The method is:

A. Indirect method

B. Direct method

C. Relative bioavailabilty

D. Absolute bioavailabilty

508. Pharmacodynamic methods are complementary to pharmacokinetic methods.

b. Pharmacokinetic methods are non-complementary to pharmacodynamic methods.

Which of the following statement is correct:

A. a and b

B. Only b

C. Only a

D. None of the above

509. When there is an increase in dose as well as absorption rate, the peak plasma concentration will:

A. increase

B. No effect on Cmax

C. decrease

D. None of the above

510. In plasma level-time studies, the peak plasma concentration increase with increase in dose which further:

A. Decrease absorption

B. Decrease peak time

C. Increase peak time

D. None of the above

511. For oral and intravenous route relation, the mathematical expression for extent of bioavailability is :

A. F= [AUC] oral D IV / [AUC] IV D oral

B. F= [AUC] IV D oral / [AUC] oral D IV

C. F= [AUC] oral D oral / [AUC] IV D oral

D. F= [AUC] IV D IV / [AUC] IV D oral

512. Which is the correct mathematical equation for determining bioavailability from peak plasma concentration at steady-state Css,max ?

A. Fr = (Css , max)std D std τ test / (Css , max)test Dtest τstd

B. Fr = (Css , max)std D test τ std / (Css , max)std Dtest τstd

C. Fr = (Css , max)test D std τ test / (Css , max)std Dtest τstd

D. Fr = (Css , max)test D std τ test / (Css , max)std Dtest τstd

513. Rate of absorption is not necessary in:

A. Single dose method

B. Multiple dose method

C. both

D. None of the above

514. The principle for urinary excretion studies used to access bioavailabilty is:

A. Urinary excretion of unchanged drug is directly proportional to plasma concentration of drug.

B. Urinary excretion of unchanged drug is inversely proportional to plasma concentration of drug.

C. Plasma concentration of drug is directly proportional to urinary excretion of drug

D. Urinary excretion of unchanged drug is equals to plasma concentration of drug.

515. Bioavailability can be identified by urinary excretion data only when the dose administered is excreted unchanged in urine, which should be:

A. 40% B. 70%

C. 50% D. 20%

516. Thiazide diuretics and sulphonamides are an example of in urinary excretion studies:

A. Drugs having urine at site of action

B. Drugs extensively excreted unchanged in urine

C. both

D. None of the above

517. Examples for drugs that have urine as site of action in urinary excretion studies are:

A. Sulphonamides B. diuretics

C. cephalosporin D. nitrofurantoin

518. For the calculations , the concentration of metabolites excreted are never counted because :

A. Drug may undergo presystemic metabolism

B. Degradation of drug may occur

C. Resistance of drug may occur

D. It can't bind to appropriate receptor

519. Analysis of unchanged drug in the collected sample

2. Collection of urine at regular intervals for time-span equal to 7 biological half-times

3. Determination of drug overall excreted

Which of the following methods used in urinary excretion studies are correct?

A. A and c B. B and c

C. Only a D. A and b

520. Frequent sampling of urine is very necessary in beginning after administration of dose because:

A. To note rate rate of urinary excretion

B. To note rate of absorption

C. both

D. None of the above

521. To have a valid result in urinary excretion studies, the fraction excreted unchanged in urine should:

A. increase B. constant

C. decrease D. None of the above

522. Parameters analyzed in urinary excretion data identified through single dose are:

A. (DxU /dt)max and (tU)max

B. (DxU /dt)max ; XU∞ and (tU)max

C. (tU)max and XU∞

D. (DxU/dt)max and (t)max; XU∞

523. In maximum urinary excretion rate, the plot between rate of excretion versus midpoint time of urine collection period, the graph of this plot:

A. decreases B. Remains constant

C. increases D. None of the above

524. As the rate of absorption increases,the value of Cmax in maximum urinary excretion rate ,

A. decreases B. increases

C. constant D. none

525. The value of tUmax in urinary excretion data increases when :

A. Rate of absorption increases

B. Rate of urinary excretion decreases

C. Cmax increases

D. Rate of absorption decreases

526. Estimation of bioavailability by urinary excretion method has high degree of variability and is less reliable than those obtained from plasma concentration time profile.

Estimation of bioavailability by urinary excretion method has low degree of variability and is obtained from plasma concentration time profile.

Which of the following is true?

A. Both a and b B. Only b

C. Only a D. None of the above

527. The bioavailability of few drugs apart from plasma and urine studies can be determined by:

A. Assay of biological fluids
B. Assay of antibiotics
C. both
D. None of the above

528. Salivary excretion can be used in case of which drug?

A. cephalosporin B. nimesulamide
C. minoxidil D. theophylline

529. Which method is based on observing clinical response to a drug formulation given to patient suffering from disease ?

A. Acute pharmacological response method
B. Therapeutic response method
C. Urinary excretion method
D. none

530. Which studies are used in therapeutic response method:

A. Topical anti-fungal agents
B. Anti-viral agents
C. Anti-protozoic agents
D. Anti-malarial agents

531. Which of the following is used in ulcer therapy:

A. cimetidine B. thiopene
C. benzaldehyde D. sucralfate

532. Which method can assimilate biological availability of drug from its formulation:

A. In vivo test
B. In vivo in vitro correlation
C. In vitro dissolution test
D. none

533. What are the following factors required in in-vitro drug dissolution tests?

A. Factors relating to dissolution fluid and apparatus
B. Fators relating to disintegration time
C. Factors relating to IVIVC
D. none

534. Dissolution apparatus can offer various agitation variables like:

A. Mild, non-uniform
B. Non-turbulent, fats, uniform
C. Turbulent, fast, non-uniform
D. Mild, non-turbulent, uniform

535. In an ideal dissolution apparatus which of the following contents are right:

1. Prevents evaporation of dissolution medium
2. Temperature maintained at 30°C
3. Maintains sink conditions
4. Agitation is fast

A. 1. and 2. B. 2. and 4.
C. 1. and 3. D. All of the above

536. Dissolution apparatus can be classified on absence or presence of sink conditions. The types are :

A. Closed compartment and open compartment
B. 1 compartment and 2 compartment apparatus
C. Rotating paddle and rotating basket apparatus
D. Continuous flow through and flow-through cell apparatus

537. Closed compartment apparatus is operated under which conditions:

A. Sink conditions
B. Non-sink conditions
C. both
D. None of the above

538. Rotating paddle apparatus is example of which dissolution apparatus?

A. Continuous flow- through
B. Open compartment
C. Closed compartment apparatus
D. Flow through cell apparatus

539. Beaker type apparatus consists of which of the following apparatus:

A. Reciprocating cylinder
B. Paddle over disc
C. Reciprocating disc
D. Rotating basket

540. Continuous flow through are operated under which conditions :

A. Non-sink B. sink
C. both D. none

541. In open-compartment apparatus the dosage is contained in:

A. pillar B. compartment
C. post D. column

542. Dialysis system can be defined as:
A. Poorly aqueous solution drugs for which maintenance of sink conditions require huge volume of dissolution fluid
B. They are freely soluble drugs operated in sink conditions
C. They are aqueous soluble drugs operated under non-sink conditions
D. None of the above

543. Which of the following are official test apparatus according to USP :
A. Rotating paddle apparatus (apparatus 2)
B. Rotating paddle apparatus (apparatus 1)
C. Reciprocating cylinder apparatus (apparatus 1)
D. Flow through cell apparatus (apparatus 1)

544. Name an apparatus which was first described by Pernarowski :
A. Rotating paddle apparatus
B. Flow through cell apparatus
C. Cylinder apparatus
D. Rotating basket apparatus

545. Dissolution apparatus according to USP is comprised of?
A. A set of cylindrical flat bottomed glass vessels
B. Reservoir for dissolution medium and pump that forces dissolution medium through cell holding test sample
C. Cylindrical glass vessel with hemi-spherical bottom
D. Sample holder

546. In rotating basket apparatus according to USP, the cylindrical basket for holding dosage form is made of how many meshes?
A. 20 B. 18
C. 40 D. 22

547. The cylindrical basket in apparatus 1 according to USP is held centrally. The distance from bottom is:
A. 4cm B. 2cm
C. 3cm D. 6cm

548. The metal parts of rotating basket apparatus are made of :
A. SS 316 B. SS 308
C. SS 418 D. SS 238

549. In rotating paddle apparatus the rotating basket is replaced by :
A. paddle B. Acrylic rod
C. cylinder D. disc

550. Levy and Hayes introduced a method for dissolution known as:
A. Rotating basket apparatus
B. Reciprocating disc apparatus
C. Rotating paddle apparatus
D. Paddle over disc apparatus

551. In rotating paddle apparatus the dosage form is kept on a plate.
b. In rotating paddle apparatus, the dosage form is allowed to sink to the bottom.
Which is true?
A. Only a B. Only b
C. both D. None of the above

552. Capsules and other floatable forms are prevented from floating due to the help of?
A. plates B. reservoirs
C. stirrers D. sinkers

553. Cylindrical flat-bottomed glass vessels with reciprocating cylinders are present in which dissolution apparatus ?
A. Flow through cell apparatus
B. Cylinder apparatus
C. Reciprocating cylinder apparatus
D. Reciprocating disc apparatus

554. Which formulations are used for dissolution test in reciprocating cylinder apparatus?
A. Tablets B. Capsules
C. Pellets D. All of the above

555. The bead-type formulations in reciprocating cylinder apparatus are which kind of drug delivery system?
A. Control-release
B. Target release
C. Sustain release
D. Modified release

556. Flow-through cell apparatus for dissolution medium consists of :
A. matrix B. reservoir
C. pump D. cell

557. The closed mode for dissolution medium in flow-through cell apparatus consists of fluid which :

A. Continuously replenish

B. agitated

C. Is re-circulated

D. None of the above

558. Tablets / capsules/ granules that are to be tested in dissolution medium of flow through cell apparatus are kept in :

A. chamber

B. basket

C. Vertically mounted dissolution cell

D. Flat bottom glass vessel

559. The fresh solvent to pump in flow through cell apparatus has to be pumped between range of:

A. 240-960ml/h

B. 200-940l/h

C. 240-960min/se

D. 200-940m/s

560. Sink conditions are easy to maintain during dissolution.

2. This can be performed only in non-sink conditions.

3. Automation of this apparatus is difficult.

Which of the following state is correct for flow through cell apparatus?

A. 1. and 3. B. Only 1.

C. 1. and 2. D. 2. and 3.

561. Evaluation of which products can be done through paddle over disc apparatus?

A. transdermal B. oral

C. nasal D. All of the above

562. The product in paddle over disc apparatus is held by:

A. disc B. rod

C. cylinder D. basket

563. Trandermal products can be evaluated through which dissolution apparatus?

A. Cylinder apparatus

B. Flow through cell

C. Rotating basket

D. None of the above

564. The sample in cylinder apparatus is held in what?

A. basket B. Teflon cylinder

C. Ss cylinder D. Ss rod

565. The sample used in cylinder apparatus is mounted on?

A. Acrylic porous plate

B. Non-porous plate

C. Spring holder

D. Inert porous cellulosic material

566. Reciprocating disc apparatus are used for evaluation of which products?

A. implants

B. Non-disintegrating control release oral preparation

C. Orally disintegrating tablets

D. Chewable tablets

567. At which temperature the dissolution test is carries out in reciprocating disc apparatus?

A. 37°c B. 32°C

C. 45°c D. 25°C

568. The frequency of reciprocating in apparatus 7 according to USP is :

A. 30cycles/min

B. 50cycles /min

C. 42cycles/min

D. 120cycles/min

569. Which of the following are used as reciprocating holders in apparatus 7-

A. Basket, cylindrical disc, cylindrical vessel

B. Spring holder, Teflon cylinder, cylindrical vessel

C. Acrylic rod, angled disc, Teflon cylinder

D. A and B

570. Spring holder and angled disc are examples of :

A. Reciprocating holders

B. Dissolution cell

C. Rotating basket

D. Reciprocating cylinder apparatus

571. Acrylic rod, Teflon cylinders and reciprocating disc are examples of which dissolution apparatus according to USP-

A. Apparatus 1 B. Apparatus 4

C. Apparatus 5 D. Apparatus 7

572. The difference between apparatus 5 and apparatus 2 according to USP is that:

A. Apparatus 5 has disc attached to padde

B. Apparatus 5 has a disc placed below rotating paddle

C. Apparatus 2 doesn't have rotating cylinders

D. All of the above

573. Conventional tablets can be tested in which dissolution apparatus -

A. Apparatus 7 B. Apparatus 4

C. Apparatus 3 D. Apparatus 1

574. Transferal formula can be tested in which dissolution apparatus :

A. Paddle over disc/cylinder/ reciprocating disc

B. Reciprocating cylinder, paddle over disc

C. Paddle over disc / cylinder

D. Cylinder, reciprocating cylinder, paddle over disc

575. In reciprocating cylinder test which of the following formulated drug is used -

A. Controled-release formula

B. Formulation containing poorly soluble drug

C. Powders

D. All of the above

576. The poorly soluble drugs are generally tested in dissolution apparatus :

A. 6 B. 1

C. 3 D. 4

577. What should be the dissolution methodology for immediate release products of BCS class II :

A. Single point

B. Multiple point

C. Multiple point if NLT 85% Q in 15 min

D. Single point if NLT 85% Q in 15 min

578. The dissolution methodology based on BCS classification is for which kind of products -

A. Sustain release B. Control release

C. Immediate release D. Moderate release

579. Which BCS class has same dissolution methodology for immediate release products :

A. Class I and IV B. Class I and II

C. Class II and III D. Class I and III

580. The multiple point dissolution methodology for BCS class I is only when:

A. Q=85% in 15min B. Q<85% in 25min

C. Q>85% in 10min D. Q<85% in 15min

581. The dissolution acceptance criteria for S1 stage should be -

A. Dosage units equal or greater than Q+5%

B. Dosage units equal or greater than Q+15%

C. Dosage unit less than Q-5%

D. Dosage unit less than Q+5%

582. The "Q" in dissolution acceptance criteria generally stands for -

A. % of drug content dissolved in given solvent

B. % of drug content dissolved in given time period

C. % of solvent used during time period

D. % of solvent used to dissolve drug content

583. Second stage for dissolution criteria must consist of :

A. Average of 12 dosage units equal to OR greater than Q

B. Average of 6 dosage units equal to OR greater than Q

C. Average of 12 dosage units less than Q

D. None of the above

584. No dosage unit is less than Q-15%.

The following statement is criteria for which stage?

A. S1 B. S3

C. S2 D. None of the above

585. What is the number of dosage units tested in S3 stage of dissolution acceptance criteria :

A. 6 B. 24

C. 12 D. 6

586. What should be the dissolution acceptance criteria having 12 dosage units that are to be tested:

A. 3 dosage unit less than Q-15%

B. dosage unit less than Q-15% and no dosage unit less than Q-25%

C. 2 dosage unit less than Q-15% and no dosage unit less than Q-25%

D. 3 dosage unit less than Q-15%

587. The in vitro dissolution profile of rest drug product and approved drug product are compared and can be useful in :

A. Development of new drug

B. Demonstrate equivalent after change in formulation of drug product

C. Both

D. None

588. Which of the following is an equation for difference factor f1 :

A. f1= {[Σnt=1 (Rt-Tt(] / Σ nt=1 Rt ×100

B. f1= {[Σnt=0 (Rt-Tt(] / Σ nt=0 Rt ×100

C. f1= {[Σnt=n-1 (Rt-Tt(] / Σ nt=n-1 Rt ×100

D.f1= {[Σn=0t=1 (Rt-Tt(] / Σ n=0t=1 Rt ×100

589. F2= 50 × log{[1+1/n Σnt=1 (Rt – Tt)2]-0.5 100} is the mathematical expression for :

A. Difference factor

B. Comparison

C. Similarity

D. Equality

590. Name a method which is used for comparison of dissolution profile by identifying f1 and f2 :

A. Model independent method

B. In vitro drug dissolution

C. Model dependent method

D. Therapeutic response method

591. What is the minimum dissolution time points that is measured for evaluation of dissolution profile :

A. 4 B. 3

C. 1 D. 12

592. What is the following conditions are true for evaluation of dissolution profile :

1. Minimum 5 dissolution points should be measured.

2. The standard deviation for mean of any product should not be more than 10%.

3. One mean value not more than > 80% dissolved for each product.

A. 1 and 2 B. 2 and 3

C. Only 2 D. Only 3

593. What is the number of products to be tested both test and reference for evaluation of dissolution profile:

A. 12 B. 10

C. 8 D. 15

594. Therapeutic efficacy of any drug can be speculated through :

A. In vitro dissolution test

B. In vivo dissolution test

C. IVIVC

D. None

595. In-vitro in-vivo correlation can be defined as:

A. Mathematical framework describing relationship between rate and extent of dissolution of dosage with respect to drug absorbed in plasma concentration.

B. Mathematical framework describing relationship between distribution and rate at which drug is dissolved.

C. Both

D. None.

596. What is the alternate method for in vivo bioavalability studies performed in humans :

A. IVIVC

B. In vitro dissolution test

C. Dissolution profile

D. Bio equivalence studies

597. How can a correlation be developed between bioavailability and dissolution testing :

A. Modifying bioavailabilty

B. Developing linear relationship between in vivo bioavailability and in vitro dissolution

C. Having single dissolution rate

D. All of the above

598. Which of the following is a linear in Vitro in vivo correlation :

A. Correlation based on dissolution rate

B. Correlation based on distribution time

C. Correlation based on urinary excretion data

D. Correlation based on extent of absorption

599. What is the in vivo plasma data parameter for specific amount of drug that is to be dissolved in in-vitro dissolution :

A. λ_{max} B. C_{max}

C. t,time D. K_a

600. Which of the following are factors that correlate in vitro dissolution with Plasma data :

1. **Amount dissolved at specific time point - fraction absorption**
2. **Specific amount of drug to dissolve - Ka**
3. **Mean dissolution time - mean absorption time**

A. 1 and 2　B. 2 and 3
C. All of the above　D. 1 and 3

601. D50 effect can be identified through which of the following IVIVC parameter :

602. Which theory can determine the relationship of mean dissolution time and mean residence time:

A. Statistical moments
B. Pharmacological response
C. Both
D. None

603. Give an example in which the systemic availability doesn't depend upon dissolution characteristics of drug :

A. Thyrotropin　B. Corticosteroids
C. Oxytoxin　D. Vasopressin

604. Which IVIVC represent relationship between in vitro dissolution and in vivo rate of absorption :

A. Level A　B. LevelB
C. Level C　D. Level D

605. The graphical curve for level A IVIVC having same mathematical expression is :

A. Logarithm　B. Polynomial
C. Non-linear　D. Superimposable

606. The principle of statistical moments theory is used by which IVIVC level :

A. A　B. C
C. B　D. Multiple level C

607. The mean in vitro dissolution time in level B IVIVC can be compared to :

A. Mean in vitro dissolution time
B. Mean in Virginia o absorption rate
C. Mean residence time
D. Mean in vitro absorption rate

608. The level B of IVIVC can't be relied for justification of changes in manufacturing or modification in formula. What can be the reason behind this:

A. As correlation is not point-to-point since a number of in vivo curves will produce similar mean residence time value.
B. As correlation is point-to-point and in vivo curve produce only a mean residence time value
C. As correlation is not point-to-point since in vivo curve is only produced
D. As correlation is point-to-point since graph curve overlap

609. Which of the following can't be used for collecting data for quality C standards :

A. In vivo data　B. In vitro data
C. IVIVC　D. None

610. Which level of IVIVC is a single point correlation :

A. Level A　B. Level B
C. Level C　D. Multiple level C

611. Level C relates to which dissolution time point :

A. 1　B. 6
C. 3　D. 2

612. Which pharmacokinetic parameter is related to the dissolution time point in level C :

A. C_{max}　B. t_{max}
C. AUC　D. All of the above

613. Level C can only be useful in what parameter due to its limitations :

A. Guide in formulation development
B. In dissolution time
C. Quality assurance
D. All of the above

614. Multiple level C is a correlation in which parameter to the amount of drug dissolved at various time points:

A. One or several pharmacodynamic parameter
B. One or several pharmacokinetic
C. Only two pharmacokinetic
D. Only one pharmacodynamic

615. What are the expectations of IVIVC for BCS class I for immediate release products :

A. Dissolution rate is slower then gastric emptying rate should be slower

B. Dissolution rate is high then gastric emptying rates hould be higher

C. If dissolution rate is slower than gastric emptying rate should be high

D. Dissolution rate is high then gastric emptying rate should be slower

616. Which of following BCS class has an IVIVC expectations that in vitro dissolution rate can be similar to in Vivo dissolution rate :

A. I B. II

C. III D. IV

617. What can be the possibility of prediction IVIVC for BCS class I from dissolution data of immediate release products :

A. Yes

B. Dissolution rate increases

C. No

D. None

618. What is the IVIVC expectations for BCS class I for immediate release products :

A. Dissolution is rate determining and limited

B. Absorption is rate determining and limited

C. In vitro and in vivo dissolution rate similar

D. None

619. What is the prediction possibility of IVIVC from dissolution data for BCS class IV for immediate release products :

A. Yes B. Little IVIVC

C. No D. Level A IVIVC

620. What can be the IVIVC expectation for BCS class Ia for extended release drug products :

A. IVIVC level C B. IVIVC level A

C. No IVIVC D. Both A and B

621. IVIVC level C is expected for BCS class Ib for extended release drug products. What is the permeability of BCS class Ib :

A. Variable

B. High and site independent

C. Site dependent and narrow absorption window

D. Site dependent and high absorption window

622. What is expectation of IVIVC for BCS class IIb for extended release drug products:

A. Level A B. Little IVIVC

C. Level C D. Little or no IVIVC

623. IVIVC level A is expected for which BCS class for controlled release preparations:

A. Ib B. IIb

C. Vb : basic D. Va : acidic

624. Va : acidic the class of BCS has what kind of IVIVC expectation for controlled release products :

A. Level A B. Little or no IVIVC

C. Level C D. Level B

625. What can be the following conditions for in vivo bioavailability and bioequivalence study to not be conducted for drug products based on BCS classification :

A. High solubility and rapid dissolution

B. Narrow therapeutic window

C. Low solubility, low permeability, low dissolution

D. High solubility, low permeability, similar dissolution

626. Excipients present in dosage form are same as those present in approved drug product.

2. There should be narrow therapeutic window.

Which of the following is correct for conditions of in vivo bioavailability and bioequivalence as per BCS classification :

A. Only 2 B. Only 1

C. Both D. None

627. Which of the following are risks for conduction of bio equivalence studies :

1. Risk of bio-inequivalence

2. Risk of high therapeutic window

3. Diminished clinical safety

A. 1 and 3 B. 2 and 3

C. 1 and 2 D. All of the above

628. The comparison of drug products with specific characteristics or functions is defined as:

A. Bioequivalence

B. Physical equivalence

C. Pharmaceutical equivalence

D. Equivalence

629. Name a term which elicits that two or more drug product contain same chemical substance as an active ingredient in same amount :

A. Chemical equivalence
B. Bio equivalence
C. Equivalence
D. Pharmaceutical equivalence

630. Pharmaceutical equivalence can be defined as:

A. Have identical dosage form
B. Two or more drugs products identical in strength, quality, purity, dissolution, disintegration
C. Two or more drugs products identical in exipients, quality, purity, dissolution, disintegration
D. Two or more drugs products Having same chemical substance as active ingredient

631. Pharmaceutical equivalence can have two or more drug product identical in various prospects expect from :

A. Strength B. Dissolution
C. Exipients D. Active ingredient

632. Which term denotes that drug substance in two or more identical dosage form reaches systemic circulation at same relative rate to same relative extent :

A. Therapeutic equivalence
B. Pharmacological equivalence
C. Bioequivalence
D. Physical equivalence

633. How bio equivalence can be indicated when observed the bioavailability of two or more drug products :

A. When statistically significant different observed
B. When statistically insignificant different observed
C. Without statistically significant different observed
D. A and C

634. Therapeutic equivalence is term that indicates two or more drug product containing :

A. Different therapeutic but identical pharmacology
B. Same therapeutic active ingredient having identical pharmacological effect
C. Different pharmacological and control disease
D. Can't control disease to same extent as therapeutic

635. Bioequivalence studies can be scrutinized through which demonstration :

A. In vivo B. IVIVC
C. In vitro D. Both A and C

636. What is the sequence for assessing in-vivo bio equivalence studies :

A. Oral immediate release products with systemic action, non-oral immediate -release products, modified -release products
B. Modified release products, Oral immediate release products with systemic action, oral immediate -release products,
C. Oral immediate release products with systemic action, modified -release products
D. non-oral immediate -release products, Oral immediate release products with systemic action, modified -release products

637. Which of the following statements are true for oral immediate -release products with systemic action:

A. 1 and 3 B. 2 and 3
C. 1 and 2 D. All of the above

638. When in vitro dissolution studies are used instead of in vivo bioequivalence. These can be known as:

A. Exemptions
B. Biowaivers
C. Both A and B
D. Statistical moment theory

639. Which of the following conditions for biowaivers is correct :

1. Ratio between active substance and exipients are same
2. Under same test condition, in vivo dissolution rate is same
3. Quantitative composition is different
4. Pharmacokinetics are linear

A. 1 and 2 B. 1 and 4
C. 2 and 4 D. 3 and 4

640. Which of following test designs are used in bioequivalence experimental study design :

A. Completely randomized design
B. Micronization
C. Confidence interval approach
D. Molecular encapsulation

641. Name a bioequivalence experiment study design where subject as well as block are same

A. randomized block design
B. Latin square design
C. Cross over design
D. Completely randomized design

642. When one or more administration are induced in a patient with a specified or randomized pattern. This is known as -

A. randomized block design
B. Completely randomized design
C. Latin square design
D. Change over design

643. Cross over design has fall out which is :

A. Potential for distortion due to carry over
B. Sources of variability between subjects are excluded from experiment error
C. No effects shown even after preceding treatment
D. None of the above

644. The term "continuous trial" in bioequivalence experimental study design is referred as :

A. Where treatment is assigned at random interval
B. Experiment where subjects remain on treatment from start of experiment till the end
C. Where treatment is discharged at random interval
D. None of the above

645. Latin square design can be ellicited as :

A. 2-factor design with one observation in each cell
B. 2-factor design with two observation in each cell
C. 1-factor design with one observation in each cell
D. 4-factor design with two observation in each cell

646. Which of the following are commonly used bioequivalence studies in Latin square design :

A. Randomized, block, cell
B. Cross over, column, block
C. Block, cross over, repeated measure
D. Randomized, cross over, balanced

647. When various treatments are under observation in Latin square design, what will be the degree of freedom for experiment error :

A. Smaller
B. Constant
C. Larger than necessary
D. Non - error

648. In which kind of statistical interpretation the data is tested for different within and between treatment and control group :

A. Latin square design
B. Randomized block design
C. Confidence interval approach
D. Analysis of variance

649. What is the statistical difference for ANOVA between pharmacokinetic parameters :

A. More than 1 in 20
B. Equal to 0.05
C. Less than 1 in 20
D. Greater than 0.05

650. The level of statistical significance is indicated by:

A. Mean difference B. C_{max}
C. AUC D. Probability p

651. In which probability the difference between drug products ain't considered statistically significant :

A. $P \geq 0.05$ B. $P \leq 0.05$
C. $P \geq 0.005$ D. $P \leq 0.005$

652. Name a statistical interpretation of bioequivalence data where determined if bioavailability from test product too low or high in comparison to reference :

A. Analysis of variance
B. Micronization
C. 2 one-sided test procedure
D. Cross over design

653. What should be the ratio of a 90% confidence interval of a means of 2 drug products :

A. Greater than 20% B. Equal to 20%
C. Within ± 20% D. Less than ± 20%

654. What is the set value when log transformed data are used in 2 one-sided test procedure :

A. 80-125% B. 80-120%
C. 85-125% D. 85-120%

655. The confidence limits used in 90% confidence interval are also known as :

A. Carriers
B. Student's t distribution
C. 2 one-sided test procedure
D. Bioequivalence interval

656. Which of the following factors are responsible for having a poor bioavailability of drug:

A. Fast dissolution rate
B. High permeability
C. Poor permeability and solubility
D. High absorption and solubility

657. BCS classification was including permeability and solubility of drugs was developed by whom :

A. Amidon and coworkers
B. European Medicine Agency
C. What and Benet
D. FDA

658. The class I of BCS classification enlightens which class of drugs :

A. Low solubility / high permeability
B. Low solubility / low permeability
C. High solubility / low permeability
D. High solubility / high permeability

659. What kind of drugs are available in class IV BCS classification :

A. Who readily absorb orally
B. Poorly absorbed orally with solubility and permeability limitation
C. Variable absorption with permeability limitation
D. Variable absorption with solubility limitation

660. High solubility / low permeability is shown by which class of BCS class:

A. I B. IV
C. III D. II

661. Which class of drug is not sphered in BCS classification :

A. V B. II
C. IV D. I

662. Class V drugs of BCS classification include poor absorption of drugs due to :

A. Poor oral absorption
B. Poor GI stability
C. Poor permeability
D. Poor solubility

663. Name a drug that can be given when having a poor GI stability as such in class V of BCS class :

A. Metformin B. Taxol
C. Nicardipine D. Omeprazole

664. What are the challenges faced for control-release drug delivery system by BCS class I :

A. Absorption of released drug is rapid
B. Absorption of released drug is slow
C. GI poor stability
D. Permeability problem

665. Which drugs are used in class I BCS classification :

A. Minoxidil B. Propranolol
C. Lansoprazole D. Nimesulamide

666. Naproxen is example of which BCS class :

A. IV B. V
C. II D. III

667. Which of the following drugs fall on account of class III drugs :

A. Insulin, cimetidine, metformin
B. Carbamazepine, nifedipine, nicardipine
C. Metformin, taxol, minoxidil
D. Diltiazem, metroprolol, propranolol

668. Which of the following drugs are correct as per class IV of BCS classification :

A. Nifedipine B. Furosemide
C. Ranitidine D. Omeprazole

669. As class V drugs of BCS classification are metabolically and chemically unstable. What are the certain measures that are held onto account to improve their stability :

A. Enhance presystemic metabolism

B. Improve solubility and dissolution rate

C. Enhance GI permeability

D. Prodrug design and lipid technology

670. What is the parameter that co-relate to solubility / dissolution and permeability of BCS class:

A. Disintegration number

B. Permeability number

C. Absorption number

D. Dose %

671. What is the pH range where a high solubility drug can be soluble in 250ml of water:

A. 1-7 B. 1-8

C. 7-12 D. 2-6

672. What is the labelled amount at which the drug is dissolved in USP apparatus :

A. =85% B. ≤ 85%

C. >85% D. ≥ 85%

673. Drugs having high permeability and high absorption number belongs to which BCS class :

A. III and IV B. V

C. I and II D. II and III

674. High dissolution number belongs to which BCS class with low permeability :

A. IV B. III

C. II D. I

675. Solubility can be determined through various methods are :

A. Mass balance

B. Tilting box method

C. Shake flask method

D. Capillary tube merhod

676. What should be the pH range for the determination of solubility in aqeuous media :

A. 1-7.5 B. 4-6

C. 2-8 D. 5-12

677. Which of the following is a method used in determining the extent of absorption in permeability determination:

A. Titration

B. In vitro permeation experiment across epithelial cell monolayer

C. Mass balance

D. In vivo intestinal perfection study

678. Which of the following are methods used in detection of intestinal permeability:

A. Absolute bioavailabilty

B. In vivo in situ intestinal perfusion study

C. In vivo permeation across epithelial cell monolayer

D. In vitro in situ intestinal perfusion study

679. What is the rpm for USP apparatus 1 :

A. 250 B. 50

C. 70 D. 100

680. Name an equipment in which the process of micronization can be done :

A. Ball mill B. Fluid energy mill

C. Planetary mixer D. Freeze drying

681. Give an example for drug whose bioavailability can be increased by process of micro-melting:

A. Vasoprasil

B. Chloramphenicol

C. Acetazoline

D. Griseofulvin

682. What is the size of particles where in process of nanonization :

A. 100-500nm B. 300-800nm

C. 200-600nm D. 400-800nm

683. Give an example of drug used in nanonisation process for enhancement of bioavailability :

A. Amphotericin B B. Ciprofloxacin

C. Nystatin D. Furosemide

684. Nanosuspension can be defined as:

A. Dispersion of drug nanocrystal in liquid

B. Dispersion of Nano drug liquid in liquid

C. Non-aqueous media in water

D. None

685. What are the various technologies used in the preparation of nanoparticles :

A. Nanosuspension
B. Micro-milling
C. Molecular dispersion
D. Pearl milling

686. Those fluids which have greater temperature and pressure than critical temperature and critical pressure and having properties of both a liquid and gas are called :

A. Spray freezing into liquid
B. Supercritical fluid
C. Molecular dispersion
D. Critical Micelle concentration

687. Name a technique which involves atomization of aqueuos, organic, aqeuos - organic cosolvent solution, aqueous organic emulsion or suspension containing drug that is directly compressed gas:

A. Spray freezing into liquid
B. Evaporative precipitation into aqueous solution
C. Supercritical fluid recrystallization
D. Nano structured lipid carrier

688. Which of the following fall into the category of cryogenic liquid:

A. Helium
B. Ethane
C. Carbon dioxide
D. Argon and hydrofluoroethers

689. Name a process through which the frozen particles are then obtained as dry free-flowing powders:

A. Crystallization
B. Cryogenization
C. Lyophillization
D. Nano structured lipid carrier

690. Which solvent decreases the time of drying for lyophillization process:

A. Acetonitrile B. Acetoacetate
C. Ether D. Sodium benzoate

691. Due to spray freezing into liquid the dissolution rate has increased. What can be the reason behind this :

A. Have metastable polymorphs
B. Nano structured lipid carriers
C. Microionized polmorphs
D. Amorphous Nano structured aggregates

692. The rapid phase separation for lipophilic drug so that they nucleate and grow Nano and micro particles. This process is known as :

A. CMC
B. Spray freezing into liquid
C. Evaporative precipitation in aqueous solution
D. Supercritical fluid

693. EPAS also stands for:

A. Electronic protocol application software
B. Evaporative precipitation in aqueous solution
C. Evaporative precipitation for amorphous solid
D. Evaporative pseudo amorphous state

694. In EPAS, what inhibits the crystallization of growing particles for enhancing dissolution:

A. Hydrosol
B. Lyophilic stabilizer
C. Hydrophobic stabilizer
D. Hydrophilic stabilizer

695. Surfactants are generally introduced into any system because they're helpful as:

A. Enhance disintegration
B. Enhance dissolution rate
C. Increase solubility
D. Enhance particle size

696. Surfactants can only be used when they have concentration:

A. Below CMC B. Equal to CMC
C. Above CMC D. None

697. Which one of the following is an example of nonionic Surfactants :

A. Tween 80
B. Sodium laurel sulphate
C. Polysorbate
D. Sodium dodecyl sulphate

698. Which one of the following drug is an example with increase in bioavailability due to use of Surfactant :

A. Terbutaline B. Diphenhydramine
C. Spironolactone D. Chlorpropamide

699. Salt forms are generally used instead of original drug as they improve :

A. Dissolution
B. Disintegration
C. Permeability
D. Solubility and dissolution

700. Give an example of an alkali metals salt of acidic drug:

A. Penicillin B. Chloramphenicol
C. Atropine D. Ofloxacin

701. What is the example for strong acid salts of basic drugs:

A. Penicillin B. Salbutamol
C. Atropine D. Phenylephrine

702. Name some inert polymers which impairs the formation of crystals or precipitation of drug:

A. Nylon B. Polyethylene glycol
C. Teflon D. Polyurethane

703. Which of the following factors are not responsible for enhancement of bioavailability by enhancement of drug solubility:

A. Solvent deposition
B. Alteration of pH of drug micro environment
C. Use of amorphous, solvates
D. Use of metabolism inhibitors

704. When poorly aqueous soluble drug dissolved in organic solvent by mixing it rapidly with non-solvent to effect precipitation. The product so formed is called as:

A. Solvent deposition
B. Hydrosol
C. Glass solution
D. Mixed crystals

705. Name a poorly aqueous soluble drug used in solvent deposition for enhancement of bioavailability:

A. Nifedipine B. Hexamine
C. Nicardipine D. Acetylcholine

706. Bentonite can enhance dissolution rate of poor water soluble drugs by:

A. Maintain solubility
B. Maintain concentration gradient
C. Maintain permeability
D. All of the above

707. When 2 components crystallize in a homogeneous one phase system, it is known as :

A. Glass solution
B. Hydrosol
C. Molecular dispersion
D. Glass dispersion

708. Melts are systems that are generally prepared through:

A. Lyophillization B. Solution
C. Dispersion D. Fusion

709. When resulted solid solution formed is homogeneously transparent and brittle system such solution are called as:

A. Glass solution
B. Molecular dispersion
C. Mixed crystals
D. Glass dispersion

710. When drug molecules substitute for carrier in its crystal lattice. Such systems are called as:

A. Substituional crystalline solid solution
B. Discontinuous solid solution
C. Continuous solid solution
D. Interstitial crystalline solid solution

711. Interstitial crystalline solid solution case occurs when the size of drug molecule is

A. Greater than 40%
B. 40% or less
C. Greater than 50%
D. 20% or less

712. Which of the following is an example of eutectics:

A. Griseofulvin B. Paracetamol - urea
C. Indomethacin D. All of the above

713. Eutectic can also be called as eutectic melts because:

A. Made by fusion method
B. Same as solid solution
C. Both
D. None of the above

714. Among the following which dissolution rate for griseofulvin is highest as solid solution :

A. Microionized Drug
B. Eutectic mixture
C. Solid solution
D. Coarse drug

715. Name a method through which solid dispersion are prepared :

A. Fusion
B. Melt
C. Glass dispersion
D. Co-precipitate

716. How does solid dispersion differ from solid solution:

A. Drug precipitate out in crystalline form
B. Drug precipitate out in amorphous form
C. Drug precipitate out in solvate form
D. None

717. Co-evaporates is another name for which kind of systems:

A. Glass dispersion
B. Solid solution
C. Eutectic melt
D. Solid dispersion

718. If the solid dispersion formed have glassy materials, they're known as:

A. Glass suspension
B. Glass melt
C. Glass solution
D. Glass mixture

719. Various derivatives of cyxlodextrins along with hydrophobic drugs havea capability to form which kind of complexes:

A. Lipid drug conjugate
B. Molecular inclusion complexes
C. Co-evaporate complex
D. Molecular complex

720. Olihosaccharides produces from starch in molecular encapsulation with cyclodextrins have which kind of shape:

A. Bucket
B. Chair
C. Bakset
D. Hat

721. What is the mean diameter for solid lipid nanoparticles:

A. 500-1000nm
B. 100-1000nm
C. 400-800nm
D. 100-500nm

722. Name a compound which facilitate drug transportation across biomembrane:

A. Penetration enhancers
B. Pore transport
C. Bioadhesives
D. Carrier transport

723. The release of drugs in stomach is inhibited by enteric coating. Why?:

A. As polymers are insoluble in gastric fluid
B. As polymers are soluble in gastric fluid
C. Due to high permeability in GI fluid
D. Due to low permeability in GI fluid

724. Which of the following drug can be improved by enteric coating due to gastric instability :

A. Caffeine
B. Sodium salicylate
C. Erythromycin
D. Sodium benzoate

725. Which of the following is completing agent used to enhance drug stability in GI :

A. Omeprazole
B. Ephrine
C. Penicillin - G
D. Nicotinamide

726. What is the range of bioavailability when cyclosporin drug is administered undergoing intestinal metabolism:

A. 20-30 %
B. 30-40%
C. 10-20%
D. 10-30%

727. Which is the powerful inhibitor for enzyme CYP3A4 and also increase bioavailability :

A. Orange juice
B. Apple cider
C. Grapefruit juice
D. Lime juice

728. The non-existant invasive measurement of in vivo hepatic CYP3A4 activity is also known as :

A. Permeation enhancer
B. Erythromycin breath test
C. P-gp mediated efflux of cyclosporine
D. CYP3A4 inhibitors

729. Disintegration apparatus consists of which assembly for tablets and capsules:

A. Cylindrical basket
B. Glass plate
C. Basket rack
D. Cylindrical vessel

730. How many cylindrical glass tubes are present in basket rack disintegration apparatus:

A. 8 B. 12
C. 6 D. 5

731. Which of the following length and diameter of basket rack disintegration apparatus is correct :

A. 77.5 ± 2.5mm long, 21.5mm internal diameter
B. 72.5 ± 2.5mm long, 15mm internal diameter
C. 76.5 ± 3.5mm long, 20mm internal diameter
D. 77.5 ± 2.5cm long, 21.5cm internal diameter

732. What is the diameter of plastic plates that holds the tubes in basket rack assembly:

A. 90 ± 2 mm in diameter
B. 90 ± 2 CM in diameter
C. 80 ± 1.5 mm in diameter
D. 100 ± 1.5 mm in diameter

733. What is the diameter of wire that is woven under the side of the lower plate:

A. 0.615 ± 0.045 cm
B. 0.620 ± 0.25 mm
C. 0.615 ± 0.045 mm
D. 0.456 ± 0.35 mm

734. The plates in basket rack assembly are held rigidly at 77.5mm apart with help of

A. SS cylinder B. Metal column
C. SS cell D. Vertical metal rod

735. The plate and rod in basket rack assembly are further attached to device and raised and lowered simultaneously with a frequency of :

A. 30-32 cycles / min
B. 40-45cycles / min
C. 28-32cycles / min
D. 50-52cycle / min

736. What is the breadth and diameter of disc for each in basket rack assembly:

A. 20.7 ± 0.15 mm thick in diameter and 9.5 ± 0.15 mm thick
B. 25.7 ± 0.25 mm thick in diameter and 6.5 ± 0.1 mm thick
C. 20.7 ± 0.15 cm thick in diameter and 9.5 ± 0.15 cm thick
D. 20.5 ± 0.5 mm thick in diameter and 7.5 ± 0.2 mm thick

737. What's the density for cylindrical discs for tubes in basket rack assembly:

A. 1.5-1.2 B. 1.4-1.8
C. 1.18-1.20 D. 1.12-1.45

738. What is the temperature at which the thermostatic arrangement maintain the temperature of basket rack assembly:

A. 32° ± 2° B. 35° ± 2°
C. 37° ± 2° D. 40° ± 2°

739. The enteric coated tablets are each added to tube and suspended in a beaker containing 0.1M hydrochloric acid which are then operated for:

A. 2 hr B. 4 hr
C. 1hr D. 1.5hr

740. The liquid in the second operation for enteric coated tablets is replaced by:

A. Phosphate buffer, pH-7.2
B. Mixed phosphate buffer, pH-6.8
C. Acidic buffer, pH-4.5
D. Sodium buffer, pH-5.6

741. What is the height and diameter for apparatus for disintegration of pessaries and suppositories:

A. 60mm high, 52mm internal diameter
B. 60cm high, 52cm internal diameter
C. 50mm high, 82mm internal diameter
D. 80mm high, 42mm internal diameter

742. The Stainless Steel discs used in disintegration apparatus for pessaries and suppositories are separated by what distance:

A. 40mm B. 50mm
C. 30mm D. 20mm

743. For compressed pessaries to support the metal device, the hook end is used in which direction:

A. Upward B. Sideways
C. Straight D. Downward

744. The apparatus for moulded pessaries and suppositories is held at what distance below the surface of water:

A. 100mm B. 90mm
C. 80mm D. 60mm

745. In case of insoluble powders what happens once the disintegration is complete:

A. The component parts remain on surface
B. The component parts are distributed
C. The component parts dissolve
D. The component parts sink to the bottom

746. What is the temperature of water used for compressed pessaries:

A. 36°-37° C B. 32°-33° C
C. 30°-32° C D. 35°-36° C

747. The humid atmosphere is maintained when one compressed pessary is kept on the upper perforated disc and the apparatus is covered by:

A. Plastic plate
B. Stainless Steel plate
C. Glass plate
D. Glass disc

748. The disintegration for compressed pessaries is completed when either there is no residue left or when :

A. The remained residue consists of soft mass with no solid core
B. Remained residue has been distributed
C. Remained residue sinks to the bottom
D. None of the above

749. All parts of the dissolution apparatus that comes in contact with dissolution medium or preparations are generally:

A. Chemically inert B. Can absorb
C. Stable D. Forms a thin layer

750. What is the grading of metal materials used in dissolution apparatus :

A. SS 316 B. SS 320
C. SS 215 D. SS 420

751. The cylindrical vessel used in apparatus 1 of dissolution test as per IP is made up of:

A. Cadium glass
B. Germanium glass
C. Borosilicate glass
D. Silicon glass

752. What is the inner diameter of cylindrical vessel used in dissolution apparatus 1 as per IP :

A. 98-100mm B. 85-95mm
C. 96-105mm D. 98-106mm

753. What is the position of the axis of shaft with the vessel of dissolution apparatus 1 as per IP:

A. 3mm B. 1mm
C. 2mm D. 5mm

754. What is the temperature used for maintaining dissolution medium in apparatus 1 as per IP:

A. 32.5°-35.5° C B. 40.5°-42.5° C
C. 35.5°-38.5° C D. 36.5°-37.5° C

755. In dissolution apparatus 2 as per IP the paddle is replaced by:

A. Beaker B. Basket
C. Cylinder D. Rod

756. The lower detachable part of basket in dissolution apparatus 2 is made up of :

A. Stainless Steel
B. Glass
C. Welded-steam cloth
D. Silicon

757. What is the thickness of wire present at the lower detachable part of basket in dissolution apparatus 2:

A. 0.2 mm B. 0.356mm
C. 0.75mm D. 0.254mm

758. The basket in dissolution apparatus 2 for use of acidic media is plated with:

A. 2.5mm layer of gold
B. 5.5mm layer of Stainless Steel
C. 3.5mm layer of copper
D. 2.0mm layer of silver

759. What is the distance between the inside bottom of vessel and basket in dissolution apparatus 2:

A. 36-38mm B. 35-40mm
C. 23-27mm D. 25-30mm

760. Before subjected to testing the dissolution medium should be :

A. Deaerated B. Nitrification
C. Carbonated D. None of the above

761. What is the average pore diameter of membrane filter disc used in dissolution apparatus:

A. 0.1 micrometer B. 2.0 micrometer
C. 1.0 micrometer D. 3.0 micrometer

762. Which medium is added to buffer stage of method A in modified - release dosage forms:

A. 0.1M hydrochloric acid
B. 0.2 M trisodium phosphate dodecahydrate
C. 0.2 M disodium hydrogen phosphate
D. 0.1 M trisodium phosphate dodecahydrate

763. At what pH is the medium maintained in buffer stage of method A in modified - release dosage forms:

A. 6.8 ± 0.05 B. 4.8 ± 0.5
C. 6.8 ± 0.2 D. 7.8 ± 0.05

764. Which buffer is added in buffer stage of method B for modified - release dosage forms:

A. pH 6.8 phosphate buffer
B. pH 7.3 phosphate buffer
C. pH 7.8 phosphate buffer
D. pH 5.6 phosphate buffer

765. What is acceptance criteria for level A_1 for modified - release dosage forms:

A. No individual value exceeds 25% dissolved
B. No individual value exceeds 20% dissolved
C. No individual value exceeds 10% dissolved
D. No individual value exceeds 5% dissolved

766. What is the acceptance criteria for level A_3 for modified - release dosage forms :

A. The average value of 12units is not more than 10% dissolved
B. The average value of 24units is not more than 10% dissolved
C. The average value of 6units is not more than 10% dissolved
D. The average value of 24units is not more than 25% dissolved

767. What is the acceptance criteria for level B_1 for modified - release dosage forms:

A. No unit is less than D+10%
B. No unit is less than D+15%
C. No unit is less than D+5%
D. No unit is less than D+25%

768. The average value of 24units is equal to OR greater than D and not more than 2 units are less than D-15% and no unit is less than D-25%.

The following statement is an acceptable criteria for which level of modified release dosage forms:

A. Level A_1 B. Level B_1
C. Level A_3 D. Level B_3

769. What is the % deviation for uncoated and film coated tablets with 80mg or less as an average weight:

A. 20 B. 5
C. 30 D. 10

770. What is the average weight for capsules, granules and powders (singld-dose) with 10% deviation:

A. Less than 300mg B. 250mg and more
C. More than 300mg D. More than 80mg

771. What is the % deviation for pessaries and suppositories:

A. 10 B. 5
C. 7.5 D. 3.5

772. What is the acceptance limit for tablets, powders, suspensions for injection and ophthalmic inserts with average content of:

A. 85-115% B. 75-95%
C. 90-100% D. 85-110%

773. The preparation will fail to comply with test if any single preparation from tablets, powders, suspension for injection and ophthalmic inserts is outside of limit :

A. 75-85% B. 95-125%
C. 75-125% D. 85-110%

774. The apparatus for friability contains a drum which is made of:

A. Glass B. Plastic
C. Stainless Steel D. Synthetic polymer

775. What is the diameter and depthness of drum present in friability apparatus as per IP:

A. 283-291 mm diameter, 36-40mm depthness

B. 263-271 mm diameter, 36-45mm depthness

C. 280-290mm diameter, 35-40mm depthness

D. 183-191mm diameter, 26-42mm depthness

776. What is the outer diameter of central ring present in the drum of friabilator as per IP:

A. 36.5-37.5mm B. 24.5-25.5mm

C. 40.2-42.5mm D. 30.2-32.5mm

777. What is the speed of friabilator drum that is attached to horizontal axis of the device as per IP:

A. 26±2 rpm B. 28±2 rpm

C. 25±1 rpm D. 30±2 rpm

778. What should be the weight of tablets taken into the friability apparatus with an average weight and of 0.65gm or less tablets:

A. 10gm B. 6.5gm

C. 0.65gm D. 7.5gm

779. How many times is the friabilator drum rotated with inserted tablets within as per IP:

A. 200 B. 50

C. 100 D. 250

780. What is net weight of any single container with a labeled amount of 50g or less for preparations like ointments, creams, pastes, granules and powders for oral liquids:

A. Not less than 91% and not more than 109%

B. Not less than 95.5% and not more than 104.5%

C. Not less than 90% and not more than 100%

D. Not less than 80% and not more than 120%

781. What is the nominal mesh aperture for a sieve having coarse powders:

A. 1700 micrometer

B. 1680 micrometer

C. 1500 micrometer

D. 1800 micrometer

782. What is the nominal mesh aperture for moderately coarse powders with not more than 40% by weight:

A. 355 micrometer B. 250 micrometer

C. 170 micrometer D. 300 micrometer

783. What is the size of superfine powders with not less than 90% of number of particles:

A. Not less than 15micrometer

B. 20micrometer

C. Not less than 10micrometer

D. Not more than 10micrometer

784. 45 micrometer is the nominal mesh aperture with not more than 40% by weight is for which grade of powders:

A. Very fine powder B. Superfine powder

C. Microfine powder D. Fine powder

785. 355micrometer is the nominal mesh aperture size of a sieve through which powders will pass:

A. Coarse powders

B. Moderately coarse powders

C. Fine powders

D. Moderately fine powders

786. What is the nominal mesh aperture size for moderately coarse powders:

A. 710micrometer B. 510 micrometer

C. 250micrometer D. 1600 micrometer

787. Which of the following is not included in 4 central compartment of tdds?

A. The drug candidate

B. Release patterns

C. Patch design

D. The skin

788. The characterstics of an ideal transdermal drug delivery system are:

A. Agent independent

B. Selected delivery profile

C. Targeting

D. All of the above

789. IDDS has the capability of changing which of the following:

A. Rate of delivery B. Quantity of delivery

C. Size of delivery D. Both A and B

790. The speed of drug release by transdermal patch as compare to stratum corneum

A. Fast B. Slow
C. Same D. Very fast

791. Drug release trough TDDS goes into:

A. Blood circulation
B. Gastrointestinal tract
C. Liver
D. None of the above

792. The range for daily dose of TDDS?

A. 10mg/ml or less B. 10-20 mg/ml
C. 20-30 mg/ml D. 30-40 mg/ml

793. As compare to oral route bioavailability of TDDS is:

A. Very high B. High
C. Equal D. Low

794. The thickness of stratum corneum layer is

A. 5-10 μm B. 10-20 μm
C. 15-20 μm D. 20-25 μm

795. The outer most layer of skin is

A. Stratum germinativum
B. Stratum spinosm
C. Stratum granulosm
D. Stratum corneum

796. The drug used in TDDS must have molecular mass in between

A. 10-100da B. 100-200da
C. 200-750da D. 700-1000da

797. Stratum corneum lipid of human is consist of

A. Sterols B. Triglycerides
C. Fatty acid D. All of the above

798. "Removal of the upper three epidermal layers result into water loss and an enhanced of the trasndermal permeability" Concept wsas given by:

A. Monash and Blank
B. Wertz and Downing
C. Modison etal
D. None of the above

799. Relative surface area (%)of transfollicular pathway is:

A. 0.5 B. 10
C. 0.7 D. 0.1

800. Relative surface area (%)of intercellular pathway is:

A. 0.1 B. 10
C. 0.7 D. 0.6

801. Relative surface area (%)of transcellular pathway is:

A. 70.0 B. 0.1
C. 90.0 D. 99.0

802. Which statement is true for transfollicular pathway:

A. High relative surface area ,long diffusion pathway
B. Low relative surface area , short diffusion pathway
C. High relative surface area,Short diffusion pathway
D. Long relative surface area, long diffusion pathway

803. Most embedded protein present in dermis is:

A. Collegen B. Elastin
C. Albumin D. Globuline

804. Vascular layer of skin is:

A. Stratum corneum
B. Stratum spinosm
C. Stratum gralosome
D. Dermis

805. Innermost layer of epidermis is:

A. Stratum corneum
B. Stratum spinosm
C. Stratum granulosm
D. Srtatum germinativum

806. The fastest route of absorption through skin is

A. Transcellular B. Intercellular
C. Transfollicular D. None of the above

807. The rate of skin permeation can be expressed mathematically by the equation:

A. dq/dt=Cp(Ps-Cr)
B. dq/dt=Cr(Ps-Cp)
C. dt/dt=Ps(Cp-Cr)
D. dq/dt=Ps(Cp-Cr)

808. The principal transport mechanism in mammalian skin is:

A. Active diffusion B. Passive transport
C. Passive diffusion D. Active transport

809. The factor that control the percutaneous absorption:

A. Physiochemical properties of penetrants
B. Physicochemical properties of drug delivery system
C. Physiochemical and pathological condition of the skin
D. All of the above

810. Three major variables account for difference in the rate at which the drug permeate the skin:

A. The Concentraation of the drug in the vehicle
B. The diffusivity of the drug through the stratum corneum
C. Both A and B
D. None of the above

811. Product of metabolism of drug hydrocortisone:

A. Oestrone
B. Cartisone
C. 5 Alpha-Dihydrotestestrone
D. Testestrone

812. Product of metabolism of drug oestradiol:

A. Cartisone
B. Testestrone
C. Oestrone
D. 5 alpha-Dihydrotestestrone

813. Product of the metabolism of drug testosterone:

A. Castisone
B. Testestrone
C. 5 Alpha-Dihydrotestestrone
D. Oestradiol

814. The most significant physiological factor that affect the rate and extent of precuteneous absorption is:

A. Patient age
B. Location on the body
C. Hydration state
D. None of the above

815. The permeation across hydration skin of corticosteroids and caffeine is:

A. Low B. Very low
C. High D. No penetration

816. Increase hydration of stratum corneum cause:

A. Decrease in porosity
B. Increase in porosity
C. Close product cell
D. Increase density of cell

817. Occulsion effectively reduce the irreversible binding capacity of:

A. Stratum corneum
B. Stratum granulosome
C. Stratum germinosm
D. Stratum spinosm

818. Site of transdermal patch affect the:

A. Rate of percutaneous absorption
B. Extent of percutaneous absorpation
C. Time of Percutaneous absorption
D. Both A and B

819. Which of the following came variation in permeability?

A. Amount of surface lipids
B. Stracking of cell
C. Difference in nature of cell
D. All of the above

820. Skin of which of the following area is less permeable to drug?

A. Palms B. Chest
C. Soles D. Scrotum

821. Disruption in the continuity of stratum corneum result in increase in trasansdermal permeability the reason for this is:

A. Decrease in cell layer
B. Increase vascoconstrition
C. Increase vasodilation
D. Decrease lipid content

822. Which of these reduce the reservoir effect of skin?

A. Anion surfactant
B. Cationic surfactant
C. Both A and b
D. None of the above

823. Which of the following is the most metabolically active layer of skin?
A. Viable dermis
B. Viable epidermis
C. Viable hypodermis
D. All of the above

824. What is the reason behind the permeability enhancement by application of anionic surfactant?
A. Modification of stratum germination
B. Modification of stratum spinosm
C. Modification of lipid content
D. Denaturation of dermal protein

825. Composition of drug delivery system affect which of the following?
A. Rate of drug release
B. Extent of drug release
C. Permeability of stratum corneum
D. Both A and C

826. Transdermal permeability of flucisnolone acetomide in human whole abdominal skin increase with:
A. Increase in volume fraction of propylene
B. Decrease in volume fraction of sodium
C. Decrease in particle of the filucinolene
D. All of the above

827. Which of the Following cause alteration in percuteaneous absorption due to modification in diffusion barrier?
A. Penetration enhancer
B. Sonophorosis
C. Iontophresis
D. All of the above

828. Which of the following increase the skin permeability?
A. Ethanol B. Hexanol
C. Octanol D. None of the above

829. Which of these reason is true for increase in permeability by lower alcohol?
A. Addition of more hydrophilic cosolvent
B. Extraction capacity of lipids
C. Both A and B
D. None of the above

830. Which of the following markedly increase the skin permeability?
A. Aryl methyl sulphoxide
B. Diethyl sulphoxide
C. Decyl methyl sulphoxide
D. All of the above

831. Which of these is the mode of action of DM50?
A. Displacement of bound water
B. Delamination of horny layer
C. Extraction of stratum corneum lipid
D. All of the above

832. Surfactant also alter of increase the transdermal permeation of some drug by?
A. Increase Pore size
B. Decreasing surface tension
C. Both A and B
D. None of the above

833. The terms nature moisturizing factor is used for which compound?
A. Sulphoxides B. Glycols
C. Pyrrolidones D. All of the above

834. Which of the following is mode of action of Azones?
A. Protein Extraction
B. Lipid extraction
C. Displacement of bound water
D. Ion –pairing

835. Which type of drug permeation is facilitate by long chain alkyl amines?
A. Anion drug B. Cationic Drug
C. Both A and B D. None of the above

836. Which of the following technique is used to determine the effect of treatment on stratum corneum by fatty acids?
A. Diffrential scanning calrimety
B. Infrared spectroscopy
C. Both A and B
D. High performance liquid Chromatography

837. The cis –unsaturated analoges cause disorder of lipids in ectracellular region of stratum corenum and this change is related with:
A. Action of surfactant
B. Increased drug flux
C. Decrease permeation
D. None of the above

838. Which of these technique use electrical potential to facilitate the drug permeation across the skin?

A. Iontophorsis B. Sonophorosis
C. Electrophoeris D. None of the above

839. Skin is permselective to passage of which type of ion?

A. Negative B. Positive
C. Natural D. None of the above

840. Which type of floco is induced by ionophorosis?

A. Laminar flow B. Turbulent Flow
C. Convective Flow D. All of the above

841. Pathway of elctrotransport in iontophoresis is:

A. Lipodal B. Aqueous
C. Both A and B D. None of the above

842. Which of these compound is more efficiently delivered from anode in iontophoresis?

A. Positively charged
B. Negatively charged
C. Neutral substance
D. None of the above

843. Large molecule are suitable Candidate in iontophoresis because of their:

A. Potency
B. Requirement in high dose
C. Increased distribution
D. None of the above

844. In iontophoresis which type of current is applied between two electrode placed on skin?

A. Constant B. Variable
C. Pulsed D. Both B and C

845. Which of the reversible electrodes is used in ionotophoresis?

A. Pt electrode B. Ag electrode
C. Cu electrode D. Zu electrode

846. Reversible electrode is used in iontophoresis because of:

A. Fast motion of ion
B. Easily release of ion
C. Present hydrolysis
D. None of hte above

847. The passage of 0.5 mA?cm2 across human skin requires a voltage of:

A. 1-10 V B. 5-15 V
C. 2-12 V D. 6-20 V

848. Which of the following is major mechanism of transport for larger compound?

A. Electroporation B. Electro osmosis
C. Both A and B D. None of the above

849. Which of these is physical method of enhancement of skin permeation?

A. Electroporation B. Sonophoresis
C. Laser ablation D. All of the above

850. In which of the technique high voltage pulse is used?

A. Sonophoresis B. Electroporation
C. Laser – ablation D. None of the above

851. In electroporation how much volt of pulse can induce permeation enhancement of diverse compound?

A. 200 V B. 150 V
C. 100 V D. 50 V

852. The degree of enhancement achieved invitro is related to:

A. Applied voltage B. Number of pulses
C. Duration of Pulses D. All of the above

853. In which technique ultrasound based delivery of drug is possible?

A. Sonophoresis B. Iontophoresis
C. Electroporation D. Laser ablation

854. In which technique high powered pulses are utilize and vapourise away the stratum corneum?

A. Electroosmosis B. Electroporation
C. Laser-Abration D. None of the above

855. In which of the technique pores are created by high voltage pulse?

A. Iontophoresis B. Electroporation
C. Sonophoresis D. None of the above

856. In which technique discrete permeable windows are created by high powdered pluse?

A. Laser abration B. Ionophoresis
C. Electroporation D. Sonophoresis

857. In which technique minimal inrasive methodologics are designed to short circuit the banner function of the stratum corneum?

A. Sonophoresis B. Ionophoresis
C. Both A and B D. Laser ablation

858. Which of the prodrug are the most extencively studied derivative used for optimization dermal delivery?

A. Alpha-acyloxyalkyl
B. Beta-acyloxyalkyl
C. Beta-alkoxyalkyl
D. None of the above

859. Which of the group is used to introduce water solubility into acyl portion of the prodrug?

A. Tertiary amino B. Alkoxyl group
C. Alcoxy group D. Both A and B

860. Which of the Following neuropeptide are located in the pilosebaceous unit of human skin?

A. Vaccular intenstinal peptides
B. Neuro tunctional peptides
C. Propiomelanocortin peptides
D. Both A and B

861. POMC exerts important immunoleegulatory effect bly anatogonizing the function of which cytokines?

A. TNF- Alpha B. Interleukin
C. Interleukin D. All of the above

862. Which of the following is taken comideration for the polymer which are used in the preparation of component in the preparation of component of TDDS

A. Molecular weight
B. Physical character
C. Chemical functional
D. All of the above

863. Which of the polymer is widely used in preparation of transdermal devices?

A. EVA polymer B. Polyvnyl carbonate
C. Polyacrylo nitirte D. All of the above

864. One to which of the following Reason permeation of drug is poor?

A. Low molecular weight
B. High O/W partitioning
C. Different chemical functionality
D. None of the above

865. Which of the following is considered as penetration enhancer?

A. Surface active system
B. Two component system
C. Lipophilic system
D. All of the above

866. Which of these greatly enhance the permeability of hydrophilic drugs?

A. Surface active agents
B. Two component system
C. Lipophilic system
D. None of the above

867. Two component system are mainly composed of:

A. Oleic acid and glycerol
B. Gallic acid and glycerol
C. Oleic acid and propylene glycol
D. Gallic acid and propylene glycol

868. Which of thereis important for pressure sensitive adhesive ?

A. Physically and chemically compatible with drug
B. Moisture resistence
C. Non-irritant to skin
D. All of the above

869. Which of these is category of pressure sensitive adhesive ?

A. Polyneo butylenes B. Butyl rubber
C. Both A and b D. None of the above

870. Which of the homopolymer is used as pressure sensitive agent ?

A. Polyisobutylene B. Butyl rubber
C. Isoprenoids D. None of the above

871. Butyl rubber is a copolymer of:

A. Synthetic rubber
B. Polyisobutylene
C. Monoisobutylene
D. None of the above

872. Which of these in structure of pressure sensitive adhesive is responsible for low permeability of gas , air and moisture?

A. Double bond B. Central atom
C. Side group D. None of the above

873. Butyl rubber used in pressure sensitive adhesive differentiate on the basis of :
A. Molecule weight
B. Number of isoprene unit per 100 monomer
C. Physical parameter
D. Both A and B

874. Which of these stabilizer is used in butyl rubber when used in pressure sensitive adhesive?
A. BHT
B. Mono thio carbonate
C. Zinc diprophyl
D. None of hte above

875. POlisobutylene differ from butyl rubber in:
A. Alternative bonds
B. Low molecular weight range
C. Terminal unsaturation
D. None of the above

876. Which of the following does not contain stabilisers?
A. High Molecular weight polyisotutylenes
B. Low molecular weight Polyisobutylene
C. Both A and B
D. None

877. The pressure sensitive acrylic adhesive derive their pressure sensitivity form:
A. Acrylic Ether B. Acrylic ester
C. Acrylic acid D. None of the above

878. Which of the monomer is commonly used in pressure sensitive adhesive?
A. Ethyl hexyl acrylate
B. Butyl acrylate
C. Acrylic acid
D. All of hte above

879. Which of these property of pressure sensitive adhesive is related to Tg?
A. Stickiness B. Tuckiness
C. Ped adhesion D. None of the above

880. Which technique is used to improve cohesiveness using monomer?
A. Hydrophobicity B. Copolymerization
C. Solid dispersion D. None of the above

881. Which of the polymer have good tack property?
A. Butyl acrylate B. Ethyl hexyl acrylate
C. Both A and B D. None of the above

882. Silicon pressure sensitive adhesive is med because of:
A. Flexibility
B. Temperature resistance
C. Both A and B
D. None of the above

883. Phenyl based silicon adhesive are available in viscocity range?
A. 2000-4000 cp B. 6000-25000 cp
C. 100-1000 cp D. 30000-45000 cp

884. For the preparation of test laminate in laboratory which process is used?
A. Transfer coating process
B. Transfer peeling process
C. Transfer tacking process
D. None of the above

885. Pressure sensitive adhesive can be evaluated on the basis of:
A. Shear strength B. Peal adhesion
C. Both A and B D. None of the above

886. Non- traumatic removal of tdds from skin depend on which property?
A. Stracking B. Peel adhesion
C. Shear strength D. None of the above

887. The force required to remove tape in TDDS expressed in:
A. Ounce/inch B. Ounce/cm
C. Mg/inch D. Mg/cm

888. Which of the following testis not used to determine tack property?
A. Thumb rolling ball
B. Quick – stick
C. Probe – adherence
D. All of the above

889. Rolling ball tack test is used to measure?
A. Hardness of system
B. Softness of polymer
C. Stickiness of system
D. None of the above

890. In rolling ball tack test the diameter of ball is:
A. 6/15 B. 7/16
C. 8/20 D. 4/14

891. Ball used in rolling ball tack test is made of which substance?

A. Glass B. Iron
C. Stainless steal D. None of the above

892. In quick stick test for tack property tape is pulled away from substance at which temperature?

A. 90.C B. 120.C
C. 60.C D. None of the above

893. In quick stick test the speed of pulling tape form substance is:

A. 10 inches/min B. 12 inches/min
C. 14 inches/min D. 16 inches/min

894. In measurement of shear strength adhesive coated tape is applies on:

A. Glass plates
B. Stainless steel plate
C. Plastic plate
D. None of the above

895. In membrane moderated TDDS the drug Polymer matrix is suspended in viscous fluid that form:

A. Paste like suspension
B. Viscous liquid
C. Clear solution
D. None of the above

896. The rate of drug release in membrane moderated TDDS can be tailored by varying the:

A. Permeability coefficient
B. Polymer composition
C. Thickness of rate controlling membrane
D. All of the above

897. Transdermal scop transdermal patch used for:

A. Morning sickness
B. Angina pectoris
C. Motion sickness
D. None of the above

898. In adhesive dispersion type TDDS medicated adhesive is spreaded to backing membrane by which method

A. Solution film casting
B. Solvent film casting
C. Both A and B
D. None of the above

899. Nitrodur system is used for:

A. Angina pectoris
B. Hypertension
C. Nyocardical infraction
D. None of the above

900. In micro reservoir TDDS drug reservoir is formed by suspending the drug solid in:

A. Aqueous solution
B. Lipophilic solution
C. Both A and B
D. None of the above

901. Which of the following is the process movement of solvent form lower concentration of solute towards higherconcentration of solvent across a semi-permeable membrane?

A. Diffusion B. Osmosis
C. Imlulution D. Plasmolysis

902. Which of the following first reported osmotic effect in 1748

A. Abbe nollent
B. Hildeluand and scott
C. Pfeffer
D. None of the following

903. Which of the following had been the pioneer of quantitative measurement of osmotic effect ?

A. Abbe Nollent
B. Hildelerand and scott
C. Pfeffer
D. None

904. Which of the following postulated that the osmotic pressure of sugar is directly proportional to the solution concentration and absolute temperature?

A. Abbe Nollent
B. Hildeluand and scott
C. Both A and B
D. Pfeffer

905. Which of the following established the anology between the pfeffer result and the ideal gas laws?

A. Van't hoff
B. Higuchi
C. Hixson – Gowell Wle root
D. Nonoe

906. Which of the following equation established the analogy between the pfeffer and ideal gas laws?

A. Pie= RT In(Po/P)

B. Pie+

C. y = mx + C

D. None of the above

907. What will be the effect of osmotic pressure for soluble solutes?

A. High B. Extremely high

C. Low D. Extremely low

908. Which of the following equation is used for rate of water flow?

A. π=RT In [Po/p] / V

B. π=n2RT

C. Dv/Dt = A0 Δπ/1

D. None of the above

909. Which of the following includes stauerman reflection coefficient:

A. π=RT In [Po/p] / V

B. Dv/Dt = A0 Δπ/1

C. π=n2RT

D. None of the above

910. Which of the following is used to account for derivation from complete semi-permeability character of membrane?

A. Stanerman reflection coefficient

B. Higuchi

C. Both A and B

D. None of the above

911. Which of the following may act as an osmogen and shows good aqueous solubility:

A. Potassium chloride pump

B. Alzet pump

C. Both A and B

D. None of the above

912. Which of the following is employed semi-permeable polymer for the preparation of osmotic pumps?

A. Cellulose acetate

B. Amylone triacetate

C. Agar acetate

D. All of the above

913. Which of the following is employed as selectively permeable membrane for the preparation of osmotic pump?

A. Lactic acid B. Glycolic acid

C. Both A and B D. None of the above

914. Which of the following is important criteria for the selection of semi-permeable polymer?

A. Solubilty B. Permeability

C. Both A and B D. None of the above

915. Which of the following polymer are used in the formulation development of osmotic system for making drug containing matrix core?

A. Ethyl cellulose

B. Vinyl pyrrolidone

C. Carboxy methyl cellulose

D. All of the Above

916. Which of the following is the important criteria for the selection of hydrophilic and hydrophobic polymer?

A. Solubility of drug

B. Amount of drug to be released from the pump

C. Rate of drug to be released from the pump

D. All of the above

917. Which of the following polymer are used for the pumps containing moderately water soluble drugs?

A. Swellable B. Non- swellable

C. Both A and B D. None of the above

918. Swellable Polymer will _________ the hydrostatic pressure inside the pump.

A. Increase

B. Increase than stable

C. Decrease

D. Decrease than stable

919. The non – swellable polymer are employed for which type of drugs?

A. Highly water soluble drugs

B. Moderately water soluble drugs

C. Water insoluble

D. None of the above

920. Which of the following hydrogels are used because of the osmogenic nature?
A. Sodium carboxy methyl cellulose
B. Ethyl cellulose
C. Vinyl pynolidone
D. All of the above

921. Which of the following is a hydrophilic polymer?
A. Carboxy methyl cellulose
B. Ethyl cellulose
C. Wax material
D. All of the above

922. Which of the following is the material with the ability to draw water into the porous network of delivery device?
A. Bending agent B. Wicking agent
C. Osmogen D. Flux regulators

923. A wicking agent is
A. Swellable B. Non Swellable
C. Both A and B D. None of the above

924. Which is the following is characterized by having the ability to undergo phyrisoption
A. Flux regulators B. Bending agent
C. Wicking agent D. None

925. Which of the following is form of absorption where the solvent molecules loosely adhare to surface of the wicking agent?
A. Physisorption
B. Chemisorption
C. Facetilated absorption
D. None of the above

926. For bioactive agent with ________ solubility, the wicking agent aids in the delivery of partially solubilized bioactive gent through the passage way in the semi-permeable coating?
A. High B. Extremely high
C. Low D. Extremely low

927. Which of the following act as the swellable wicking agent?
A. Kaolin B. Alumina
C. SLS D. Both A and B

928. Which of the following is a non-swellable wicking agent?
A. SLS B. PVP
C. Colloidal silica D. All of the above

929. Which of the following solubilizing Agent are classified into 3 group?
A. Swellable B. Non-swellable
C. Both A and B D. None of hte above

930. Which of the following inhibit crystal formation of the formation of the drugs or act by complexation with the drugs?
A. PVP
B. PEG 8000
C. Alpha, Beta, Gama-Cyclodesrine
D. All of the above

931. Which of the following inhibit is a high HCl micelle forming surfactant, mainly anionic surfactants?
A. SLS B. PEG -8000
C. PVP D. All of the above

932. Which of the following are the essential ingredient of the osmotic formulation?
A. Fructose
B. Sucrose
C. Sodium phosphate
D. All of the above

933. Which of the following is the HLB value of sodium oleate?
A. 18 B. 20
C. 17.9 D. 16.9

934. Which of the following is the HLB value of solution trioleate?
A. 2 B. 3.4
C. 3.8 D. 1.8

935. Which of the following solvent are suitable for making polymer solution used for manufacturing the wall of the osmotic device?
A. Carbon- tetrachloride
B. Acetates
C. Poly-butylene
D. None of the above

936. Which of the following will lower the temperature of the 2nd order phase tiansitions of the wall?

A. Plasticizer B. Surfactant
C. Blocking agent D. None of the above

937. Which of the following drug will lower the temperature of the 2nd order phase transition of the wall?

A. Benzoates B. Sorlution loeate
C. PVP D. None of the above

938. Which of the following are pre-selected to increase or decrease the liquid flux?

A. Plasticizer B. Flux regulator
C. Wicking agent D. None of the above

939. Which of the following are the agents which increase the permeability to fluid?

A. Hydrophobic B. Hydrophilic
C. Both A and B D. None of the above

940. The tract which has been largely used for the treatment of obstructive airways diseases?

A. Digestive tract
B. Respiratory tract
C. Urinary tract
D. Elimentary tract

941. For optimum effect the particle size should be:

A. <5.0 μm B. >5.0 μm
C. >10.0 μm D. >47.5 μm

942. The choice area design of inhalation delivery system are predisposed by:

A. Target patient population
B. Clinical objective to be met
C. Physiochemical properties of the drug
D. All of the above

943. Which of the following is a type of inhalation delivery system:

A. Nebulizers B. MDIS
C. DPIS D. All of the above

944. Which of the following is used for acute care of non ambulatory patient:

A. MDIS B. Nebulizers
C. DPIS D. None of the above

945. Which of the following is used for patient having coordination or dexterity problems?

A. Nebulizers B. MDIS
C. DPIS D. None of the above

946. Which of the following is used for local anaesthesia for bronchoscopy?

A. DPIS B. MDIS
C. Nebulizers D. All of the above

947. The activated fate of which substance after their passage through the pulmonary circulation is:

A. Epinephrine B. Bradykinin
C. Dopamine D. Angiotensin – 1

948. The unaffected fate of which substance after their passage through the pulmonary circulation is:

A. Dopamine
B. Bradykinin
C.Angiotensin
D. Epinephrine

949. The removed fate of which substance after their passage through the pulmonary Circulation is:

A. Dopamine B. Bradykinin
C. Angiotensin D. Epinpherine

950. The nebulizers are largely designed with:

A. Non Aqueous Solution
B. Aqueous Solution
C. Emulsion
D. Both A and B

951. The cosolvents which are used in nebulizers are:

A. Glycerine B. Ethanol
C. Propylene glycol D. All of the above

952. The factor which should be considered while developing the nebulizer solution are:

A. Solubility B. Isoelectric PH
C. PKa D. All of the above

953. The Ph of the nebulizer solution should be ideally:

A. Higher than 5.0 B. Lower than 5.0
C. 5.0 D. None of the above

954. Aerosol upon activation emit:
A. Fine liquid dispersion
B. Fine solid particle
C. Gaseous particle
D. Both A and B

955. Aerosol differ from most of the dosage form in their dependence upon the function of:
A. Container B. Valve assembly
C. Components D. All of the above

956. Which of the following term is used to reffering the whole aersol product?
A. Aerosol container
B. Pressurizes container
C. Pressurized package
D. None of the above

957. Pressure is applied to the aerosol system by using :
A. Liquid propllent B. Gaseous propllent
C. Solid propllent D. Both A and B

958. Upon activation of valve assembly of the aerosol which of the following exert pressure?
A. Drug solution B. Propllent
C. Excipient D. All of the above

959. The physical form in which content are emitted is depended upon:
A. Formulation of product
B. Amount of propellent
C. Type of valve employed
D. Both A and B

960. Aerosol product are designed to expel their content as:
A. Dry spray
B. Fine mist
C. Stable or breaking foam
D. All of the above

961. Aerosol used for inhalation therapy must contain particle in which form?
A. Fine liquid mist
B. Wet spray
C. Stable foam
D. Coarse solid particle

962. Which of this particle size is optimum for used in aerosol system to deliver it to bronchioles?
A. 2 µm B. 4 µm
C. 6 µm D. 9 µm

963. Which of this particle size is optimum for used in aerosol system to deliver it to alveolar ducts and alveoli?
A. 6 µm B. 2 µm
C. 0.5 µm D. 4 µm

964. In dermatological spray intended for deposition skin particle size should be:
A. Coarse B. Fine
C. Very fine D. Moderate coarse

965. Aerosol used to provide on air – borne mist are termed as:
A. Stable spray
B. Space spray
C. Breaking form spray
D. None of the above

966. In aerosols space spray are used to deliver:
A. Coarse mist B. Dry mist
C. Fine mist D. Air borne

967. Which of the following product is not apart of space spray?
A. Room deodorizer B. Space insecticide
C. Perfumes D. Room disinfectant

968. Particle size of airbone mist used in space sprays is:
A. <100 µm B. >100 µm
C. <150 µm D. >50 µm

969. A one second burst form a typical aerosol space spray will produce how many particles?
A. 120 million B. 140 million
C. 100 million D. 50 million

970. Aerosol in which ingredient is intended to surface is termed as:
A. Surface coating B. Surface sprays
C. Space sprays D. Both A and B

971. Which of the following product is included in surface sprays?
A. Room deodrizer
B. Cosmetic hair laquer
C. Room disinfectant
D. Space pesticide

972. Which property of container protect aerosol drug from adversely affect by light?

A. Amber bottle B. Opaque
C. Both A and B D. None of the above

973. Physical form and particle size of product of aerosol contribute to:

A. Delivery of drug B. Potency of drug
C. Efficacy of drug D. All of the above

974. An aerosol formulation consist of which these component parts:

A. Product concentration
B. Drug solution
C. Propellent
D. Both A and C

975. Which type of propellet serve the dual role of propellent and vehicle for product concentrate?

A. Compressed gas
B. Liquefied gas
C. Natural gas
D. All of the above

976. Which of the following non – Liquefied compressed gas used in aerosol as propellent?

A. Nitrogen B. CFC
C. HFC D. Carbonmaooxide

977. Which of the following is most used liquefied gas in propellent in aerosol?

A. propane B. CFC
C. HFC D. Ethane

978. Which of the following propellent is not gas at room temperature?

A. Fluorinated Hydrocarbon
B. Carbondioxide
C. Nitrogen
D. None of the above

979. Which of the following is used to made fluorinated hydrocarbon liquefied?

A. By cooling below their boiling point
B. By compressing the gas at room temperature
C. By heating the gas at high temperature
D. Both A and B

980. At which temperature diflueomethone gas will form a liquid?

A. -10* F B. -15*F
C. -5*F D. -22*F

981. As propellant meet the air it immediately evaporates due to:

A. Drop in temperature
B. Drop in humidity
C. Drop in pressure
D. Rise in temperature

982. Depending upon the formulation product concentration product concentrate leave the aerosol Container as:

A. Airborne Liquid drops
B. Airborne drug particle
C. Airborne gaseous praticle
D. Both A and B

983. The gas propellent can be in aerosol to enhance:

A. Solubility of drug
B. Delivery of medicine
C. Carrier ability
D. All of the above

984. Which of the following is not a example of aerosol?

A. Nasal inhalers B. Surface spray
C. Space spray D. Aerated fossil

985. Which of the following property of propellant is important for aerosol?

A. Molecular weight
B. Liquid density
C. Flash point
D. All of the Above

986. The pressure of aerosol is critical and controlled by:

A. Amount of propellant
B. Amount of material
C. Nature of material
D. All of the above

987. Which of the following aerosol consist of greater proportion of propellant?

A. Space spray B. Surface coating
C. Aerosol form D. Surface spray

988. Amount of propellant contain in space spray is:

A. 70% B. 90%
C. 85% D. 65%

989. Space sprays usually operate at pressure between:

A. 25-30 p sig B. 30-40 p sig
C. 45-55 p sig D. 10-20 p sig

990. Surface sprays operate at pressure between:

A. 10-20 p sig B. 25-55 p sig
C. 60-80 p sig D. 05-20 p sig

991. Amount of propellant present in foam aerosol is:

A. 5-10 % B. 15-20 %
C. 80-90 % D. 30-40 %

992. Amount of aerosol present in surface spray is:

A. 30-60 % B. 80-95 %
C. 10-25 % D. 5-20 %

993. Form aerosol considered as:

A. emulsion B. Lotion
C. Suspension D. Sprays

994. Liquefied propellant does not dissolve in which formation?

A. Aqueous B. Non-aqueous
C. Gaseous D. None of the above

995. When the valve is activated the active ingredient leave the container in the form of:

A. Mist B. Form
C. Dry particle D. Liquid

996. To achieve which of these properties blend of the various liquefied gas propellant are generally used?

A. Solubility B. Bioavailability
C. Vapour pressure D. Flash point

997. Which of the following propellant do not used in ability to form HCL with water?

A. Dichlodifluromethane
B. Tertahydrofuromethane
C. Dichlotertaflurometane
D. Trichloromonofulromethane

998. One to which reason influence of the recipient tissue must evaluated?

A. Irritating effect
B. Change in absorption
C. Change in site of action
D. All of the above

999. In aerosol absorption pattern of drug may change due to:

A. Increase solubility
B. Decreased vapour pressure
C. Increased dissolution
D. None of the above

1000. Individual who utilize an inhalation aerosol and sensitive to propellant may exhibit:

A. Respirotoxic effect
B. Cardiotoxic effect
C. CNS toxicity
D. All of the above

1001. Which of these phases are present in two phase system?

A. Liquid and solid phase
B. Solid and vapour phase
C. Vapour and liquid phase
D. None of the above

1002. Which of the following is not present in three phase system?

A. Water miscible liquid propellant
B. Highly aqueous product concentration
C. Vapour phase
D. Both A and B

1003. Which of the following has greatest density in three phase aerosol?

A. Liquefied drug solution
B. Liquefied propellant
C. Aqueous layer
D. Solid phase

1004. Which type of gas will result in emission of the product in aerosol?

A. Gas soluble in product concentrate
B. Gas settle in product concentrate
C. Gas insoluble in product concentrate
D. None of the above

1005. Which of the following propellent gas is used due to their inert nature?

A. CFC B. CO2
C. Nitrogen D. Helium

1006. Which of the following gas is used with the product that are suceptible to oxidation in aerosol?

A. CFC B. Nitrogen
C. Nitrous oxide D. CO2

1007. Which of these propellant does not contribute adversely to smell or taste of aerosol product?

A. CO2 B. CO
C. Nitrogen D. Helium

1008. Which of the following propellant is use when aerosol product is derived in the form of spray or form when expel?

A. CO2 B. Nitrogen
C. Nitrous oxide D. Both A and B

1009. In which type of propellant aerosol system pressure is diminished as product is used?

A. Liquefied gas B. Compressed gas
C. Natural Gas D. Both A and b

1010. Which of this propellant gas is slightly soluble in liquid phase?

A. CO2 B. Nitrogen
C. CFC D. Propane

1011. Which of the metal is not used in the manufacture of aerosol container?

A. Stainless steel B. Aluminium
C. Tinplated steel D. Copper

1012. The selection of aerosol container is based on:

A. Adaptability to production method
B. Compatability with product component
C. Ability to with stand pressure
D. All of the above

1013. Coating of which material is provided to glass container of aerosol to render them more resistance to accidental breakage?

A. Plastic B. Stainless steel
C. Teflon D. Copper

1014. Which of the following coating present the scatthering of glass fragments?

A. Polymer coating B. Plastic coating
C. Metal coating D. None of the above

1015. Which of the following metal is used for certain small volume container aerosol?

A. Tin plate steel B. Aluminium
C. copper D. Stainless steel

1016. Which of this metal in aerosol limitation of high cost?

A. Aluminium B. Stainless steel
C. Plastic D. Copper

1017. Which of the following container material reduce the efficacy of drug?

A. Stainless steel B. Glass
C. Plastic D. Tin plated steel

1018. Which of the following is not used in manufacturing of valve?

A. Rubber B. Plastic
C. Aluminium D. Tin plated steel

1019. Which of the following device used in inhaler for the patent who faces inability to use inhaler?

A. Meter pipe B. Spacer
C. Meter valve D. None of the above

1020. Which of the following is the advantage to use extended device between aerosol container and patient mouth?

A. Reduce aerosol velocity
B. Decrease droplet size
C. Increase time of evaporation
D. All of the above

1021. Aerosol for topical use should deliver at distance of:

A. 4-6 inches B. 2-5 inches
C. 6-8 inches D. 9-11 inches

1022. Which of the following extended device is used with most pressurized aerosol canister?

A. Fisons
B. Brethancer inhaler
C. Nitroease inhaler
D. Allen and hanburg's

1023. To which of the following propellant numerical designation 114 is provided?

A. Difloroethane
B. Octaflurocyclobutanane
C. Dichlorotetrafulroethane
D. Chloropentafluroethane

1024. In which form are dosage from are given to treat chronic illness?

A. Tablet B. Capsule
C. Pills D. All of the above

1025. Which of the following is OTC product?
A. Tablet B. Aerosol
C. Oiltments D. All of the above

1026. What fluctuate the drug plasma level?
A. API
B. Vehicle
C. Concentration of drug
D. None of the above

1027. Which of the following is modes of drug delivery?
A. Targeted delivery
B. Controlled release
C. Modullated release
D. All of the above

1028. What's the objective of targeted delivery system?
A. Deliver drug to specific cell, tissue and organs
B. To reach at specification
C. To modify the release time
D. None of the above

1029. What's the objective of controlled release drug delivery system?
A. Delivery at specific tissue
B. To deliver API at predetermined speed
C. To modify the release time
D. All of the above

1030. What's objective of modulated release drug delivery system?
A. Deliver at specific tissue
B. To deliver API at predetermined rate
C. To release drug at variable rate controlled by environmental condition
D. All of the above

1031. In which year sustained release system were used?
A. 1950 B. 1980
C. 1910 D. 1960

1032. By which route of drug administration 1st sustained release system was used?
A. Oral route B. Parentral
C. opthalmic D. None of the above

1033. Which type of tablet was used as 1st sustained release system?
A. Composed tablet
B. Enteric coated tablet
C. Chewable tablet
D. Double compassion tablet

1034. What are examples of other slow release system?
A. Encapsulated pellets or beads
B. Tablet composed
C. Capsule
D. None of the above

1035. Which of the following is slow release system?
A. Drug embedded in matrix
B. Effervesenct tablet
C. capsule
D. None of the above

1036. In which of the field were sustained drug delivery system was used?
A. Pharmaceutical B. Agriculture
C. genetics D. All of the above

1037. What was a drawback of sustained delivery system?
A. They were affected by environmental condition
B. They do not get affected by acidic pH
C. Design off an tablet
D. All of the above

1038. What was advantages of controlled release system?
A. Independent of environment
B. Design of system
C. Concentration of API
D. Both A and B

1039. The term "smart" was given by whom to controlled release system?
A. Chien and robinson
B. Heilman
C. Banker
D. Nono of the above

1040. The term "targeted" was given by whom to controlled release system?
A. Golberg B. Sefton
C. Horbert D. None of the above

1041. The term "Therapeutic" was given by whom to controlled release system?
A. Heilman B. Herbert
C. Chien D. Relsomsor

1042. What is principle of controlled release system?
A. Advanced engineering
B. Blood volume
C. Plasma concentration
D. None of the above

1043. Where controlled release system having sensor
A. Yes
B. According to release pateern
C. Depend on drug
D. No

1044. 1st self programmed controlled release system was by:
A. Banker
B. Sefton
C. Horbett
D. None of the above

1045. In which way rate controlled delivery system is programmed?
A. Active
B. Passive
C. Self
D. None of the above

1046. Who made metered insulin pump and in which year?
A. Sefton 1984
B. Horbell 1984
C. Banker 1984
D. None of the above

1047. 1st active self programmed therapeutic controlled system was made by whom and in which year?
A. Hobett 1984
B. Sefton 1984
C. Chein and robinson 1956
D. None of the above

1048. Which of the following equation represent zero order release delivery system?
A. dMt/dt=k
B. dMt/dt=K(Ho=Ht)
C. dMt/dt=KMo e-kt
D. dMt/dt=K/t

1049. Which of the following equation represent 1st order release?
A. dMt/dt=k
B. dMt/dt=K(Mo-Mt)
C. dMt/dt=K/t
D. None of the above

1050. What is the basic idea of controlled drug delivery?
A. Alter pharmacokinetic and pharmcodynamic of bioactives
B. Modifying molecule structure
C. Physiological parameters - alternations
D. All of the above

1051. What is primary objective of controlled drug delivery?
A. Ensure safety and enhance efficacy of drug
B. Improved patient compliance
C. Both A and B
D. None of the above

1052. Which of the following things affect controlled drug release?
A. Better modification
B. Control of plasma drug level
C. Reduction in dosing frequency
D. All of the above

1053. What is the prime parameter for development of a controlled delivery system?
A. Therapeutic index
B. Drug concentration
C. Dosing frequency
D. None of the above

1054. Which of the following scientist gave relation between therapeutic index and dosing interval?
A. Sefton
B. Theeuwes and Bayne
C. Horbett
D. None of the above

1055. Which of the following equation represents relation between dosing interval of therapeutic index?
A. I<Ty2(InTI)/In2
B. dMt/dt=K/t
C. dMt/dt=Kmoe-Kt
D. None of the above

1056. It is mandatory to dose the patient at intervals shouter than the half life?
A. Yes
B. No
C. Dependent on toxicity
D. None of the above

1057. How dosing interval are extended?
A. Either by manipulation drug molecule
B. Reduce rate of elimination
C. Release rate of a dosage form alteration
D. All of the above

1058. Which of the following are the factors affecting the design of controlled release products?

A. Physiocochemical properties of drug
B. Route of administration
C. Acute /chronic therapy
D. All of the above

1059. Which of the following physiochemical properties of drug affect designing of controlled release of drug?

A. solubility
B. Stability
C. Partition coefficient
D. All of the above

1060. Do route of administration affect the design of controlled release product?

A. Always B. Some times
C. Never D. None of the above

1061. spleen influences the performance of

A. Controlled release
B. Sustained release
C. Both of the above
D. Delayed release

1062. Who Un wanted side effect can be minimised?

A. By delivering the maximum fraction of applied does reaching the target site
B. Wealized delivery
C. Inducing novel carrier
D. All of the above

1063. Which step in drug availability form conventional delivery system is rate limiting step?

A. Absorption of drug across a biological membrane
B. API concentration
C. Plasma level concentration
D. None of the above

1064. Which of the following equation represents maintenance of dose calculation?

A. MD=Css.CL.I/f B. Ro=F.MD/I
C. Rel=Kcl.Css.Vd D. None of the abo

1065. Which of the following equation represents amount of drug required for controlled release system conventional steady state?

A. MD=Di+Der
B. Ro=Ra
C. Rel=MDKel
D. MD control gel=MDFconven.0.693.I/T1/2

1066. Which kind of dose gives a flat plateau?

A. Loading dose B. Single dose
C. Multiple dose D. None of the above

1067. Which of the following equation represent total dose?

A. MD=di+der B. MD=Css.CL.I/F
C. Rel=MD.Kel D. None of the above

1068. Primary controlled released system achieved by which of the following factor?

A. Diffusion B. Degradation
C. Swelling D. All of the above

1069. When diffusion occurs?

A. When bioactive agent passes through the polymer
B. Movement of particle from higher concentration to lower concentration
C. Both A and B
D. All of the above

1070. Which of the following is a slow dissolve drug?

A. Digoxin B. Salicylamide
C. Griseofulvin D. All of the above

1071. Which of the following are important parameters to assess the therapeutic efficacy of any drug?

A. Pharmacokinetic
B. Pharmacodynamic
C. Both A and B
D. None of the above

1072. Which of the following terms describe about absorption, distribution, metabolism of dimnasion?

A. Pharmacokinetic
B. Pharmacodynamic
C. Both a and B
D. All of the above

1073. Which of the following terms describes about pharmacological and toxicological profile of drug?
- A. Pharmacokinetic
- B. Pharmacodynamic
- C. Both A and B
- D. Pharmacovigilance

1074. Which was the 1st pharmacokinetic model have been put forward for studies of drug targeting via either IV or intra asterial route?
- A. Himmustein And Lutz
- B. Notari
- C. Wagner
- D. Weiss

1075. What was the name of 1st pharmacokinetic model for study of drug targeting will either IV or IA route?
- A. Hypothesis
- B. Compartment
- C. Physiological Models
- D. None of the above

1076. Which system of body works to control the amount and time of endogenous chemical release for optimal physiological response?
- A. Homeostasis
- B. Feedback Mechanism
- C. Both A and B
- D. None of the Above

1077. Which of the following are module features of drug for sustained and controlled delivery
- A. Larger Dose
- B. Poor absorption
- C. Nero Therapeutic Index
- D. All of the above

1078. By which factors frequency of administration and doses regimen are determined?
- A. Biological Half Life
- B. Therapeutic Index
- C. Plasma Drug Concentration
- D. Both A and B

1079. Which of the following scientist gave idea for determining frequency of administration and doses regimen?
- A. Stella and reamcy
- B. Horbett
- C. Sefton
- D. Chein and Robinson

1080. Which of the following formula represents therapeutic index?
- A. Ms – Ktn
- B. dv/ dt = Alp (IDT-DP) / L
- C. dm/dt = (dv/dt) C
- D. TI = MTDD / MED

1081. Which of the following is drawback of conventional drug delivery system?
- A. In ability to take therapeutic benefits of those Drug, which either have a shorter therapeutic index
- B. Very short elimination half life
- C. Both A and B
- D. None of the above

1082. According the which model it was assumed 1, 2 or more functional components are arranged in parallel?
- A. Hypothetical
- B. Compartment
- C. Physiological response
- D. None of the above

1083. Which of the following model were used with term open?
- A. One compartment model
- B. Two Compartment model
- C. Multiple Compartment model
- D. All of the above

1084. Which of the following equation represents Zero order absorption followed by first order dimention?
- A. Cp=FKo (e-ketT-1)e-kcl+/ K el Vd
- B. Cp=FKo (e-ketT-1)e-kcl+/ Vol (Ka-Kel)
- C. Both A and B
- D. None of the above

1085. Which of the following equation represents mean residence time?
- A. MRT =∫_0^(∋∞)tcdt/ ∫_0^∞▒cdt=aumc/auco
- B. MRT = MRT oral – MRT IV
- C. MAT – 1/ka
- D. MAT = T/2

1086. In which of the following dry powder is used as an doses form

A. MDIS
B. DPIS
C. Nebulizer
D. None of the above

1087. Most commonly used plant part for tincture preparation is........................

A. Dried Roots B. Stems (Dried)
C. Flowers (Dried) D. Dried Leaves

1088. Tincture of Orange is produced by the process of....................................

A. Infusion B. Maceration
C. Decoction D. Percolation

1089. The term maceration is derived from the Latin word macerare meaning.................

A. To Dissolve B. To crush
C. To soak D. To boil

1090. In which extraction process, very less quantity of menstrum is required?

A. Reserved Percolation
B. Percolation
C. Counter Current Extraction
D. Continuous Hot Percolation

1091. Solvent mixture in the form of menstruum is not allowed in which extraction process?

A. Maceration B. Double Maceration
C. Triple Maceration D. Both B&C

1092. Enzyme degradation of active principles of plant extract is possible in...........................

A. Acidic and Basic Medium
B. Aqueous and Dilute Alcohol
C. Only in basic Medium
D. None of the above

1093. Name the extraction process where vegetable drugs are treated with cold water and boiling water for a short time.

A. Spirit B. Infusion
C. Tincture D. Percolation

1094. The term " Galenicals" is associated with which process

A. Drying B. Packaging
C. Extraction D. Size reduction

1095. Which of the following is observed during extraction process?

A. Heat Transfer B. Mass Transfer
C. Fluid Transfer D. Energy Transfer

1096. According to WHO, a plant used for extraction must be free from

A. Fibres B. Trichomes
C. Aflatoxins D. Microorganisms

1097. Heat sensitive chemical components are not extracted by............................ process.

A. Digestion B. Soxhelation
C. Decoction D. Maceration

1098. .... is designated as Father of Chromatography.

A. Aristotle
B. Mikhail Semyonovich Tswett
C. Antonie Philips van Leeuwenhoek
D. Alexander Von Humboldt

1099. Defatting of plant parts is majorly caused by which solvent?

A. Acetone B. Ether
C. Petroleum Ether D. Chloroform

1100. What is the nature of the Silica Gel which is used as stationary phase in TLC?

A. Acidic
B. Both Acidic and Basic
C. Basic
D. None of the above

1101. Leaching by immersion of crude materials is also known as.............................

A. Expression B. Percolation
C. Maceration D. Infusion

1102. Expression is a .... extraction process.

A. Chemical B. Biotechnological
C. Physical D. Biological

1103. .... process is preferred for extraction of unorganised crude materials.

A. Percolation B. Maceration
C. Compression D. Expression

1104. Commonest disadvantage of using alcohol as a solvent in extraction is it's .....

A. Neutrality B. Cost
C. Toxicity D. All of the above

1105. Commonly used solvent in infusion is...........

A. Boiling water B. Boiling alcohol
C. Regular Water D. Chilled Water

1106. Tincture of Lemon is produced by which process?

A. Soxhlet Extraction
B. Simple Maceration
C. Percolation
D. Digestion

1107. Concentrated infusion of Orange is produced by ....

A. Maceration
B. Simple Maceration
C. Double Maceration
D. Percolation

1108. Volume of menstruum required for double maceration is calculated by which formula?

A. Volume of menstruum required for first maceration=Total Volume of menstruum-Volume to be retained by Drug/2 +Volume to be retained by the drug.
B. Volume of menstruum required for 2nd maceration=Total Volume of menstruum – Volume of menstruum used in first maceration
C. Only Option 1 is correct.
D. Both 1st and 2nd options are correct.

1109. One Fourth volume of 90% Alcohol is added in finished product obtained from 1st maceration of which extraction process?

A. Double Maceration
B. Simple Maceration
C. Triple Maceration
D. Decoction

1110. Simple Maceration process is commonly applied for which types of drugs?

A. Unorganised drugs
B. Organised Drugs
C. Neither for Organised nor for Unorganised
D. For both Organised & Unorganised

1111. Concentrated infusion of Quassia is prepared by .... process.

A. Double Maceration
B. Simple Maceration
C. Triple Maceration
D. Expression

1112. Conical Percolators used in extraction process is coated inside with which material?

A. Copper B. Tin
C. Iron D. Stainless Steel

1113. Bottom/Lower Diameter of Conical Percolator is ....

A. Not greater than twice of upper diameter
B. Equal to half of upper diameter
C. Not less than half of upper diameter
D. Equal to half of upper diameter

1114. Which type of percolator is suitable for use of highly concentrated alcohol as menstruum?

A. Conical Percolator
B. Cylindrical Percolator
C. Steam Packet Percolator
D. Modified Percolator

1115. Drugs which active constituents are not freely soluble in solvent can be extracted through ....

A. Soxhelation B. Maceration
C. Digestion D. Simple Maceration

1116. Fixed oils are extracted out through which of the extraction method?

A. Decoction
B. Perfusion
C. Contineous hot percolation
D. Double Maceration

1117. Syphon tube is present in which type of extraction method apparatus?

A. Percolator
B. Soxhlet apparatus
C. Counter current extractor
D. Digestor

1118. What is the function of siphon tube which is present in soxhlet apparatus?

A. It contains boiling solvent
B. It helps to maintain the temperature
C. It is a glass body in which crude drug is placed
D. It helps in the extraction of active constituents

1119. Which drug would block the soxhlet apparatus when its extraction is done by this method?

A. Orange peel B. Caffiene
C. Fennel D. Clove

1120. Which of the below is limitation for continuous hot percolation process?

A. Only cold mixture of solvent is used
B. Thermostable compounds are used
C. Only pure solvent can be used
D. Gum and resins are also extracted

1121. When a drug is extracted by heating at a particular pressure name the process?

A. Digestion
B. Percolation
C. Decoction
D. Countercurrent extraction

1122. In soxhelation process .... solvent or .... mixtures are used.

A. Mixture, cold mixture
B. Benzene, hydrocarbons
C. Pure, constant boiling
D. Polymers, hydrocarbons

1123. Immunogens are smaller in size in which range their molecular weight belongs to ....

A. 10,000-70,000 B. 1000-10,000
C. 20,000-80,000 D. 1000-50,000

1124. Which of the below are example of inhalant allergens?

A. Mites B. Mould spores
C. Dander D. All of the above

1125. Pollen allergens have many apertures the adject biological term used for that is ....

A. Acolpate B. Psilate
C. Multicolpate D. Echinate

1126. Biological tern used for spiny pollen allergen is ....

A. Silate B. Echinate
C. Granulate D. Cophate

1127. Timothy grass pollens diameter ranges from ....

A. 15-45 μ B. 0.5-10 μ
C. 45-80 μ D. 0.05-100 μ

1128. Different characterstics of entomophilous pollens are except ....

A. Scented plants
B. Upto 200 μ in diameter
C. Adhesive
D. All of the above

1129. Natural source of injectant allergens produced by ....

A. Alfalfa B. Rice flour
C. Citrus D. Hornets

1130. Anaphylactic shock is the severe symptom caused by which type of alleregn?

A. Ingestant allergen
B. Pollen allergens
C. Inhalant allergens
D. Injectant allergens

1131. The north American plant sumjac responsible for contact dermatitis belongs to which family?

A. Ancardiaceae B. Umbelliferaceae
C. Scrophulariaceae D. Myrtaceae

1132. Phenolic compound which cause contact allergy the allergenic component called ....

A. Ivy B. Uricosuric
C. Urushiols D. Uric crystals

1133. Plants which give rise to contact allergic reaction except

A. Ruta graveolens B. Alfalfa
C. Osage orange D. May-apple

1134. Allergy caused by metabolic product of living organisms is produced by.............

A. Infectant allergens
B. Contactant allegens
C. Injectant allergens
D. Pollen allergens

1135. Which type of allergens do not produce localized effect to one organs through blood?

A. Injectant allergens
B. Contactant allergens
C. Ingestant allergens
D. Infectant allergens

1136. Predisposing factors which make person hypersensitive to allergens except
A. Psychic Influences
B. Endocrine gland dysfunction
C. Hepatic dysfunction
D. Alveoler dysfunction

1137. Pressure and temperature conditions for supercritical fluid extraction of pyrithrins
A. 500C, 250 bar B. 100 0C, 280 bar
C. 700C, 380 bar D. 1100C, 280 bar

1138. Advantages of CO2 gas in supercritical fluid extraction are ....
A. Sterile B. Non-explosive
C. Bacteriostatic D. All of the above

1139. CO2 gas behave like supercritical fluid at critical point of .... pressure and .... temperature.
A. 100 bar, 1000C
B. 150 bar, 1500C
C. 73.83 bar, 31.060C
D. 80.73 bar, 42.020C

1140. What is the advantage of carbon-di-oxide in supercritical fluid extaction?
A. Low polarity B. Non-polar
C. High polarity D. Ionic

1141. Temperature and pressure requied for extraction of caffeine from coffee by supercritical fluid extraction method is ....
A. 20-400C, 60-90 bar
B. 400C, 160 bar
C. 40-800C, 200-300 bar
D. 500C, 250 bar

1142. Solvent used for extraction of carotenoids and essential fatty acids is...........................
A. Alcohol B. Oil
C. Butylene glycol D. Propylene glycol

1143. What is the ratio of herb and menstrum for preparation of cassia alata leaf extract?
A. 5:1 B. 15:1
C. 10:1 D. 20:1

1144. The resultant product of solvents action on raw material is known as
A. Solution B. Extracts
C. Suspension D. None of the above

1145. Biophenolic fractions, vitamins, terpenes and amino acid is extracted by using various solvents except
A. Alcohol B. Propylene glycol
C. Phenol D. Water

1146. What is the limit for glycosidic extracts is in its rational form?
A. 1:10 B. 4:10
C. 2:10 D. 5:10

1147. The Ph of cosmetic extracts ranges from
A. 5-7 B. 8-10
C. 7-8 D. 4-8

1148. What is the composition of arithritis tincture?
A. Pepper, willow bark
B. Cardamom, alcohol
C. Alcohol, ginger
D. Cardamom, yellow gentian

1149. Effect of ingestant allergens is
A. Organ specific B. Localised
C. Non-localised D. None of the above

1150. Cardamom and yellow gentian tincture is used for
A. Poor appetite B. Digestive problem
C. Arthritis D. Heart tonic

1151. What is the composition of tincture which is used to treat digestive problem?
A. Pepper, 70% alcohol
B. Ginger, 90% alcohol
C. Cardamom, gentian
D. Ginger, 70% alcohol

1152. Wild sunflower and thyme tincture is used for
A. Arithritis B. Poor appetite
C. Bronchitis D. Nausea

1153. What is the family of inula helenium?
A. Roseaceae B. Fabeaceae
C. Liliaceae D. Astereaceae

1154. Which solvent used in supercritical fluid extraction is?
A. Carbon di oxide B. Propane
C. Acetone D. All of the above

1155. Which one of the below herb act as insect repellent

A. Carica papaya
B. Cymbopogon flexusus
C. Cuminum cyminum
D. All of the above

1156. What is the ratio of herb and menstrum for preparation of zanthoxylem spp. soft ectract?

A. 2:1 B. 8:1
C. 5:1 D. 12:1

1157. From which family weldelia calendulacea belongs to ....

A. Liliaceae B. Solanaceae
C. Ruteaceae D. Compositae

1158. Propane used as solvent in supercritical fluid extraction process, at what temperature and pressure it act as supercritical fluid?

A. 369.8 K, 4.25atm
B. 304.1 K, 7.39atm
C. 512.6 K, 8.09atm
D. 573.9 K, 6.14atm

1159. What is the ratio of herb and menstrum for preparation of weldelia calendulacea soft extract?

A. 1:2 B. 8:1
C. 5:1 D. 8:2

1160. Co-solvents used in supercritical fluid extraction is ....

A. Propane
B. Trichlorofluoromethyane
C. Propylene
D. All of the above

1161. What is the viscosity of supercritical fluid?

A. 100-1000kg/m3 B. 100 kg/m3
C. 1000 kg/m3 D. 10,000 kg/m3

1162. Which step is involved in supercritical fluid extraction?

A. Extraction and expansion
B. Solvent conditioning
C. Separation
D. All of the above

1163. The herbal feed partical size range in super critical fluid extraction is ....

A. 0.5mm-3mm B. 5mm-10mm
C. 0.1mm-1mm D. 10mm-50mm

1164. Super critical fluid extractin technology is applied to ....

A. Extracting nicotine and caffeine
B. Cleaning wafers
C. Drying aerogels
D. All of the above

1165. What is the ratio of herb and menstrum for preparation of viburnum spp.dry extract?

A. 5:1 B. 6:1
C. 8:1 D. 12:1

1166. For primary size reduction of leaves, stems, barks, roots, kernels and shells which equipment is suitable?

A. Hammer mill
B. Jaw crusher
C. Magnetic seperator
D. Belt conveyor

1167. Soft extract of wedelia calendulaceae is used in

A. Deobstruent
B. Uterine haemorrhage
C. Cephalic lesion
D. All of the above

1168. What is the beneficial use of exhausted herb discharge?

A. Biochemical gas production
B. Underground dumping to prevent its harmful effects
C. Food for aquatic animals
D. Production of nitrogen gas

1169. Which equipment is used to remove iron trash from the feed, which is feeded in size reduction equipment?

A. Belt conveyor
B. Jaw crusher
C. Magnetic separator
D. Hammer mill

1170. What does the term miscellae means ....

A. The substance form at critical temperature and pressure
B. Solution containing extracted substances
C. Ionic substances
D. Foaming agents

1171. White spirit when used as menstrum its boiling point is allowed in range is........

A. 40-60C B. 80-110C
C. 60-80C D. 160-196 0C

1172. When tolune used as menstrum its boiling point recommended is ....

A. 80.10C B. 80.730C
C. 98.400C D. 110.620C

1173. Which filtration equipment used in continuous herbal extraction process?

A. Enclosed filter press
B. Meta filter
C. Nutch filter
D. Leaf filter

1174. At what temperature volatile solvent recovery is possible.

A. -5-100C B. 5-100C
C. 10-150C D. 10-500C

1175. What is the ratio of herb and menstrum for preparation of aristolochia indica dry extract?

A. 10:1 B. 8:1
C. 12:1 D. 15:1

1176. Extraction does not involve one of the following component?

A. Solvent B. Vapour
C. Crude solids D. Active constituent

1177. Alcohol is unable to dissolve ....

A. Sugar B. Gums
C. Waxes D. All of the above

1178. What is the ratio of herb and menstrum for preparation of blepharis edulis dry extract?

A. 4:1 B. 6:1
C. 8:1 D. 10:1

1179. Which part of aegle marmelos used to prepare its dry extract?

A. Unripe dried fruit B. Root
C. Ripe dried fruit D. Bark

1180. Compound tincture of cardamom is prepared by a process called ....

A. Double maceration
B. Triple maceration
C. Percolation
D. Continuous percolation

1181. Belladonna tincture prepared by percolation due to its

A. Therapeutic value of drug
B. Chemical properties of constituents
C. Nature of crude drug
D. None of the above

1182. Which process utilise soxhlet extractor?

A. Continuous hot percolation
B. Infusion
C. Simple percolation
D. Double aceration

1183. Tincture contain drug and menstrum in ratio

A. 1:2 B. 1:3
C. 1:4 D. 1:5

1184. Liquid extracts contain drug and menstrum in ratio of

A. 1:1 B. 1:2
C. 2:1 D. None of the above

1185. Infusions are generally used when crude drug is .... in nature.

A. Hard B. Soft
C. Woody D. Prickle

1186. Chamomile infusion is prepared by using which infusion method?

A. Cold infusion B. Hot infusion
C. Pot infusion D. None of the above

1187. The process of boiling drug with water for 10-15 min is called ....

A. Decoction B. Percolation
C. Infusion D. Maceration

1188. Unorganised drugs are usually extracted by a process called ....

A. Decoction B. Percolation
C. Infusion D. Maceration

1189. In which extraction process crude drug is imbibed initially by soaking into menstrum for few hours?

A. Double maceration
B. Triple maceration
C. Simple maceration
D. Infusion

1190. Which method is used for extraction of volatile nature active constituents of drugs?

A. Pot infusion B. Cold infusion
C. Decoction D. Percolation

1191. What is the effect of saturated vapour pressure in volatile solvent recovery?

A. Solvent condenses
B. Solvent evaporated
C. Solvent filter easily
D. All of the above

1192. Which type of dryer is suitable for free flowing and non-hygroscopic material?
A. Tray dryer B. Vaccum dryer
C. Spray dryer D. Freeze dryer

1193. Atomization of feed is done in which type of drying process?
A. Tray dryer B. Vaccum dryer
C. Spray dryer D. Freeze dryer

1194. What is the ratio of herb and menstrum for preparation of acacia Arabica dry extract?
A. 5:1 B. 10:1
C. 15:1 D. 20:1

1195. What is the ratio of herb and menstrum for preparation of juglans regia dry extract?
A. 5:1 B. 10:1
C. 15:1 D. 20:1

1196. Which part of rhamnus purshiana is used to prepare its dry extract?
A. Bark B. Stem
C. Root D. Rhizome

1197. The fluidized mixture of .... and .... comes out from the bottom of spray dryer and introduced in a cyclone separator.
A. Air, powder B. Liquid, vapours
C. Liquid, powder D. Solid, vapours

1198. Changes occur in properties of spray dried product
A. Color change B. Decrease density
C. Decrease potency D. No effect

1199. Correct statement for allergenic extract except
A. Used for diagnosis
B. Treat allergenic diseases
C. Produces allergy
D. Suspension of allergens

1200. What is the chemical nature of allergen?
A. proteinous B. Glycoproteinous
C. Both of the above D. None

1201. What is the range of allergen molecular weight?
A. 10,000-20,000 B. 20,000-40,000
C. 5000-40,000 D. 40,000-80,000

1202. Allergenic substance constitute ....
A. One allergen
B. One type of allergen
C. More than one allergen
D. Poisonous substances

1203. What is the composition of allergenic extract which is used for diagnosis?
A. Glycerine B. Phenol
C. Saline D. All of the above

1204. What is the ratio of herb and menstrum for preparation of rheum spp. Dry extract?
A. 2:1 B. 3:1
C. 4:1 D. 5:1

1205. What is the ratio of herb and menstrum for preparation of ricinus communis root dry extract?
A. 5:1 B. 10:1
C. 15:1 D. 20:1

1206. At what concentration phenol act as preservativein allergenic extract.
A. 0.4% B. 0.04%
C. 0.7% D. 0.8%

1207. What is the Ph of allergenic extract used in diagnosis of allergy?
A. 7 B. 7.5
C. 7.5 D. 8

1208. Pollinosis is caused by which allergen?
A. Inhalant allergen
B. Ingestant allergen
C. Infectant allegen
D. Contactant allergen

1209. Diagnostic extracts prepared from various allergenic extracts except
A. Dandelion B. Barley
C. Mustard D. Rhizopus

1210. Which of the below fungal extract used for diagnosis and treatment of allergenic reactions?
A. Penicillium species
B. Juniper
C. Gladiolus
D. Orchard grass

1211. Dust mites belongs to which species?
A. Spectabilis B. Dermatophagoides
C. Dorsata D. Nearctica

1212. What is the ratio of herb and menstrum for preparation of viburnum spp.soft extract?
A. 5:1 B. 6:1
C. 8:1 D. 10:1

1213. Soft extract of withania somnifera is used for............
A. Aphrodisiac
B. Alopecia
C. Uterine menorrhagia
D. Hair oil

1214. Insect allergy occur due to except one
A. Insect bite
B. Inhalation of insect scales
C. Inhalation of insect hair
D. Substance released by insect

1215. What are the symptom of insect allergy?
A. Asthma B. Urticaria
C. Cardiac arrest D. All of the above

1216. Pollen extract prepared from..........
A. Epidermophyton
B. Gladiolus
C. Helminthotsporium
D. Alternaria

1217. Which of the below belongs to order hymenoptera?
A. Insects B. Fungi
C. Eucalyptus D. Dandelion

1218. Which of the below insect produce insect allergy?
A. Mosquitos B. Mites
C. Honeybee D. All of the above

1219. Food extracts prepared from
A. Arrowroot B. Sunflower seed
C. Beef liver D. All of the above

1220. Which food produces food allergy?
A. Yeast B. Banana
C. Apricot D. All of the above

1221. Allergen sterilization done by
A. Boiling B. Filtration
C. Refrigeration D. All of the above

1222. Which of the below insect cause insect allergy?
A. Red ant B. Honeybee
C. Wasps D. All of the above

1223. Which step is involved in preparation of allergenic extract?
A. Drying B. Defatting
C. Dissolution D. All of the above

1224. Necessary condition required during extraction is ....
A. Aseptic area B. Temperate area
C. Refrigerated area D. Polluted area

1225. What is the ratio of herb and menstrum for preparation of valerian wallichii soft extract?
A. 4:1 B. 5:1
C. 6:1 D. 8:1

1226. Which part of zanthoxylum spp. used to prepare its soft extract?
A. Bark B. Root
C. Leaves D. Rhizome

1227. Which part of urginea indica used to prepare its soft extract?
A. Bulbs B. Seeds
C. Root D. Leaves

1228. Allergenic extract sterility test performed for
A. Aerobic micro-organisms
B. Anaerobic micro-organisms
C. For both a and b
D. None

1229. Standards of allergenic extracts expressed in form of
A. Weight/volume B. Volume/volume
C. Weight/weight D. All of the above

1230. Standards of allergenic extracts expressed in form of
A. Pollen units
B. Protein-nitrogen units
C. Total nitrogen units
D. All of the above

1231. What is the ratio of herb and menstrum for preparation of urtica dioica soft extract?
A. 2:1 B. 4:1
C. 6:1 D. 8:1

1232. What is the chemical name of allergen whose source is rhus?
A. Helenin B. Urushiol
C. Phorbol D. Parthenin

1233. What is the chemical name of allergen whose source is coleus forskohlii?

A. Helenin B. Urushiol
C. Phorbol D. Parthenin

1234. What is the chemical name of allergen whose source is derris elliptica?

A. Allicin B. Rotenone
C. Pyrethrein D. Geraneol

1235. What is the chemical name of allergen whose source is Bulgarian rose oil?

A. Allicin B. Rotenone
C. Pyrethrin D. Geraneol

1236. What is the chemical name of allergen whose source is chrysanthemum cinerariaefolium?

A. Allicin B. Helenin
C. Pyrethrin D. Geraneol

1237. What is the storage condition required for allergenic extract?

A. -6-10C B. 2-80C
C. 250C D. 270C

1238. What is the chemical name of allergen whose source is congress grass?

A. Helenin B. Urushiol
C. Phorbol D. Parthenin

1239. What is the chemical name of allergen whose source is podophyllum peltatum?

A. Podophylotoxin B. Allicin
C. Pyrethrin D. Geraneol

1240. Which solvent is used for removal of fat from allergenic substance?

A. Petroleum ether B. Phenol
C. Alcohol D. Benzene

1241. What is the ratio of herb and menstrum for preparation of withania somnifera dry extract?

A. 5:1 B. 1:5
C. 1:2 D. 12:1

1242. Which part of trigonella foenumgraecum is used to prepare its dry extract?

A. Leaves B. Root
C. Seeds D. Stem

1243. In preparation of allergenic extract defatting process takes place for

A. For 24-72 hours B. For 12 hours
C. For 1 hours D. For 2 hours

1244. Early spring pollinating trees, which produce inhalant allergen except

A. American elm B. Butter nuts
C. Slippery elm D. Red maple

1245. Grasses which produce inhalant allergens except

A. Black walnuts B. Orchard grass
C. Timothy D. Johnson grass

1246. Late spring pollinating trees, which produce inhalant allergen except

A. Black walnut B. Bermuda grass
C. White oak D. Red oak

1247. What is the thickness of stationary phase in thin layer chromatography?

A. 0.02-0.08mm B. 0.2-0.25mm
C. 2-4mm D. 2-8mm

1248. What is the length of stationary phase glass plate?

A. 8 cm B. 10 cm
C. 18 cm D. 20 cm

1249. What is the ratio of herb and menstrum for preparation of tinospora cardifolia dry extract?

A. 8:1 B. 10:1
C. 12:1 D. 15:1

1250. At what temperature TLC plate is activated

A. 500C B. 700C
C. 100-1050C D. 1500C

1251. How much time is required to activate cellulose TLC plate?

A. 10min B. 30min
C. 45min D. 60min

1252. Which method is used to measure the ash?

A. Ether ash B. Phenol ash
C. Sulphated ash D. All of the above

1253. Determine the amount of material that remains after ignition, is termed as

A. Total acid value B. Total ash value
C. Protein content D. Water content

1254. Total ash consists of

A. Carbonates B. Silicates
C. Phosphates D. All of the above

1255. What is the composition of infusion prepared for cold?

A. Peppermint leaves, alfalfa leaves, lemon balm

B. Peppermint, orange rind, dandelion

C. Peppermint leaves, cinnamon, blassoms

D. Liquorice, sweet violet, cinnamon

1256. What is the composition of infusion prepared for de-toxification?

A. Alfalfa, romaine leaves, cinnamon stick

B. clover blossoms, cinnamon stick, orange rind

C. Liquorice balm, alfalfa leaves

D. lemon balm, alfalfa leaves

1257. What is the composition of infusion prepared for vitamins /

A. Rose hips, cinnamon stick, lemon balm

B. Filaree, peppermint leaves, alfalfa

C. Alfalfa, dandelion, romanine, parsley, celerytops, mint

D. Indian mallow, alfalfa, liquorice

1258. What is the composition of infusion prepared for vitamin c?

A. Mint, alfalfa, parsley, peppermint

B. Colver blossoms, cinnamon

C. Cinnamon, liquorice

D. Rose hips, cinnamon stick, lemon balm, lemon rind

1259. What is the composition of infusion prepared for stress?

A. Abuthilon indicum, sidacordifolia, liquorice, holy basil, ashwagandha

B. Mint, alfalfa, dandelion, parsley

C. Cinnamon, liquorice, sweet violet flower

D. Peppermint, dried lemon balm, alfalfa

1260. What is the composition of infusion prepared for antitussive?

A. Indian mallow, country mallow, mint

B. Cinnamon, liquorice, sweet violet flower

C. Filaree, dandelion, romainee

D. Clover blossoms, orange rinel, mint

1261. What is the composition of infusion prepared for indigestion?

A. Ginger, honey

B. Ginger, berries

C. Calumba, sweet flag

D. Ashwagandha

1262. What is the composition of decoction prepared for relieving menstrual pain?

A. Senna pods, ginger

B. Carydalis, cinnamon

C. Calumba, sweetflag

D. Ashwagandha root

1263. What is the composition of decoction prepared for constipation?

A. Senna pods, ginger

B. Carydalis, cinnamon

C. Calumba, sweetflag

D. Prickly ash berries

1264. What is the composition of decoction prepared for anaemia?

A. Senna pods, ginger

B. Astragalus, angelica

C. Calumba, sweetflag

D. Prickly ash berries

1265. What is the ratio of herb and menstrum for preparation of symplocos racemosa soft extract?

A. 2:1 B. 3:1

C. 4:1 D. 5:1

1266. Which part of taraxacum officinale is used to prepare its extracts?

A. Roots and rhizome

B. Stem

C. Fruit

D. Bark

1267. What is the herb and menstrum ratio for preparation of strebulus as per dry extract?

A. 8:1 B. 10:1

C. 12:1 D. 15:1

1268. What is the composition of decoction prepared for bronchial asthma?

A. Ashwagandha root

B. Cinnamon, corydalis

C. Senna pods

D. Coleus pods

1269. What is the composition of decoction prepared for cough?

A. Calumba B. Senna pods
C. Schisandra D. Corydalis

1270. What is the composition of decoction prepared for poor circulation?

A. Astragalus
B. Ginger, prickly ash berries
C. Ashwagandha root
D. Senna pods

1271. What is the composition of decoction prepared for stress?

A. Ashwagandha root
B. Corydalis
C. Senna pods
D. Calumba

1272. What is the ratio of herb and menstrum for preparation of terminalia chebula pericarpdry extract?

A. 1:1 B. 2:1
C. 3:1 D. 4:1

1273. Which part of tinospora cardifolia is used to prepare its dry extract?

A. Leaf B. Stem
C. Root D. Fruit

1274. Liquid extract of zea mays gives in cardiac infaraction because it posses ....

A. High content of unsaturated acids
B. Low content of unsaturated acids
C. High content of saturated acids
D. Low content of saturated acids

1275. Determination method for gingerols

A. GLC
B. HPLC
C. Gravimetric method
D. All of the above

1276. Soft extract of zingiber officinaleis used in.................

A. Antiallergic B. Migraine
C. Hypothermic D. All of the above

1277. What is the ratio of herb and menstrum for preparation of taraxacum officinale soft extract?

A. 1:1 B. 2:1
C. 3:1 D. 4:1

1278. What is the main function of fragaronine, which is taken in form of soft extract of zanthoxylum spp.?

A. Antisickling activity
B. Carminative action
C. Hypocholestemia
D. Reduce urinary sodium level

1279. Viburnum spp. Extracts are used in ....

A. Infantile enuresis
B. Ovarian and uterine pain
C. Sedative
D. All of the above

1280. Which one of the below drug show adaptogenic and restogenic effects?

A. Valerian wallichii B. Viburnum spp.
C. Vitex negundo D. Xanthoxylum spp.

1281. What is the ratio of herb and menstrum for preparation of urginea indica soft extract /

A. 4:1 B. 5:1
C. 8:1 D. 12:1

1282. Soft extract of urtica dioica used as ....

A. Diuretic B. Emmenaoggue
C. Astringent D. All of the above

1283. What is the ratio of herb and menstrum for preparation of tribulus terrestris dry extract?

A. 6:1 B. 7:1
C. 8:1 D. 10:1

1284. What is the ratio of herb and menstrum for preparation of trikuta soft extract?

A. 4:1 B. 5:1
C. 10:1 D. 12:1

1285. Tinospora cardifolia dry extract is used as ....

A. Diuretic B. Anaemia
C. Demulcent D. All of the above

1286. Which part of pueraria tuberose is used to prepare its dry extract?

A. Root B. Seeds
C. Leaf D. Rhizome

1287. What is the ratio of herb and menstrum for preparation of pterocarpus santalins wood dry extract?

A. 1:1 B. 2:1
C. 3:1 D. 4:1

1288. What is the biological name of heartwood?
A. Pterocarpus santalinus
B. Pterocarpous marsupium
C. Rouwolfia vomitoria
D. Rouwolfia serpentina

1289. What is the ratio of herb and menstrum for preparation of pueraria tuberose dry extract?
A. 1:1 B. 5:1
C. 10:1 D. 15:1

1290. What is the ratio of herb and menstrum for preparation of trigonella foenumgraecum dry extract?
A. 1:1 B. 5:1
C. 10:1 D. 15:1

1291. Which part of symplocos racemosa is used to prepare its soft extract?
A. Bark B. Stem
C. Rhizome D. Root

1292. What is the ratio of herb and menstrum for preparation of Eugenia aromaticum dry extract?
A. 5:1 B. 6:1
C. 7:1 D. 8:1

1293. Tephrosia purpurea dry extract is udes as ....
A. Blood purifier B. Chologogue
C. Laxative D. All of the above

1294. Saraca indica extracts are used as ....
A. Uterine sedative
B. Leucorrhoea
C. Menorrhagia
D. All of the above

1295. What is the ratio of herb and menstrum for preparation of silybum marianum dry extract?
A. 5:1 B. 6:1
C. 7:1 D. 8:1

1296. What is the ratio of herb and menstrum for preparation of triphala dry extract?
A. 4:1 B. 5:1
C. 6:1 D. 7:1

1297. Trigonella foenumgraecum dry extract is used to treat ....
A. Cellulitis B. Nephritis
C. Dieresis D. Bronchitis

1298. Sapindus trifoliatus soft extract used in
A. Cosmetics B. Induce abortion
C. Cleanse hair D. All of the above

1299. Which part of saussurea lappa is used to prepare its soft extract?
A. Stem B. Bark
C. Root D. Leaf

1300. Strebulus asper dry extract is used for treatment of ....
A. Sickle cell anaemia
B. Elephantitis
C. Anaemia
D. All of the above

1301. What is the ratio of herb and menstrum for preparation of solanum spp.soft extract?
A. 1:1 B. 5:1
C. 10:1 D. 15:1

1302. From which family vitex negundo belongs to
A. Rutaceae B. Compositae
C. Verbenacea D. Solanaceae

1303. From which family ricinus communis belongs to
A. Rhamnaceae B. Euphorbiaceae
C. Polygonaceae D. Apocyanaceae

1304. What is the pH of ajmaline, which stimulates and controls peripheral nervous system?
A. 6.0 B. 7.0
C. 8.0 D. 9.0

1305. Dry extract of triphala used in ....
A. Piles B. Laxative
C. Headache D. All of the above

1306. What is the ratio of herb and menstrum for preparation of tribulus terrestris soft extract?
A. 2:1 B. 4:1
C. 5:1 D. 10:1

1307. Soft extract of randia dumentorum contains ....
A. Saponins B. Triterpene
C. Tannins D. All of the above

1308. From which family quercus infectoria belongs to ....
A. Rubiaceae B. Apocyanaceae
C. Fagaceae D. Rhamnaceae

1309. What is the ratio of herb and menstrum for preparation of piper longum soft extract?

A. 4:1 B. 5:1
C. 6:1 D. 7:1

1310. Plumbago zeylenica dry extract prepared from root is used as ....

A. Stimulant B. In Piles
C. Appetizer D. All of the above

1311. Plumbago rosea extract from leaf is used in ....

A. Prevention of pregnancy
B. Astringent preparation
C. Bronchitis
D. Diuretics

1312. What is the ratio of herb and menstrum for preparation of psoralea corylifolia dry extract?

A. 5:1 B. 10:1
C. 15:1 D. 20:1

1313. Dry extract of pueraria tuberose is used as ....

A. Hypoglycaemic agent
B. Anti-tubercular
C. Antibacterial
D. All of the above

1314. Which part of quercus infectoria is used to prepare its dry extract ?

A. Fruit B. Galls
C. Seed D. Root

1315. Which part of randia dumentorum is used to prepare its soft extract?

A. Gel B. Bark
C. Fruit D. Root

1316. Quercus infectoria dry extract is used as ....

A. Acute diarrhoea
B. Haemmorhoids
C. Astringent
D. All of the above

1317. What is the ratio of herb and menstrum for preparation of saraca indica soft extract ?

A. 5:1 B. 8:1
C. 10:1 D. 12:1

1318. What is the ratio of herb and menstrum for preparation of santalumalbum wood soft extract?

A. 8:1 B. 12:1
C. 15:1 D. 25:1

1319. Which part of tribulus terrestris is used to prepare its extract?

A. Fruit B. Leaf
C. Bulbs D. Root

1320. What is the ratio of herb and menstrum for preparation of thymus vulgaris soft extract?

A. 4:1 B. 5:1
C. 6:1 D. 8:1

1321. What is the ratio of herb and menstrum for preparation of saussurea lappa soft extract /

A. 4:1 B. 5:1
C. 6:1 D. 8:1

1322. Randia dumentorum soft extract used in ....

A. Anti-aging B. Anti-acne
C. Anti-wrinkles D. All of the above

1323. Which part of psoralea corylifolia is used to prepare its dry extract?

A. Root B. Stem
C. Seeds D. Bark

1324. What is the ratio of herb and menstrum for preparation of plumbago indica oil soluble extract?

A. 12:1 B. 15:1
C. 18:1 D. 20:1

1325. Piper cubeba soft extractis used as ....

A. Carminative B. Uritheritis
C. Diuretic D. All of the above

1326. Which part of piper spp. Is used to prepare its extract?

A. Rhizome B. Fruit
C. Bulb D. Root

1327. What is the ratio of herb and menstrum for preparation of paedaria foetida dry extract?

A. 7:1 B. 8:1
C. 9:1 D. 10:1

1328. What is the ratio of herb and menstrum for preparation of terminalia belericapericarp dry extract?

A. 1:1 B. 2:1
C. 3:1 D. 4:1

1329. Portulaca oleracea dry extract is used in ....

A. Cardiovascular B. Antiscorbiotic
C. Antiulcer D. All of the above

1330. Which part of prunus puddum is used to prepare it soft extract?

A. Bark B. Rhizome
C. Root D. Nut

1331. What is the ratio of herb and menstrum for preparation of phyllanthus amarus soft extract?

A. 3:1 B. 5:1
C. 7:1 D. 10:1

1332. Which part of passiflora incarnate used to prepare its soft extract?

A. Root B. Bark
C. Stem D. Leaf

1333. Which one of the below is family of phyllanthus niruri?

A. Passifloraceae
B. Rubeaceae
C. Euphorbeaceae
D. Plumbaginaceae

1334. Chemical constituents present in dry extract of paedaria foetida.

A. Nitrogen compounds, alkaloids, tannins
B. Essential oil, alkaloids, sulphur compounds
C. Tannin, essential oil, nitrogen compounds
D. Essentialoil, resin, tannin

1335. Commonly used plant part for tincture preparation is ....

A. Dried root B. Dried flowers
C. Dried stem D. Dried leaves

1336. By which process tincture of raspberries is produced ....

A. Maceration B. Percolation
C. Infusion D. Decoction

1337. What is the ratio of herb and menstrum for preparation of quercus infectoria dry extracts?

A. 2:1 B. 4:1
C. 6:1 D. 8:1

1338. Ocimum sanctum soft extract is used as ....

A. Expectorant B. Antipyretic
C. Carminative D. All of the above

1339. Moringa oleifera extract is used as ....

A. Source of vitamin C
B. Source of vitamin K
C. Source of vitamin B
D. Source of vitamin A

1340. Alcoholic extract of leptadenia rticulata is used as ....

A. Antiviral B. Antihelminthic
C. Antibacterial D. All of the above

1341. Which drug extract stops the mammary gland secretions?

A. Juglans regia
B. Lawsonia alba
C. Leptadenia reticulate
D. Olea europaea

1342. Which part of acacia concinna used to prepare its dry extract?

A. Pods B. Bark
C. Root D. Rhizome

1343. Which drug extract contains alpha and beta asarone?

A. Acacia Arabica
B. Acorus calamus
C. Aconitum root
D. Achyranthus aspera

1344. What is the ratio of herb and menstrum for preparation of tephrosia purpurea dry extract?

A. 1:1 B. 8:1
C. 9:1 D. 10:1

1345. Juglans regia dry extract is used as ....

A. Mild cathartic
B. In hepatic dysfunction
C. Dyspepsia
D. All of the above

1346. Aegle marmelos leaves extract is used as ....
A. Bronchodilator
B. Antidiabetic
C. Oxytocic
D. Abortifacient

1347. Which one of the below herb is the most suitable nutrient for diabetics?
A. Amygdale dulcis
B. Aloe vera
C. Acacia Arabica
D. Amomum subulatum

1348. What is the ratio of herb and menstrum for preparation of aloe vera dry extract?
A. 8:1 B. 10:1
C. 12:1 D. 15:1

1349. Which drug extract contains alpha and beta phallandrene?
A. Allium ceppa B. Allium sativum
C. Amygdale dulcis D. Anethum sowa

1350. What is the ratio of herb and menstrum for preparation of randia dumentorum soft extract?
A. 1:1 B. 2:1
C. 3:1 D. 4:1

1351. Psoralea corylifolia dry extract is used as ....
A. Anti-inflammatory
B. Anti-bacterial
C. Anti-helminthic
D. All of the above

1352. Piper nigrum soft extracts is used as ...
A. CNS depressent
B. CNS stimulant
C. Reduce saliva secretion
D. Increase saliva secretion

1353. Andrographics paniculata soft extract used as ...
A. Antifilarial B. Antibacterial
C. Antiviral D. Antifungal

1354. What is the ratio of herb and menstrum for preparation of saraca indica dry extract?
A. 6:1 B. 8:1
C. 10:1 D. 12:1

1355. Picrorhiza kurroa extracts is used as ...
A. Antiperiodic B. Mild laxative
C. Anti spasmodic D. All of the above

1356. Acorus calamus soft extract is used as:
A. Emetic B. Antihelminthic
C. Antispasmodic D. All of the above

1357. From which category does alpha and beta asarone belongs to
A. Essential oil B. Resin
C. Alkaloid D. Tannin

1358. What is the ratio of herb and menstrum for preparation of lawsonia alba oil soluble soft extract?
A. 10:1 B. 20:1
C. 30:1 D. 40:1

1359. Adhatoda vasika soft extract is used as ...
A. Expectorant B. Uterine stimulant
C. Bronchodilator D. All of the above

1360. What is the ratio of herb and menstrum for preparation of rhamnus pushiana dry extract?
A. 1:1 B. 2:1
C. 3:1 D. 4:1

1361. Apium graveolens soft extract is used as
A. Sedative B. Urinary antiseptic
C. Antirheumatic D. All of the above

1362. What is the ratio of herb and menstrum for preparation of nardosytachys jatamansi soft extract?
A. 8:1 B. 10:1
C. 12:1 D. 15:1

1363. Annona squamosa extract is used as:
A. Emetic B. Insecticide
C. Astringent D. All of the above

1364. Which drug extract is used externally to relieve spasm and pain of annul fistula?
A. Annona squamosa
B. Apium graveolens
C. Atropa belladonna
D. Arachis hypogaea

1365. What is the ratio of herb and menstrum for preparation of taraxacum officinale dry extract?
A. 2:1 B. 3:1
C. 4:1 D. 5:1

1366. Which drug leaf dry extract is used as insecticide?
A. Azadiracta indica
B. Acacia Arabica
C. Bergenia ligulata
D. Annona squamosa

1367. Herpestis monieri soft extract is used as
A. Antistress
B. Hysteria
C. Nervous breakdown
D. All of the above

1368. From which family boerhaavia diffusa belongs to
A. Acanthaceae
B. Nyctaginaceae
C. Bixaceae
D. Chenopodiaceae

1369. What is the ratio of herb and menstrum for preparation of cucurbita maxima dry extract?
A. 10:1 B. 15:1
C. 20:1 D. 25:1

1370. What is the ratio of herb and menstrum for preparation of piper betle soft extract?
A. 8:1 B. 12:1
C. 15:1 D. 20:1

1371. Atropa belladonna extract is used as ...
A. Anticholinergic B. Antihidrotic
C. Antiasthamatic D. All of the above

1372. Which drug soft extract restores memory, enhances power of speech and poetic imagination?
A. Bacopa monnieri
B. Annona squamosa
C. Bergenia ligulata
D. Azadiracta indica

1373. Which drug powder and extract used externally in wounds?
A. Bergenia ligulata
B. Berberis spp.
C. Bacopa monnieri
D. Herpestis monnieri

1374. What is the ratio of herb and menstrum for preparation of moringa oleifera leaf extract/
A. 5:1 B. 10:1
C. 15:1 D. 20:1

1375. Which drug extract contains saponin becoside a and b, which stimulates memory?
A. Bergenia ligulata
B. Berberis spp.
C. Bacopa monnieri
D. Herpestis monnieri

1376. Beta vulgaris rich in ...
A. Iron B. Zinc
C. Vitamin D. All of the above

1377. What is the ratio of herb and menstrum for preparation of momordica charantia dry extract?
A. 5:1 B. 10:1
C. 15:1 D. 20:1

1378. Which drug extract contain alpha and beta boswellic acid?
A. Bixa orellana B. Brassica spp.
C. Blepharis edulis D. Boswellia serrata

1379. Which one of the below act as potential binding agent in pharmaceutical formulations?
A. Cassia angustifolia B. Cassia alata
C. Cassia fistula D. Cassia auriculata

1380. Celastrus panniculatus extract is act as.
A. Antiseptic B. Anticonvulsant
C. Spasmolytic D. All of the above

1381. What is the ratio of herb and menstrum for preparation of ocimum sanctum oleoresin extract?
A. 10:1 B. 12:1
C. 15:1 D. 20:1

1382. What is the refractive index of celastrus oil?
A. 1.26 B. 1.28
C. 1.47 D. 1.58

1383. What is the ratio of herb and menstruum for preparation of butea frondosa flower extract?
A. 2:1 B. 4:1
C. 6:1 D. 8:1

1384. What is the ratio of herb and menstrum for preparation of butea monosperma seed extract?
A. 2:1 B. 4:1
C. 6:1 D. 8:1

1385. What is the ratio of herb and menstrum for preparation of celastrus seed extract?

a. 10:1
b. 15:1
c. 20:1
d. 25:1

1386. What is the ratio of herb and menstrum for preparation of achyranthes as per a soft extract

A. 10:1
B. 8:1
C. 6:1
D. 4:1

1387. GRID layout, loop layout, spin layout, free flow layout are the part of which layout?

A. Stores layout
B. Packaging layout
C. Manufacturing layout
D. Quality layout

1388. The product layout, process layout and fixed position layout are the part of?

A. Plant layout
B. Pilot plant
C. Stationary layout
D. Stores layout

1389. Processing and material handling are less required in

A. Product layout
B. Process layout
C. Both a and b
D. Stationary layout

1390. Diversified product can be used in

A. Product layout
B. Process layout
C. Fixed position layout
D. Stationary layout

1391. Production center in process layout are

A. simple
B. Complex
C. both
D. Intermediate

1392. In product layout floor space is less required in compared to..........................?

A. Process layout
B. Stationary layout
C. Fixed layout
D. None of the above

1393. Size function layout may be affected by ..

A. Nature of the product
B. Size of output
C. Nature of manufacturing system
D. Localization of plant

1394. Factors affecting plant layout are-

A. Nature of product
B. Size of output
C. Manufacturing system
D. All the above

1395. The holes of sieve trey are arrested in triangular pitch have diameter

A. 10 to 15 times the hole diameter
B. 1.5 to 2 times
C. 2.5 to 5 times
D. 5 to 10 times

1396. Significant amendemente to the manufacturing process.

A. evaluated
B. Should be validated
C. specification
D. Both B & C

1397. For the development of production formulation process, equipment train & specification what required-

A. GMP
B. GLP
C. CDCSO
D. WHO

1398. All critical feature of a process must be identified why it required?

A. It assure that product are good
B. Evaluation of product
C. Provide assurance that the process is under control
D. None of this

1399. The effectiveness of the pilot plant is determined by-

A. The ease with which new product into routine production
B. Relationship between other group
C. High rate production & less error
D. All of the above

1400. The basic space requirement for pilot plant is:

A. Administrand information process
B. Physical testing area
C. Standard pilot plant equipment floor space
D. All of the above

1401. In the physical testing area all should required except :-

A. Bench top space
B. Equipment
C. Qualified person
D. Storage

1402. For the solid dosage form, semisolid product, liquid preparation & sterile product which space requirement are best?

A. Physical testing area
B. Standard pilot plant equipment floor space
C. Information process
D. Quality formulation

1403. The review of the formula is important in:
A. Scale up process
B. Modification of formulation during scale up
C. Both a & b
D. Experimental production batches

1404. The one of the most responsibilities of pilot plant fuction is:
A. Evaluate alternate supplies
B. Approval & validation of active excipients & raw material
C. Continuing technical support
D. Understand the perspective of production

1405. The stability of finished product can be evaluated relative to standard product can be:
A. Suppliers requirement
B. Performance in the formulation
C. Stability of finished product
D. Both b & c

1406. The pilot plant equipment shoulb be able to:
A. Experiment trial B. Not too small
C. Too large D. Both a & b

1407. The ease of clearing is required in case of (mostly):
A. Multiple product are used to manufactured
B. Single product manufactured
C. Small scale formulation
D. None of these

1408. The evaluation of the processing equipment help to the determined?
A. True capability of equipment
B. Quality of technical support
C. Reliability of large production
D. All of these

1409. The equipment & process should be choose for:
A. To produce batch at frequency
B. Provide economically utilization
C. Experimental trials
D. None of these

1410. The evaluation of the process critically & the optimise its performance based on:
A. Product evaluation
B. Process evaluation
C. Equipment evaluation
D. Product & process evaluation

1411. The purpose of process validation is:
A. Increased production growth
B. Validate product quality
C. Assure the quality product at various critical stage
D. For economical consideration

1412. Changes in formula quality of the ingredient or equipment these required:
A. Permission for regulatory
B. Relevant processing equipment
C. Revalidation required
D. Personal responsibilities

1413. The master manufacturing procedure contain:
A. Weight sheet of each chemical
B. Processing directions
C. SOP"s guidlines
D. All of the above

1414. The addition rates, mixing time, mixing speed, temperature include:
A. Batch record direction
B. Batch production record
C. Master formula
D. WHO directions

1415. Batch manufactured of drug designed the-
A. Half life of drug B. Shelf life
C. Expirary duration D. Dose of the drug

1416. Consistent product quality maintaining by
A. Periodic revalidation
B. Monitoring test
C. GMP procedure
D. All of these

1417. For the chamber on the edge of the hole required
A. Engraving operation
B. Counter sinking operation
C. Facing process
D. None of these

1418. The process of removing the metal by a cutter is
A. Down milling B. Counter sinking
C. Under milling D. Batch milling

1419. Downmilling is rotated-
A. Against the travel of the wordpiece
B. In the same direction of travel
C. Parallel to the axis of rotation
D. Perpendicular to the axis

1420. Which one is not the element of a single point cutting tool?
A. Fillet B. Lip angle
C. shank D. Rake

1421. Manufacturing good classified on the basis of
A. Primary: costelly & consumer
B. Primary, secondary & tertiary
C. Essential: market & standard
D. Consumer capital & defence

1422. The following aspect is help ease and efficiency of product performance
A. Functional aspect
B. Operational aspect
C. Durational aspect
D. None of these

1423. The functional aspect of product is concerned with
A. Market sell of the product
B. Critically operation and long procedures
C. Simplicity to operate and easy to understand
D. Revalidate and evaluate the SOPs

1424. Standardization helps in
A. Interchangability of the product
B. Quality and quantity evaluation
C. Maintaining critical data
D. Processing of product

1425. In which type the manufacturing cost may be 90 UP
A. standardization B. diversification
C. simplication D. All of these

1426. The welding method which is used for joining the metal sheets
A. Arc welding
B. Gas welding
C. Resistance welding
D. Hydrogen welding

1427. Pilot plant scale up process is-
A. High speed production
B. Reserve curioocity
C. Development of laboratory
D. Transformed a formula in large scale

1428. The study of the formula to determine its ability to withstand batch scale and process modification
A. Production process
B. Quality development
C. Process scale up
D. Pilot plant scale up

1429. Pilot plant scale up must include-
A. Close examination of formula
B. Review of relevant processing equipment
C. Formula must economical and simple
D. None of the above

1430. The physical space required and layout should be taken during pilot plant for
A. Short termefficiency
B. Adequate physical and chemical specifications
C. Short term and long term efficiency
D. High speed production

1431. For successful product scale up which factor required
A. Training
B. Reporting relationship
C. Responsibility of personnel
D. All of these

1432. An operation of enlarging a hole through a certain distance; the drilled surface is,
A. Counter sinking B. Counter boring
C. Under cutting D. Engraving

1433. A channel or orifice connecting the runner to the impression is said to be
A. Gate B. Cavity
C. Insert D. Slide core

1434. Product development and design is the primary step of
A. Production planning
B. Capacing planning
C. Material required planning
D. None of the above

1435. In production the following is the source for developing new or improveproduct
- A. Research and development department
- B. Other competitive products in the market
- C. Consumer suggestion and complaints
- D. All of the above

1436. The main objective of the product is
- A. Utilising existing manpower
- B. To monopolise the market
- C. To provide a new look
- D. The substandard substitutions

1437. Specification is ultimate objective of variety reduction of
- A. Product B. Process
- C. Equipment D. Standard

1438. The followin is the process of stock control
- A. Standardisation B. Both a and b
- C. Simplication D. Specification

1439. The following is the durability aspect of a product
- A. Efficiency of the product
- B. Easy of understand
- C. Ease with which a product can be maintained
- D. All of the above

1440. For good natural ventilation the type of building preferred-
- A. Flare proof B. Saw tooth
- C. High bay D. Monitor

1441. Space available in vertical and horizontal direction is most effectively unified these principles
- A. Minimum distance
- B. Cubic space utilization
- C. Flow
- D. Flexibility

1442. All the processing equipment and machine are arranged sequence in
- A. Product layout
- B. Process layout
- C. Fixed position layout
- D. Combination layout

1443. Which layout manufacture standard product in large quantity
- A. Combination layout
- B. Fixed position layout
- C. Product layout
- D. Process layout

1444. In case of low volume of non standard production preferred
- A. Fixed position layout
- B. Product and process layout
- C. Process layout
- D. Product layout

1445. Fixed position layout help in
- A. Ship manufacturing
- B. Multiple processing
- C. Process evaluation
- D. None of these

1446. The graphic representation of all production activities on shop floor are
- A. Template
- B. Flow process chart
- C. Operation process chart
- D. All of the above

1447. The art for designing of prototype using the data technique are
- A. Scale up
- B. Approval
- C. Product designing
- D. Method changes

1448. Market requirement consideration help in adjustment
- A. Raw materialrequirement
- B. Production rate
- C. Production changes
- D. Equipment

1449. Appropriate recorder and reporter are issued to support-
- A. Produce validation
- B. GMP procedures
- C. Marketing procedures
- D. GMP evaluation

1450. Reporting responsibilities are-
- A. R and D group separate staffing
- B. Formulator who developed product
- C. Production support
- D. All of the above

1451. In personal requirement should have-
- A. Scientists with experience in pilot plant
- B. Well trained and knowledge
- C. Knowledge of computer and electronics
- D. All of the above

1452. Basic space requirement in plant for
- A. Administration and information processing
- B. Physical testing area
- C. Equipment floor space and storage area
- D. All of the above

1453. Top space for routinely used for all except
- A. Physical testing are
- B. Product evaluation
- C. Storage area
- D. Computer and operator

1454. Intermediate sized and full scale production equipment is essential
- A. Process evaluation
- B. validate the scale up
- C. Evaluate the effect of scale up
- D. None of the above

1455. The manufacturing of all type of dosage from needed
- A. Production plant
- B. Discreet pilot plant space
- C. Small storage room
- D. Intermediate scale up

1456. Approved area and unapproved area are the type of or-
- A. Production area
- B. Evaluation area
- C. Storage area
- D. Cleaning area

1457. The purpose of each ingredient and its contribution in final product see in-
- A. Evaluation of formula
- B. Validation of formula
- C. Review of the formula
- D. None of the above

1458. Change in ingredient particles size, morphology affect the
- A. Bulk density
- B. Static charges and rate of solubility
- C. Flow properties
- D. All of the above

1459. Equipment used in pilot plant must have property excepta
- A. Economical and simpleest
- B. Relevant to production size
- C. Too small
- D. Ease of cleaning

1460. For determination of production rates must consider
- A. Future market trends
- B. Requirement of patients
- C. Industrial budget
- D. All of the above

1461. Heating and cooling rate, order of mixing, drying temperature are parameter of
- A. Product evaluation
- B. Process evaluation
- C. Market evaluation
- D. GMP evaluation

1462. Why to carry out process evaluation?
- A. Knowledge of inprocess and finished product quality
- B. Process optimization and validation
- C. For assure product availability at various critical stages
- D. All of the above

1463. Weight sheet, manufacturing produse and processing and sampling direction are important aspect
- A. Master manufacturing process
- B. SOPs
- C. GMP consideration
- D. Process of evaluation

1464. Transfer of analytical method to QA make sure-
- A. Proper analytical instrumentation
- B. Proper testing process
- C. Proper packaging process
- D. None of these

1465. Primary objective of pilot plant is-
- A. The physical and chemical stability
- B. For scale up the product manufacturing
- C. Both a and b
- D. For fulfill the market needs

1466. Stability studies also done in-
A. Finished package
B. Cleaning products
C. Equipment
D. None of these

1467. Statistical quality control techniques are based on the theory of
A. Departmentation B. Probability
C. Quality assurance D. R and D

1468. Under the apprenticeship act only industries employing
A. More than 200 worker to recruit apprentices
B. More than 500 workers have to recruit
C. More than 100 worker have to recruit
D. Not less than 200 workers to recruit

1469. Standing order which are statutory are applicable to-
A. All industries employing more than 500 workers
B. More than200 workers
C. Moreover than 100 worker
D. Not more than 100 workers

1470. Acceptance sampling is widely used in
A. Mass production
B. Mass weighting
C. Mass analysis
D. None of these

1471. The technique of valve analytical can be applied to
A. Certain item B. Quality product
C. Raw material D. Any item

1472. The term value in valve analysis refers to
A. Utility of the sample
B. Utility of the product
C. Utility of the final compound
D. Both a and b

1473. Material handling and plant location is analysed by
A. Ongoing value chart
B. Travel chart
C. Processing chart
D. WHO chart

1474. Work cost implies
A. Secondary +primary cost
B. Primary cost+factory expenses
C. Secondary cost+factory expenses
D. None of these

1475. Motion study involve analysis of
A. Action of analysis
B. Action of operator
C. Action of equipment
D. Action of chemical

1476. In which of the following layout the line need to the balanced
A. Processing layout
B. Product layout
C. Quality layout
D. None of these

1477. Which of the following layout is suited for the mass production
A. Production layout
B. Processing layout
C. Quality layout
D. Both a and b

1478. Which of the following layout is suited job production
A. Production layout B. Processing layout
C. Quality layout D. None of these

1479. The employees provident fund act is applicable to
A. The industries not notified by Government
B. The industries notified by Government
C. For all production industries
D. Only for pharmaceutical industries

1480. In current assets include
A. Production plants
B. Manufacturing plants
C. Government industries
D. None of these

1481. In ABC control study policy, maximum attention is given to
A. Those items which consume less money
B. Those items which consume more money
C. Which are required extreme environment
D Which are not applicable to industrial use

1482. In which case of drying and equipment cost are relatively high
A. Freeze drying operation
B. Tween shell blenders
C. Vacuum drying operation
D. Double core system

1483. For the tablet coating mostly use equipment in large scale
A. Standard coating pan
B. Perforated coating pan
C. Fluidized bed coater
D. All of the above

1484. In coating layout, optimum drying is achieved by
A. Adela Cota
B. Air suspension coating
C. Pellegriri system
D. Perforated coating

1485. During coating process which air introduced
A. Cooled air
B. Heated air
C. Room temperature air
D. Extremely freeze air

1486. The conventional wet granulation process require yield
A. Free flowing granulation
B. High amount of product
C. High concentration
D. None of these

1487. In scaling up a dry blending operation special attain required in all except
A. Blender loads
B. Mixing speed
C. Blender type
D. Blending time

1488. The mixing time also be important for
A. Compresibility of granules
B. Compresibility of finished blend
C. For all in process blend
D. Compresibility of the tablets

1489. In plant processing,excessive mixing time cause
A. Degrade the expiration
B. Fracture fragile excipient
C. Decompose the excipient
D. None of these

1490. The blender efficiency affect by
A. The blender speed
B. Blender time
C. The blender load
D. Blender type

1491. Overload of blender in scale up retqrd the
A. Free flow or granulation
B. Increase the blanding time
C. Decrease the blender of efficiency
D. All of the above

1492. In tablet plant production, dry granulation requires
A. Slugging
B. Drying
C. Cooling
D. Compression

1493. The pilot point scientist pay particular attention on
A. Force used for slugging operation
B. Diameter of the puncher
C. Size and screening operation
D. All of these

1494. In Case of high speed graduation machine require
A. Indused die feed system
B. Fast feed system
C. Fastfeed system
D. Wet granules

1495. During speed production cappingdefect reduced by
A. Add lubricant
B. Slow down the press speed
C. Add high amount of binder
D. None of these

1496. During mixing the intraptment of air cause
A. Physical and chemical stability changes
B. degradation of product
C. Increase the volume of bulk
D. Change in excipient ratio

1497. Duringscale up processing,air entrapment removed by
A. Pycnometer
B. Versatore
C. Adding salt
D. UV visible

1498. In emulsionmanufacturing air entrapment also caused by
- A. Low shear mixer
- B. High shear mixer
- C. Medium shear mixer
- D. Excess products concentration

1499. Major problem between simple liquid and semi solid productsscale up
- A. Drying equipment
- B. Collecting equipment
- C. Storage equipment
- D. Mixing equipments

1500. The two bin System is concerned with
- A. Ordering procedure
- B. Evaluating in procedure
- C. Validation procedure
- D. None of these

1501. Bin card used in
- A. Production
- B. Discarding
- C. Stores
- D. Layout process

1502. Work study comprises following man techniques
- A. Method study and process control
- B. Market study and work measurement
- C. Method study and work measurement
- D. Evaluate in the processstudy

1503. Process which follow by company to design and develop container for particular product classified as
- A. Guranteer
- B. Warranties
- C. Labelling
- D. Packaging

1504. An ongoing activity of system support is
- A. Assisting uses
- B. Adopting the system to new requirement
- C. Recovering the system
- D. All of these

1505. Process design or redginn is most important when
- A. Current performance is adequate
- B. You have a significant competitive advantage
- C. Competitive priorities have charged
- D. The cost of inputs remain stable

1506. A management consultancy is an example of
- A. High volume /high variety
- B. Low volume/low variety
- C. High volume/low variety
- D. Low volume/high variety

1507. All of the following classified according to service process expect
- A. Customer satisfaction
- B. Customer contact
- C. Service of goods information
- D. Service flexibility to customer service

1508. The highest eligibility of equipment in which of the production system
- A. Customer satisfaction
- B. Batch
- C. Services of goods, information
- D. Service flexibility to customer service

1509. In case of low variety and large volume mix theseis
- A. Less contact duration
- B. Above customisation
- C. Short customer transaction
- D. Small volume or customers exchanger

1510. Which one the following is increasing process flexibility
- A. Mass/ continuous/ batch/ project
- B. Project/batch/mass /continuous
- C. continuous/ mass /project/ batch
- D. continuous/mass/batch/project

1511. What is the characteristics of service shops
- A. Staff discretion, degree of customisation, customer contact
- B. Orientation of project
- C. Customer transaction in short time
- D. Service organisation of the customer need

1512. Solid phulera photo mast process accept
- A. Standard products and large scale production
- B. The product are manufactured to order of customer
- C. Product bailed on equipment and operation
- D. None of these

1513. The object of desire activity
- A. To provide services product which satisfy the customer
- B. To assure the product is efficient and effective
- C. Decrease the post of product
- D. To provide product on order of customer

1514. Process design hair in port 10th role in order design activities caused
- A. For service the process are important
- B. Cost of product less than cost of process
- C. Customer needs are fulfill by design
- D. Product manufacturing is expensive

1515. Process type work on
- A. Mass service same ti other
- B. Batch and service shopper carry same level
- C. Jobbing process differ from higher service
- D. Service shopper have less volume then professional service

1516. Composition of Similar machine are found in
- A. Project
- B. Jobbing
- C. Batch
- D. All of the above

1517. Flexible manufacturing have important role in which operation
- A. Project
- B. Validation
- C. Low volume and high variety
- D High volume and low variety

1518. The relation between product and process design
- A. Separate
- B. Incomplete
- C. Inter-related
- D. None of these

1519. The production time generally maximum in which layout
- A. Process
- B. Product
- C. Design
- D. All of these

1520. The fixed cost are
- A. Salary of production employees
- B. Cost of packaging material
- C. Cost of packaging material
- D. Both a and b

1521. All of following example of continuous process industry except
- A. Steel plant
- B. Sugar plant
- C. Oil refineries
- D. None of these

1522. Which of following help in assist the choice of layout
- A. WHO guideline
- B. GMP guideline
- C. Break even analysis
- D. PQ chart and GMP guideline

1523. All of following example of element of TQM except
- A. Leadership
- B. Perceived quality
- C. Employees empowerment
- D. Customer focus

1524. Cement plant is mostly use in
- A. Continuous production
- B. Batch process
- C. Flow shop
- D. Job shop

1525. Process selection have important role in
- A. Leading
- B. Planning
- C. Organisation
- D. Controlling

1526. Primary product layout is preferred for
- A. Receptive processing
- B. Short time processing
- C. Intermittent process
- D. Both Aand B

1527. Which of the following pump is used for handling of corrosive liquid?
- A. Turbine pump
- B. Peristatic pump
- C. Valve pump
- D. Air binding pump

1528. Breakdown analysis consists of
- A. Fixed and variable cost
- B. Fixed Cost
- C. Sales revenue cost
- D. None of these

1529. The time when industry will undergo loss are represents by
- A. Breakeven point
- B. Bridge point
- C. Breaking point
- D. Breakeven analysis

1530. Work study Concerd with
A. Improving present method and finding standard time
B. Analysis standard time and improving it
C. Done the improving process
D. None of these

1531. Basic tool in work study is
A. Stop watch
B. Scale
C. Process manufacturing
D. Both a andb

1532. Work study is most useful where-
A. Production activities are involved
B. Packaging activities are work
C. All quality check are performed
D. The major method is forbidden

1533. Work sampling observation are taken on the basis of
A. According to review of formula
B. Table of random numbers
C. Table of mixed procedures
D. Not done in numbers

1534. Process layout is employed for
A. Continuous production
B. Both c and d
C. Batch production
D. Ethical production

1535. For a product layout the material handling equipment must be designed as
A. Special purpose for particular application
B. For all purpose applications
C. Not for packaging purposes application
D. None of these

1536. Product layout is employed for
A. Batch production
B. Both c and d
C. Continuous production
D. For product estmation

1537. The process layout is the best suited where
A. Few number of standard units
B. Few number or non standardised unit
C. For all unit production
D. None of these

1538. The low unit cost can be obtained by..................
A. Product layout B. Packaging layout
C. Process layout D. All of these

1539. F.W.Taylor introduced a system of working known as ....
A. Functional organization
B. Process Organization
C. Multi product organizations
D. None of these

1540. Templates are used for ....
A. Product layout B. Process layout
C. Planning layout D. Removing layout

1541. Routing Prescribed the ....
A. Flow of material in the product
B. Manufacturing of material
C. Removing contamination in plant
D. None of these

1542. Father of industrial engineering is ....
A. Charak B. Gantt
C. Aristotle D. Galen

1543. The grouping of activities into organizational unit are called ....
A. Quality checking B. Departmentatio
C. Production D. Washing

1544. Which of the following is independent of sales forecasts ....
A. Productivity B. Market activity
C. Quality D. Product growth

1545. Gantt chart are used for
A. Quality schedules
B. Production schedule
C. Manufacturing schedule
D. None of these

1546. In inventory control the economic order quantity is the ....
A. Optimum lot size
B. Optimum market size
C. Both a and b
D. Optimum quality product

1547. The designers made up by ....
A. The designer creativity
B. Marketing growth
C. Customer satisfaction need
D. Need to revenue

1548. Design process of getting is all except ....

A. Revenue B. Cost
C. Speed D. Adaptabality

1549. Ki sector 4 service design accept

A. Staff raining cost
B. Customer need
C. Alternative products
D. Intangible components

1550. Efficiency in service operation is difficult because of

A. Dependability
B. Intra functionalvariability
C. Demand variables
D. Intangible components

1551. Continuous process involved

A. Extremely low variety and high volume
B. Small quantities
C. Specially made
D. Skill requirements

1552. Service vs consists of following accept

A. Supporting goods
B. Fasciliting good
C. Explicit services
D. Implicit services

1553. The process collection and product the designer ....

A. Financial decisions
B. System decision
C. System design
D. System operation

1554. Poor quality also effects ....

A. Cost of product B. Productivity
C. Profitability D. All of these

1555. Transportation process is a ....

A. Qualitative process
B. Qualitative
C. Scientific
D. All of these

1556. Which of thefactorare regional for location planning

A. Row material
B. Labour consideration
C. Market
D. Attitudes

1557. Which of the primarily part of location decision

A. Marketing strategy
B. Growth factor
C. Financial aspects
D. Both a and b

1558. Paper mill are use switch process

A. Continuous flow
B. Batch flow
C. Job shop
D. Flow shop

1559. Call home depot lohar not operating type

A. Goods production
B. Storage/ transportation
C. Entertainment
D. All of the above

1560. Technology choice also affects

A. Cost B. Union activity
C. Productivity D. Quality

1561. Measurement at various tranformation process for control purposes are

A. Plans B. Directions
C. Controls D. Feedback

1562. Manufacturingwork transport to other countries is called

A. Down sized B. International
C. Out scored D. None of these

1563. Service corporation are not follows

A. Intangible output
B. High labourcontact
C. High customer contact
D. Measurement of productivity

1564. What is the recent trend in present business

A. Pollution control
B. TQM
C. Supply chain management
D. Bothb and c

1565. An Assembly line is a

A. Jobing process
B. Batch process
C. Mass process
D. Continuous process

1566. Which one of the following phrases means a mass processed type

A. Low volume, high variety
B. Finished goods are usually made to order
C. Process are design to perform a wide variety of activities
D. High fixed cost, low variable cost

1567. The code of federal regulation content requirement for the

A. cGMPfor finished pharmaceuticals
B. cGMP for in process pharmaceutical
C. cGMP for raw material
D. cGMP for active pharmaceuticals

1568. The objective of plant layout is to

A. To provide quality product
B. Physical arrangement that most economical
C. Use minimum number of equipment
D. None of the above

1569. Importance of plant layout is

A. Minimise material handling and time,cost
B. Easy production flow
C. It is long term commitment
D. All of the above

1570. Pharmaceutical manufacturing operation security follow which guideline

A. GMP B. MCC
C. CDCSO D. WHO

1571. Adequate security measure are essential to protect installation from

A. Authorised person
B. In person
C. Unauthorised person
D. Out person

1572. Which of the following measures may be appropriate

A. Aperimeter fence of good quality
B. Adequate security lightning
C. Limited and restricted access
D. All of the above

1573. Factories are inspected on an annual basis by the

A. National occupational safety Association
B. World Health Organisation
C. National commodity organisation
D. None of the above

1574. Good Pharmaceutical wholesaling practice dear with the issue except

A. Storage of finished product
B. Maintenance of store and warehouse
C. transportation of finished
D. Legal guideline on industrial safety

1575. Pharmaceutical audit are the type of axcept

A. Internal audits B. Quality audits
C. External audits D. Regulatory audits

1576. Regulatory audit of South Africa which also for security of plant

A. MCC B. USFDA
C. TGA D. CDCSO

1577. The main objective of internal audit are

A. To assist the internal controlsystem
B. Review of organisational
C. Safeguarding the assets
D. All of the above

1578. SOP on storage of finished productcomes under

A. Store and warehouse
B. Production
C. Quality assurance
D. Quality control

1579. Acceptable criteriais

A. Unacceptable quality level
B. Acceptable quality level
C. Estabilized criteria level
D. None of the above

1580. Acceptable quality level Equipment qualification, product validation and SOPs comes under

A. GMP consideration
B. GLP consideration
C. Manufacturing and evaluation
D. Product processing

1581. Advantage of of GMP consideration

A. Readily observe scale-up
B. Supplies of drug and excipient
C. Equipment installation and maintenance
D. All of the above

1582. Dry granulation done by
A. Rotatory compactor
B. Chilsolator
C. Planetarymixer
D. Both a and b

1583. Wet granulation work on
A. Liquid binding theorem
B. Newet theorem
C. Diffusion coefficient
D. Noyes Whitney theorem

1584. For lactose as diluent and which granulation is best
A. Dry granulation
B. Wet granulation
C. Direct compression
D. Botha and c

1585. For pilot plant which equipment are used for particle size reduction
A. Oscillating granulator mechanicalseive
B. Hammer mill
C. Screening device
D. All of the above

1586. During scale-up weight variation and motting occurs due to
A. Too small particle size
B. Too large particle size
C. Wet particle
D. Fluffy particle

1587. To fine particle size during scale up cause
A. Weight variation
B. Capping
C. Orange peel defect
D. Both a and b

1588. Drug content information is affected by all except
A. Granulation B. Blending
C. Excipient D. API

1589. In scale up separation and mixing occurs due to the all except
A. Particle size and shape
B. Mixing speed and blender load
C. Hardness and density
D. Low dose active ingredient

1590. In pilot plant equipment over loading in Blender cause all except
A. Retard freeflow
B. Reduce efficiency
C. Content un-uniformity
D. None of these

1591. required evaluate because
A. Poor flow properties
B. Poor wetting of raw material
C. Decrease in moisture of content
D. Not compressed proper

1592. How many tons pressure required compared to normal tablet press
A. 5 ton B. 15 ton
C. 4 ton D. 11 ton

1593. During the which formulation consideration the sticking and weight variation are done
A. Tablet B. Capsule
C. Injection D. Cream/Semi solid

1594. In plant layout the glatt system is used for
A. Tablet punching
B. Coating process
C. Tablet packaging
D. Powder mixing

1595. During scale up the coating Apparatus are used all except
A. Perforating coating pan
B. Glatt system
C. Rotating dryer
D. Pelligriny system

1596. For pilot plant scale up capsule on high speed the Powder blend have
A. Uniform particle size
B. Bulk density
C. Sufficient cohesiveness
D. All of these

1597. For hard gelatin capsule all machine use except
A. Elli Lilly B. Zanasi
C. Dosatore D. None of these

1598. In case of capsule overly lubricated granular cause
A. Extended disintegration
B. Dealing disintegration
C. Control disintegration
D. Programmed disintegration

1599. Humidity affect the moisture content of
A. granulation
B. On the empty gelatin capsule
C. Coating materials
D. Both a and b

1600. During scale up the empty gelatin capsule storage condition have
A. 15 to 25 Celsius B. 25 to 35 Celsius
C. 37 to 38 celsius D. 0 to 25 Celsius

1601. At low humidity capsule become
A. Brittle B. Hard
C. Swells D. Sticks

1602. Adequate size and suitable mixing ability is required for
A. Solid dosage scale up
B. Liquid orals
C. Gaseous dosage form
D. Parenterals

1603. Liquid Pharmaceutical equipment mostly Fabricated from
A. Stainless steel B. Aluminium plate
C. Iron fabric D. None of the above

1604. Stainless steel react with acidic Pharmaceutical liquid the problem minimised by
A. Pressurization B. Colorization
C. Passivation D. Fabrication

1605. During metallic construction the interaction with metallic surface can be minimised by
A. Taflon coating B. Glass coating
C. Sodaline coating D. Both a and b

1606. During paranteral product the scale of equipment
A. Tankare
B. Piping and filtration
C. Ancillary equipment for liquid mixing
D. All of the above

1607. Suspension require more attention during scale up because
A. High Shear mixing equipment
B. Vibrating feed system
C. Uniformity dispersed
D. All of the above

1608. In case of plant mixing at too speed result cause
A. Physical stability
B. Chemical stability
C. Hydration of agents
D. Physical and chemical stability

1609. Vacuum unit versator having screen of 150 mesh with
A. 200 Micron B. 150 Micron
C. 100 Micron D. 80 Micron

1610. Mixing homogenizing and filling equipment are required in
A. Emulsion scale B. Suspension
C. Capsules D. I.V. fluids

1611. The aspects of the scale up of semisolid products
A. Viscosity B. Product quality
C. Surface tension D. Refractive index

1612. Molten mass and molten base are prepared in case
A. Semisolid preparation
B. Liquid preparation
C. Suppository
D. Creams

1613. Scale up and manufacture of a product is need done in
A. Contract manufacture
B. Product processing
C. Product specialised technique
D. None of these

1614. For the scale up and post approval changes of new drug approved by
A. FDA B. CDCSO
C. WHO D. PCI

1615. The size of batches is gradually increased in
A. Scale up B. SUPAC
C. Pilot plant D. Product plant

1616. Force SUPAC the FDA approved help in
A. safety and effectiveness
B. Regulatory burden
C. Adverse effect study
D. Market study

1617. SUPAC IR MR SS are designed for
A. FDA guideline for SUPAC
B. WHO guideline for SUPAC
C. SUPAC related to moderately release
D. None of these

1618. SUPAC-SS stands for
A. Semisolid dosage form
B. Semisolid dosage form
C. Non sterile semi solids
D. Standard semi solid

1619. The guideline provide recommendation for post approval change in
A. Component or composition
B. Site of manufacture
C. Scale up manufacture
D. All of the above

1620. The effectiveness of layout evolution consists of
A. Three components
B. One components
C. Two components
D. Four components

1621. The chances of material storage or move and
A. 80%
B. 20%
C. Depend on use
D. 50%

1622. Quality of plant location is evaluated by
A. High weight method
B. Equal weight method
C. Environmental method
D. None of these

1623. High number of industrial reason meanslocation quotient is
A. less than Unity
B. Higher than Unity
C. Zero
D. Equal to the unity

1624. Transportation cost based on
A. Median and gravity
B. Gravity and break even analysis
C. Medium median and multi facility location
D. Break even analysis and multi facility location

1625. The reason of inefficiency handling of material
A. Increase volume turnover
B. Overcrowding
C. Increase material handling
D. None of these

1626. Different arrangement layout "short fat" have an advantage
A. Simple handling of material
B. Control material flow
C. Low requirement of capital
D. Higher robustness arrangement

1627. There is not considered as arrangement advantage of "short fat"
A. Mix flexibility high
B. High volume flexibility
C. Less montaneus work
D. Lower Capital requirement

1628. The degree and destination of flow usually seen in
A. QFD matrix
B. Slow record chart
C. Decision tree
D. Flow diagram

1629. Heating, ventilation and air conditioning required in which layout
A. Parenteral layout
B. Tablet layout
C. Solid dosage form
D. For all layout

1630. which is necessaryfor paranteral product processing
A. Ventilation
B. HEPAfilter
C. Aspects condition
D. All of the above

1631. Phone 99.99% efficiency which filter is required
A. HEPA filter
B. Laminar flow
C. ULPA filter
D. Turbulent flow

1632. For manufacturing of parenteral the condition required
A. Personal
B. Documentation
C. Scheduling
D. Preparation of facilities

1633. In parenteral product scale up the flow of material done in which direction
A. Storage to aseptic area
B. Clean area to aseptic area
C. Aseptic area to storage supply
D. Controlled clean environment to aseptic area

1634. The filling and sealing in parenteral production done in
A. Under control environment
B. Under terminal processing
C. In aseptic process
D. None of these

1635. Filling and sealing machine are stored in
A. Class A area B. Class 1000 area
C. Class 10000 area D. Class D area

1636. Preparation of solution and component done in which operation layout
A. Class 100 area B. Class 10000 area
C. Class C area D. Class 100000 area

1637. Class A and B comes under
A. ISO 5 B. ISO 7
C. ISO 8 D. ISO 10

1638. The low risk of contamination in which layout
A. Class A area B. Microbiology layout
C. Class B area D. Class 100000 area

1639. In aseptic preparation class D works for
A. Sealing of cardboard
B. Transportation
C. Solution filtration
D. Handling of component after washing

1640. The operation of plastic container done in
A. Grade pay with ISO 5
B. Grade C with ISO 7
C. Grade D with ISO 8
D. Grade A with ISO 8

1641. The microbe and particle size NMT 0.5-5 micometer have more than 10000 in which grade
A. Grade A B. Brade B
C. Grade D D. Grade C

1642. according to WHO for raw material dispensing done in which background
A. Class A B. Class C
C. Closed system D. Local protection

1643. Lymphilization operation done in
A. Tablet processing B. Parenteral process
C. Pallet processing D. Drying process

1644. Site selection of parenteral production facility done in
A. Basic factor
B. Pharmaceuticalsimportant factor
C. Labour availability
D. Both a and b

1645. Basic parental plant requirement are
A. Raw materials
B. Transportation availability
C. Market proximity
D. All of the above

1646. Due to lack of environmental the cause are all except
A. Potential contamination
B. Material degradation
C. Physical and chemical instability
D. Labour availability

1647. In a plant layout area planning depend on
A. Type of production
B. Container size
C. Environmental control needs
D. All of these

1648. Sterilization and depyrogeneration of in container before filling require in
A. Aseptic filling process
B. For container cleaning
C. For storage
D. Both a and b

1649. In terminal sterilization the accumulation insegregation area required for
A. Storage of product
B. Product transferred to the next step
C. Both a and b
D. Filling and sealing

1650. In parenteral compounding area close to the filling line for ease transfer problem
A. Liquids B. Emulsion
C. Suspension D. Semi solids

1651. In which feeling,homogeneous mixture is maintained
A. Vaccines
B. Suspension
C. Insulin preparation
D. All of these

1652. Peeping, reservoir and pump system used for high fillingrate
A. Suspension B. Liquids
C. Lozengea D. None of these

1653. Is per GMP environmental control zone grouping by
A. As per cGMP
B. As per gazette of India
C. Face per WHO
D. Both a and b

1654. According tocGMP the number of zone
A. 7 zone B. 6 zone
C. 3 zone D. 10 zone

1655. According to cGMP zone 5 follows ....
A. General production
B. Warehouse
C. Weighing mixture and transfer area
D. Filling area

1656. Filling area comes under ....
A. Zone 1 B. Zone 2
C. Zone 6 D. Zone 7

1657. According to gazette of India
A. Colour zone B. Black zone
C. 3 zone D. None of these

1658. White zone in parenteral layout are
A. Filling of parental B. Filtration
C. Clean area D. Contaminated

1659. Weighing the solution infiltration zone is ....
A. White zone B. Grey zone
C. Black zone D. Zone 4

1660. .... zone is worst area from contamination viewpoint.
A. White zone
B. Grey zone
C. Black zone
D. White and grey zone

1661. For pproduction the space required in parenteral are
A. 1018 square meter
B. 1716 square meter
C. 11094 square meter
D. 7606 square meter

1662. For warehouse requirement space required is ....
A. 45.1% B. 30%
C. 20% D. 10%

1663. Lowest space requirement in parenteral department is for ....
A. Quality control B. Production
C. Administration D. Maintenance

1664. Quality space required in parenteral are ....
A. 7606 square meter
B. 1018 square meter
C. 1700 square meter
D. 80 square meter

1665. The Efficiency of HEPA filter used for aseptic filling is ....
A. 99.99% B. 100%
C. 99.9 7% D. 70%

1666. For parenteral layout, adjacent rooms of different grades should have ....
A. Pressure difference 22 to 30 Pascal
B. 20 to 30 humidity changes
C. 10 to 15 pascals pressure difference
D. 5 degree Celsius changes in temperature

1667. Epoxy paint are used in ....
A. Solid dosage form layout
B. Parenteral layout
C. Semisolid layout
D. For all plants

1668. In maximum plant layout the air flow is ....
A. 100 to 120 fit/m B. 60 to 80 fit/m
C. 20 to 90 fit/m D. None of these

1669. For coating of stainless steel the material used is ....
A. Providence pthalate
B. Ethyl cellulose
C. Silver and Zinc containing zeolite matrix
D. Zeolite and gold coating

1670. In pharmaceutical industry the phenomenon which considered in layout ....
A. Market earning B. Customer demand
C. Productivity D. Both B and C

1671. For solid dosage form the type of layout followed ....

A. Circular flow B. Parallel flow
C. Cross overflow D. All of the above

1672. For tableting area pressure maintained is (in pascals) ....

A. 10 B. 15
C. 20 D. 30

1673. Humidity maintenance are sensitive for production of ....

A. Oral cavity tablet
B. Effervescent tablet
C. Thermolabile tablet
D. Hypodermic tablet

1674. The environmental condition for hard gelatin capsule(humidity/ temperature) is ....

A. Not more than 25 percent / 35degree cent
B. NMT 25%/NMT 25 dc
C. 20-25% RH /25 dc
D. 40% RH / 20 dc

1675. The environmental condition for soft gelatin capsule is ....

A. 22 25 percent RH / 30 degree centigrade
B. 10 to 15% RH / 40dc
C. 20-25% RH/25 dc
D. 20-40% RH /25 dc

1676. The basic installation requirements for uncoated tablets is ....

A. 60 square meter B. 20 square meter
C. 30 square meter D. 10 square meter

1677. Ancillary area required for coating section are ....

A. 50 square meter B. 30 square meter
C. 20 square meter D. 10 square meter

1678. Suppository, inhaler, capsule and ophthalmic required area are

A. 25 square feet B. 35 square feet
C. 30 square feet D. 20 square feet

1679. The equipment which are work both granulator with drawing

A. Diosena granulator
B. Gral mixer
C. Marumerizer
D. Twin shell processor

1680. Manufacturing area required for cream are

A. 60 square metre
B. 27 square metre
C. 25 square metre
D. 40 square metre

1681. Highest area layout required in cream which are

A. Filling area
B. Packaging and labeling
C. Manufacturing area
D. Storage Area

1682. Quantitative layout of cream have plant capacity

A. 100 tube per day
B. 1000 tube Par day
C. 10,000 tubes per day
D. 100000 tube per day

1683. Topical preparation plant shell have air filter at least ....

A. 15 Micron filter B. 10 Micron filter
C. 20 Micron filter D. None of these

1684. In topical preparation the manufacturing area temperature are ....?

A. Not more than 20 degree centigrade
B. 37 degree centigrade
C. Cold temperature
D. Not more than30 dc

1685. The product layout have advantage of ....?

A. High flexibility
B. Low raw material cost
C. Low capital cost
D. Low cost variable in per unit

1686. Which layout required in equipment installation?

A. Product layout
B. Process layout
C. Fixed position layout
D. Both a and b

1687. Which of the following is a non absorbable suture?

A. Polypropylene B. Vicryl
C. Cutgut D. Polydioxanane

1688. **Surgically used suture material polydioxanane.**
   A. A non-absorbable and remain encapsulated
   B. Undergoes hydrolysis and complete absorption
   C. Undergoes phagocylesis and enzymatic degradation
   D. Is specifically used for heart values of synthetic

1689. **PDS is absorbed within**
   A. 7 days B. 21 days
   C. 100 days D. 225 days

1690. **The surgenon who introducecatgut is surgery was.**
   A. Astley Cooper B. Lord Lister
   C. Johan hunter D. Syme

1691. **Which of the following is not absorbable suture?**
   A. Catgut B. Polyglactin
   C. Polyamide D. Polyester

1692. **Which of the following is ideal time to removal of scalp suture.**
   A. 3days B. 5 days
   C. 7 days D. 10 days

1693. **Catgut is prepared from submucosal layer of the intestine of.**
   A. Cat B. Human
   C. Sheep D. Rabbit

1694. **Vicryl, the commonly used suture material is a.**
   A. Homopolymer of polydiozanone
   B. Homopolymer of glycolide
   C. Co-polymer of glycolide and lactide
   D. Homopolymer of lactide

1695. **Who is still used in surgical procedure -**
   A. Mucose B. Catgut
   C. Gut D. Ammonia

1696. **What is received from the small intestine serosal or submucosal layer of ruminants (cow, sheep, goats)?**
   A. Collagen B. Intestine
   C. Horse D. Ligature

1697. **The catgut and violin is made from whom.**
   A. Intestine of human
   B. Plastic
   C. Glass
   D. Intestine of the sheep

1698. **Which of these is used in absorbable?**
   A. Hydrogen
   B. ammonia
   C. Suture and ligature
   D. carbon

1699. **First 7.5 m intestine was selected to make.**
   A. Violin
   B. surgical gut preparation
   C. Nonabsorbable
   D. Absorbable

1700. **What is the first process of the selection and washing in the catgut.**
   A. Glass B. washing
   C. Clean the intestine D. Gut

1701. **For what the smooth ribbon is selected.**
   A. Water B. Surgical gut
   C. Ligature D. Mucose

1702. **How many layer are there gut formed.**
   A. Four layers B. Two layers
   C. 10 layers D. One layers

1703. **Which of these layer gut?**
   A. Submucous B. Intestine
   C. Collagen D. Gut

1704. **With whom increase the tensile strength?**
   A. Ligature
   B. Collagen
   C. Orienlation of fibres
   D. Plastic

1705. **What type of polish is made on dry thread?**
   A. Mechanical type B. chemical type
   C. Physical type D. Biological type

1706. **What is a highly important part of the manufacturer of good quality surgical gut?**
   A. Cleaning B. Ligature
   C. Finishing D. Mucus

1707. **Who's may be sterilized by Heat chemicals of ionizing radiation?**
   A. Gut B. Absorbable
   C. Polyamide D. None

1708. Which process of sterilisation is iodine used?
A. Physical process B. Biological process
C. Chemical process D. Microbial

1709. What did the process of sterilisation start?
A. 1960 B. 1961
C. 1962 D. 1951

1710. By whom can the enzymes be digest quickly
A. Chromic gut B. Intestine
C. Collagen D. Ligature

1711. How are surgical gut cause tissue reaction in small size
A. More B. Less
C. Many D. Few

1712. Whom leukocytes in the area also increase in number?
A. Tissue reaction B. Tissue size
C. Tissue shap D. Tissue length

1713. What is formed in the wound after surgical incision?
A. WBC B. RBC
C. Blood and lymph D. Body

1714. With whom does surgical gut repair?
A. Gut B. Suture
C. Ligature D. Tissue

1715. Which is surgeon choose the gut?
A Collagen
B. Intestine
C. Plain and chromic gut
D. Non polar

1716. Surgeon never uses which suture?
A. Collagen
B. Tissue is more stronger than
C. Tissue is less stronger than
D. Tissue / ligature

1717. Which machine uses the temperature and pressure of the steam for disinfection?
A. Laminar air flow B. Autoclave
C. Oven D. Water jet

1718. What is purpose of CDDS?
A. Stronger of clean equipment
B. Storing sterile equipment
C. Providing sterile equipment to the operation theater
D. Pharmacy of the operation theater.

1719. What is sterilized in dry conditions?
A. Implant B. Gauze
C. Scalpel D. Cannula

1720. Which of the following chemicals are used to treat the instrument made out of polymers?
A. Hydrochloric acid, saline solution.
B. Saline solution
C. Ethylene, ozone, hydrogen
D. Silver cyanide

1721. What is the commonest method of sterilization?
A Dry heat sterilization
B. Heat sterilization
C. Autoclave
D. Water jet

1722. What is the source of suture?
A. Physical B. Chemical
C. Natural\synthetic D. Collagen

1723. Who is structure of monufilament?
A. Suture material B. Gut
C. Nylone D. Surgical

1724. Surgical used suture material polydioxanone.
A. Is non absorbable and remain encapsulated
B. Undergoes hydrolysis and complete absorption
C. Undergoes phagocytosis and enzymatic degradation
D Is specifically used for heart values or synthetic grafts

1725. Which of the following is a delayed absorbable synthetic suture material?
A. Chromic catgut B. Vicryl
C. Silk D. Nylone

1726. Which one of the following is used as preservative for packing catgut suture?
A. Isopropyl alcohol B. Colloidal iodine
C. Glutaraldehyde D. Hydrogen peroxide

1727. Suture material used for laparascopic choledechotomy repair.

A. Silk B. Catgut
C. Polyethylene D. Vicryl

1728. Catgut is preserved in

A. Glutaraldehyde B. Isopropyl alcohol
C. Iodine D. Certrimide

1729. Raw material used in nylone suture is.

A. Polyethylene theraphthelate
B. Polyamide polymer
C. Polyester polyester
D. Polybutylene terephthalate

1730. On the needle suture attachment.

A. To straighten the suture
B. Synthetic absorbable suture
C. Do not place any tension
D. Do not pull or stretch

1731. Selected to correspond to the size and strength of the tissue to be sewn.

A. Ligature method B. Ligature
C. Suture size D. Surgical gut

1732. Used for most spectacular skin colosures

A. 6-0 and 7-0 B. 1 and 0
C. 3-0 and 4-0 D. 4-0 and 5-0

1733. Suture size, material, and type and size of needle.

A. Knots of monofilament
B. Synthetic absorption suture
C. Nonabsorbable suture
D. Most important information on the suture box

1734. Free -tie, suture ligature, reel - tie, and the instrument tie.

A. Ligature methods B. The needle holder
C. Ligature reel D. Suture size

1735. Digested by body enzymes that attack the suture strand, eventually destroying it.

A. Absorbable suture
B. Synthetic absorbable suture
C. Natural absorbable suture
D STSR should arrange the suture

1736. What is the type of suturefate?

A. Absorbable /nonabsorbable
B. Ligature
C. Mucous
D. Collagen

1737. How many coating of sutures

A. 3 B. 2
C. 1 D. 4

1738. What is the natural source of absorbable sutures?

A. Catgut / fascia lata / collagen
B. Cotton
C. Ramine
D. Plastic

1739. What is the natural source of non absorbable sutures?

A. Plastic / glass B. Catgut
C. Silk /cotten D. Paper

1740. What is the synthetic source of absorbable suture?

A. Polyglycolic acid B. Catgut
C. Ammonia D. Water

1741. What is the synthetic source of nonabsorbable suture?

A. Nylone / polyamide
B. Glass
C. Plastic
D. Water

1742. What is the disadvantage of monofilament?

A. Polyester
B. Handling and knotting
C. No, capillarity
D. No bacterial harbours

1743. What is advantage of monofilament?

A. Smooth surface
B. Stretch
C. Nick or cimp in material
D. Catgut

1744. What are the absorbable of monofilament?

A. Polymide
B. Polydiaxanone
C. Polyester
D. PVDF suture

1745. What is nonabsorbable of monofilament?

A. Ammonia B. Polyglactin
C. Hydrogen D. Polypropylene

1746. **What is the advantage of monufilament?**
A. Bacterial harbours B. Tissue trauma
C. Good handling D. Gut

1747. **What is the disadvantage of monufilament?**
A. Capillary action B. Hot air oven
C. Good konting D. Glass rod

1748. **What is absorbable of multifilament?**
A. Cotton B. Glass
C. Polyglycolic acid D. Linen

1749. **What is non absorbable of multifilament?**
A. Polyglactin 910 B. Bottle
C. Paper D. Silk

1750. **How many days of vicryl wound support?**
A. 10 days B. 100day
C. 1000 days D. 250days

1751. **How many days of monocryl wound support?**
A. 300 days B. 40days
C. 20 days D. 100days

1752. **How many days of coated vircryl wound support?**
A. 20 days B. 200 days
C. 50 days D. 30 days

1753. **How many days of PDS -II wound support?**
A. 50 days B. 70 days
C 60 days D. 40days

1754. **What is the typical use of vicryl?**
A. Skin / oral B. Ligature
C. Fascia D. Glass

1755. **What are the typical uses of monocryl?**
A. General B. Oral
C. Ligature / mucosa D. Opthelmic

1756. **What are typical uses of coted vircyl?**
A. Ligature B. Ophthalmic
C. Oral D. Skin

1757. **What is the typical use of PDS - II?**
A. Fascia B. Ligature
C. General D. Mucosa

1758. **How many days of vicryl mass absorption?**
A. By 52.days B. By 42 days
C. By 62 days D. By 41days

1759. **How many days of monocryl mass absorption?**
A. 90-120 days B. 91-120 days
C. 20-90 days D. 90-911 days

1760. **How many days of coated mass absorption?**
A. 51-55 days B. 70-90 days
C. 57-81days D. 56-70 days

1761. **How many days of PDS-II mass absorption**
A. 181-120 days B. 180-210 days
C. 120-222days D. 180-220days

1762. **What are the adorable sutures made of?**
A. Animal intestine B. Plastic
C. Glass D. Non

1763. **Who is collagen converted?**
A. Collagen B. Gelatin
C. Intestine D. Gut

1764. **What is the brand name of poliglecapron 25?**
A. Gut B. Intestine
C. Monocryl D. Normal

1765. **What is the brand name of polyglactin 910?**
A. Monocryl B. Vicryl
C. Dexon D. Gelatin

1766. **What is brand name of Polyglycolic acid?**
A. Vicryl B. Gut
C. Dexon D. Intestine

1767. **What are brand names of Polydioxanane?**
A. Monocryl B. Vicryl
C. PDS-II D. Collagen

1768. **How are tissue reactivity of polydioxanane?**
A. Normal B. Minimal
C. Collagen D. Tissue

1769. **How is tissue reactivity of plain catgut?**
A. Minimal B. Severe
C. Monocryl D. PDS-II

1770. How are tissue reactivity of chromic catgut

A. Severe B. Minimal
C. Moderate D. Normal

1771. How are tissue reactivity of poliglecapron -25

A. Shap B. Normal
C Minimal D. Poor

1772. How is the tissue reactivity of Polyglycolic acid?

A. Minimal B. Monocryl
C. Normal D. Gelatin

1773. How is knot security of plain catgut

A. Normal B. Poor
C. Good D. Bed

1774. How is knot security of chromic catgut?

A. Poor B. Good
C. Gelatin D. Gut

1775. How are knot security of polyglecapron - 25

A. Minimal B. Poor
C. Ligature D Good

1776. How is knot security of polyglactin 910?

A. Ligature B. Gut
C. Good D. Good

1777. How are knot securities of Polyglycolic acid?

A. Fair B. Poor
C. Good D. None

1778. How are knot security of polydioxanane

A. Fair B. Gut
C. Ligature D. Good

1779. What are sutures means?

A. Seam or sweet B. Salt or sew
C. Sweet or seam D. Sew or seam

1780. What is the chemical agent amongst the given options?

A. Dry
B. Heat
C. Alcohol / metallic salts
D. Sunlight

1781. What is physical agent?

A. Sunlight B. Alcohol
C. Dry D. None

1782. How many types of sterilization method is there for surgical sutures.

A. 5 B. 2
C. 6 D. 1

1783. How is needle point geometry of teper point?

A. Suited to soft tissue
B. Sample
C. Hard shop
D. Long tissue

1784. How is needle point geometry of revers cutting?

A. Very sharp B. Blunt
C. Simple D. None

1785. How is needle point geometry of conventional cutting?

A. Suited to tissue
B. Cuts rather than dilates
C. Opthelmic surgery
D. Normal size

1786. How are needle point geometry of spatula

A. Very sharp B. Long tissue
C. Suited to tissue D. Opthelmic surgry

1787. Catgutis ....

A. Natural B. Synthetic
C. Semisolid D. None

1788. What is catgut made out of?

A. Carbon B. Fiber
C. Purified collagen D. Tissue

1789. What is downside of using catgut?

A. Purified water
B. Variable absorption and loss of tensile strength
C. Enzymes
D. None

1790. How is catgut degraded?

A. Enzymatically B. Collagen
C. Tissue D. Plastic

1791. How quick does chromic catgut lose tensile strength?

A. 2% tensile strength
B. 0% tensile strength at 2-3 weeks
C. 4% tensile strength 5 weeks
D. 1%

1792. How quick does chromic catgut lose in the stomach?
A. 5% at 6 hours in the stomach
B. 1% at 12 hours in stomach
C. 0% at 24 hours in the stomach
D. None

1793. How quick does chromic catgut lose in the urinary bladder?
A. 0% at 7 days in the bladder
B. 0% at 2 days in the bladder
C. 1 % at 2 days in the bladder
D. 5% at 1 days in the bladder

1794. How long does it take for chromic catgut to be completely absorbed?
A. 2-3 days
C. Unpredictable but approximately 14-80 days
C. 2-5days
D. 3-6 days

1795. How well does chromic catgut handle?
A. Fair B. Hard
C. Vicryl D. Soft

1796. What are some contraindications for using chromic catgut
A. Normal conditions B Hydrolysis
C. Harsh conditions D. None

1797. What are the trade name for polyglactin 910
A. Vicryl B. Hydrolysis
C. Natural D. None

1798. How is Vicryl / polyglactin 910 degraded?
A. Synthetic B. Vicryl
C. Hydrolysis D Polymer

1799. In what type of environment does vircyl / polyglactin 910 lose it's tensile strength more rapidly.
A. In a alkaline environment
B. Saline environment
C Natural environment
D. None

1800. What are vicryl rapide?
A. Vicryl is no rapidly
B. Vicryl is a slow absorbed rapidly
C. Vicryl is absorbed very rapidly
D Vircyl is smooth

1801. What is the tensile strength of vicryl at 2 weeks
A. 50% at 2-3 weeks B. 55% at 5 weeks
C. 60% at 3-4 weeks D. 56% 2-3 weeks

1802. What is the tensile strength of vicryl rapide at 2 weeks
A. 1 % at 2 weeks B. 2% at 2 weeks
C. 0% at 2 weeks D 4% at 2 weeks

1803. What is vicryl completely absorbed?
A. 45-70days B. 60-70 days
C. 55-60 days D. 56-70 days

1804. When is vicryl rapide completely absorbed?
A. 41 days B. 42days
C. 44 days D. 88days

1805. What degree of tissue reactivity does vicryl cause?
A. Minimal B. Monufilament
C. Monoclonal D. None

1806. How is vicryl'S handling?
A. Batter C. Poor
B. Good D. Very good

1807. How is Vicky'S knot security?
A. Fair B. Good
C. Monocryl D. Poor

1808. What is the trade name for poliglecaprone 25?
A. Minimal B. Monocryl
C. Monoclonal D. Synthetic

1809. Is poliglecaprone 25/ monocryl?
A. Synthetic B. Minimal
C. Natural D. None

1810. Is poliglcaprone 25/ mononal monofilament / multifilament?
A. Monofilament B. Minimal
C. Multifilament D. None

1811. Piloglecaprone 25/monocryl absorbable / nonabsorbable?
A. Absorbed B. Nonabsorbed
C. Nonabsorbable D. Absorbable

1812. How is poliglecaprone 25 degraded?
A. Hydrolysis B. Carbon
C. Alkaline D. Monomer

1813. In what environment does poliglecaprone 25/ monocyl lose it's tensile strength?
A. Minimal B. Hydrolysis
C. Alkaline D. Minimal

1814. Does poliglecaprone 25 have a high or low intial breaking strength?
A. Low B. High
C. Medium D. None

1815. At what time is poliglecaprone 25 at 50% tensile strength?
A. 2-3 weeks B. 2-5 weeks
C. 3-6 weeks D. 1-2 weeks

1816. When is poliglecaprone 25 / monocyl completely absorbed?
A. 119 days B. 22 days
C. 220 days D. 18 days

1817. How is poliglecaprone 25/ monocryl's tissue reactivity?
A Minimal B. Small
C. Monomal D. Large

1818. How does poliglecaprone 25 / monocryl handle?
A. Medium B. Good
C. Fair D. None

1819. How is poliglecaprone 25 / monocryl's knot security?
A. Large B. Good
C. Small D. Fair

1820. What is the generic name for PDS-II?
A. Polidioxanone B. Polymer
C. Hydrolysis D. Isomers

1821. How is polydioxanone / PDS-II degraded?
A. Alkaline B. Carbon
C. Polymer D. Hydrolysis

1822. In what environment does polydioxanone PDS-II lose it's tensile strength most rapidly?
A. Basic environment
B. Weak base environment
C. Acidic environment
D. Weak acid environment

1823. When is the tensile strength of PDS-II 50%?
A. 1-3 weeks B. 2-5 weeks
C. 4-5weeks D. 5-6 weeks

1824. When is PDS-II completely absorbed?
A. 170 days B. 171 days
C. 160 days D. 180 days

1825. How much tissue reactivity is noted with PDS-II?
A Minimal B. Acidic
C. Monomal D. Basic

1826. How does PDS -II handle?
A. Fine B. Poor
C. Good D. None

1827. What is the generic name for prolene?
A. Polymethayl B. Polypropylene
C. Polymer D. None

1828. How quickly is prolene absorbed?
A. Lack of hydrogen bonds
B. Lack of alkaline bond
C. Lack of hydrolyzable bond
D. Lack of chemicals

1829. What is the nylon nature?
A. Synthetic B. Minimal
C. Natural D. None

1830. Is nylon?
A. Monufilament B. Monofilament
C. Multifilament D All the above

1831. Is nylon susceptible to hydrolysis?
A. No B. Good
C. Less D. Yes

1832. When does nylon have 50% tensile strength?
A. 11weeks B. 10 weeks
C. 8 weeks D. 12 weeks

1833. What is the trade name for polymerized caprolactam?
A. Braunamide B. Bromide
C. Amide D. All the above

1834. What are triclosan?
A. Antioxidants B. Analgesic
C. Antibiotics D. Monomal

1835. What do suture with the word "PLUS" refer to?
A. Having an antibiotic coating
B. Antioxidants coating
C. Having an analgesic coating
D. None

1836. What are skin glues?
A. Absorbable B. Natural
C. Nonabsorbable D. Synthetic

1837. What are the basic principles of sutures?
A. Purification B. Adsorption
C. Absorption
D. Minimize amount used

1838. What is the source of catgut sutures?
A. Mammalian intestinB. Small intestine
C. Long intestine D. None

1839. Why is cutgut packaged in alcohol?
A. To maintain temperature
B. To maintain acidic nature
C. To maintain pliability
D. To maintain basic nature

1840. Catgut rate of strength less?
A. Pliability B. Basic
C. Acidic D Unpredictable

1841. Can catgut be resterilized by heat?
A. No, the protein in it will denature
B. Polycaprolate
C. Number of cell
D. Mammalian intestine

1842. Is dexon S coated
A. Yes B. Large
C. No D. Small

1843. Dexon -ll is coated with?
A. Polymer B. Polycaprolate
C. Alcohol D. Monufilament

1844. How long does it take for silk to be absorbed?
A. 5 years B. 1 years
C. 2 years C. 3 years

1845. Review : rapid absorbable suture that is natural
A. Chromic gut B. Monufilament
C. Sheep intestine D. Polycaprolate

1846. Review : absorbable long lasting synthetic suture
A. Monofilament B. Sheep intestine
C. Polymer D. None

1847. What layer should you bury knot in?
A. Intrauterine B. Intravenous
C. Subcutaneous D. Polycaprolate

1848. What are the types of needles on most sutures?
A. Swaged needles B. Large needles
C. Small needles D. None

1849. Catgut sutures are made from?
A. Goat intestine
B. Hair
C. Sheep / cattle initma
D. Cat

1850. Catgut tensile strength duration
A. 4-7 b B. 4-6 b
C. 4-8 b D. 3-4 b

1851. Chromic gut lastes for......
A. 10-15 d B. 10-11 d
C. 12-13d D. 10-14 d

1852. At what agle should the needle enter the skin
A. 90 degrees B. 50 degrees
C. 80 degrees D. 75 degrees

1853. To what severity is the tissue reaction of all nature suture type
A. Inflammatory reaction
B. Mild
C. Moderate except steel is the least
D. None

1854. How is vicryl tissue reaction?
A. Mild B. Natural
C. Synthetic D. Inflation

1855. What are the major classes of sutures material?
A. Synthetic Vs natural
B. Plain gut
C. Inflammatory reaction
D. None

1856. Absorbable suture material replacement healthy tissue as a result of what?
A. Polymer reaction
B. Basic reaction
C. Inflammatory reaction
D. Acidic reaction

1857. Suture material can be manufactured by what
A. Synthetic or animal sources
B. Biological source
C Natural sources
D. Chromic gut

1858. What are the 2 type of catgut
A. Synthetic, natural
B. Simple, natural
C. Plain, chromic
D. Plain, synthetic

1859. Plain catgut is absorbed in low many days?
A. 7-10 B. 7-9
C. 4-5 D. 9-10

1860. Dexon degraded rapidly in what type of environment?
A. Acidic B. Natural
C. Alkaline D. None

1861. Vicryl degraded rapidly in what type of environment?
A. Alkaline B. Acidic
C. Weak base D. Natural

1862. What species do we not see as many tissue reaction when using monocryl?
A. Cow B. Elephant
C. Cats D. Dog

1863. What species do we not see as many tissue reaction when using PDS?
A. Dog B. Cow
C. elephant D. Cat

1864. If Nonabsorbable suture are left in the body too long what could happen?
A. Hydrolysis
B. Absorption
C. They can get buried and can become encysted
D. None

1865. When should Nonabsorbable suture be taken out?
A. 7-14 days B. 7-9 days
C 6-9 days D. 5-6 days

1866. What is cotton?
A. Natural fibers B. Absorbable
C. Synthetic fibers D. None

1867. How to prevent dehiscence?
A. Natural fibre B. Synthetic
C. e- collar D. Acidic

1868. Disadvantage of wire?
A. Poor handling B. Poor product
C. Expensive D. None

1869. Suture material sizes are measured how?
A. Ought B. Large
C. Expensive D. Weight balance

1870. What number ought is used for eyelid surgery?
A. >6-1 B. >6-0
C. < 6-0 D. 1-2

1871. What number ought is used for small animals?
A. 3-0 B. 1-0
C. 2-0 D 4-0

1872. What number ought is the avg size used?
A. 5-0 B. 1-0
C. 2-0 D. 2-3

1873. Suture needle very in what
A. Size B. Shape
C. Length D. None

1874. What are the pros of using eyed needle?
A. Reusable B. Size
C. Shap D. More expensive

1875. What are the cons of using eyed needle?
A. Ear
B. Suture is threaded thru an eye
C. Mouth
D. None

1876. What are the pros of using swaged / seeded needle)
A. Readily available B. More expensive
C. Small needle D. all of these

1877. What are the cons of swaged / swedged?
A. Chief B. Low cost
C. More expensive D. None

1878. How are the staplers named?
A. Abbreviation of their designed function
B. Suture
C. Abbreviation
D. Catgut

1879. Rate of catgut absorbable suture can be affected by
A. Cold B Fever
C. Swaiting D. Vomiting

1880. How many times of gastrointestinal stapler (GAI)
A. One B. Four
C. Two D. five

1881. What are use thoracoabdominal stapler (TA)
A. Heart B. Kidney
C. Lung resection D. Mouth

1882. What are the used of ligate and divide stapler (LDS)
A. Tissue
B. Blood vessels ligature
C. Lung
D. Opthelmic surgery

1883. What are the 1/4 curved needle used for?
A. Opthelmic surgery B. Lung
C. Heart surgery D. None

1884. What is the 3/8 and 1/2 curved needle used for?
A. Heart surgery
B. Popular in general surgery
C. Opthelmic surgery
D. Lung

1885. Minimum number of throws for suturing?
A. 5 B. 3
C. 4 D. 1

1886. What are the numbers of throws normally placed when suturing?
A. 4 B. 3
C. 6 D. 5

1887. What are glucomer 631(biosyn)?
A. Nonabsorbable B. Monufilament
C. Absorbable D. Minimal

1888. How can you overcome "memory" In suture?
A. Gelatin
B. Stretch, wipe off preserving fluid if catgut
C. Monomer
D. Metallic

1889. Which suture material is least likely to cause inflammation?
A. Silk B. Starch
C. Metallic D. Acacia

1890. Which suture type is preferred for opthelmic procedure?
A. Metallic B Silk
C. Silver D. Carbon

1891. How many times can Nonabsorbable suture be autoclaved without less of tensile strength
A. 4 times B. 2 times
C. 8 times D. 3 times

1892. What is tissue adhesive?
A. Nexaband B. Cyanoacrylate
C. Gauze sponge D. None

1893. What tissue adhesive is used for doclaw surgery?
A. Metallic B. Cyanoacrylate
C. Nexaband D Silver

1894. How much blood a 4.4 hold?
A. 6-10 ml B. 5-10 ml
C. 7-10 ml D. 4-9 ml

1895. What are the method of homeostasis?
A. Gauze sponges B. Nexaband
C. Hydrogen D None

1896. When can Chemical cauterization be used for homeostasis?
A. Toenails B. Stomach
C. Mouth D. Hand

1897. No sutures is perfect , but all suture can -
A. Uniform in shape
B. Lenagh
C. Uniform in size and diameter
D. Metal

1898. After how long should skin sutures be removed
A. 12-13 days B. 4-6 days
C. 10-14 days D. 6- 10 days

1899. What suture material is most likely to leave a scar?
A. Silver B. Carbon
C. Gold D. Metal

1900. What is the advantage of treating catgut with chromic salts?
A. Easy procedure
B. Low cost
C More constant resorption rate
D. None

1901. How long does it chromic catgut to absorb?
A. 30 days B. 5 days
C. 10 days D. 40 days

1902. What are the application of ligature?
A. Circumferential ligature
B. Homostasis
C. Transfixation
D. None

1903. What is the type of ligature?
A. Circumferential B. Transfixation
C. Miller's knot D. All the above

1904. What can the Miller knot be used in lieu of?
A. Homostesis
C. Circumferential ligature
B. Miller knot
D. Ligature

1905. How should a curved homostate point in the three - clamp technique?
A. Point up towards the ovary
B. Kidney
C. Point up towards the lung
D. None

1906. What ligature is used for the second ligature?
A. Miller 'S knot
B.. Tissue
C. Transfixation ligature
D. Circumferential

1907. Where is the circumferential ligature placed?
A. Most proximally on the pedicle
B. Tissue
C. Distally on pedicle
D. None

1908. Where are the transfixing knot applied?
A. Ligature
B. Cells
C. Tissue
D. Applied most distally on pedicle

1909. What are "thumb to thumb "used for?
A. metal B Cell
C. Tissue D. All ligature

1910. Which direction should the curved homostate be facing in a OHE?
A. Pointing Towards the ovary
B. Pointing toward the kidney
C. Pointing toward the lung
D. None

1911. Where is the second ligature placed?
A. Between the 1st tissue
B. Between the 3rd ligature
C. Between the 1st ligature
D. Between the 3rd tissue

1912. Where is the pedicle transacted?
A. Between the middle and distal homostats
B. Between the lung
C. Between the tissue
D. Between the 1st tissue

1913. Absorbable synthetic suture are made from what?
A. Polymer B. Polyglycolic acid
C. Monomer D. Polyglycolytic

1914. What are the components of a suture
A. Suture stand, surgical needle
B. Glassrod
C. Beaker
D. Funnel

1915. How suture strand chemicals degradation occurs?
A. Hydrogen bond
B. Hydrolysis of ester bond
C. Carbon compound
D. Alkaline

1916. What are all multifilament suture are coated?
A. Yes B. Good
C. No D. None

1917. What is the purpose of the suture package?
A. Maintain the product
B. To maintain temperature
C. Maintain the area
D. To maintain sterility during storage.

1918. What are the important of braided polymers?
A. Decrease overall strength
B. Increase the temperature
C. increase overall strength
D. None.

1919. Why are ceramic not used for suture?
A. Acidic nature B. They are brittle
C. Basic nature D. They are hard

1920. What are the qualities of the ideal skin substitutes

A. inexpensive B. Hydrolysis
C. expensive D. Good

1921. What are 2 ways a suture is absorbable

A. Enzymatic breakdown or hydrolysis
B. Reductions or hydrolysis
C. Oxidation or reductions
D. Breakdown or oxidation

1922. What are the most type of sutures?

A. Synthetic
B. Nonabsorbable
C. Natural absorbable suture
D. Monufilament

1923. What is the anatomy of a suture needle?

A. Point, needle length
B. Shape
C. Needle size
D. Small needle

1924. What are 1/4 and 3/8 needle used for

A. Taper B. Superficial use
C. Cutting D. Surface use

1925. What are the 2 type of points?

A. Taper or cutting B. Superficial use
C. Size or shape D. None

1926. Surgical gut is AKA?

A. Sheep B. Catgut
C. Dog D. Cow

1927. This is produced from the submucosa of sheep and dog intestines?

A. Catgut B. Ligature
C. Suture D. Intestines

1928. Plain catgut is absorbed in how long?

A. 2-3 days B. 1-2 days
C. 4-5 days D. 3-5 days

1929. Chromic cat guy is absorbed in how long?

A 4-6 days B. 14-16 days
C. 10-15 days D. 1-5 days

1930. Polyglycolic acid is AKA?

A. Catgut B. Dexon
C. Nylon D. Carbon

1931. How long does Polyglycolic acid lost?

A. 14-21 days B. 10-15 days
C. 12-21 days D. 15-19 days

1932. Dexon is less reactive that what other suture?

A. Catgut B. Ligature
C Suture D. Monufilament

1933. PDS is better for what type of wound?

A. Fast healing
B. Increase reaction
C. Wounds that heal slowly
D. None

1934. How long does it take for PDS absorb?

A. 170 days B. 140 days
C. 160 days D. 180 days

1935. Poliglecaprone and glycomer 631 and used for what type of wound?

A. Fast healing wound
B. Catgut
C. Slow healing
D. None

1936. Poliglecaprone and glycomer 631 are mostly used where?

A. Suture B. Intestines
C. Chromic gut D. Gut

1937. How long poliglecaprone and glycomer 631 does lose?

A. 7-14 days B. 8-10 days
C. 7-12 days D. 10-15 days

1938. A stitch that is tied and cut before placing another stich is called

A. Halting B. Noncontinuous
C. Continuous D. Interrpted

1939. Wound of the following is NOT a consideration for suture selection?

A. Blue color B. Wound color
C. Red color D. Black color

1940. What type of needle is used for wound and laceration care?

A. Large needle
B. A revers cutting needle
C. Small needle
D. None

1941. When are tapered needle used

A. To stitch soft tissue
B. To stitch soft cell
C. To stitch long tissue
D. To stitch hard cell

1942. What size suture should be used for scalp?

A. 5-0 B. 1-0
C. 3-0 D. 2-0

1943. What type of sutures material should be used when closing a facial wound?

A. Cotton B. Nylon
C. Catgut D. Sheep

1944. What are sutures needle made of?

A. Iron B. Steel silver
C. Copper D. Stainless / carbon

1945. Cuts longer than ___usually require structures

A. 0.5 inch B. 0.4 inch
C. 0.6 inch D. 0.3 inch

1946. What is the standard needle holder size?

A. 2 inches B. 1 inches
C. 3 inches D. 4 inches

1947. How long does it generally take for sitches to heal after surgery?

A. 3 days to 3 weeks
B. 4 days to 3 weeks
C. 2 days to 3 weeks
D. 1 days to 3 weeks

1948. Which of the following is not an interrupt suture?

A. Polyamide B Interlocking
C. Cotton D. None

1949. What is nylon also referred to as?

A. Polymer B. Interlocking
C. Monomer D. Polyamide

1950. Name the member of the nylon family?

A. Metallic
B. Absorbable
C. Aliphatic or aromatic nylon
D Nonabsorbable

1951. What are the properties of nylon?

A. Easy to dry B. Hard dry
C. Soft dry D. None

1952. What are nylon used for -

A. Shape B. Stocking and tights
C. Size D. Length

1953. What was the first commercial produced synthetic Fiber

A Nylon B. rubber
C. Cotton D. Glass

1954. " Nylons " were an upgrade from the silk stocking women wore at the time when were " nylons "first introduced?

A. 1937 B. 1958
C. 1964 D. 1939

1955. Where did nylon make it's dobut?

A. 1939 New York B. 1939 USA
C. 1939 India D. None

1956. What year did dupont sell the nylon business

A. 2002 B. 2004
C. 2003 D. 2005

1957. What happened when supplies of the latest in women's hosiery ran short??

A. Cotton were
B. Nylon were provoked
C. Riots were provoked
D. None

1958. Nylon has _____of cross section

A. Variety B. Suture
C. Catgut D. Ligature

1959. What is the specific gravity of nylon?

A. 1.3g/cc B. 1.4g/cc
C. 1.2g/cc D. 1.5g/cc

1960. How is nylon strength?

A. Poor B. Medium
C. Excellent D. Good

1961. What are nylon absorbency

A. 2.8-4.8 low B. 2.1-4.1 low
C. 2.3-4.8 low D. 3.1-4.8 low

1962. Nylon is ___it melts spun

A. Carbon B. Plastic
C. Cotton D. Thermoplastic

1963. How many effect of heat?

A. 300 F melt B. 200 F melt
C. 302 F melt D. 100 F melt

1964. How is nylon acid?

A. Poor B. Good
C. Medium D. Excellent

1965. What are nylon sunlight

A. High B. Less
C. Low D. Fast

1966. What is nylon dimension stability?

A. Good B. Excellent
C. Poor D. None

1967. What are nylon abrasion resistance

A. Poor B. Medium
C. Good D. Excellent

1968. Nylon is easy ___fiber, most nylon items are machine washable.

A. Care B. Careless
C. Poor D. Good

1969. Manufactured Fiber in which the Fiber forming substance is " any long chain "

A. Polymer B. Polyester
C. Monomer D. Cotton

1970. Polyester forms ___ kind of appearance.

A. Any kind B. Polymer
C. Manykind D. Ester

1971. Engineering to resemble several types of natural fibers

A. Polymer B. Polyester
C. Monomer D. Ester

1972. Polyester was famous in the ____

A. 1956 B. 1958
C. 1623 D. 1953

1973. What is the polyester gravity?

A. 1.38g B. 1.39g
C. 1.28g D. 1.36g

1974. What is polyester effect of heat?

A. 324F melt B. 323F melt
C. 325 F melt D. 235F melt

1975. Polyester shrinks from Flame and will ___

A. Metallic B. Good
C. Melt D. Poor

1976. What is polyester sunlight?

A. Good B. Poor
C. Excellent D. Low

1977. What is polyester dimensional stability?

A. Excellent B. High
C. Poor C. Low

1978. How are polyester abrasion resistance

A. Good - good B. Low - low
C. Good - high D. Low - good

1979. Polyester trademark : weliman has more than ____tradmark

A. 11 B. 8
C. 16 D. 10

1980. What are polyester trademark -

A. Invista cool MAX B. Coolmax
C Invista cool D. Invista heat

1981. This fibres has the lowest density

A. Filament B Cotton
C. Olefin D. None

1982. Which of these fabrics is most likely to exhibit yarn slippage?

A. Smooth filament
B. Smooth filament yarns in a stain
C. Smooth ligature
D. Heat

1983. What two things cause permanent flattering of the yarns?

A. Heat and pressure
B. Humidity and cool
C. Heat and humidity
D. Cool and pressure

1984. What is the only reliable test to ID synthetic Fibers?

A. Metling point test
B. Temperature maintain
C. Solubility test
D. Loss activities

1985. What are the 2nd most used Fiber in the country?

A. Cotton B. Nylon
C. Carbon D. Rubber

1986. Which Fiber has a red -like shape with a smooth surface:

A. Nylon B. Monomer
C. Polymer D. Carbon

1987. Which of the following is a delayed absorbable synthetic suture material?

A. Chromic catgut B. Vicryl
C. Silk D. Nylon

1988. Which Chemical Stabilizer Is Used In Syrup?
A. Amaranth B. Glycerine
C. Both A and C D. Sorbitol

1989. Which Preservative is generally Used In Syrups?
A. Benzoic Acid B. Chloroform
C. Sedatives D. Sodium Benzoate

1990. Linctuses Are Generally Used For?
A. Sedative B. Nasals
C. Relief of Cough D. Both A & B

1991. What Is Specific Gravity Of Sugar Syrup U.S.P?
A. 1.31 B. 1.80
C. 2.0 D. 2.30

1992. What Is Specific Concentration Of Syrup USP?
A. 60% w/v B. 85% w/v
C. 65% w/v D. 70% w/v

1993. Which Type condition Prescribed Mixtures?
A. Acute Condition
B. Normal Condition
C. Constipation Condition
D. All Of The Above

1994. Which Type Mixture Solution Remove Finger Prints?
A. Silver Nitrate B. Pollutant
C. Cynoacrylates D. Aluminium Flax

1995. Which Are Diffusible Drug Mixture In 90ml Method?
A. Magnesium Carbonate
B. Quinine Sulphate
C. Bismuth Carbonate
D. All Of The Above

1996. Which Chemical Stabilizer Is Used In Mixtures?
A. Ascorbic Acid
B. Antioxidant
C. Sodium Salicylate
D. Atmospheric Oxidant

1997. Which Type Aromatic Water Is Used In Mixtures?
A. Volatile B. Anise Water
C. Peppermint Water D. Caraway Water

1998. Which Type Sweetening Agent Used In Mixture?
A. Syrup
B. Glycerol
C. Chloroform Water
D. Peppermint Water

1999. Which Mixtures Used In Liquorice (Masking Agent)
A. Certain Mixture B. Liquid Extract
C. Alkaline Extract D. Orange

2000. Which Preservative is Used in Mixture?
A. Flavouring Agent B. Chloroform
C. Benzoic Acid D. Vegetable Extract

2001. Which Dose To Preferred For Child in Syrup
A. (Age In Year)/(Age+12)×Adult Dose
B. (Age In Year)/20×Adult Dose
C. Both A&B
D. None Of The Above

2002. Which One Firstly Introduced Solubilisation?
A. M.E. Aulton B. S.N.Sharma
C. M.C.Bain D. All Of Above

2003. Complexation Formula Is-
A. X[DxCy] B. St=D+X(DxCy)
C. Both A And B D. All Of Above

2004. Commonly Use OF Stability In Drug
A. Viscosity B. Clarity
C. Oranoleptic D. Viscolizers

2005. Which Methods Use In Preparation Of Aromatic Water?
A. Distillation B. Dissolution
C. Both A&B D. None Of The Above

2006. Camphor Is Which Type Substance Is Soluble
A. Water B. Alcohol
C. Rose Water D. Dill Water

2007. Through Which Route Elixirs are to be taken?
A. Oral Route B. Nasal Route
C. Rectal Route D. All of The Above

2008. Which Tinctures are Used as Sedative And Hypnotic?
A. Compound Cardamom Tincture
B. Opium Tincture
C. Compound Opium Tincture I.P.
D. Compound Benzoin Tincture

2009. Which Tincture is Used In Carminative?
A. Compound Benzoin Tincture
B. Compound Cardamom Tincture
C. Camphorated Opium Tincture I.P.
D. Compound Benzoin Tincture

2010. Which Type Used In Citric Acid Syrup?
A. Analgesic And Antiseptic
B. Antihistamine
C. Both A And B
D. As A Flavouring Vehicle

2011. Codeine Phosphate Syrups I.P BPC Use As
A. As A Flavoured Vehicle
B. Analgesic And Antitussive
C. Antihistamine
D. All Of The Above

2012. Chlopheniramine Maleate Syrup Usp used as-
A. As A Haematic Tonic
B. Antihistamine
C. Analgesic
D. Antitussive

2013. Which Type treatment Used In Piperazine Citrate Syrup Usp Is
A. Haematinic Tonic B. Analgesic
C. Pinworm D. Round Worm

2014. Which Type Treatment Used In Compound Ferrous Phosphate Syrup BPC

2015. Which Type Treatment Used In Gargles?
A. Cough B. Flavouring Agent
C. Artificial Flavours D. Throat Infections

2016. Which Type Of Solution Are Gargles?
A. Aqueous B. Non Aqueous
C. Suspension D. All Of Above

2017. Type of Substances are Gargles?
A. Oily Substance B. Water Substance
C. Pharynx D. All Of Above

2018. Which Type Suspension In Gargles?
A. Aspirin
B. Alcohol
C. Phenolphthalein
D. Chloroform Water

2019. Which is Use of Digitalis Tincture?
A. Cardio tonics B. Anticholinergic
C. Emetics D. Flavouring agent

2020. Which Type Use Is Belladonna Tincture?
A. Anti cholinergic B. Emetics
C. Flavouring Agent D. Flavouring Agent

2021. Which is the use Of Impecana Tincture
A. Emetics B. Flavouring Agent
C. Cardio tonics D. Anticholinergic

2022. Tincture Is Mainly Use As_
A. Animal Drug
B. Potent Drug
C. Therapy Drug
D. All Of Above

2023. Which Type Methods of Preparation of Tincture?
A. Maceration B. Percolation
C. Both A & B D. All Of Above

2024. Why is Glycerine added In Elixirs?
A. Increasing Stability
B. Increasing Solubility
C. Flavouring Agent
D. As Preservatives

2025. Which Preparation to Commonly Use in Elixirs?
A. Aromatic Elixir NF
B. Phenobarbital Elixir
C. Terpintypdrute Elixir USP
D. All Of The Above

2026. Which Type of Preparation Method Use in Non –Medicated Elixir?
A. Aromatic Elixir NF
B. Phenobarbital Elixir
C. Terpintydrute Elixir USP
D. All Of Above

2027. Which Type of Method Use In Medicated Elixir?
A. Aromatic Elixir NF
B. Phenobarbital Elixir
C. Terpintydrute Elixir USP
D. All Of Above

2028. Which Type of Method to Made Up To Codeine Elixir?
A. Phenobarbital Elixir
B. Aromatic Elixir NF
C. Terpintypdrute Elixir USP
D. All Of Above

2029. Which Type Solution Use In Spirits?
A. Hydrochloric Solutions
B. Alcoholic Solution
C. Chloroform Solution
D. All Of The Above

2030. Which Was The First Spirit Brand?
A. Brandy B. Whisky
C. Alcoho l D. All OF The Above

2031. Which Is The Type Of Generally Contain Spirits?
A. High Concentrated Of Alcohol
B. Chloroform Spirits
C. Aromatic
D. Volatile Substance

2032. Which Are Use Of Internally OF Spirits?
A. Medicinal Value B. Flavouring Agent
C. Inhalation D. None Of Above

2033. Simple Methods Of Preparation Of Spirits is ....
A. Chemical Reaction
B. Distillation
C. Simple Dissolution
D. All of the above

2034. Which Synonym of Aromatic Spirits?
A. Spirit oF Sulvolatile
B. Spirit
C. Nuthmecy Oil
D. All of the above

2035. Which Method Use in Majority of the Spirits
A. Chemical Reaction
B. Simple Dissolution
C. Sal Volatile
D. All Of The Above

2036. Which Type of Use of Aromatic Spirit of Ammonia?
A. Stimulant
B. Pharmaceutical Aid
C. Both A And B
D. None Of The Above

2037. Which Type Use of Chloroform Spirit?
A. Flavouring Agent
B. Colouring Agent
C. Both A And B
D. None of the above

2038. Which Type Use Of Industrial Methylated Spirit?
A. Solvent B. Colour
C. Flavour D. None Of the Above

2039. Which Type Solution used in Drops
A. Aqueous Solution B. None Aqueous
C. Soluble D. None of the above

2040. What is the Diameter of Drops for External Use?
A. 4mm B. 5mm
C. 3mm D. 6mm

2041. Which Type of Preparations Use In Liniment?
A. Monophasic B. Biphasic
C. Semisolid D. Solid

2042. Which Type Apply In Liniment In Our Body
A. Unbroken Skin B. Broken Skin
C. Friction D. All Of Above

2043. Which Type of Product are Liniments?
A. Soapy B. Oily
C. Tablet D. Both A&B

2044. Normally Use Of Liniments --
A. Antiseptic B. Locul Action
C. Both A And B D. None of the Above

2045. Which Use Is Camphor Liniment?
A. Counterirritant B. Antiseptic
C. Both A & B D. None of the Above

2046. What is the use of Turpentine Liniment?
A. Rubefacient B. Counterirritant
C. Both A&B D. None of the above

2047. Which Are Uses Of Soap Liniment?
A. Detergent B. Mild Local Irritant
C. Eye D. All of above

2048. Where is Lotion applied generally?
A. Skin B. Hair
C. Eye D. All of above

2049. Which Form to Use in Gargles
A. Concentrated Form
B. Non Aqueous Form
C. Aqueous
D. Non concentration

2050. What is the use of Calamine Lotion
A. Local Astringent B. Antiseptic
C. Anti sunburns D. Scabies

2051. Which Type OF Use In White Lotion (NF)
A. Psychotics B. Antiseptic
C. Local Anti Agent D. Both A & B

2052. Which Type Solution Use In Mouthwash?
A. Aqueous
B. Non Aqueous
C. Concentrated Solution
D. Both A & B

2053. Which Percentage Dissolve Boric Acid In Mouth Washes
A. 60% B. 70%
C. 80% D. 50%

2054. Which Type Compound Use In Mouth washes ?
A. Zinc Sulphate B. Zinc chloride
C. Sodium Chloride D. None Of Above

2055. Which Type Solution In Use Of Mouthwashes?
A. Alcoholic Solution B. Aqueous Solvent
C. Both A & B D. None Of The Above

2056. Which Type Use Solvent In Throat Paints ?
A. Solvent B. Viscous Solvent
C. Both A & B D. None of the above

2057. Which Are Mainly Example Of Throut Paints
A. Glycerin
B. Liquid Paraffin
C. Both A&B
D. None of the above

2058. Which Type Bassed Process On Throat Paints?
A. Glycerin
B. Liquid Paraffin
C. Both A & B
D. None of the above

2059. Which Type Solution Is Use In Eye Drops?
A. Oil Solution B. Water Solution
C. Alcohol D. Both A And B

2060. Which Type Form Is Use In Eye Drops?
A. Free Form Foreign Particles
B. Irritating Effect
C. Both A And B
D. None of the above

2061. Which One Important Property Of Eye Drops?
A. Partitioning B. Ophthalmic
C. Eye D. None Of Above

2062. What are the essential criteria for Eye Drops?
A. Isotonic With Lachrymal Secretion
B. Lachrymal With Secretion
C. Isotonic
D. Lachrymal Secretion

2063. In Which Type Substance Are Eye Drops?
A. Antimicrobial
B. Anti-Inflammatory
C. Meiotic Drugs
D. Neostigmine Sulphate

2064. In Which Percentage is Benzalkconium Chloride used In Eye Drop Preparation?
A. 0.002% B. 0.01%
C. 0.05% D. 0.1%

2065. Which Percentage Chlorohexidin Acetate Used In Eye Drop Preparation
A. 0.01% B. 0.002%
C. 0.05% D. 0.1%

2066. Which Parentage Cetrimide Preservative Used In Eye Drop Preparation?
A. 0.05% B. 0.002%
C. 0.01% D. 0.1%

2067. Which Percentage Chlorobutanol As Preservative Used In Eye Drop Preparation?
A. 0.5% B. 0.002%
C. 0.01% D. 0.1%

2068. Which Percentage Chlorocresol As Preservatives Used In Eye Drops Preparation?
A. 0.05% B. 0.002%
C. 0.01% D. 0.1%

2069. Which Percentage Methyl Hydroxy Benzoate as Preservative Used In Eye Drop preparations?

A. 0.1% B. 0.5%
C. 0.05% D. 0.002%

2070. In Which Type Use of Methyl Hydro Benzoate in Eye Drop Preparation?

A. Self – Sterilising Vehicles Preservative
C. Both A & B
D. None of the above

2071. Which Percentage of Methyl Alcohol Preservative Used In Eye Drop Preparation?

A. 0.1% B. 0.5%
C. 0.05% D. 0.002%

2072. Which Type Role Of Viscosity In Eye Drop Preparations?

A. Free From Adverse Reaction
B. Increasing Viscous
C. Both A And B
D. None Of Above

2073. What Kind Of System Is Emulsion?

A. Biphasic B. Monophasic
C. Both A & B D. Heterogeneous

2074. What Is The Name Of The Outer Phase Of Emulsion?

A. Dispersion Medium
B. External Phase
C. Continuous Phase
D. All Of Above

2075. What Kind Uses Of Emulsion?

A. Masking The Disagreeable Taste of Oil
B. Oil-In-Water Emulsion
C. Liquid Paraffin
D. Olive Oil Enhance

2076. Which Type Oral Liquid Formulation Which Whold Be Considered As An Orphrynayral Formulation?

A. Elixir B. Syrup
C. Linctuses D. Mouthwashes

2077. Which Type Of The Oral Dosage Form?

A. Tablet B. Nebulizer
C. Transdermal D. Aerosol

2078. Which Type Inhalation Use Of Dosage Form?

A. Aerosol
B. Substances Administration
C. Tablet
D. Nebulizer

2079. Which Are The Type of Parenteral Dosage Form?

A. Lotion
B. Tablet
C. Pressurized Metered
D. Transdermal Implant

2080. Which Type Of Property Measure The Resistance Of Liquid Flow

A. Viscosity B. Density
C. Volume D. Solubility

2081. Which One Name Of Embrocation In Pharmaceutical Liquid Dosage Form Studies For

A. Elixir B. Colloidions
C. Liniment D. Oleoivitanins

2082. Which Is The Indicator Used In Complex metric Titration?

A. Crystal Violet B. Brilliants Green
C. Cetechol Violet D. None Of Above

2083. Which Type Major Impurities Of Bicarbonate?

A. Alkaline Water B. Acidic Water
C. Hard Water D. None Of Above

2084. Which Type Preparations Use In Solution?

A. Simple Dissolution B. Chemical
C. Extraction D. Solubility

2085. Which Type Solution Use In Simple Dissolution?

A. Calcium Hydron
B. Adrenaline Hydraction
C. Morphin Hydrochloride
D. All Of Above

2086. Which Solution Use In Chemical Reaction?

A. Aluminium Subcetute
B. Adrinaline Hydration
C. Morphine Hydrochloride
D. All Of Above

2087. Which Solution Use In Extraction Preparation?

A. Liquid Extraction B. Tinctures
C. Solution D. All Of Above

2088. Which Type Use In Morphine Hydro Chloride Solution?

A. Antiseptic B. Source of Iodine
C. Analgesic D. Topical Antinfective

2089. Which Type Used In Weak Iodine Solution I.P?

A. Source of Iodine B. Antiseptic
C. Anti-infective D. All of above

2090. Which Type Use In Aqueous Iodine Solution IP?

A. Anti-Infective B. Source Of Iodine
C. Antiseptic D. All Of Above

2091. Which Type Use In Povidone Iodine Solution IP?

A. Topical Anti Infective
B. Antiseptic
C. Source of Iodine
D. All of above

2092. How many times Purified Water is Shaken In Aromatic Water Preparations?

A. 500 Times B. 600 Times
C. 1000 Times D. 100 Time

2093. Which Way to use Spray Solution?

A. Throat B. Nose
C. Skin D. Eye

2094. Which Principle Use In Dosage Form?

A. Predictable Therapeutic
B. Acceptability
C. Both A & B
D. None Of Above

2095. How Many Phase In Monophasic Liquid Dosage Form?

A. 1-Phase B. 2-Phase
C. Both A & B D. All Of Above

2096. The Specific H.L.B Value Of Acacia In Emulsifying Agent Is?

A. 8 B. 3.8
C. 4.7 D. 16.7

2097. The Specific H.L.B Value Of Glycerol Monostearate In Emulsifying Agent Is?

A. 3.8 B. 4.7
C. 8 D. 14.9

2098. The Specific HLB Value Of Sorbitol Monosterarte In Emulsifying Agent Is?

A. 4.7 B. 16.7
C. 14.9 D. 8

2099. The Specific HLB Value of Polysorbate 20 In Emulsifying Agent Is?

A. 4.7 B. 14.9
C. 16.7 D. 8

2100. The Specific HLB Value of Polysorbate 60 In Emulsifying Agent Is?

A. 4.7 B. 14.9
C. 16.7 D. 8

2101. Specific HLB Value of Polysorbate 80 In Emulsifying Agent Is?

A. 8 B. 15.0
C. 16.7 D. 14.9

2102. Specific HLB Value of Sodium Lauryl Sulphate In Emulsifying Egent Is?

A. 8 B. 40.0
C. 16.7 D. 14.9

2103. Specific HLB Value of Sodium Oleate as Emulsifying Agent Is?

A. 40.0 B. 18.0
C. 8 D. 16.7

2104. Specific HLB Value of Tragacanth as Emulsifying Agent Is?

A. 40.2 B. 16.7
C. 13.2 D. 18.0

2105. Specific HLB Value of Triethanolmine Oleate In Emulsifying Agent Is?

A. 12.0 B. 18.0
C. 16.7 D. 32.2

2106. What Is The Noyes-Whitney Equation?

A. dc/dt=kS(Cs-Ct)
B. dc/dt=(Cs-Ct)
C. dc/dt
D. dc/dt=kS

2107. The Specific and one of Main Advantage of Powders?

A. Powders Are one of the Oldest Dosage Form and are used Both Internally and Externally
B. The Dispensing of Powder is a Time Consuming
C. Both A and B
D. All of above

2108. The Specific and one of Main Disadvantage of Powders?

A. The Dispensing of Powder Is A Time Consuming
B. Powders are one of the Oldest Dosage Form and are used both Internally and Externally
C. Both a and b
D. All of above

2109. Cut the required number of Powder Papers In Suatable Size Is

A. 100×100 B. 150×150
C. 120×100 D. 120×120

2110. Translate The Following Letin Term Liquor Into English?

A. A Solution B. A Capsule
C. A Powder D. A Mouth Wash

2111. Translate The Following Latin Term Charta Into English?

A. A Powder B. A Solution
C. A Mouthwash D. A Cream

2112. Trnaslate the following Letin Term Nebula into English?

A. A Paste B. A Spray Solution
C. Nasal Drops D. A Pill

2113. Trnaslate the Following Letin Term Pilula into English?

A. A Pill B. A Spray
C. A Tablet D. A Paste

2114. Translate the following Latin Term Tabella into English?

A. A Tablet B. A Pill
C. A Solution D. A Lotion

2115. Translate the following Letin Term Addendus into English?

A. To be added B. To be applied
C. To be Taken D. To be given

2116. Translate The Following Letin Term Pasta Into English?

A. A Paste B. A Pill
C. A Lotion D. A Solution

2117. Translate The Following Letin Term Signa Into English?

A. Label B. To be taken
C. To be given D. To be used

2118. Translate The Following Letin Term Dandus Into English?

A. To be added B. To be given
C. To be mixed D. Let apply

2119. Translate the following Letin Term Applicat into English?

A. Let Apply B. To be apply
C. To be taken D. To be used

2120. Translate the Following Letin Term Anti Cibos into English?

A. After Meal B. Before Meal
C. Between Meal D. As Directed

2121. Translate the Following Letin Term Post Cibos Into English?

A. Before Meal B. After Meal
C. As Directed D. Between Meal

2122. Translate the following Letin Term Inter Cibos into English?

A. After Meal B. Before Meal
C. Between Meal D. As Directed

2123. Translate the following Letin Term Lente into English?

A. Slowly B. At Night
C. Every Night D. At Morning

2124. Translate The Following Letin Term Statim into English?

A. Slowly B. Immediately
C. Every Night D. At Night

2125. Translate the following Letin Term Sextis Horis into English?

A. Every Night B. Immediately
C. Every Six Hours D. Every Two Hours

2126. Translate the Following Letin Term Omni Hora into English?

A. Every Hour
B. Every Two Hours
C. Every Three Hours
D. Every Four Hours

2127. Trnaslate the following Letin Term Omni Quatra Hora into English?
A. Every Hour
B. Every Two Hours
C. Every Three Hours
D. Every Fourth Hours

2128. Trnaslate The Following Letin Term Singulis Horis Into English?
A. Every Hour
B. Every Two Hours
C. Every Three Hours
D. Every Four Hours

2129. Translate the following Letin Term Alternis Horis into English?
A. Every hour B. Every two hours
C. Every three hours
D. Every four hours

2130. Translate the following Letin Term Tertis Horis into English?
A. Every hour
B. Every two hours
C. Every three hours
D. Every four hours

2131. Translate the Following Letin Term Quartis Horis into English?
A. Every hour
B. Every two hours
C. Every three hours
D. Every four hours

2132. Translate The Following Letin Term Omni Mane Into English?
A. Every morning B. Every night
C. At night D. Break fast

2133. Translate The Following Letin Term Omni Nocta into English?
A. Every morning B. Every night
C. At night D. Break fast

2134. Translate The Following Letin Term Nocte Into English?
A. Every morning B. Every night
C. At night D. Break fast

2135. Translate the following Letin Term Jentaculum into English?
A. Every morning B. Every night
C. At night D. Break fast

2136. Translate The Following Letin Term Auris Dexter Into English?
A. To right ear B. To left ear
C. To the body D. To the throat

2137. Translate The Following Letin Term Auris Laevus into English?
A. To right ear B. To left ear
C. To the body D. To the throat

2138. Translate the following Letin Term Brachis into English?
A. To right ear B. To left ear
C. To the body D. To the throat

2139. Translate the following Letin Term Jugulo into English?
A. To right ear B. To left ear
C. To the body D. To the throat

2140. The specific formula of density?
A. Density = weight/volume
B. Weight = density ×volume
C. Volume = weight/density
D. All of above

2141. Specific percentage of alcohol use in dilute alcohol is?
A. 80% B. 90%
C. 95% D. 50%

2142. Calculate the volume of 2 kg of glycerin the density of glycerin is 1.25g/ml
A. 1600ml B. 1700ml
C. 1500ml D. 1650ml

2143. Calculate the weight of 250 ml of alcohol whose density is 0.816 g/m
A. 204.0 g B. 270.0g
C. 250.0g D. 200.0g

2144. Calculate the weight of 150 ml of sulphuric acid whose density is 1.8 g/m
A. 270.0 g B. 204.0g
C. 200.0g D. 250g

2145. Calculate the weight of 1.5 litre of fixed oil whose density is 0.9624 g/ml
A. 1443.6g B. 1650.4g
C. 1555.6g D. 1750.5g

2146. Calculate the amount of 95 per cent alcohol required to prepare 400 ml of 45 cent alcohol

A. 190 ml B. 200ml
C. 180ml D. 300ml

2147. Calculate the volume of 95 per cent alcohol required to prepare 600 ml of 60 per cent alcohol

A. 442.10 ml B. 379 ml
C. 190 ml D. 200 ml

2148. Calculate the volume of 95 per cent alcohol required to prepare 600 ml of 70 per cent alcohol (using alligation mathod)

A. 442.10 ml B. 379 ml
C. 190 ml D. 200 ml

2149. Calculate the real strength of 30° o.p. and 40°u.p.

A. 34.23% v/v B. 66.53° o.p.
C. 1.753 D. 22.71° o.p.

2150. How many proof gallons are contained in 5 gallon of 70% v/v alcohol?

A. 6.135 gallons of proof spirit
B. 7.135 gallons of proof spirit
C. 8.135 gallons of proof spirit
D. 4.444 gallons of proof spirit

2151. Calculate the meq wt of calcium (ca++) given gram-atomic wt of calcium = 40.08

A. 20.04 mg B. 30.04 mg
C. 40.04 mg D. 50.04 mg

2152. Calculate meq of na+ and cl^- in solution that contains 409.5 mg of nacl/100 ml

A. 7 mEq B. 8 mEq
C. 9 mEq D. 5 mEq

2153. Express 0.9% Sodium Chloride can be expressed in terms of milliequivalent per litre

A. 154 mEq/Litre B. 155 mEq/Litre
C. 152 mEq/Litre D. 160 mEq/Litre

2154. Mouthwash are generally use-

A. Buccal Cavity B. Anti Bactirial agent
C. Both A & B D. All of above

2155. Calculate the number of grains required to make 8 oz of a 4 per cent solution and label with direction for preparing a quart of a 1 in 2000 solution?

A. 80 Times B. 50 Times
C. 90 Times C. 40 Times

2156. Calculate the Quantity of Sodium Chloride required preparing 400ml of a 0.9% solution?

A. 3.6g B. 4.6g
C. 7.7g D. 5g

2157. Prepare 400ml Of a 5 Per Cent Solution and Label with A Direction for preparing 2 litre

A. 20 ml B. 100ml
C. 30ml D. 90 ml

2158. Prepare 500 ml of a 1 In 4000 solution from the 1 in 800 solution

A. 100 ml B. 20 ml
C. 30ml D. 90 ml

2159. How much of a 5 Percent will be required to prepare 600 ml of a 1 In 800 Solution

A. 15 ml B. 20 ml
C. 30 ml D. 100 ml

2160. What will be the dose for a child of 5 years if the adult dose of a drug is 400 mg?

A. 117 mg B. 13.3 mg
C. 80 mg D. 33 mg

2161. What is the dose for an 8 month old infant if the if the average adult dose of a drug is 250 mg

A. 117 mg B. 13.3 mg
C. 80 mg D. 33 mg

2162. Calculate the dose for a (i)9 months old infant;(ii)a child of 5 year age; and (iii)a boy of 16 years age when the adult dose of a drug is 100 mg

A. 117 mg B. 13.3 mg
C. 80 mg D. 33 mg

2163. Calculate the dose for a child that has a body surface area of 0.57 m2, when the adult dose of a drug is 100 mg

A. 117 mg B. 13.3 mg
C. 80 mg D. 33 mg

2164. Convert 120° f into °C

A. 48.9°c B. 86°c
C. 23°c D. 88°c

2165. Convert 30°C into °f

A. 86°f B. 87°f
C. 90°f D. 50°f

2166. Write the formula of calculate the amount of theobroma oil present in medicated suppositories

A. 10/100×b=c gramme
B. 60/100×b=c gramme
C. 20/100×b=c gramme
D. 50/100×b=c gramme

2167. write the formula of calculate the amount of medicament present in medicated suppositories

A. 40/100×b=d gramme
B. 10/100×b=d gramme
C. 50/100×b=d gramme
D. 100/100×b=d gramme

2168. Write the formula of displacement value of medicament

A. D/(a-c)
B. A/(b-c)
C. Dy/(d-x)
D. A/(d-c)

2169. Chose the following formula of benzene?

A. C_6H_6
B. C_6H_5COOH
C. $C_6H_5CH_2OH$
D. C_6H_5OH

2170. Chose the following formula of benzoic acid?

A. C_6H_6
B. C_6H_5COOH
C. $C_6H_5CH_2OH$
D. C6H5OH

2171. Chose the following formula of benzyl alcohol?

A. C_6H_6
B. C_6H_5COOH
C. $C_6H_5CH_2OH$
D. C_6H_5OH

2172. Chose the following formula of phenol?

A. C_6H_6
B. C_6H_5COOH
C. $C_6H_5CH_2OH$
D. C_6H_5OH

2173. Chose the following formula of pyrocatechol?

A. $C_6H_4(OH)_2$
B. $C_6\ H_3(OH)_3$
C. CCL_4
D. $CHCL_3$

2174. Chose the following formula of pyrogallol?

A. $C_6H_4(OH)_2$
B. $C_6\ H_3(OH)_3$
C. CCL_4
D. $CHCL_3$

2175. Chose the following formula of Carbon Tetra Chloride?

A. $C_6H_4(OH)_2$
B. $C_6\ H_3(OH)_3$
C. CCL_4
D. $CHCL_3$

2176. Chose the following formula of chloroform?

A. $C_6H_4(OH)_2$
B. $C_6\ H_3(OH)_3$
C. CCL_4
D. $C_6H_4(OH)_2$

2177. Chose the following formula of methylene chloride?

A. $C_6H_4(OH)_2$
B. CH_2Cl_2
C. CCL_4
D. $C_6H_4(OH)_2$

2178. Write the cation exchange method?

A. H-resin+m++x-+h2o→m-resin+h++x-+h2o
B. M-resin+h++x-+h2o
C. Resin-nh2+h++x-+h2o→resin-nh2.hx+h2o
D. H-resin+m++x-+h2o

2179. Write the anion exchange method?

A. H-resin+m++x-+h2o →m-resin+h++x-+h2o
B. M-resin+h++x-+h2o
C. Resin-nh2+h++x-+h2o→resin-nh2.hx+h2o
D. H-resin+m++x-+h2o

2180. Which type vehicle is used in medicated syrups?

A. Non medicated vehicle
B. Flavoured vehicle
C. Both a and b
D. None of above

2181. Which type medium is Cherry syrup?

A. Acid medium
B. Base medium
C. Both a and b
D. None of the above

2182. Which type cocoa syrup use as --

A. Administering bitter tasting drugs to children
B. Administering bitter tasting drugs to adult
C. Administering bitter tasting drugs to old person
D. All of above

2183. In simple syrup preparations which present use sucrose-

A. 90%
B. 95%
C. 80%
D. 85%

2184. Chose the right stokes equation?

A. Dx/dt=d2(pi-pe)g/18n
B. Dx/dt=d(pi-pe)/18n
C. Dx/dt=d(pe)g/18n
D. Dx/dt=d(pi-pe)g/18

2185. Write the Young's formula use in doses proportionate method

A. (age in years)/(age in years+12)×adult dose

B. (age in years)/(age in years)×adult dose

C. (age in years)/12×adult dose

D. (age in years)/20×adult dose

2186. Write the Dilling's formula use in doses proportionate method

A. (age in years)/(age in years+12)×adult dose

B. (age in years)/(age in years)×adult dose

C. (age in years)/12×adult dose

D. (age in years)/20×adult dose

2187. Write the Clark's formula use in doses proportionate to body weight?

A. =(childof weight in kg)/70×adult dose

B. =(surface area of child)/(surface area of adult)

C. =(childof weight in kg)/70

D. =(surface area of child)/(surface area of adult)×100

2188. Write The Formula Use In Doses Proportionate To Surface Area?

A. =(Child Of Weight In Kg)/70×Adult Dose

B. =(Surface Area Of Child)/(Surface Area Of Adult)

C. =(Child Of Weight In Kg)/70

D. =(Surface Area Of Child)/(Surface Area Of Adult)×100

2189. Which Type Preparations Is Liniments?

A. Solid Preparations

B. Liquid Preparations

C. Semi Solid Preparations

D. Gaseous Preparations

2190. Which Chemical Stabilizer Is Used In Liniments ?

A. Glycerin B. Sorbitol

C. Both A And B D. All Of Above

2191. Which Flavouring Agent Is Used In Liniment?

A. Tinctures B. Fruit Juices

C. Essence D. Syrup

2192. Chose The Example Of Monophasic Liquid Dosage Form Meant For Internal Use

A. Syrup B. Lotion

C. Liniment D. MouthWash

2193. Chose The Example Of Monophasic Liquid Dosage Form Meant For External Use

A. Lotion B. Syrup

C. Mixture D. Elixir

2194. Define The Monophasic Liquid Dosage Form In One Word?

A. One Phase Preparations

B. Biphasic Preparations

C. Three Phase Preparation

D. All Of Above

2195. What Dose The Term Mixture Mean?

A. Combination Of Two Substanc

B. Mixing Substance

C. Both A And B

D. All Of Above

2196. The Specific pH Of Nasal Spray Is?

A. 4.5-6.5 B. 6.5-7.0

C. 0.025-0.015 D. 3.0

2197. The Specific pH Of Syrup Is?

A. 4.5-6.5 B. 6.5-7.0

C. 0.025-0.015 D. 3.0

2198. The Specific pH Of Mixture is?

A. 4.5-6.5 B. 6.5-7.0

C. 0.025-0.015 D. 3.0

2199. The Specific pH Of Liniments is?

A. 4.5-6.5 B. 6.5-7.0

C. 0.025-0.015 D. 3.0

2200. The Specific pH Of Lotion is?

A. 4.5-6.5 B. 6.7-7.4

C. 2.89-7.83 D. 2.0

2201. The Specific pH Of Mouthwash is?

A. 4.5-6.5 B. 6.7-7.4

C. 2.89-7.83 D. 2.89-7.83

2202. The Specific pH Of Ear Drops is?

A. 4.5-6.5 B. 6.7-7.4

C. 2.89-7.83 D. 2.0

2203. The Specific pH Of Nasal Drop is ?

A. 4.5-6.5 B. 6.7-7.4

C. 2.89-7.83 D. 2.0

2204. The Specific Boiling Point Of Syrup is?
A. 78.3°C B. 100°C
C. 99.61°C D. 103.8°

2205. The Specific Boiling Point Of Mixture is ?
A. 78.3°C B. 100°C
C. 99.61°C D. 103.8°C

2206. The Specific Boiling Point Of Linctuses is?
A. 78.3°C B. 100°C
C. 99.61°C D. 103.8°C

2207. The Specific Boiling Point Of Liniment is?
A. 78.3°C B. 100°C
C. 99.61°C D. 103.8°C

2208. The Specific Boiling Point Of Gargles is ?
A. 100°C B. 78.3°C
C. 103.8°C D. 99.61°C

2209. The Specific Boiling Point Of Throat Paint Is ?
A. 103.8°C B. 10.4°C
C. 99.61°C D. 100°C

2210. The Storage Condition Of Mixtures is?
A. Dispensed In Plain Glass Bottle
B. Dispensed In Normal Paper
C. Dispensed In Plastic Containe
D. All Of Above

2211. The Storage Condition Of Elixirs is?
A. Air Tight Glass Bottle Having Screw Caps
B. Dispensed In Plain Glass Bottle
C. Dispensed In Plastic Container
D Dispensed In Normal Paper

2212. The Storage Condition Of Liniments is?
A. Air Tight Containers
B. Dispensed In Plain Glass Bottle
C. Dispensed In Plastic Container
D. Dispensed In Normal Paper

2213. The Storage Condition of Lotion?
A. Air Tight Containers
B. Dispensed In Plain Glass Bottle
C. Dispensed In Plastic Container
D. Dispensed In Normal Paper

2214. The Storage Condition Of Throat Paints?
A. Air Tight Containers In Cool Place
B. Dispensed In Plain Glass Bottle
C. Dispensed In Plastic Container
D. Dispensed In Normal Paper

2215. The Storage Condition Of Douches is?
A. In A Cool Place
B. Dispensed In Plain Glass Bottle
C. Dispensed In Plastic Container
D. Dispensed In Normal Paper

2216. The Storage Condition Of Ear Drops is?
A. Well-Filled And Air Tight Containers
B. Dispensed In Plain Glass Bottle
C. Dispensed In Plastic Container
D. Dispensed In Normal Paper

2217. Chose The Following Main Aim Of Nasal Spray
A. Reduce Nasal Congestion
B. Treat Infections
C. Both A And B
D. All Of The Above

2218. Chose The Following The Uses Of Douches
A. As Preservatives
B. Vaginal Solution
C. As Chemical Stabilizer
D. All Of Above

2219. Chose The Following The difference Between Lotion And Liniment
A. Lotion-External Application Without Friction Liniment-External Application With Friction
B. Lotion-External Application With Friction Liniment-External Application Without Friction
C. Both A And B
D. All Of Above

2220. Chose The Following Main Aim Of Syrup?
A. As Flavoured Substances
B. As Preservative
C. As Chemical Stabilizer
D. All Of Above

2221. Chose The Following Main Aim Of Mixture
A. Acute Condition Use
B. As Chemical Stabilizer
C. As Flavoured Substances
D. As Preservative

2222. Chose The Following Main Aim Of Elixir?
A. Antibiotic
B. Antihistamines
C. Sedative
D. All Of Above

2223. Chose The Following Main Aim Of Linctuses?
A. Expectorant Action
B. Sedative
C. Antibiotic
D. Antihistamines

2224. Chose The Following Main Aim Of Liniment?
A. Expectorant Action
B. Penetration Medicament
C. Antibiotic
D. Antihistamine

2225. Chose The Following Main Aim Of Gargles?
A. Antihistamine
B. Expectorant Action
C. Treat Throat Infection
D. Antibiotic

2226. Chose The Following Main Aim Of Mouth Wash?
A. The Buccal Cavity
B. Expectorant Action
C. Treat Throat Infection
D. Antibiotic

2227. Chose The Following Main Aim Of Throat Paint?
A. The Buccal Cavity
B. Expectorant Action
C. Treat Throat Infection
D. Antibiotic

2228. Chose The Following Main Aim Of Douche?
A. The Buccal Cavity
B. Expectorant Action
C. Treat Throat Infection
D. Vaginal Solution

2229. Chose The Following Main Aim Of Nasal Drops ?
A. The Buccal Cavity
B. Expectorant Action
C. Cause Lipoid Pneumonia
D. Vaginal Solution

2230. Chose The Following Main Aim Of Nasal Spray?
A. Retain The Nasal Solution In The Droplet Form In The Nasal Tract
B. Expectorant Action
C. Cause Lipoid Pneumonia
D. Vaginal Solution

2231. Chose The Following The Uses Of Mixture?
A. Indigestion, Diarrhoea
B. Expectorant Action
C. Cause Lipoid Pneumonia
D. Vaginal Solution

2232. Chose The Following The Uses Of Syrup?
A. Sweet Viscous Preparations
B. Expectorant Action
C. Cause Lipoid Pneumonia
D. Vaginal Solution

2233. Chose The Following The Uses Of Elixer ?
A. Antibiotics
B. Expectorant Action
C. Cause Lipoid Pneumonia
D. Vaginal Solution

2234. Chose The Following The Uses Of Linctuses?
A. Expectorant Action
B. Antibiotics
C. Cause Lipoid Pneumonia
D. Vaginal Solution

2235. Chose The Following The Uses Of Liniment ?
A. Expectorant Action
B. Antibiotics
C. Penetratipon Of Medicament
D. Vaginal Solution

2236. Sodium Sulfite is an effective antimicrobial preservative, against fungi at a concentration of ....
A. 0.1% w/v
B. 0.3% w/v
C. 0.5% w/v
D. 0.7% w/v

2237. Saponification value of Stearic Acid is ....
A. 220–240
B. 180–200
C. 250–270
D. 200–220

2238. Empirical Formula of Triethanolamine is ....
A. $C_6H_{15}NO_3$
B. $C_{12}H_{20}O_7$
C. $C_{57}H_{104}O_6$
D. $C_{20}H_{40}O_4$

2239. In I.P. 2018, the pyrogen test has been replaced by.................................. test

A. bacterial exotoxin
B. bacterial count
C. bacterial endotoxin
D. bacterial inhibition

2240. The International Pharmacopoeia is published by the ....

A. Royal Pharmaceutical Society of Great Britain
B. World Health Organization
C. American Pharmaceutical Association
D. Council of the Pharmaceutical Society

2241. The United States Pharmacopoeia was originally published in the year.......................

A. 1888 B. 1907
C. 1864 D. 1820

2242. The first National Formulary (NF) was published in ....

A. 1860 B. 1888
C. 1905 D. 1864

2243. .... is a reference book for the use of medical practitioners and dispensing pharmacists of Britain.

A. British Pharmacopoeial Codex
B. National Formulary
C. British Pharmaceutical Codex
D. British Pharmacopoeia

2244. The Merk index is .... Compendia.

A. Non-Official B. Medical
C. Private D. Official

2245. The first edition of the Merck's Index was published in the year ....

A. 1898 B. 1899
C. 1889 D. 1890

2246. DailyMed is an online information resource that contains more than .... drug listings.

A. 42,000 B. 92,000
C. 82,000 D. 102,000

2247. ....contains information on prescription and over-the-counter medications written in English language.

A. DailyMed
B. Drug Enforcement Administration
C. Centers for Disease Control and Prevention
D. Medline Plus

2248. The Centers for Disease Control and Prevention is the online resource for ....information.

A. prescriptions B. vaccine
C. package inserts D. regulations

2249. The ....website can provide updates on new medication approvals and drug recalls.

A. Daily Med
B. Drug Enforcement Administration
C. FDA
D. MedlinePlus

2250. ....contains full-text versions of medical and pharmacy texts.

A. STAT!Ref
B. Access Pharmacy
C. Lexicomp
D. Micromedex

2251. .... is an online database providing drug information with over 1700 drug monographs.

A. DailyMed
B. Access Pharmacy
C. Lexicomp
D. Medline Plus

2252. ......is a tertiary resource designed to provide information to the health care professional about clinical inquires.

A. Access Pharmacy B. Daily Med
C. Micromed D. Lexicomp

2253. Which of the following websites is a portal for international clinical trials?

A. www.clinicalevidence.com
B. apps.who.int/trialsearch/
C. www.clinicaltrials.gov
D. www.controlled-trials.com

2254. Which website will provide the best resource to find clinical trials in a particular disease in United States?

A. www.clinicaltrials.gov
B. WebMD
C. www.fda.gov
D. www.controlled-trials.com

2255. ....offers the best choice to look for the most recent studies and publications.

A. Up To Date. B. Google.
C. www.fda.gov D. PubMed

2256. ....gives an inclusive record of national and even some local clinical procedure.

A. Google
B. WebMD
C. www.guideline.gov
D. www.controlled-trials.com.

2257. In ....more than 28,000 givers write systematic reviews committed to compile up-to-date, accurate in order about the effects of health care.

A. U.S. Food and Drug Administration (FDA)
B. Cochrane Library
C. Clinical Evidence
D. PubMed

2258. ....associates to 1500 organizations to search for health information for a patient.

A. Healthfinder B. Mayo Clinic
C. DailyMed D. WebMD

2259. .... contains more than 150,000 records on herbals.

A. Mantis B. Arrcbase
C. Napralert D. TCMLARS

2260. More than 760,000 citations about Dietary supplements are available in ....

A. Extract Databas
B. IBIDS
C. Mantis
D. Wanfang Database

2261. Which of the following is an easily searched database for both generic and brand name of drugs?

A. MEDLINEPlus
B. DailyMed
C. Drugs A to Z
D. NetWellness

2262. Journal publications on drug-related subjects, reports of clinical drug trials, case reports, and pharmacological research are ....sources of drug information

A. Primary B. Tertiary
C. Secondary D. Accessory

2263. Review articles, meta-analyses, indexes, abstracts and combinations of abstracts and full-text reprints consists of ....sources of drug information.

A. Primary B. Tertiary
C. Secondary D. Accessory

2264. Drug information provided by manufacturers is..................................... information.

A. Primary or Secondary
B. Secondary or Tertiary
C. Primary or Tertiary
D. Secondary or Accessory

2265. Formulary manuals, standard treatment manuals, textbooks, general reference books, drug bulletins, and drug compendia are examples of.................... source of information.

A. Secondary B. Tertiary
C. Accessory D. Primary

2266. A Drug has a minimum of .... different names.

A. 03 B. 02
C. 04 D. 05

2267. A chemical name is given to the drug in harmony with regulations of chemical taxonomy established by.............................

A. IUCAC B. IUPEC
C. IUPAK D. IUPAC

2268. IUPAC stands for....................................

A. International Union of Pure with Applied Chemistry
B. International Uniform of Pure and Applied Chemistry
C. International Union of Pure and Applied Chemistry
D. Intercountry Union of Pure and Applied Chemistry

2269. .... is a short name given to a drug which is not subjected to proprietary rights.

A. Non-Proprietary Name
B. Brand Name
C. Proprietary Name
D. IUPAC Name

2270. The other term used to designate Non-Proprietary Name of drugs is.....................

A. Brand Name B. Generic Name
C. Common Name D. Chemical Name

2271. ....assigns International Non-proprietary Names (INN) to pharmaceutical substances.

A. IUPAC B. WHO
C. ICH D. USP

2272. Which Pharmacopoeia has been recognized by The Federal Food, Drug and Cosmetic (FDC) Act?

A. United States Pharmacopoeia / National Formulary (USP/NF)
B. British Pharmacopoeia (BP)
C. European Pharmacopoeia
D. All of them

2273. Which of the following is actually a drug compendium (list of items)

A. International Pharmacopoeia
B. City pharmacopoeia
C. PharmacopoieaAmstelredamensis
D. Martindale: The Extra Pharmacopoeia

2274. Formularies are the books containing ....

A. Lists of drugs approved for use by a particular hospital, health plan or government
B. Information for the preparation of drugs
C. Lists of drugs approved by the US Food and Drug Administration (FDA)
D. Information about the therapeutic uses of drugs.

2275. Health finder associates to .... organizations to search for health information for a patient.

A. 1500 B. 400
C. 1200 D. 1260

2276. The word viscosity was suggested by Bingham and Crawford

A. Hazard and Mic
B. Cristiano and leo
C. Einstein and Newton

2277. Rheology is used to describe

A. Flow of liquids and the deformation of solid
B. Study of crystal
C. Flow of semisolid
D. Formation of solid

2278. Which property measures the resistance of a liquid to flow?

A. Density B. Viscosity
C. Volume D. Solubility

2279. Fluidity is defined as

A. Directly proportional to viscosity
B. Inversly proportional to viscosity
C. Square of viscosity
D. Two times of viscosity

2280. The unit of viscosity is ?

A. Dynes B. Poise
C. Cm/sec D. m/sec

2281. Which one is not in the class of Non-newtonian flow system ?

A. Plastic B. Pseudo plastic
C. Dilatant D. Polythene

2282. Viscosity of castor oil at 20 °C?

A. 2000 B. 1000
C. 50 D. 5000

2283. Viscosity of Chloroform at 20 °C?

A. 0.563 B. 0.666
C. 0.452 D. 0.545

2284. Viscosity of ethyl alcohol at 20 °C ?

A. 1.19 B. 1.11
C. 1.2 D. 2

2285. Viscosity of glycerin at 20 °C?

A. 200 B. 100
C. 400 D. 500

2286. Viscosity of olive oil at 20 °C?

A. 100 B. 300
C. 460 D. 400

2287. Viscosity of water at 20 °C?
A. 1.0019 B. 1.212
C. 1.6001 D. 1.464

2288. Viscosity of a gas increases with
A. Increase in temperature
B. Decreases in temperature
C. At constant Temperature
D. None of them

2289. In Newtonian Law of flow
A. Shear stress is directly proportional to rate of shear
B. Shear stress is inversly proportional to rate of shear
C. A & B both
D. None of them

2290. Which equation represent plastic flow?
A. U= (F-f)/G B. U=(F-G)/f
C. BOTH A&B D. None of the

2291. The material which follows plastic flaw also known as
A. Bingham bodies B. Pseudo bodies
C. Dilatant bodies D. None of them

2292. Type of flow in which viscosity increases when the substance agitated is
A. Plastic B. Pseudoplastic
C. Dilatant D. Thixotropy

2293. Non-Newtonian flow can be described by using
A. None of them Shear viscosity
B. Apparent viscosity
C. True viscosity
D. None of them

2294. Dilatant material are often termed as
A. Shear thickening system
B. Shear thinning system
C. Shearing system

2295. Which substance follows Non-Newtonian flow
A. Water B. Glycerin
C. Solution of syrup D. Emulsion

2296. Which of the following substance consider as Newtonian fluid in molten state but at room temperature consider as Non-newtonian fluid
A. Vaseline B. Glycerin
C. Colloidal solution D. None of them

2297. Which of the following is time dependent
A. Plastic flow B. Pseudoplastic flow
C. Dilatant flow D. Thixotropy

2298. Which of the following is time independent
A. Thixotropy B. Rheopexy
C. Plastic flow D. None of them

2299. Which of the following curve does not pass through origin
A. Plastic flow
B. Pseudoplastic flow
C. Dilatant flow
D. Thixotropy

2300. Which of the following are also known as shear thinning material
A. Plastic flow B. Pseudoplastic flow
C. Dilatant flow D. Thixotropy

2301. Pseudoplastic flow is characterized as a reverse phenomenon of
A. Dilatant flow B. Plastic flow
C. Newtonian flow D. None of these

2302. Viscometer is used to determine
A. Viscosity B. Surface tension
C. Both D. None of them

2303. Which of the following is single point viscometer?
A. Cup and bob
B. Cone and plate
C. Ostwald viscometer
D. None of them

2304. Which of the following is multi point viscometer?
A. Ostwald viscometer
B. Ostwald viscometer
C. Cup and bob
D. None of them

2305. Which of the following viscometer is used for non-newtonian fluids?
A. Ostwald viscometer
B. Falling sphere viscometer
C. Cup and bob
D. Capillary viscometer

2306. Applications of viscosity ?
A. Manufacturing of dosage forms
B. Identification of disease
C. Standards of liquids
D. All of them

2307. Which of the following is intrinsic factor?
A. Chemical nature B. Shape
C. Size D. All of them

2308. Thixotropic behavior exhibited by
A. Plastic system
B. Pseudoplastic system
C. Dilatansystem
D. A & B both

2309. In thixotropy, time takes to recover after agitation when compare to time taken for agitation
A. longer time B. Takes shorter time
C. Takes same time D. Takes double time

2310. Semi-solids obey which type of flow?
A. Newtonian flow B. Non-newtonian flow
C. A&B both D. None of them

2311. Which of the following is extrinsic factors?
A. Shape B. Molecular size
C. Molecular weight D. Pressure

2312. Deflocculated particles exhibit the flow of a type
A. Newtonian B. Dilatant
C. Plastic D. Pseudoplastic

2313. Capillary viscometer also known as
A. Ostwald viscometer
B. Falling sphere
C. Cup and bob
D. Cone and plate

2314. Disadvantage of cup & bob viscometer is
A. Application to less viscous
B. Plug flow
C. Large volume required
D. None of them

2315. Which of the following is not the advantage of cone & plate viscometer
A. The required volume is small (0.1 to 0.2 ml)
B. The cleaning and filling is easy
C. Less time required for temperature equilibrium
D. Study of flow of liquids through capillary tube

2316. Capillary tube
A. Plug flow can be minimized by
B. Increase the size of bob
C. Increase the speed of rotation of bob
D. Both
E. None of them

2317. Which of the following viscometer is rotational viscometer
A. Brookfield viscometer
B. Cup & bob
C. A & b both
D. Ostwald viscometer

2318. In which type of flow deflocculated suspension with high concentration of dispersed solid exhibits
A. Dilatant B. Newtonian
C. Plastic D. Pseudoplastic

2319. ______________ is a phenomenon in which a sol transform to a gel state more readily rather than keeping a sol at rest
A. Thixotropy B. Negative thixotropy
C. Rheopexy D. None of them

2320. _________ is defined as an isothermal & comparatively slow recovery on standing of a material of a consistency lost through shearing
A. Thixotrop B. Negative thixotropy
C. Rheopexy D. None of them

2321. The plastic flow behaviour can be explained by
A. Apparent viscometer
B. Area of hysteresis loop
C. Hysteresis loop
D. Yield value

2322. The behaviour of pseudoplastic can be explained by
A. Apparent viscosity
B. Area of hysteresis loop
C. Hystetresis loop
D. Yield value

2323. In which system that undergoes gel to sol transformation is known as
A. Elastic B. Deformation
C. Shear thickening D. Shear thinning

2324. At rest the thixotropy behavior of pseudoplastic system exhibit in
A. Gel B. Sol
C. Wax D. Lotion

2325. In which term viscosity is expressed ?
A. Drug stability B. Rheology
C. Drug solubility D. Drug diffusion

2326. On shaking magnesia magma transform state from sol to
A. Sol B. Gel
C. Paste D. Lotion

2327. The principle involved in falling sphere viscometer is based on
A. Hoeppler viscometer
B. Macmichael viscometer
C. Stormer viscometer
D. A&B both

2328. S.I. unit of kinematic viscosity is expressed as
A. M2/s B. m/s
C. cm/s D. cm2/s

2329. Newtons equation for the flow of a liquid is
A. F=mG B. F=nG
C. G=nF D. None of them

2330. Example of brook-field viscometer is
A. Cone and plate B. Extrusion
C. Rotating sphere D. Rotating spindle

2331. Which of the following viscometer is not used as multiple-point viscometer?
A. Cube& bob B. Cone& plate
C. Redwood D. Brookfield

2332. Which of the following viscometer is not used as single-point viscometer?
A. Ostwald B. Falling sphere
C. Redwood D. Brookfield

2333. One 134entipoises is equal to
A. 0.001 poise B. 0.1 poise
C. 0.01 poise D. 1 poise

2334. Unit of kinematic viscosity is
A. Poise B. Stokes
C. Dyne D. Centipoise

2335. A plastic material was found to have yield value of 5000 dynes/cm2 At shearing stresses above the yield value F was found to increases linearity with G, If the rate of shear was 150 sec when F was 7800 dynes/cm2, calculate U the plastic viscosity of the sample
A. 18.67 poise B. 18.67 stokes
C. 20.54 poise D. 22.3 poise

2336. The greater the thixotropy the ____________ is physical stability of suspension
A. Lower B. Equal
C. Higher D. None of them

2337. In plastic flow, more the flocculated suspension, the ____________ will be yield value
A. Lower B. Equal
C. Higher D. None of them

2338. In plastic flow, more the flocculated the suspension the higher will be the
A. Yield value
B. Apparent viscosity
C. Hysteresis loop
D. Area of hysteresis loop

2339. Yield value indicates the
A. Degree of flocculation
B. Force of deflocculation
C. Force of flocculation
D. Degree of deflocculation

2340. In which of the following is not having importance of rheology in pharmacy
A. Emulsion B. Tablet coating
C. Powder D. Pastes

2341. Absolute viscosity divided by the density of liquid at specific temperature is known assess.
A. Kinematic viscosity
B. Thixotropy
C. Viscoelasticity
D. Psychorheology

2342. In pseudoplastic substance, the viscosity is decrease with increase in _______
A. Rate of shear B. Rate of stress
C. Force D. Shearing stress

2343. Dilatant type of flow is inverse of
A. Plastic B. Pseudoplastic
C. Thixotropy D. Negative thixotropy

2344. The shear stress is increased, the bulk of system expands or dilates is termed as
A .Plastic B. Expandable
C. Dilatant D. Pseudoplastic

2345. Which of the following graph shows Newtonian flow

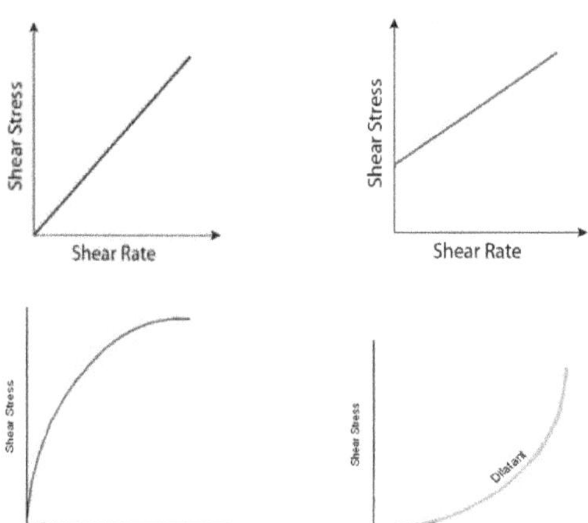

2346. Which of the following graph shows plastic flow

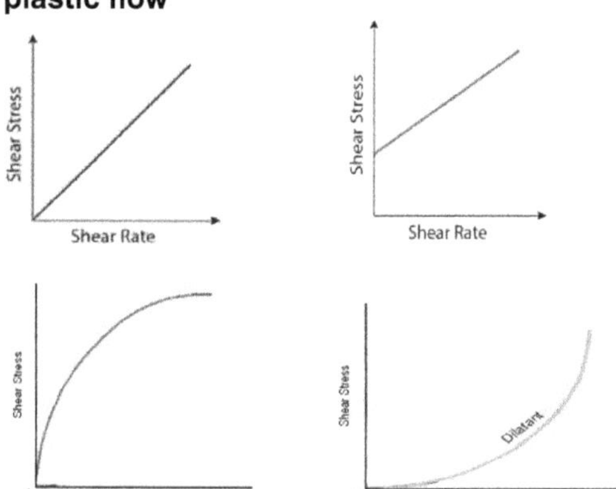

2347. Which of the following graph shows pseudoplastic flow

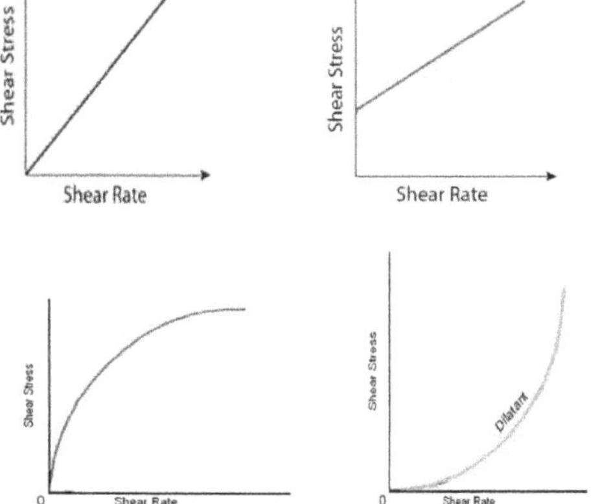

2348. Which of the following graph shows dilatant flow

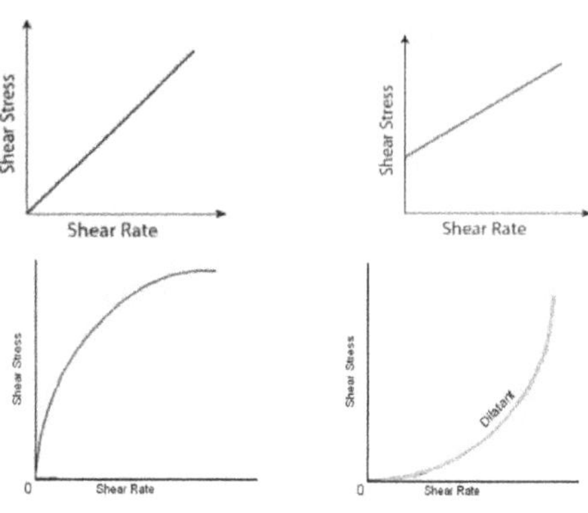

2349. Blood is a

A. Newtonian fluid B. Dilatant
C. Pseudoplastic D. Casson plastic

2350. Which of the following is actual name of viscometer?

A. Capillary tube B. Plate and cone
C. Cup and bob D. All of them

2351. In Brookfield viscometer, the viscosity produce which force

A. Torque force B. Vander wall force
C. Contact force D. Nuclear force

2352. In Brookfield viscometer, the viscosity produce torque which is directly proportional to

A. Shearing rate B. Shear stress
C. Thixotropy D. Negative thixotropy

2353. Ferranti-shirley viscometer is an example of a ____________

A. Plate and cone
B. Cup and bob
C Capillary tube viscometer
D. Broookfield viscometer

2354. In Ferranti-shirley viscometer, which of force is produced on cone?

A. Contact force
B. Gravitational force
C. Torque force
D. Nuclear force

2355. Drawback of cone & plate viscometer is

A. Plug flow B. Temperature effect
C. Both D. None of them

2356. Why the cone & plate viscometer advantage over cup and bob type instrument

A. Rate of shear is variable

B. Rate of shear is constant throughout entire sample

C. Temperature is constant

D. None of them

2357. Which property measures resistance of liquid to flow

A. Density B. Viscosity

C. Volume D. Solubility

2358. Which of the following is correct definition of pseudoplastic liquid

A. A liquid which becomes less viscous when the rate of shear increases

B. A liquid which becomes more viscous when the rate of shear increases

C. A liquid which becomes less viscous as the rate of shear decreases

D. A liquid which becomes more viscous when the rate of shear decreases

2359. The role of xanthan gum in liquid formulation

A. Regulate ph

B. Control viscosity

C. Enhance solubility

D. Enhance stability

2360. Newtons law of flow

A. Flow rate is directly proportional to applied stress

B. Rate of flow is inversely proportional to applied stress

C. Rate of flow is directly proportional to the square of applied stress

D. Rate of flow is doubled of applied stress

2361. Fluids that abide newtons law are known as __________

A. Newtonian fluids

B. Non-newtonian fluids

C. Real fluids

D. Ideal fluids

2362. Fluids that do not abide Newton's law are known as ________

A. Newtonian fluids

B. Non-newtonian fluids

C. Ideal fluids

D. Real fluids

2363. Difference in velocity between two planes of liquids separated by a distance is known as ______

A. Rate of shear B. Shearing stress

C. Degree of shear D. None of them

2364. Which is not type of non-newtonian flow

A. Plastic B. Pseudoplastic

C. Dilatant D. Thixotropy

2365. Yield value F indicates

A. e Flocculation B. F Deflocculation

C. V Void volume D. L Low consistency

2366. Which one of the following is not a example of pseudoplastic flow

A. Tragacanth B. Sodium alginate

C. Glycerin D. Methyl cellulose

2367. Pseudoplastic flow happens with ____________

A. Polymer solution

B. Monomer solution

C. Suspension

D. Bingham bodies

2368. In thixotropy, hysteresis loop means

A. Area of hysteresis

B. Up-down curve of thixotropy system

C. Up curve of thixotropy system

D. Down curve of thixotropy

2369. Rheological properties of a pharmaceutical system can influence the selection of

A. Processing equipments used in manufacturing

B. Dose

C. Drug

D. Formulation

2370. Milk is a ________ fluid

A. Viscous B. Elastic

C. Visco-elastic D. Extraneous

2371. Property of fluid that describe its internal resistance is known as

A. Viscosity B. Friction

C. Resistance D. Internal energy

2372. Which of the following are non-newtonian material which are time dependent?
A. Shear thickening
B. Rheo-pectic
C. Shear thinning
D. Plastic

2373. Rheo-pectic is also known as
A. Negative thixotropy
B. Anti-thixotropy
C. Viscoelastic
D. A & B both

2374. Dispersed system consist of particulate matter are known as____________
A. Continuous phase
B. Dispersed phase
C. Dispersion phase
D. Dispersion medium

2375. In dispersed system colloidal particles are dissolved in
A. Dispersion medium
B. Dispersed phase
C. Dispersed medium
D. None of them

2376. Dispersion System is classified into
A. 4 types B. 3 types
C. 2 types D. 6 types

2377. The color of colloidal dispersion is related to
A. Size of particles
B. Shape of particles
C. Weight of particles
D. A & B Both

2378. Particle size range of Molecular dispersion.
A. Less than 1 nm B. 1 nm to 0.5 μm
C. 0.5 μm to 1 μm D. 1 μm to 2 μm

2379. Particle size range of Colloidal dispersion
A. Less than 1 nm B. 1 nm to 0.5 μm
C. 0.5 μm to 1 μm D. 1 μm to 2 μm

2380. Particle size range of Coarse dispersion
A. Less than 1 nm B. 1 nm to 0.5 μm
C. 1 nm to 5 nm D. Greater than 0.5 μm

2381. In Colloidal dispersion, particles are visible in
A. Simple Microscope
B. Ordinary Microscope
C. Electron Microscope
D. Not Visible

2382. RBC is an example of
A. Molecular Dispersion
B. Colloidal Dispersion
C. Coarse Dispersion
D. None of them

2383. Example of Colloidal Dispersion
A. Natural Polymer
B. Synthetic Polymer
C. Colloidal Silver Sols
D. All of them

2384. Oxygen is an example of
A. Molecular Dispersion
B. Colloidal Dispersion
C. Coarse Dispersion
D. None of them

2385. Which Dispersion system is not visible in electron microscope
A. Molecular Dispersion
B. Colloidal Dispersion
C. Coarse Dispersion
D. All of them

2386. Arsenic trisulfides change color from red to yellow when particle size is
A. Increased
B. Doubled
C. Reduced
D. Diffused

2387. When particle size reduced, the antimony color changes from red to
A. Brown B. Violet
C. Green D. Yellow

2388. The technique Separation of colloidal particles from molecular particles is
A. Dialysis B. Cellophane
C. Collodian D. Sieving

2389. Name the semipermeable membrane is used for dialysis ?
A. Cellophane
B. Proton exchange membrane
C. Dialysis membrane
D. None of them

2390. The Process of removal of charged particles from colloidal dispersion system is known as
A. Dialysis B. Electro Dialysis
C. Haemodialysis D. Peritoneal dialysis

2391. Dialysis is occurs in
A. In-Vivo B. In-vitro
C. Both D. None of them

2392. Cromoglycic acid is used for
A. GIT disorder
B. Heart attack
C. Control asthmatic attack
D. Paralysis

2393. Colloidal copper is used in
A. Syphilis B. T.B.
C. Malaria D. Cancer

2394. Colloidal silver chloride is used as
A. Fungicide B. Germicide
C. Bactericide D. Anti-Protozoal

2395. ______ are Important natural colloids found in the body
A. Protein B. Glucose
C. RBC D. WBC

2396. Brownian movement of particles prevent
A. Diffusion B. Oxidation
C. Sedimentation D. Adsorption

2397. Which one of the following substance that belong to colloidal system is
A. Blood B. Sand
C. Milk D. Glucose

2398. Scattering of Light in colloidal system is known as
A. Brownian motion
B. Coagulation
C. Electrophoresis
D. Tyndall Effect

2399. Blood is a
A. Sol B. Foam
C. Solution D. Aerosol

2400. Colloidal system are classified into
A. 4 groups B. 3 groups
C. 5 groups D. 7 groups

2401. Hydroxyethyl starch is used as
A. Protein substitude
B. Vitamin
C. Plasma Substitude
D. Fat

2402. Examples of Lyophilic colloids are
A. Gold B. Insulin
C. Sulfer D. Micelles

2403. Rubber is the
A. Lyophilic colloid
B. Lyophobic colloid
C. Association colloid
D. Micelles

2404. Lyophilic means
A. Solvent-hating B. Solvent-Loving
C. Amphiphiles D. Solvent-repelling

2405. Example of Lyophobic colloids
A. Gold B. Silver
C. Arsenic sulfide D. All of them

2406. In which of the following special method's is used for preparation of colloids
A. Lyophobic colloids
B. Lyophilic colloid
C. Association colloid
D. Solvent-Loving colloids

2407. In which method of preparation of Lyophobic colloids, coarse particles are reduced in size
A. Condensation method
B. Dissolution method
C. Dispersion method
D. Distribution method

2408. The required conditions for the formation of Lyophobic colloid by condensation involve
A. Saturation B. Unsaturation
C. Supersaturation D. None of them

2409. Any colloid consists of a solid dispersed in a gas is known as ___________
A. Sol B. Foam
C. Aerosol D. Smoke

2410. __________is the colloidal suspension with solid particles in the liquid medium
A. Sol B. Foam
C. Aerosol D. Smoke

2411. Aerosol consists the small particles of liquid or solid dispersed in ___________

A. Solid B. Gas
C. Liquid D. Semi-Solid

2412. Amphiphile means

A. Water-loving
B. Fat-loving
C. Water-loving and Fat-Loving
D. Water-hating

2413. Example of micelle formation

A. Soap added to water
B. Water added to glycerine
C. Water added to milk
D. Salt added to water

2414. The number of monomers required for the formation of micelles (Aggregation)

A. 10 B. 20
C. 30 D. 50 or more than 50

2415. The concentration of monomer at which micelles form

A. CMC B. MMC
C. CCM D. BMC

2416. What is critical micelle concentration ?

A. The maximum amount of concentration required for micelle formation
B. The minimum amount of concentration required for micelle formation
C. The maximum amount of concentration not required for micelle formation
D. The minimum amount of concentration not required for micelle formation

2417. Genenions reduces (CMC)

A. Overall negative charge
B. Overall Positive charge
C. Neutral charge
D. No effect

2418. Sodium lauryl sulfate is used as

A. Wetting agent
B. Surfactant
C. Reducing agent
D. Sweetening agent

2419. Viscosity__________with increase in the concentration of amphiphile

A. Increases B. Decreases
C. Constant D. None of them

2420. Critical micelle concentration is reduced by the addition of

A. Surfactant B. Wetting agent
C. Electrolyte D. Bulking agent

2421. The ultra microscope is developed by

A. Harry Kane
B. Zsigmondy
C. Robert
D. Thomas Edison

2422. Drawback of ultra microscope

A. Not useful in scattering phenomena
B. It does not resolve lyophilic colloids
C. Not useful for colloidal particles
D. Not useful for coarse particles

2423. The scattering of light in colloidal dispersed system is known as the __________

A. Tyndall effects B. Brownian motion
C. Micelles D. None of them

2424. Tyndall effects is first described by

A. John Tyndall B. Micheal Tyndall
C. Micheal faraday D. Edison

2425. Uses of Light Scattering

A. Determining the molecular weight
B. Determine shape and size
C. A & B Both
D. Colour

2426. Light Scattering is used for study of

A. Protein B. Association colloids
C. Lyophobic sols D. All of them

2427. Brownian motion was studied by

A. Robert brown in 1827
B. Robert brown in 1817
C. Albert brown in 1827
D. Albert brown in 1817

2428. Which one of the following is optical properties of colloid

A. Brownian motion
B. Light Scattering
C. Sedimentation
D. Osmosis

2429. Brownian movements depends upon
A. Particles size
B. Viscosity of solution
C. Nature of colloid
D. A & B Both

2430. In Brownian movement smaller the particle size lesser the viscosity of solution ______the motion of particles
A. Slower
B. Reduce
C. Faster
D. None of them

2431. Minimum size required to observe Brownian motion
A. 10 μm
B. 5 μm
C. 3 μm
D. 9 nm

2432. _______is a direct result of Brownian movement
A. Scattering of light
B. Sedimentation
C. Diffusion
D. Osmosis

2433. Higher the HLB value of surfactant, more ______it is
A. Lipophilic
B. Hydrophilic
C. Amphoteric
D. None of them

2434. Lyophilic colloids has
A. Weak Tyndall effect
B. Strong Tyndall effect
C. No Tyndall effect
D. None of them

2435. Lyophobic colloids has
A. Weak Tyndall effect
B. Strong Tyndall effect
C. No Tyndall effect
D. None of them

2436. Why preparation Lyophobic colloids is difficult ?
A. Due to higher affinity towards solvent
B. Due to lower affinity towards solvent
C. Due to higher dissolution rate
D. Due to lower dissolution rate

2437. Gold number is used to measure protective ability of
A. Hydrophobic colloid
B. Association colloid
C. Hydrophilic colloid
D. All of them

2438. Breakdown of aggregates into particles of colloidal size is known as
A. Peptization
B. Diffusion
C. Disintegration
D. Distribution

2439. Lower the gold number, higher the
A. Peptization
B. Defensive ability
C. Protective ability
D. Coligative ability

2440. Gold number of gelatine is
A. 0.005 – 0.01
B. 0.1
C. 0.1-0.2
D. 2

2441. Gold number of Tragacanth is
A. 0.005 – 0.01
B. 0.1
C. 0.1-0.2
D. 2

2442. Gold number of albumin is
A. 0.005 – 0.01
B. 0.1
C. 0.1-0.2
D. 2

2443. Gold number of Acacia is
A. 0.005 – 0.01
B. 0.1
C. 0.1-0.2
D. 2

2444. The Krafft point is the temperature at which solubility of the surfactant equal to
A. Peptization
B. CMC
C. Diffusion
D. BMC

2445. Below Krafft point increase in concentration of surface-active agent leads to
A. More formation of Micelles
B. Peptization
C. Precipitation
D. Complexation

2446. Which compound forms a colloidal solution in water
A. NaCl
B. Glucose
C. Fructose
D. Starch

2447. Which of the following is not a solution
A. Blich
B. Carbonated beverages
C. Smoke
D. Salt Water

2448. Fick's law is used for

A. Sedimentation
B. Diffusion
C. Brownian motion
D. Osmotic Pressure

2449. Which law is used for diffusion

A. Stoke's law   B. Nernst's law
C. Fick's law   D. Henry law

2450. van'thoff equation is used to calculate

A. Molecular weight of colloidal solution
B. Molecular weight of colloidal dilute solution
C. Molecular weight of any solution
D. Concentration

2451. Viscosity is identified by which law

A. Stoke's law   B. Nernst's law
C. Fick's law   D. Henry law

2452. Which type of filtration colloidal particles are separated

A. Convention filter paper
B. Ultra-filters
C. Cloth filter
D. Quantitative filter paper

2453. Which of the following is hydrobhopic

A. Gum   B. Sulfur
C. Gelatin   D. Acacia

2454. Which of the following is not a property of lyophilic sols

A. It can be prepared directly by mixing dispersion phase and dispersion medium
B. viscosity of dispersed phase same as that of dispersed medium
C. It is reversible
D. Its particles do not carry charge

2455. The emulsifier of milk is

A. casein   B. Fat
C. lactose   D. Lactic acid

2456. Soap water removes grease by

A. Adsorption
B. Coagulation
C. Emulsification
D. Absorption

2457. Curd is an example of

A. sol   B. foam
C. Gel   D. Aerosol

2458. Which colloid is used for eye disease treatment

A. colloidal sulphur
B. colloidal silver
C. colloidal gold
D. colloidal antimony

2459. Which of the following easily form colloidal solution

A. Associated colloidal
B. Hydrophilic colloidal
C. Hydrophobic colloidal
D. Amphoteric colloidal

2460. Emulsion is a colloidal of a

A. Gas in liquid
B. Liquid in liquid
C. Liquid in gas
D. Gas in solid

2461. How can we determine solution is colloidal or not

A. By tyndall effect
B. By sedimentation
C. By hund's rule
D. By diffusion

2462. In electrodialysis diffusion of ions or molecules is

A. Enhanced   B. Reduced
C. Constant   D. No effect

2463. In electrodialysis diffusion of ions or molecules is enhanced by applying

A. Heat   B. Potential difference
C. voltage   D. None of them

2464. Full form of cmc

A. Critical micelle concentration
B. Constant micelle concentration
C. Colloidal micelle concentration
D. Coarse micelle concentration

2465. Amphiphile molecules or ions shows affinity for

A. Polar Solvent   B. Non -polar solvent
C. A & B Both   D. None of them

2466. Molecules or ions which have affinity for both polar and non polar solvent is known as

A. Hydrophilics   B. Lipophilics
C. Amphiphiles   D. None of them

2467. Spherical micelles exists at
A. CMC B. Above CMC
C. Below CMC D A & B both

2468. Laminar Micelles exists at
A. CMC B. Above CMC
C. Below CMC D. A & B both

2469. __________ micelles only exists at above CMC
A. Laminar B. Spherical
C. Colloidal D. Coarse

2470. DLVO Theory describes Stability of
A. Lyophobic Colloid
B. Lyophilic colloid
C. Hydrophilic colloid
D. Amphiphiles

2471. Stability of Lyophobic colloid is described by
A. Tyndall Effect B. Fick's Law
C. DLVO Theory D. Stoke's Law

2472. In DLVO Theory, Attractive force due to
A. Nuclear Force
B. Van derwaal force
C. Electric double layer
D. Frictional force

2473. In DLVO Theory, Repulsive force due to
A. Nuclear Force
B. Van der waal force
C. Electric double layer
D. Frictional force

2474. In DLVO Theory, Due to vanderwaal force which force occurs
A. Attractive force
B. Repulsive force
C. Both
D. None of them

2475. Sodium Lauryl sulphate is
A. Lyophobic colloid
B. Association colloid
C. Lyophilic colloid
D. Hydrophilic colloid

2476. Which of the following Zwitter ionic colloid
A. Cetrimide
B. Lecithin
C. Poly oxyethylene lauryl ether
D. None of them

2477. In association colloids, sodium lauryl sulphate is
A. Anoinic type colloid
B. Non-ionic type colloid
C. Cationic type colloid
D. Ampholytic type colloid

2478. Which one is Non-ionic type colloid (association colloid)
A. Sodium lauryl sulphate
B. Cetyl trim ethyl ammonium bromide
C. Poly oxyethylene lauryl ether
D. Lecithin

2479. Lyophobic colloid mainly depends (Stability) on the presence of
A. Solvent B. Charge
C. Valency D. Power

2480. Precipitation power of an ion on a dispersed phase of opposite charge increases with increase in the
A. Charge of the ion
B. Hydration
C. Precipitation
D. Complexation

2481. According to schulze-Hardy rule, Higher the valency, ______ the precipitation power
A. Lower
B. Greater
C. No relationship between them
D. None of them

2482. When two oppositely charged hydrophobic colloid mixed, result in precipitation due to neutralization of charge is known as
A. Coacervation
B. Protection
C. Mutual Precipitation
D. Sensitization

2483. When high amount of hydrophilic colloid, makes the hydrophobic colloid more stable towards electrolytes is known as

A. Coacervation
B. Protection
C. Mutual Precipitation
D. Sensitization

2484. When two opposite charged hydrophilic colloid mixed, result in a colloid rice layer separate called

A. Coacervation
B. Protection
C. Mutual Precipitation
D. Sensitization

2485. When Acacia (-ve charged) and gelatine (+ve charged) mixed, is an example of

A. Protection
B. Sensitization
C. Coacervation
D. Mutual Precipitation

2486. Turbidity is determined by

A. Electrophoresis
B. Spectroscopy
C. Electron Microscope
D. Turbidometer

2487. Nephelometer is used to determine

A. Precipitation B. Complexation
C. Turbidity D. Gold Number

2488. Movement of liquid relative to a fixed solid under influence of electric field is known as

A. Electro-osmosis
B. Electrophoresis
C. Streaming potential
D. Sedimentation Potential

2489. Movement of charged dispersed phase through a liquid medium upon applying potential difference is known as

A. Electro-osmosis
B. Electrophoresis
C. Streaming potential
D. Sedimentation Potential

2490. Colloidal particles flow is an example of

A. Newtonian flow
B. Non-Newtonian flow
C. Pseudoplastic flow
D. None of them

2491. Dispersion of particles are thermodynamically__________

A. Stable B. Unstable
C. Partially stable D. None of them

2492. Dispersions are thermodynamically unstable due to

A. Aggregation B. Settlement
C. A & B Both D. Presence of charge

2493. The difference in potential between actual surface and electro neutral region is known as

A. Nernst Potential
B. Zeta Potential
C. Electro Kinetic Potential
D. None of these

2494. In Zeta potential, potential occurs at

A. Interface B. Actual surface
C. Shear plane D. None of these

2495. The potential difference between shear plane and electro neutral region is known as

A. Nernst Potential
B. Zeta Potential
C. Electro thermodynamic Potential
D. None of these

2496. In Facilitated diffusion, which of the following used as carrier

A . Carbohydrate B. Protein
C. Fat D. Liquid

2497. In simple diffusion, Rate of diffusion is directly proportional to the

A. Dissolution
B. Pressure gradient
C. Concentration gradient
D. Gradient

2498. Lecithin is a __________surfactant

A. Cationic B. Anoinci
C. Zwitterionic D. Non-ionic

2499. Which of the following is coarse dispersion ?

A. Oxygen B. Silver
C. RBC D. Polymer

2500. In colloids the Tyndall effect due to
A. Brownian motion
B. Scattering of light
C. Sedimentation
D. Diffusion

2501. In Colloids which effect occurs due to scattering of light in particle
A. Direct effect
B. Tyndall effect
C. Sedimentation effect
D. Indirect effect

2502. The term 'colloid' means
A. Sol-like
B. Gel-like
C. Glue-like
D. Sticky

2503. Iron dextran injection (BP) is used for treatment of
A. Intramuscular use
B. Anemia
C. Germicidal
D. Cancer

2504. Iron Sorbitol injection (BP) is used for
A. Intramuscular use
B. Anemia
C. Germicidal
D. Cancer

2505. Iron dextran injection is an example of
A. Non-ionic hydrophobic sol
B. Non-ionic hydrophilic sol
C. Non-ionic hydrophobic gel
D. Ionic hydrophobic sol

2506. Iron dextran injection contains
A. Dextran complexes with ferric ions
B. Sorbitol, dextran complexes with ferric ions
C. Dextran, citric acid complexes with ferric ions
D. Dextran, sorbitol and citric acid

2507. Iron sorbitol injection contains
A. Dextran complexes with ferric ions
B. Sorbitol, dextran complexes with ferric ions
C. Dextran, citric acid complexes with ferric ions
D. Dextran, sorbitol and citric acid complexes with ferric ions

2508. Uses of colloids are
A. In Therapy
B. As a coating agent
C. As a Excipient
D. All of them

2509. Which of the following colloid used as excipient
A. Hydroxy ethyl starch
B. Synthetic polymer
C. Colloidal copper
D. Sorbital

2510. Colloidal acacia is used as
A. Viscosity Enhancer
B. Emulsifying agent
C. Solubilizing agent
D. Wetting agent

2511. Diffusion Rate in colloidal dispersion is
A. Rapid
B. Slow
C. Very Fast
D. None of these

2512. Colloidal gold has a
A. Red Colour
B. Violet Colour
C. Blue Colour
D. Brown Colour

2513. Coarse dispersion of gold appears
A. Red Colour
B. Violet Colour
C. Blue Colour
D. Brown Colour

2514. Which of the following dispersion does not show Tyndall effect ?
A. Molecular dispersion
B. Colloidal dispersion
C. Both
D. None of them

2515. Spherical particles of gold shows red colour, while the disc like particles of gold gives
A. Red Colour
B. Violet Colour
C. Blue Colour
D. Brown Colour

2516. Shape of Colloids affects
A. Colour
B. Viscosity
C. A & B Both
D. None of these

2517. Platinum colloids used as a
A. Anti-Cancer
B. Catalyst
C. Anti-Syphilis
D. Emulsifying agent

2518. In Colloidal dispersion, Larger the surface, ________ the solubility of drug

A. Lower B. Slower
C. Greater D. A & C Both

2519. Colloidal Acacia possess ________charge on their surface

A. Positive B. Negative
C. Neutral D. A & B Both

2520. Colloidal gelatin possess ________ charge on their surface

A. Positive B. Negative
C. Neutral D. A & B Both

2521. Colloidal tragacanth posses ________charge on their surface

A. Positive B. Negative
C. Neutral D. None of these

2522. Antacids produce ________charged particles

A. Negative B. Positive
C. A & B Both D. Neutral

2523. Which of the following has highly charged particles

A. Lyophobic colloids
B. Lyophilic colloids
C. Association colloids
D. A & B Both

2524. Lyophilic colloids are thermodynamically ____________

A. Unstable B. Stable
C. Partially stable D. None of these

2525. Lyophobic colloids are thermodynamically ____________

A. Unstable B. Stable
C. Partially stable D. None of these

2526. When water is used as a medium, the system are termed as

A. Hydrophilic dispersion
B. Lyophilic dispersion
C. Hydrophobic dispersion
D. Association colloids

2527. Which of the following method of preparation of Lyophobic colloid involves Mechanical dispersion ?

A. Dispersion Method
B. Condensation Method
C. A & B Both
D. None of these

2528. Which of the following is used as stabilizing agent

A. Gums B. Gelatin
C. Soap D. All of them

2529. Which of the following is used as peptizing agent

A. Glycerine B. Sugar
C. Lactose D. All of them

2530. In peptization, which of the following is removed ?

A. Surfactants
B. Flocculating agent
C. Deflocculating agent
D. A & B Both

2531. In peptization, which of the following is removed ?

A. Electrolytes
B. Flocculating agent
C. Deflocculating agent
D. A & B Both

2532. In peptization, which of the following is added

A. Surfactants
B. Flocculating agent
C. Deflocculating agent
D. A & C Both

2533. In Lyophobic colloids, which of the following is Dispersion method of Preparation ?

A. Addition of Non-Solvent
B. Chemical Methods
C. Peptization
D. A & B Both

2534. In Preparation of Lyophobic colloids, Electric arc method is suitable for

A. Non-Metal B. Metal
C. Polymers D. Amples

2535. Crystallization technique is used for

A. Purification B. Stablization
C. A & B Both D. None of these

2536. Purification is done by

A. Crystallization B. Peptization
C. Condensation D. Evaporation

2537. Which of the following factor affects viscosity of colloids

A. Shape of dispersed particles
B. Type of colloids
C. Affinity of particles to the medium
D. All of them

2538. Sedimentation is influence by

A. Vander Waals force
B. Gravitational Force
C. Contact Force
D. Magnetic Force

2539. Colligative properties are not used in determination of Molecular weight of colloidal particles excepts

A. Sedimentation B. Viscosity
C. Osmotic Pressure D. Diffusion

2540. Micromeritics is the science and technology which deals with

A. Large Particles B. Small Particles
C. A & B Both D. None of these

2541. Unit of Fluidity is

A. Poise B. Poise -1
C. Centipoise D. Centipoise -1

2542. Generally, Non-Newtonian Fluids are expressed as

A. Apparent Viscosity
B. Kinematic Viscosity
C. Yield Value
D. A & B Both

2543. On Increasing temperature, Viscosity of gas

A. Increases B. Decrease
C. Constant D. A & B Both

2544. Example of pseudoplastic flow

A. Tragacanth B. CMC
C. Na-CMC D. All of them

2545. Water is an Example of

A. Newtonian flow
B. Plastic flow
C. Pseudoplastic flow
D. Dilatant

2546. Ultrasonic shear Rheometer is used for study of

A. Carbohydrate B. Fat
C. Protein D. Vitamins

2547. Example of anti-Thixotropy

A. Bentonite B. MagnesiaMagma
C. Polymers D. A & B Both

2548. Ointment, gel and creams shows

A. Dilatant flow B. Plastic flow
C. Pseudoplastic flow D. Newtonian flow

2549. Which one is correct Gibb's Phase Rule

A. E + C = P + 2 B. E + 2 = P + C
C. E + P = C + 2 D. E - C = P - 2

2550. If Phase Volume ratio is 5%. Then flow will be

A. Newtonian B. Pseudoplastic
C. Plastic D. Dilatant

2551. If Phase Volume ratio is 50%. Then flow will be

A. Newtonian B. Pseudoplastic
C. Plastic D. Dilatant

2552. If Phase Volume ratio is 74%. Then flow will be

A. Newtonian B. Pseudoplastic
C. Plastic D. Dilatant

2553. In Dilatant flow, If shear rate is increased, then viscosity is

A. Also Increased B. Decreased
C. A & B Both D. Constant

2554. Printing INK is an Example of

A. Newtonian flow B. Plastic flow
C. Pseudoplastic flow D. Dilatant flow

2555. In Fick's First law, the particles diffuse from

A. Higher to Lower Concentration
B. Lower to Higher Concentration
C. Both A & B
D. None of these

2556. The Study of Kinetic Properties of Colloidal dispersions is important for

A. Predicting the stability of a system
B. Determining the Molecular weight of Particles
C. Studying the transport Kinetic of colloidal particles
D. All of them

2557. The Brownian movement can be viewed by

A. Telescope B. Simple Microscope
C. Light Microscope D. All of them

2558. __________works against the gravitational force

A. Sedimentation B. Brownian Motion
C. A & B Both D. None of them

2559. By increasing viscosity of medium, Brownian motion will be

A. Increased B. Decreased
C. A & B Both D. Constant

2560. As the particle increases, the velocity of the particles___________

A. Increased B. Decreased
C. A & B Both D. Constant

2561. In which of the following diffusion rate is very fast

A. Gelatin B. Albumin
C. Gel D. Salts

2562. Soap forms __________ solution in alcohol

A. True B. Colloidal
C. A & B Both D. Semi-Solid

2563. Zeta potential can be determined by

A. Zeta meter B. Microscope
C. Electrophoresis D. None of these

2564. In Electrophoresis, when potential is applied across the electrodes, the particles migrate towards

A. Oppositely charged electrodes
B. Negative charged electrodes
C. Positive charged electrodes
D. All of them

2565. In Electrophoresis, the potential gradient across the electrode increases, the velocity of migration of a particles

A. Also Increases B. Decreased
C. Constant D. A & B Both

2566. Donnan membrane equilibrium is used to enhance the

A. Absorption of drugs
B. Solubility of drugs
C. Diffusion of drugs
D. Elimination of drugs

2567. Donnan membrane equilibrium is used for which drug

A. Sodium Salicylate
B. Potassium benzyl penicillin
C. Both A & B
D. None of them

2568. Which of the following method is used for purification of colloids

A. Dialysis B. Electrodialysis
C. Ultrafiltration D. All of these

2569. Which of following is electrical property of colloids

A. Light Scattering
B. Viscosity
C. Donnan Equilibrium
D. Diffusion

2570. Dust is an Example of

A. Foam B. Sol
C. Aerosol D. None of these

2571. Which of the following gold number shows highest protective ability

A. 0.5 B. 0.005
C. 0.01 D. 0.1

2572. Why plug form is not observed in cone and plate viscometer

A. Cleaning and filling of sample is easy
B. Rate of shear is independent of radius
C. Shear can be maintained uniformly
D. Temperature can be maintained uniformly

2573. Rate of shear and shearing stress for Newtonian system can be represented by

A. Simple curve B. Compound curve
C. Flow curve D. None of them

2574. In Emulsion dispersed phase is also referred as:

A. Internal phase B. Continuous phase
C. External phase D. None of the above

2575. In oil-in-water type of Emulsion dispersed phase is?

A. Oleaginous B. Aqueous
C. Both (a) and (b) D. None of the above

2576. Which of the following is necessary to prepare a stable emulsion:

A. Suspending agent
B. emulsifying agent
C. Viscocity builder
D. All of the above

2577. Depending upon constituent which route of administration is suitable for semi-solid emulsion:
A. Orally B. Rectal
C. Topical D. All of the above

2578. From which route liquid of emulsion cannot be prepared?
A. Parental B. Oral
C. Rectal D. Topical

2579. Which route is suitable for administering potatabledox of emulsion
A. Parental B. Topical
C. Oral D. Rectal

2580. Which of the following property of particle make the oil globules more readily absorbed:
A. Particle size B. Particle shape
C. Density D. None of the above

2581. Choice of emulsion for external application on skin is based on
A. Nature of surfactant
B. Nature of therapeutic agent
C. Nature of medium
D. None of the above

2582. Which of the following factor affect the choice of emulsion for external application of skin
A. Nature of Therapeutic agent
B. Disagreeability of emollient
C. Tissue softening effect
D. None of the above

2583. Which reason is responsible for more even application of emulation on skin
A. Thin film of sebum
B. Thick film of sebum
C. Both (a) and (b)
D. None of the above

2584. Which of the following factor affect the process of emulsification:
A. PH of the phase
B. Relative proportion of internal phase
C. Relative proportion of external phase
D. All of the above

2585. Which of the following is considered as theories of emulsification
A. Oriental Wedge Theory
B. Surface Tension Theory
C. Surface Renewal Theory
D. Both (a) and (b)

2586. Which of the following shape is considered best for liquid droplet to exposed to least amount of surface area
A. Spherical B. Angular
C. Cylindrical D. None of the above

2587. In surface tension theory surfactants are used as
A. Stabilizers B. Emulsifiers
C. Viscosity D. Both (a) and (b)

2588. In oriental wedge theory emulsifying agent orient themselves
A. At the surface
B. Within liquid
C. At junction of two liquid
D. None of the above

2589. The oriental wedge theory is based on which type of molecule
A. Hydrophilic
B. Hydrophobic
C. Liophilic
D. Both (a) and (b)

2590. Which cationic emulsifier is used as bacterial agent
A. Sodium laurylsalphate
B. Triethanol amine
C. Benzylconium chloride
D. None of the above

2591. In which phase emulsifying agent is more soluble in oriental wedge theory
A. Internal phase
B. External phase
C. Both (a) and (b)
D. None of the above

2592. In which theory of emulsification emulsifies is present at the interface
A. Surface tension theory
B. Oriental wedge theory
C. Plastic film theory
D. None of the above

2593. Phablity of film affects which of the property in plastic film theory
A. Apperence of emulsion
B. Contact force between liquids
C. Stability of emulsion
D. None of the above

2594. Which of the following is important continued emulsion stability
A. Film of emulsifier
B. Protective vedge of molecule
C. Interfacial tensier
D. Both (a) and (b)

2595. Which of the following carbohydrate is used as emulsifier
A. Acacia B. Tragacanth
C. Pectin D. All of the above

2596. Carbohydrate material form which type of colloids
A. Hydrophobic B. Hydrophilic
C. Both (a) and (b) D. None of the above

2597. Which of the following carbohydrate is used in preparation of extemporaneous emplifier
A. Acacia B. Tragencenth
C. Agar D. None of the above

2598. Which of these is used as thickening agent in acacia emulsified product
A. Tregacanth B. Agar
C. Pectin D. Both (a) and (b)

2599. Which of the following is used to provide dispersion stability in commercial spension
A. HPMC
B. Sodium CMC
C. Microcrystalline cellulose
D. None of the above

2600. Which of these potencies substance is used to produce oil-in-water emulsion
A. Gelatine B. Casein
C. Egg yolk D. All of the above

2601. Which of the followings is used as a stabilizer for O/W emulsion
A. Cetyl alcohol B. Stearyal alcohol
C. Ethyl alcohol D. Both (a) and (b)

2602. Which of these substance use as thickening agent in O/W emulsion
A. Pectin
B. Ethyl alcohol
C. Propyl alcohol
D. Glyseralmonostearate

2603. Which of the following is employed in externally used emulsion and promote W/O emulsion
A. Lipopolysaccharide B. Cholesterol
C. Both (a) and (b) D. None of the above

2604. In wetting agent which substance is responsible for the surface activity of molecule
A. Lipophlicprotiene
B. Hydrophilic proteins
C. Lipophilic carbohydrates
D. None of the above

2605. Which substance is included in anionic emulsion
A. Monovalent soap
B. Polyvalent soap
C. Organic soap
D. All of the above

2606. Medicinal agent in which phase are less imitating when incorporated in topical emulsion
A. External phase
B. Internal phase
C. Both (A) and (B)
D. None of the above

2607. Which of the following route is suitable for giving less irritating medicinal agent
A. Parental B. Oral
C. Topical D. None of the above

2608. Availability of medicinal agent in vehicle depend upon which factor
A. Miscibility in oil
B. Solubility in water
C. Both (A) and (B)
D. Nature of drug

2609. Cationic surfactant is effective over a PH range of
A. 2—5 B. 3—7
C. 6—12 D. None of the above

2610. When insoluble material is added to aqueous phase which of these substance form oil-in-water emulsion
A. Bentonite
B. Magnesium hydroxide
C. Aluminium hydroxide
D. All of the above

2611. In w/o emulsion of oleaginous phase volume dominate which substance is used

A. Veegum B. Bentanoite
C. Silica D. None of the above

2612. Which of the following property increase with increase in concentration of emulsion

A. Density B. Miscibility
C. Viscosity D. None of the above

2613. There is increase in viscosity of emulsion at certain point after which viscosity decreases sharply at these point emulsion has undergone

A. Conversion B. Inversion
C. Diversion D. None of the above

2614. Surface active agent categorized on the basis of

A. Molecular weight
B. Chemical composition
C. Molecular structure
D. None of the above

2615. HLB value is a indicative of which property of substance

A. Activity B. Polarity
C. Solubility D. None of the above

2616. Substances are assigned HLB number upto

A. 40 B. 20
C. 30 D. 25

2617. The usual HLB range is

A. 1—30 B. 5—15
C. 1—20 D. None of the above

2618. Surface active agent having HLB value of 3—6 for which type of emulsion

A. O/W emulsion B. W/O emulsion
C. Both (A) and (B) D. None of the above

2619. Oil in water emulsion are possible in which HLB range

A. 2—7 B. 8—18
C. 4—10 D. None of the above

2620. HLB value for mineral oil for W/O emulsion

A. 4 B. 10.5
C. 6 D. 9.2

2621. HLB value for mineral oil for O/W emulsion

A. 9 B. 10.5
C. 6.5 D. 4.5

2622. Tweens lies in HLB range of

A. 8—20 B. 9.8—11.8
C. 14.9—16.7 D. None of the above

2623. Span lies in the HLB range of

A. 3.5—4.5 B. 2—6.5
C. 7.5—9.5 D. None of the above

2624. HLB value for anti-foaming agent lies between

A. 3—6 B. 7—9
C. 1—3 D. 8—18

2625. HLB value of wetting agent lies between

A. 7—9 B. 1—3
C. 15—20 D. 8—18

2626. Which of these is a HLB range for emulsifier(O/W)

A. 15—20 B. 13—15
C. 8—18 D. None of the above

2627. Which of these is a HLB range for solublizers

A. 8—18 B. 7—9
C. 15—20 D. 13—15

2628. Which of the following is HLB range for emulsifier (W/O)

A. 1—3 B. 7—9
C. 8—12 D. 3—6

2629. 13—15 is a HLB range for

A. Anti-foaming B. Detergents
C. Solublizers D. None of the above

2630. Emulsifying agents minimize the surface energy through the formation of

A. Film B. Globules
C. Both(A) and (B) D. None of the above

2631. Detergents work by reducing the

A. Surface energy
B. Contact between solid and liquid
C. Surface tension
D. None of the above

2632. Which of the following method is used for preparation of emulsion in labs

A. Wedgewood method
B. Milkshake mixture
C. Hand homogenizer
D. All of the above

2633. Which of these method is used on small scale exteneparaneall prepration of emulsion

A. Dry gum method
B. Wet gum method
C. Forbell bottle method
D. All of the above

2634. In which method emulsifying agent is mixed with oil before addition of water

A. Wet gum method
B. Dry gum method
C. Bottle method
D. None of the above

2635. In which method mucilage is form on addition of emulsifying agent in water

A. Wet gum method
B. Dry gum method
C. Bottle method
D. None of the above

2636. Which of these method is used for volatile oils

A. Wet gum method
B. Dry gum method
C. Bottle method
D. None of the above

2637. Which of the method is also refered as 4:2:1 method

A. Wet gum method B. Dry gum method
C. Bottle method D. Both (A) and (B)

2638. How many part of oil is added in 4:2:1 or dry gum method

A. 2 B. 4
C. 1 D. None of the above

2639. Which type of emulsifier is used as dry gum method

A. Oil in water B. Water in oil
C. Both (A) and (B) D. None of the above

2640. A mortar with rough rather then smooth inner surface is used in dry gum method due to

A. Grinding action B. Small globule size
C. Both (A) and (B) D. None of the above

2641. Generally how much time is required to produce primary emulsion

A. 1 minute B. 5 minute
C. 2 minute D. 3 minute

2642. Which of the following substance should not added directly to primary emulsion

A. Alcohol B. Oil
C. Gum D. None of the above

2643. Due to which reason alcohol is not added directly to the primary emulsion

A. Breaking action
B. Film foaming action
C. Precipitating action
D. None of the above

2644. Which of these method is generally used for viscous oil

A. Dry gum B. Bottle method
C. Wet gum D. None of the above

2645. Quality of emulsion prepared by wet gum method is increased by

A. High speed stator
B. High speed rotor
C. Hand homogenizer
D. None

2646. Which type of soap are prepared by insitu soap method

A. Calcium soap B. Soft soap
C. Sodium soap D. Both (A) and (B)

2647. Which type of oil is present in calcium soaps

A. Hydrogenated oil
B. Vegetable soap
C. Mineral oil
D. None of the above

2648. Calcium soaps are which type of emulsion

A. W/O B. O/W
C. O/W D. None of the above

2649. Due to which derived property oil phase is used as external phase in ideal formulation

A. Occulation B. Skin spotning
C. Skin tightening D. Both (A) and (B)

2650. Which of these is a property of micro emulsion Optically transparent

A. Isotropic mixture
B. Stable system
C. All of the above

2651. The diameter of a droplet in the micro emulsion is

A. 10—100A. B. 100--1000 A.
C. 1000--2000 A. D. None of the above

2652. Type of micro emulsion form depend upon

A. Property of oil
B. Method of emulsion preparation
C. Surfactants
D. Both (A) and (C)

2653. To prepare transparent oil in water micro emulsion of oils which HLB range is used

A. 7—9　B. 13—16
C. 15—18　D. None of the above

2654. Surfactant that are commonly used for preparation of microemulsion for oral liquid formulation is

A. Polysorbatue 60　B. Potassium oleate
C. Gelatine　D. None of the above

2655. Which of the following statement count as the consideration for instability of emulsion

A. Formulation of globules on standing
B. Large gloubules rise on the top
C. All or part of liquid become unemulsified
D. All of the above

2656. Preparation of globules which tends to rise on top or fall to botton individually known as

A. Aggregate
B. Coalescence
C. Creaming
D. None of the above

2657. Rate of sepration of dispersed phase on an emulsion may be related to

A. Particle size of dispersed phase
B. Difference in density between phase
C. Viscocity of external phase
D. All of the above

2658. Which type of creaming take place in emulsion having internal phase of lesser density then external phase

A. Upward creaming
B. Downward creaming
C. Junctional creaming
D. None of the above

2659. Separation of which phase from emulsion termed as breaking

A. Internal phaser
B. External phase
C. Both (A) and (B)
D. None of the above

2660. Stability taste for emulsion perform at what temperature in industry

A. 50C and 400C　B. 100C and 400C
C. 60C and 500C　D. None of the above

2661. Which of these are most likely to affect or contaminate the emulsion

A. Bacteria　B. Parasite
C. Fungi　D. None of the above

2662. Which of the following is used to provide dispersion stability in commercial suspension?

A. HPMC
B. Sodium cmc
C. Microcrystine cellulose
D. None of the above

2663. Which of these pretensions substance is used to produce oil in water emulsion

A. Gelatine　B. Egg yolk
C. Casein　D. All of the above

2664. Which of the substance produce fluid like emulsion

A. Egg yolk　B. Agar
C. Gelatin　D. Acacia

2665. Which of the following is used as stabilizer for oil in water emulsion

A. Cetyl alcohol　B. Stearyal alcohol
C. Ethyl alcohol　D. Bot (A) and (B)

2666. Which of these substances use as thickening agent in oil in water emulsion

A. Pectin
B. Ethyl alcohol
C. Propyl alcohol
D. Glycerylmonostearate

2667. Cetyl alcohol is used as stabilizer for oil in water emulsion in which of the following dosage form

A. Lotion　B. Ointment
C. Laniment　D. Both a and b

2668. Which of the following is employed in externally used emulsion and promote water in oil emulsion

A. Lipopolysaccharide
B. Cholesterol
C. Both a and b
D. None of the above

2669. In wetting agent which substance is responsible for the surface activity of molecule

A. Lipophilic Protein
B. Hydrophilic Protein
C. Lipophilic carbohydrates
D. None of the above

2670. Which substance is included in anionic emulsifier

A. Monovelent soap
B. Polyvalent soap
C. Organic soap
D. All of the above

2671. Which of the following is non-ionic type of emulsifier

A. Sorbitan ester
B. Polyoxyethylene
C. Both a and b
D. None of the above

2672. Effective Ph range of non ionic surfactant

A. 3—10 B. 4—8
C. 7—12 D. None of the above

2673. Which cationic emulsifier is used as bactericidal agent?

A. Sodium lauryl sulphate
B. Triethamolamine
C. Benzyl conium chloride.
D. None of the above

2674. Due to which reason molecule oriented in oriented wedge theory

A. Size of molecule
B. Shape of molecule
C. Solublity characteristic
D. All of the above

2675. Suspension consist of which type of particle

A. Fine B. Coarse
C. Very fine D. None of the above

2676. Vehicle used in suspension should have

A. Maximum degree of drug solubility
B. Minimum degree of drug solubility
C. No drug solubility
D. None of the above

2677. Suspension are available as ________ intended for use in liquid vehicle

A. Tablet B. Dry powder
C. Dry capsule D. None of the above

2678. Which of the following is not present in drug powder used for suspension

A. Suspending agent
B. Viscosity agent
C. Dispensing agent
D. Osmotic agent

2679. Which type of drugs are formulated as dry powder intended for suspension

A. Unstable in aqueous vehicle
B. Stable in aqueous vehicle
C. Stable in non aqueous vehicle
D. None of the above

2680. Oral suspension are used to its

A. Chemical stability
B. Physical stability
C. Therapeutic stability
D. Microbiological stability

2681. Drug which are having disagreeable taste are incorporated in suspension in which form

A. Dissolved
B. Undissolved
C. Dispersed
D. None of the above

2682. Which of the following is not a derived property in pharmaceutical suspension

A. Readily redispersed
B. Settle slowly
C. Constant particle size
D. Reduce interfacial tension

2683. Which of the following is not considered in deciding ideal properties of suspension

A. Dispersed phase
B. Dispersion phase
C. Pharmaceutical adjuncts
D. Active pharmaceutical ingredients

2684. Which of the following law govern the rate of velocity of setting of particles of suspension

A. Stefan's law B. Hooke's law
C. Stoke's law D. None of the above

2685. In suspension stoke equation is derive from which type of Solution?
A. Ideal solution
B. Non-Ideal solution
C. Both (a) and (b)
D. None of the above

2686. Which type of suspension is considered best for generating stoke equation?
A. Concentrated suspension
B. Dilute suspension
C. Quasifluid suspension
D. None of the above

2687. Which type of attraction exists between particle and dispersion medium during sedimentation?
A. Physical attraction
B. Chemical attraction
C. Both (a) and (b)
D. None of the above

2695. Which of the following is one of the rapid and convenient method of producing fine drug powder for suspension
A. Micronisation
B. Micro reduction
C. Micropulverisation
D. None of the above

2696. For particle size of 1μm to 10μm which process is preffered in suspension
A. Micro B. Micronization
C. Jet milling D. Both (b) and(c

2697. Mirco pulversiation process for size reduction is mainly used for which type of suspension
A. Oral suspension
B. Parentral Suspension
C. Topical suspension
D. Both(a) and (c)

2698. In jet milling for finer particle which energy is used
A. Heat energy B. fluid energy
C. Both(a) and (b) D. none of the above

2699. Which of the following step is part of micronization
A. Polymerisation B. collision
C. Fragmentation D. Both (b) and (c)

2700. Jet milling process for five particles is used for formulation of which suspension
A. Opthelmic suspension
B. Topical suspension
C. Oral suspension
D. All of the above

2701. Which of the following drying technique can also used for producing extremely small dimension particle for suspension
A. Freeze drying B. Vaccume drying
C. Spray drying D. Spray drying

2702. Reduction of particle is good for slow sedimentstion but arise problem of
A. Formation of compact cake
B. Formation of loose cake
C. Formation of crystals
D. None of above

2703. Which of the following property affect caking of suspensoid
A. Particle size
B. Particle shape
C. Density of particle
D. Affinity of particle for medium

2704. Stable suspension of calcium carbonate consist of particle of which shape
A. Symmetrical needle shape
B. Symmetrical prism shape
C. Symmetrical sphere shape
D. Symmetrical barrel shape

2705. Which type of particles do not form cake on standing
A. Needle shape
B. Barrel shape
C. Spherical shape
D. All of the above

2706. Which of the following must prevented to avoid formation of cake
A. Agglomeration B. Redispersion
C. Stablization D. None of the above

2707. Micelles behaves as colloids when
A. Concentration is equal to CMC
B. Concentration is less than CMC
C. Concentration is more than CMC
D. They are not behaves as colloids

2708. Rigid cohesion of small particles in suspension is present by formation of
A. Less rigid particle aggregate
B. Loose particle agglomerate
C. Both (a) and (b)
D. None of the above

2709. In the formation of loose aggregates of particles which type of bond formation takes place
A. Weak particle - medium bond
B. Weak particle – suspending agent bond
C. Weak particle – particle bond
D. All of the above

2710. Particles which are loosely aggregated named as
A. Deflocculated particle
B. Flocculated particle
C. Loose agglomerate
D. None of the above

2711. Which type of particle settle more rapidly
A. Floccullated
B. Deflocculaed
C. Both (a) and (b)
D. None of the above

2712. Which type of particle is less prone to compaction
A. Deflocculated B. Rigid particle
C. Flocculated D. Both (a) and (b)

2713. Which type of particle not redispered easily by small amount of agitation
A. Deflocculated B. Flocculated
C. Loose particle D. Both (b) and (c)

2714. Which of the following is considered when method for prepration of flocculated particle is decided
A. Type of drug involved
B. Desired size of the particle
C. Type of product desired
D. Both (a) and (c)

2715. Which of the following is used as flocculating agent in oral suspension
A. Veegum B. Bentonite Magma
C. Sodium CMC D. All of the above

2716. Which of the property is altered for formation of flocs in suspension
A. Partition coefficient
B. Solubility
C. Ionisition
D. PH

2717. Electrolytes works on flocullating agent by which mechanism
A. Enhance movement of ion in Medium
B. Reduce electrical barrier between particle
C. Reduce movement of ion in medium
D. Reduce electrical barrier between medium

2718. Determined concentration of ionic and non-ionic surfactant ______ the flocculation of particle in suspension
A. Decrease
B. Increase
C. Does not have any effect
D. None of the above

2719. Rapid setting of flocculated suspension hinders which of the following
A. Redispersion of particles
B. Accurate measurement of dosage
C. Suspendability of particle
D. None of the above

2720. Which of the following is used to thicken the dispersion medium
A. Carboxymethylcellulo
B. Sodium salicylate
C. Xanthum gum
D. Both (a) and (c)

2721. Which of the following suspending agent are tested for its performance to not interfere with the theraupatic effect of medicinal substance of susoension
A. Hydrophobic colloids
B. Hydrophilic colloids
C. Polymeric substance
D. Polymeric substance

2722. Rheology is the study of
A. Viscocity of fluid
B. Flow characteristic
C. Pourability
D. None of the above

2723. Suspending must not affect which of the following property of suspension
A. Viscocity B. Stability
C. Dispersability D. All of the above

2724. Variation in solid content of a suspension intended for oral administration is depending upon which of the following factor

A. Dose of drug to be administration
B. Volume of product desired to be administered
C. Ability of medium to support concentration of drug
D. All of the above

2725. What is the convenient Measure of dose drug for adult oral suspension

A. 2 ml B. 10 ml
C. 5 ml D. None of the Above

2726. Which of the following is considered while delivering dose of pediatric suspension

A. Teaspoon full of dose
B. Tablespoon full of dose
C. Dose calibrated number of drops
D. None of the above

2727. Pediatric suspension containing antibiotic drug commonly reffered as

A. Syrups B.
C. Lotions D. None of the above

2728. Which type of flow involve constant velocity

A. Non-Newtonion B. Pseudo plastic
C. Newtonion D. All of the above

2729. Increase swar rates is characterstic of which type of flow

A. Newtonion B. Dilatant
C. Pseudo plastic D. Non-Newtonion

2730. Which of the following is not considered in newtonion flow

A. Plastic flow B. Pseudo plastic flow
C. Dilatant flow D. All of the above

2731. In which type of flow parallel layers of liquid related to flow with the bottom layer

A. Pseudopalstic B. Plastic
C. Dilatant D. None of the above

2732. Difference of velocity between two planes of liquid separated by distance is known as

A. Rate of shear B. Velocity gradient
C. Shear stress D. Both (a) and (b)

2733. If the velocity is high how it will affect the shearing stress?

A. Required lesser shearing stress
B. Required greater shearing stress
C. No effect
D. Both (a) and (b

2734. Which type of is obtained for Newtonion flow

A. Curved B. Straight line
C. Hyperbola D. Parabola

2735. In which type of flow substance is known as bingham bodies

A. Plastic flow B. Pseudo plastic
C. Dilatant D. None of the above

2736. Which of the following statement is true about plastic

A. Flow curve intersect the shearing stress axis
B. Flow cure does not pass through origin
C. Flow does not begin until shearing stress is exceeded to certain yield value
D. All of the above

2737. In plastic flow below the yield value materials are considered as

A. Rigid B. Flat
C. Elastic D. All of the above

2738. Pseudo plastic substance is also known as

A. Shear thickening system
B. Shear yielding system
C. Shear thinning system
D. None of the above

2739. On which axis molecules align themselves in Pseudoplastic flow

A. Medium axis B. Short axis
C. Long axis D. None of the above

2740. Which of the following is increased with increase in viscocity of dilatant material

A. Shear rate B. Volume
C. Density D. Both (a) and (b)

2741. Which of the following is shear thickening syste

A. Plastic B. Dilatant
C. Pseudo plastic D. Pseudo elastic

2742. Which of the following material consist of high percentage of solid formulation

A. Plastic material
B. Dilatant material
C. Pseudo plastic material
D. All of the above

2743. Which of the following is used when dispersed phase has no affinity for vehicle

A. Suspending agent
B. Thickening agent
C. Wetting Agent
D. Electrolytes

2744. Wetting agent work by Mechanism of

A. Displacing the air
B. Displacing the vehicle
C. displacing the A P I
D. Both (a) and (b)

2745. Which of the following difficulty arise in the formulation of sustained release suspension

A. Stability B. Dispersability
C. Caking D. All of the above

2746. Which of the following system is responsible for sustained release suspension

A. Pour kinetic system
B. Penn kinetic system
C. None of the above
D. Pseudo kinetic system

2747. Which of the following is useful in formulation of sustained release suspension

A. Dissolution complex
B. Dissolution diffusion complex
C. Ion exchange resin complex
D. Entraptment

2748. Which substance is used to coat particle during use of Ion exchange resin complex

A. Methyl cellulose
B. Sodium carboxymethyl cellulose
C. Hydroxymethyl cellulose
D. Ethyl cellulose

2749. Which of the following dosage for is used in prepration of extemporaneous suspension

A. Tablet B. Capsule
C. Both (A) and (B) D. None of the above

2750. Which of the following is not included in the liquid suspension for

A. Colorings B. Alcohols
C. Preservatives D. All of the above

2751. Benzyl alcohol is not used in prepration for neonatic because of risk of which disease

A. Steven Johnson syndrome
B. Hasping syndrome
C. Cushing Syndrome
D. Rett syndrome

2752. Container of suspension is designed to prevent which of the following environment problem

A. Light B. Excessive hea
C. Freezing D. All of the above

2753. Complex or coordination compounds results from

A. Lewis acid base reaction
B. oxidation reaction
C. donor acceptor mechanism
D. both (a) and (c).

2754. Which of these can act as donor in complereation

A. Metallic ion
B. Non- metallic ion
C. Both (a) and (b)
D. None of the above

2755. complex is divided into two classes depending upon

A. Acceptor B. Donor
C. adduct D. None of the above

2756. Which type of forces are included in complex formation

A. London forces
B. Vander wall forces
C. Dipole dipole attraction
D. None of the above

2757. Which of the following is important to metal complexes

A. dispersion forces
B. Hydrogen bonding
C. Co-ordinate covalence
D. All of the above

2758. Which of the following molecule act as Ligand in hexamine cobalt chloride complex

A. Chloride B. Cobalt
C. Ammonia D. None of the above

2759. In complex [CO(NH3)6]3+ Cl3- What is the coordination number of cobalt

A. 3 B. 6
C. 4 D. 5

2760. Which of these link is form between ligand and central atom when ligand donate a pair of electron

A. Hydrogen bond
B. Co-ordinate covalent bond
C. Ionic bond
D. None of the above

2761. Which of the following have an important part in coordinate compound

A. Intermolecular forces
B. Electronic structure
C. Both (a) and (b).
D. Hybridization

2762. Which of these ligand donate a pair of electron in forming a complex with metal ion

A. H2o B. H3N
C. CN D. All of the above

2763. In [N:(CN)4]2 Which of the following complex is formed

A. tetrahedral B. trigonal
C. square planar D. Octahedral

2764. In [CO(NH3)6]3+ which of the following complex is formed

A. Trigonal B. Square planar
C. Tetrahedral D. Octahedral

2765. Which of the following metal ion only form octahedral complex

A. Aluminium B. Nitrogen
C. Cobalt D. None of the above

2766. Compound in which ligand lie above a partially filled orbital are termed as

A. Inner sphere complex
B. Outer sphere complex
C. Both (a) and (b)
D. None of the above

2767. The presence of unpaired electron in a metal ion complex can be detected by

A. Nuclear magnetic resonance
B. Ultraviolet spectroscopy
C. Electron spin resonance spectroscopy

2768. Which of the metal ion form square planar complex

A. Copper B. Nickel
C. Both (a) and (b) D. Iron

2769. Which type of ligand will readily replaced by reaction with chelating agent

A. Metal ion ligand
B. Cis coordinated ligand
C. Both (a) and (b)
D. None of the above

2770. Which of the following substance is incapable of reacting with chelating agent

A. Vitamin B12 B. Bilirubin
C. Heparin D. None of the above

2771. Which of the following is the naturally occurring chelater

A. Chlorophyll B. Bilirubin
C. Histamine D. None of the above

2772. To which of the following metal human serum albumin bind with higher affinity

A. Copper B. Nickel
C. Both (a) and (b) D. zinc

2773. In the process of sequestration the chleating agent and metal ion forms

A. Water soluble compound
B. Oil soluble compound
C. Alcohol soluble compound
D. None of the above

2774. Which of the following chelating agent is used to remove calcium from hard water

A. Diethylenetriamine
B. Ethylene diamine tetra acetic acid
C. Phosphonate
D. Sodium polypartate

2775. Which of the following ligand is monodentate type

A. Pilocarpine B. Carbon monoxide
C. Ammonia D. None of the above

2776. Pilocarpine react with cobalt to form character of which geometry
A. Square planar
B. Pseudo tetrahedral
C. Tetrahedral
D. Octahedral

2777. In pilocarpine ligand the donor atom is of which Ring
A. Pyrole Ring B. Indole Ring
C. Imidazole Ring D. None of the above

2778. Procainamide form complex with cupric ion at which pH
A. 4 B. 6
C. 8 D. 3

2779. Bond distance between the components of the complex is
A. >3A B. 2A
C. 1A D. None of the above

2780. Which type of interaction exist in the charge transfer complex
A. Electrostatic interaction
B. Ionic interaction
C. diapolediapole interaction
D. None of the above

2781. Which of the following force is responsible for the stability of complex
A. London dispersion force
B. Dipole Dipole interaction
C. Both (a) and (b)
D. None of the above

2782. In trinitro benzene the intermolecular distance between two molecule is
A. 4.3A B. 5.3A
C. 2.3A D. 3.3A

2783. In charge transfer complex which of these have important contribution to complereation
A. Inductive effect B. Resonance
C. Mesomeric effect D. None of the above

2784. Organic complex that cannot be separated from their solution as definite compound, the energy of attraction between the constituent of these complex is
A. <5 kcal/mole B. >5 kcal/mole
C. <4 kcal/mole D. <3 kcal/mole

2785. Molecular complexes hacks of
A. Dipole dipole interaction
B. Vander wall forces
C. Charge transfer
D. Hydrogen bonds

2786. Which of the following complex do not show any new absorption bands
A. Charge transfer complex
B. Molecular complexes
C. Donor acceptor complex
D. Both (a) and (c)

2787. Iodine form charge transfer complex with .... in which ratio
A. 2:2 B. 3:2
C. 1:3 D. 1:1

2788. Which of these complex iron form with disulfiram
A. Charge transfer
B. Donor acceptor
C. Molecular complex
D. None of the above

2789. Which force of attraction is responsible for complex formation between caffeine and sulphonamide
A. London dispersion force
B. Vander wall force
C. Ionic forces
D. Hydrogen bond

2790. Which of these group is enter responsible for formation of complex
A. Electrophilic carbonyl oxygen
B. Nucleophilic carbonyl oxygen
C. Alkyl group
D. None of the above

2791. Caffeine for more soluble complexes with
A. Ester cation
B. Ester anion
C. Organic acid anion
D. Organic acid cation

2792. Chewable tablets formulated from caffeine - organic acid complex should provide

A. Extended Release
B. Immediate Release
C. Modified Release
D. Sustained Release

2793. Which of the following parameter is affected by complereation of drug and complereing agent

A. Drug absorption
B. Drug metabolism
C. Drug bioavailability
D. Both (a) and (c).

2794. Which of these incompatibilities may arise during formation of polymer complexes

A. Precipitation
B. Flocculation
C. Delayed biologic absorption
D. All of the above

2795. The interaction of cross povidone to many drug is due to

A. Vinyl group of cross povidone
B. Phenolic group of drug
C. Alkyl group of drug
D. None of the above

2796. Cross povidone is used as

A. Diluent B. Binder
C. Disintegrant D. Lubricant

2797. Dissolution rate of azamaline is enhanced by complereation with

A. PVP B. Caffeine
C. Polytyrene D. Iodine

2798. Complereation force in azamaline and PVP is

A. London dispersion force
B. Vander wall force
C. Hydrogen bond
D. dipole dipole interaction

2799. Which of the following is not included in inclusion compound?

A. Channel lattice B. Layer type
C. Clathrate D. Polymer complexes

2800. Which of the following is not included in inclusion compound

A. Channel lattice
B. Polymer complexes
C. Layer type
D. Clathrate

2801. Cholic acid for which type of inclusion complexes

A. Channel type B. Layer type
C. Clathrate D. None of the above

2802. Which type of complex thio urea formed with unbranched paraffin

A. Clathrate B. Layer type
C. Polymer D. Channel lattice

2803. In channel type complex of starch Iodine solution Iodine molecule entrapped within:

A. Fructose Residue
B. Amylase Residue
C. Lactose Residue
D. Glucose Residue

2804. Which of the following compound trap hydrocarbon in layer of their lattice

A. Graphite
B. Clay
C. Montmorillonite
D. All of the above

2805. Which of these is not involved in the formation of clatharates

A. Chemical bond B. Molecular size
C. Stability D. None of the above

2806. Which of the following is important about encaged compound in clathrates

A. Stability
B. Molecular size
C. Molecular structure
D. All of the above

2807. Stability of a Clathrate is due to

A. Size of structure
B. Strength of structure
C. Arrangement of structure
D. All of the above

2808. Which of these molecule cannot be trapped in cages formed by hydroquinone Clathrate

A. Methanol B. CO2
C. Ethanol D. HCl

2809. Which of these cannot used to resolve optical activity

A. Channel lattice
B. Layer type Inclusion
C. Clathrates
D. All of the above

2810. Which of these Anticoagulant drug is included in Inclusion compound in US pharmacopoeia

A. Heparin B. Warfarin sodium
C. Dicumarol D. Dabigatrin

2811. Which of these is involve in formation of Clathrate with Warfarin

A. Metyl Alcohol B. Ethanol
C. Isopropyl alcohol D. Isobutyl alcohol

2812. In monomolecular Inclusion compound which compound represent host structure

A. Polyethylene glycol
B. Niacinamide
C. Cyclodextrin
D. Carboxy methyl cellulose

2813. Cyclodextrin formed from unit of

A. Glucopyranose
B. Glucorhamnose
C. Lactorahmnose
D. Galactopyranose

2814. How many units of Glucopyranose combined to form the alpha Cyclodextrin

A. 5 B. 6
C. 8 D. 7

2815. The ability of Cyclodextrin to form inclusion compound in aqueous solution is due to

A. Ionisation of glucose unit
B. Arrangement of Glucose unit
C. Size of the glucose unit
D. All of the above

2816. Which type of Ring is formed by Cyclodextrin in inclusion compound

A. Doughnut ring
B. Spherical ring
C. Ring
D. Both (a) and (c)

2817. The molecule of Cyclodextrin is exist as

A. Flatten cube
B. edgic flattened cylinder
C. Truncated cone
D. Truncated pyramid

2818. One to which of specific interest Cyclodextrin containing polymer is used

A. Delivery of protein
B. Delivery of carbohydrates
C. Delivery of nucleic acid
D. Delivery of minerals

2819. Aziridine Ring of Mitomycin is protected from degradation in acidic solution due to interaction with

A. Alpha Cyclodextrin
B. Beta Cyclodextrin
C. Gamma Cyclodextrin
D. All of the above

2820. In Pharmaceutical dosage form Cyclodextrin is used as

A. Solubilizer B. Stabilizer
C. Both (a) and (b D. Viscosity builder

2821. Dissolution rate of which drug is increased by complereation with B – Cyclodextrin

A. Formatidine B. Metformine
C. Testosterone D. Benzoine

2822. Cyclodextrin increase or decrease the reactivity of guest molecule depending upon

A. Nature of reaction
B. Rate of reaction
C. Structure of molecule
D. Size of molecule

2823. OH group in Cyclodextrin undergo which reaction to reduce intermolecular hydrogen bonding

A. Nitration B. Alkylation
C. Cyclisation D. Isomerisation

2824. Haemolytic activity observed in some Cyclodextrin due to

A. Minimal solubility of water
B. Minimal removal of water
C. Low surface tension of water
D. All of the above

2825. Hydrophobic form of which Cyclodextrin derivative is found useful as sustained release drug carriers

A. Alpha B. Beta
C. Gamma D. All of the above

2826. Ethylated B Cyclodextrin has been used to retard the delivery of which vasodilator

A. Isosorbidedinitrate
B. Isosorbidemononitrate
C. Nitroprusside
D. Nitroglycerin

2827. Which of the reason is related to formation of complex of .... With B- Cyclodextrin

A. Mark bitter taste of drug
B. Provide stability to dosage form
C. Increase solubility of drug
D. Increase solubility of drug

2828. Zeolites and Silica gels are

A. Monomolecular inclusion compounds
B. Molecular sieves
C. Macro molecular Inclusion compound
D. Both (a) and (c)

2829. Which of these inclusion compounds is capable of ion exchange

A. Silica gel B. Zeolites
C. Dextrins D. Nicotinamide

2830. The equation of complereation is

A. M - nA = MAn
B. M+nA= MAn
C. A+Nm = AMn
D. None

2831. Which of these is correct equation for stability constant for complex formation

A. K = [MAn]\[M] [A]n
B. K = -[MAn]\[M] [A]n
C. K = [A] [M]n\ [MAn]
D. None

2832. If solution of two species A and B of equal molar concentration are mixed and if a complex form between the two species the value of additive property will pass through

A. Maximum
B. Minimum
C. No effect on additive property
D. Both (a) and (b)

2833. The concentration of which of the following is kept constant in spectro-photometric analysis

A. Ligand B. Metal ion
C. Complex D. Both (a) and (b)

2834. By using job method complex of which composition is obtained

A. 3:2 B. 1:1
C. 2:1 D. 1:2

2835. In pH titration method the addition of glycin to a solution containing cupric ion result in

A. Increase in pH B. Decrease in pH
C. No effect on Ph D. None of the above

2836. In equation M + nA = M A n quantity n donates the

A. Number of metal ion
B. Number of ligand molecule
C. Number of reactions
D. Number of complex formed

2837. For each species of complex n has a

A. Definite value
B. variable value
C. Value depend on complex
D. None of the above

2838. The value of n and p [A] at various pH values are platted the curve that is obtained is known as

A. Stability curve
B. Titration curve
C. Complereation curve
D. Formation curve

2839. Schwarzenbach method can be used as substitute of which method

A. Complereometric method
B. Gravimetric method
C. Potentiometric method
D. All of the above

2840. Lithium form complex with the Zwitterionic species of catecholamines at which pH

A. 9-10 B. 11-14
C. 7-8 D. 4-6

2841. The interaction of catecholamines with lithium depends on:

A. Dissociation of Phenolic oxygen
B. Dissociation of Phenolic oxygen
C. All of the above
D. Orientation of active group

2842. Which of these method is not used to study complexation

A. X-Ray diffraction
B. IR spectroscopy
C. HPLC
D. None of the above

2843. Caffeine interact with L-tryptophan at molar ratio of

A. 2:1 B. 1:2
C. 2:2 D. 1:1

2844. Complexation is a result of

A. Polarisation B. PI-PI Interaction
C. Both (A) and (B) D. Ionisation

2845. Caffine form complexation with which aromatic amino acid

A. L-valine B. L-tryptophan
C. L-lucin D. None of the above

2846. Binding of the catecholamine, Norepinephrine and Isoproterenol can be studied by which method

A. IR-Spectroscopy
B. X-Ray diffraction
C. Electron diffraction
D. Circular dichroism

2847. Most m-RNA consist of region of which acid

A. Polyadenylic acid
B. Galactonic acid
C. Galic acid
D. None of the above

2848. IR-Spectroscopy is used to determine which complexes in which polyfunctional bases are involved

A. Hydrogen bonded
B. Vanderwall force bonded
C. Covelent force bonded
D. None of the above

2849. Which of these bond formed by caffeine-phenol complex

A. Covalent bond B. Ionic bond
C. Hydrogen bond D. Metallic bond

2850. From IR technique Incaffiene hydrogen bonding sides are

A. Amine function B. Carbonyl function
C. Amide functioin D. Easter function

2851. Most of the complexes with caffeine are formed at which position of caffeine

A. Position 3 B. Position 4
C. Position 5 D. Position 6

2852. Least favourable position of caffeine for complexation is

A. Position 2 B. Position 3
C. Position 1 D. Position 5

2853. Which of the following titration method is used to determine 1:1 complex of uranyl-tetracycline

A. Potentiometric B. Complexometric
C. Conductometric D. Gravimetric

2854. Complexation is widely used in pharmaceutical sciences to improve which property

A. Absorption B. Solubility
C. Bioavailability D. All of the above

2855. At which wavelength adenine catechol stability constant for charge transfer complexation is measured

A. 250nm B. 560nm
C. 340nm D. 180nm

2856. In caffeine PABA complex when the caffene is added the total acid concentration of saturation is

A. 4.58*10-2mole\litre
B. 5.31*10-2mole\litre
C. 2.14*10-2mole\litre
D. 6.39*10-2mole\litre

2857. Wheniodine is distributed between water and carbondisulphide at 250c the distribution coefficient is found to be

A. 619 B. 642
C. 600 D. 625

2858. Which of these following Method is used to determined the compleseation of p- amino Benzoic acid by caffeine?

A. Distribution Method
B. Solubility Method
C. PH titration method
D. Potentiometric Method

2859. Addition of caffiene to PABA is responsible for:

A. Increase solubility of PABA
B. Increase Stability of PABA
C. Increase compleseation of PABA
D. Both A and C

2860. Absorption spectroscopy is commonly used to determine:

A. Change transfer Complex
B. Mono molecular Inclusion complex
C. Clathrates
D. None

2861. Iodine is analysed in a CCL4 the curve for this a analysis is obtain at:

A. 610 nm B. 520 nm
C. 430 nm D. 240 nm

2862. The ability of donor to donate electron is determined by its

A. Partition coefficient
B. Dielectric constant
C. Ionization potential
D. None of the above

2863. The complexation constant K is determine by use of

A. U V Spectroscopy
B. IRT Spectroscopy
C. MASS Spectroscopy
D. All of the above

2864. Distribution Method Of distributing absolute between two immiscible solvent can be used to determined

A. Ratio of ligand to metal
B. Stability constant
C. Types of complex formed
D. None of the above

2865. The Stability constant for compleration of Iodine by potassium Iodine determined by which method?

A. PH Titration Method
B. Solubility Method
C. Distribution Method
D. Both A and B

2866. In determination of solubility constant of complex of Iodine the distribution law expresses concentration of:

A. Free Iodine
B. Bound Iodine
C. Both A and B
D. Potassium Iodine

2867. The total concentration of Iodine in aqueous phase can be determined by:

A. Physical Method
B. Analytical Method
C. Chemical method
D. All of above

2868. The Stability constant for the benzoic acid caffeine at 0* C is:

A. 30.5 B. 37.5
C. 47.6 D. 28.5

2869. Which statement is true for variation in Stability constant of coffiene complex in aquous solution?

A. Coffiene Ionised in aqueous solution
B. All of the above

2870. Which of these following method is used to determine the complexarion of p-aminobenzoic acid by caffeine

A. Distribution Method
B. Solubility method
C. Ph titration method
D. Potentiometric method

2871. The ability of donor to donate electron is determined by its

A. Partition coefficient
B. Dielectric constant
C. Ionisation potential
D. None

2872. The complexation constant K is determine by use of :

A. UV-Spectroscopy
B. IR Spectroscopy
C. Mass Spectroscopy
D. All of the above

2873. Absorbece of the charge transfer band is measured at a definite wavelength, K is readily obtained by which equation

A. Henderson-hasselbalch equation
B. Benesi-hilder brand equation
C. Cran-pottermold equation
D. None

2874. Which of these method is not used to study comlexation

A. X-Ray Diffraction B. IR Spectroscopy
C. Polarography D. HPLC

2875. Complexation of caffeine with L-Tryptophan can be determined by
A. NMR Spectroscopy
B. IR Spectroscopy
C. Polarography
D. Circular dichroism

2876. Which of the following of weak force
A. Vander wall force
B. Covalent
C. Ionic bond
D. Both a and b

2877. Which force give rise to the fluidity and cohesiveness of the membrane under normal physiologic condition
A. Van der wall force
B. Ionic bond
C. London force
D. None of the above

2878. Who pointed to the analogy between human behaviour and molecular phenomenon as the molecular governed by attractive and repulsive force
A. Moelwynhughes
B. Johannes diderik vander wall
C. Fritz London
D. Peter J W debye

2879. The three dipolar forces of keesom, debye and London are called as
A. Ionic force
B. Vander wall force
C. Covalent bond
D. None of the above

2880. Hydrogen bond or hygrogen bridge was discovered by
A. Rodebush and latimer
B. Moelwynhughis
C. Latimer
D. Rodebush

2881. Which bond Is exits in between alcohol molecules carboxylic acid
A. Hydrogen bond
B. Ion ion interaction
C. London force
D. Vander wall force

2882. Freeze dry is also kmown as
A. Spray drying
B. Lipophilization
C. Tray drying
D. None of the above

2883. The process in which solid directly convert into gaseos state without melting known as
A. Condensation B. Deposition
C. Sublimation D. Both A and B

2884. The process in which non version of a vapour or gas to a liquid is known as
A. Sublimation
B. Condensation
C. Deposition
D. Mesophase

2885. Which of the following is bayles law
A. PV= k B. PK=V
C. P 1/v D. Both a and c

2886. 1 atmosphere equal to
A. 1.0133*106 dynes/ Cm3
B. 1.0133*106 dynes/ m3
C. 1.0133*107 dynes/ Cm3
D. 1.133*106 dynes/ Cm3

2887. Lighter gas diffuses more rapidly through pkorousmembreane than does a behavior one relation is discovered by
A. Graham
B. Fritz London
C. Peter j w debye
D. None of the above

2888. On which factor does the average kinectic energy (E) is depend
A. Nature of gas B. Temperature
C. Volume D. Mass

2889. A gas behaves as an ideal gas
A. Low pressure & high temperature
B. Low pressure and low temperature
C. High pressure & low temperature
D. High pressure & high temperature

2890. The concept of fugacity was introduced by
A. Lewis B. Charles darvin
C. Svartearrhenivs D. Linus pauling

2891. The temperature above which a liquid can no longer exist is known as

A. Critical temperature
B. Critical pressure
C. Supercritical fluids
D. None of the above

2892. What is critical temperature of water

A. 3000C B. 3740C
C. 6740C D. 640C

2893. Which of following gas is responsible for ozone depletion

A. Clorofloro carbon
B. Hydro floro carbon
C. Both a and b
D. None of the above

2894. Which type of drug are used in arosols

A. Non volatile drug
B. Volatile drug
C. Aromatic
D. Both A AND B

2895. In case of DNA protein etc. which route gives higher bioavalabilty in aerosols

A. Pulmonary route B. Nasal route
C. Oral route D. Both A AND B

2896. BYRON $ CLARK researched on which type of thing

A. Drug absorption from inhalation
B. Drug adsorption from inhalation
C. Drug absorption from emulsion
D. None of the above

2897. What is the specific range of pressure is there in aerosols

A. 1-6 ATM B. 1-5 ATM
C. 1-7 ATM D. 2-6 ATM

2898. CLAUSIUS – CLAPEYRAM equation based on which principle

A. realtion between vapour pressure $ absolute temperature
B. realtion between high pressure $ absolute temperature
C. realtion between low pressure $ high temperature
D. None of the above

2899. If we decreases the pressure the boiling point will be ...... ?

A. Lowered B. Both A AND B
C. increased D. None of the above

2900. If any substance have same structure but have different structure apppearance.....?

A. Habit B. Crystal
C. solid D. Polymorph

2901. Which of the following is known as electron gas?

A. Negatively charged ion in a field of furelly moving electron
B. Positively charged ion in a field of furelly moving electron
C. Negatively charged ion in a field of furelly moving electron
D. None of the above

2902. Diamond is which type of crystalline form of carbon.....?

A. metastable B. Tetrastable
C. parastable D. None of the above

2903. Which of the substance existing in four polymorphic form....?

A. Cacao butter B. Theobrama oil
C. Coca butter D. None of the above

2904. Who reported that form II of sulfameter an antibacterial agent....?

A. Khalili et al B. Aguiar et al
C. Azibi et al D. None of the above

2905. Goldberg $ becker studied which crystalline form...?

A. Tamoxifer citrate
B. Tetbedral crystal
C. polymprph
D. Pseudopolymorph

2906. The properties of polymoprhs such as enantiotropism $ momotropism are described by....?

A. Khalil et al B. Aguviar et al
C. Behme et al D. None of the above

2907. The polymorph crystal is constructed of bondimerised molecules of spiperone is described by

A. Azibi et al B. Khalili et al
C. Behme et al D. Aguviar et al

2908. The force below which the body shows 32 pg elastic properties is known as...?

A. Plastic yield B. Yield value
C. Elastic value D. None of the above

2909. The first approximation the amorphous solids are considered as…?

A. Supercooled liquid
B. Lattice form
C. Cooled liquid
D. Polymorphism

2910. X-RAY having which of the wavelength a order of inter atomic distance…?

A. 1.84 B. 1.54
C. 2 D. 1.98

2911. Which n of the following is clapeyron equation

A. (P1P2)=HvapR(1T2−1T1)
B. (P1P2)=ΔHvapR(1T1−1T2)
C. n(P2P1)=ΔHvapR(1T1−1T2)
D. n(P1P2)=ΔHvapR(1T2−1T1)

2912. Melting point of CH4

A. 95.5 k B. 90.5 k
C. 100.5 k D. 80 k

2913. Which of the following has highest melting point…?

A. 0.9988 G/CM3
B. 0.9888 G/CM3
C. 0.998 G/CM
D. NONE OF THE ABOVE

2914. What is the density of ice at 00 C

A. 0.9268 G/CM2 B. 0.9142 G/CM3
C. 0.9168 G/CM3 D. 0.9542 G/CM3

2915. WHY THE MELTING POINT of normal saturated hydrocarbons incras with increase with molecular weight

A. B/C OF VANDER WAAL FORCE
B. b/c of London force
C. b/c of ionic bond
D. None of the above

2916. The melting point of the alkanes is increase when they have _______ number of carbon atoms

A. Even number B. Equal number
C. Odd number D. Both A AND B

2917. THE MELTING point and soubilites of the xanthines in pharmaceutical interest was determined by?

A. Guttman andhiguchi
B. Khalili et al
C. Behme al
D. Aguvia et al

2918. Liquid crystalline os also known as..?

A. polumorph B. mesophase
C. Solid phase D. Supercooled phase

2919. Which of the are the types of liquid crystals

A. Nematic
B. smetic
C. Both A AND B
D. NONE OF THE ABOVE

2920. The first observation of thermotropic liquid was recoreded by ....?

A. reinitzer B. guttman
C. Khalili et al D. higuchi

2921. Which of the following is the example of liquid crystal..?

A .CHOLA B. MBBA
C.BOTH A AND B D. None of the above

2922. Generally nematic liquid crystals are sensitive to ....?

A. Electric field
B. Magnetic field
C. temperature
D. None of the above

2923. Who applied the principle of liquid crystal formation to the soulbilization $ DISSOLTUON of chlesterol

A. guttman B. bogarclus
C. higuchi D. None of the above

2924. Friedberg wrote monograph on which topic….?

A. Liquid crytals B. Solid crystals
C. amorphous D. crystalline

2925. Ibrahim studied the release of salicyclic acid as a model of ....?

A. Drug form lyotropic liquid crystalline
B. Solid phase of drug
C. Both A AND B
D, NONE OF THE ABOVE

2926. What is the uses of supercritical fluid ......?
A. Extraction
B. Crystallization
C. Both A AND B
D. NONE OF THE ABOVE

2927. Decaffination of coffee can be done by...?
A. Supercritical fluid
B. By distilation
C. filteration
D. None of the above

2928. Which of the following Is a type of thermal analysis ....?
A. DTA B. DSC
C. TGA D. All of the above

2929. Dielectric analysis is used to detect.....?
A. Momogeneity of sample
B. Dielectric constant
C. Microscopic visocity
D. viscocity

2930. All what temperature dsc measurement indicate endothermic reaction ....?
A. 1240 C B. 1200 C
C. 1100 C D. 1000 C

2931. Identity the correct phase rule equation /formula...?
A. F=C+P+2 B. F=C+P-2
C. F=C+(2+F) D. F=C-P+2

2932. Differential scanning calorimetery is measurement of
A. Heat flow
B. Pressure flow
C. Both A NAD B
D. NONE OF THE ABOVE

2933. CRYSTAL CHANGE $ eutectic formulation in frozen state can be detected by...?
A. DSC B. DTA
C. Both a AND B D. None of the above

2934. Dsc is generally used in pharmacy to establish of ...?
A. Purity B. Identity
C. Analysis D. All of the above

2935. Who formulated phase rule ...?
A. j. Wilarbgibbs B. higuchi
C. Guttman D. None of the above

2936. Thermal analysis application explored by ....?
A. Guillary associates
B. Guttman
C. J.wwillarbgibbs
D. None of the above

2937. What is gibbs phase rule gas liquid or solid..?
A. F=C-P+2 B. F=B-P+2
C. F=C-P-1 D. F=C-P+3

2938. WHAT IS THE DEGREE OF freedom at circle point for water...?
A. 2 B. 3
C. 1 D. 0

2939. Three phase system of ice water vapour to the temperature pr pressure the combination is fixed $unique is known as...?
A. Critical point
B. Supercritical point
C. Iso electric
D. None of the above

2940. At what temperature phenol $ water miscible in each other ....?
A. 66.80 C B. 65.80 C
C. 67.80 C D. None of the above

2941. At which temperature nicotine water solid liquid are miscible on together?
A. Less than 60.8 B. More than 208
C. Both A AND B D. 110

2942. Which of the following is a example of solid dispersion ?
A. Eutecticsyste m B. biphasic
C. Polyphasicsyste D. None of the above

2943. What is the freezing point of phenol-water system...?
A. 7 B. 3.5
C. 4.5 D. 3

2944. Who studied phenol water system...?
A. handmeyar B. higuchi
C. mulley D. guttman

2945. The triple point of air free water is...?
A. 0.0098 B. 0.01
C. 1 D. 0.028

2946. At what properties phenol and water will be missible at 66.8…?
A. 25% phenol, 75% water
B. 24% phenol, 76% water
C. 22% phenol, 78% water
D. None of the these

2947. What is the melting point of pure thymol../
A. 55 B. 60
C. 50 D. 40

2948. What is the melting point of pure salol…?
A. 50 B. 45
C. 60 D. 40

2949. Phenomenon in which substance exist in more than one form is ..?
A. crystalline
B. Polymorphism
C. Anisotropy
D. polycrystalinity

2950. Polymorphism refers to compound having ………?
A. Different crystal structure
B. Different stereochemistry
C. Different composition
D. All of the above

2951. Amorphous form of a drug dissolves as compared to crystalline form..?
A. slower B. faster
C. equal D. half

2952. Property of amorphous solids..?
A. No crystal structure
B. No definite melting point
C. glassy
D. All of the above

2953. Conversion of solid to gas directly is..?
A. Fusion B. Sublimination
C. Boiling D. Evaporation

2954. Conversion of ice to water by heat process with…?
A. Increase in energy decrease in entropy
B. Increase in energy increase in entropy
C. decrease in energy increase in entropy
D. Decrease in energy decrease in entropy

2955. Triple point of water…?
A. 0.0075 B. 0.01
C. 0.101 D. 0.001

2956. Heat needed to change a state of matter…?
A. Latent heat
B. Vapour heat
C. Fusion heat
D. Condensation heat

2957. Characteristics of solid…?
A. Ability of diffuse
B. Indefinite volume
C. Definite volume
D. Indefinite shape

2958. Liquid crystalline state is called as..?
A. Amorphous
B. Polymorphs
C. Mesophase
D. dispersion

2959. Repulsive $ attractive forces are equal at a distance of..?
A. 2*10 B. 3*10
C. 3*10 D. ¾*10

2960. When repulsive $ attractive forces are equal than at this position..?
A. Kinietic energy is minimum
B. Kinietic energy= potential energy
C. Potential energy is minimum
D. None of the above

2961. Large groups of molecules are associated through weak attraction knowm as…?
A. Dipole –dipole force
B. Keesam force
C. Both of the above
D. Dipole induse dipole

2962. The vander wall force are P.E OF ATTRACTION…?
A. r B. 1/r
C. 1/r D. None of the above

2963. The phase that lies betwwn liquid $ crystalline state is ..?
A. Subline phase B. mesophase
C. Solid phase D. None of the above

2964. At a constant temperature for a given mass of forces which laws relates the volume $pressure..?
A. Boyles law B. Charles law
C. Gay-lausac law D. Both a and b

2965. Mineral oil immiscible with water that process powerfull cohesive forces due to..?
A. High internal pressure
B. Low internal pressure
C. Equal pressure
D. None of the above

2966. Transition from gas to liquid $ from liquid to solid depend on ....?
A. Temperature
B. Pressure to which it is subjected
C. Both of the above
D. None of the above

2967. The temperature at which a real gas obeys the ideal gas laws over a wide range of pressure is............?
A. Critical temperature
B. Inversion temperature
C. Boyle temperature
D. Reduce temperature

2968. When molecule collides to one another oe with wall of confining vessel there is no net loss of speed this property is..?
A. plasticity B. elasicity
C. Both of the above D. None of the above

2969. The rate of diffusion of a gas is inversely proportional to the square root of the density of that gas this is that statement of ....?
A. Dalton s law B. Charles law
C. Boyle law D. Grahams law

2970. The study of fundamental and derived properties of individual and collection of particles is termed as..?
A. micromerities
B. Coarse dispersion
C. rheology
D. Colloidal dispersion

2971. THE TERMED micromerities was given by..?
A. Kozney-carman B. Dale valle
C. both D. None of these

2972. PARTICLE SIZE is measured by..?
A. poise B. micrometer
C. stoke D. none

2973. 1 Mm is____________M...?
A. 0.1 B. 0.01
C. 1 D. 0.001

2974. COARSE powder range is in between ________?
A. 0.5-10 Mm B. 50-100Mm
C. 150-1000Mm D. 10-50Mm

2975. Fine particles have apron sieve size range in between ____?
A. 0.5-10 B. 325-140
C. 100-18 D. 18-6

2976. What is cause of food poisoning....?
A. Salmonella enteridis
B. s.typhimurium
C. s.typhosa
D. Pseudomonas diminuta

2977. Diameter of an equivalent sphere undergoing sedimentation at the same rate that of asymmetric particle is termed as...?
A. Surface diameter
B. Stokes diameter
C. Volume surface diameter
D. Sieve diameter

2978. The size of stokes diameter is expressed as...........?
A. Ds B. Dsd
C. Dst D. Dsv

2979. AVERAGE particle size equation derived by....?
A. edmundson
B. Kozney-carmon
C. Dale-valle
D. None of the above

2980. General equation for the calculation of average particle size ....?
A. xn+10 B. xn2+1
C. xn+1 D. xn-1

2981. WHEN THE NUMBER OE WT OF particle lying in a certain size range is polt against the size range is termed as....?
A. Rheogram
B. Frequency distribution curve
C. Volume distribution curve
D. Histogram

2982. A method for determining the particle size is...?
A. Optical microscopy
B. Sieving method
C. Both A AND B
D. ONLY A

2983. MEASURMENT of particle volume is done by which apparatus.................?
A. microscope
B. Coulter-counter
C. Measuring cycliner
D. Both A AND B

2984. THE range of optical microscopy is ...?
A. 0.5-500Mm B. 1-200Mm
C. 50-1500Mm D. 0.2-100Mm

2985. In optical microscopy particle size is measured by........?
A. Ferret diameter
B. Martin diameter
C. Projected area diameter
D. all

2986. DISADVANTAGE of use of optical microscopy method is...?
A. Diameter is obtained from only two dimensions
B. Large amount of sample is required
C. Slow and tedious
D. all

2987. Size range of sieving method ...?
A. 0.2-100 Mm B. 15-2000Mm
C. 50-1500Mm D. 0.5-500Mm

2988. Sieving errors can be arise by ..?
A. Sieve loading
B. Duration of agitation
C. Intensity of agitation
D. all

2989. IN sedimentation method the size is expressed by.........?
A. Projected diameter
Ferret diameter
Stokes diameter
Surface diameter

2990. The rate of sedimentation is calculated by...?
A. Stoke law B. Henry law
C. Both D. None of the above

2991. For the applicable of stokes law the low of dispersion media around the particle is...?
A. Laminar B. Turbulent
C. Streamline D. Both A AND B

2992. IS REYNOLDS number is a dimensionless and is denoted by RE...?
A. TRUE FALSE B. TRUE FALSE
C. FALSE FALSE D. TRUE TRUE

2993. EVALUATION of sediment particles is done by which method...?
A. Pipette method
B. Balance method
C. Hydrometer method
D. all

2994. The range of particle size measured by conductivity method is ....?
A. 0.5-500Mm
B. 0.2-200Mm
C. 50-1500Mm
D. 1-200Mm

2995. The size of particle volume is expressed as ....?
A. Volume diameter
B. Surface diameter
C. Paricle diameter
D. Projected diameter

2996. The instrument of conductivity method is capable of counting particle upto ....?
A. 40000 B. 400
C. 4000 D. 40

2997. Advantages of coulter counted are...?
A. To study particle growth and dissolution
B. Effect of antibacterial agent on the growth of microorganism
C. Both
D. None of the above

2998. Which instrument is use to measure the particulate contamination in parental solution..?
A. HiAC INSTRUMENT
B. ROYCO INSTRUMENT
C. BOTH
D. NONE OF THE ABOVE

2999. THE HIAC/ROYCO instrument is work on the principle of...?
A. Light blockage
B. Ultracentrifugation
C. Both A AND B
D. NONE OF THE ABOVE

3000. THE COULTER MODEL N4 INSTRUMENT GIVES INFORMATION ABOUT...?
A. PARTICLE SIZE and size distribution
B. Molecular weight
C. Diffusion coeffient
D. all

3001. The shape affects which properties of powder..?
A. Only flow properties
B. Only packaging properties
C. BOTH flow and packaging properties
D. None of the above

3002. If the particle is asymmetric then the surface area per unit volume is...........?
A. Greater B. Smaller
C. Equal D. none

3003. The ratio of surface area and volume from one diameter to another is
A. Relationship between two measurements
B. Relationships of two volumes
B. Relationship between two volumes
D. No Relation

3004. If the particle is shape then the ratio of xs/xv is....?
A. 6 B. More than 6
C. Less than 6 D. None

3005. If the particle shape is asymmetric then the ratio of xs/xv is...?
A. 6 B. More than 6
C. Less than 6 D. None

3006. Methods for determining surface area are.......?
A. Adsorption method
B. Air permeability method
C. Absorption method
D. Both a and b

3007. Bet stands for
A. Brumener Emmett teller equation
B. Bismuth enotoxin test
C. Bachelor endotoxin test
D. Bioequivalence endotoxin test

3008. Types of packaging arrangement ...?
A. Only close packing
B. Only coose packing
C. Both coose and close packing
D. Other than this

3009. Powder have porosity in between ...?
A. 30-50% B. 20-40%
C. 35-55% D. 40-60%

3010. Methods for determing density is ..?
A. True density
B. Tapped density
C. Granule density
D. all

3011. Hausners ratio is...?
A. Tap density/bulk density
B. Bulk density/true density
C. Bulk density/tap density
D. Tap volume/bulk volume

3012. Frictional force in a loose powder can be calculated by..?
A. True density B. Tap density
C. Hausner ratio D. Angle of repose

3013. What kingd of flow is if angle of repose is 25...?
A. Excellent B. Good
C. Very good D. Very poor

3014. What is angle of repose of dextrose..?
A. 15 B. 20
C. 16 D. 25

3015. What is true density of starch..?
A. 1.43 B. 2.75
C. 27.5 D. 5.59

3016. What is true density of sucrose...?
A. 1.75 B. 1.6
C. 2.9 D. 10.1

3017. WHAT is density of charcoal...?
A. 2.1-2.3 B. 5.9
C. 4.9 D. 7.8

3018. Which of the following is method used in determining particle surface area..?

A. Air permeability

B. Absorption

C. conductivity

D. BOTH A AND B

3019. Which of the apparatus used in conductivity method …?

A. Counter coulter method

B. Subscine

C. A and b

D. None of the above

3020. How many particles are count per second in coulter counter method..?

A. 2000 B. 3000

C. 1000 D. 4000

3021. What is being determined by conductivity method..?

A. Particle volume

B. Particle size

C. Particle diameter

D. All of them

3022. Which of the following apparatus is used to determine particle size by gravity..?

A. Hoeppler

B. Andreason apparatus

C. Multi point viscometer

D. None of them

3023. What is the size range of particle used in sedimentation method..?

A. 1-200 B. 0.5-200

C. 50-1500 D. None of them

3024. Which of the following diameter is used to express diameter of a sphere that passes throughsieve apertor.............?

A. Dv B. Ds

C. Dst D. Dp

3025. From which material sieves are made ......?

A. Brass B. Brone

C. Stainless still D. All of them

3026. What is lower limit of paticle size in sieving method............?

A. 60 B. 10

C. 0.14 D. 50

3027. During sieving method what occurs cause size reduction of particle ....?

A. Attrition B. Compact

C. Impact D. None of them

3028. Which of the following things we can determine by optical microscopy

A. Particle size analysis in suspension

B. Particle size distribution in emulsion

C. Particle size analysis in aerosol

D. All of them

3029. Which of the following terms define it is the length of the line that bisects the image ....?

A. Martin diameter

B. Ferret diameter

C. Progeeted area

D. None of them

3030. WHICH of the following terms define as the sum of particle size divided by the no of particles..............?

A. Arithmetic mean

B. Geometric mean

C. Harmonic mean

D. NONE OF THEM

3031. _______ is NOT a physical property of drug substance being evaluated during preformulation studies?

A. Solubility

B. Degradation profile

C. Particle size distribution

D. Crystalline or amorphous nature

3032. Which of the following equation represents volume surface mean diameter?

A. $Xv = (6V/\pi)^{1/3}$ B. $Xsv = 6V/S$

C. $ds = \frac{\sqrt{\ } Ap}{\pi}$ D. $dv = dt/V$

3033. Which of the following equation represent volume weighed mean diameter?

A. $Q_0(x) = \int q0\,(x)dx$

B. $Q_r(x) = \int \quad \alpha(x)r - \frac{tq1x}{\alpha(x)xr}$

C. M_{k1r} = Mk+r-t, t/Mr-t, t

D. $X_{k,\,r} = \sqrt[K]{\ }\,Mk, r$

3034. Which of the following equation represents mean weight diameter?

A. $M_{WD}=\sum$ i=1nwix-i

B. Y=mx+c

C. $M_{WD}=\sum_{i=1}^{n} xiWi$

D. D=M/V

3035. Dissolution of a drug particle is described by

A. Drag's equation

B. Stock's equation

C. Noyes-Whitney equation

D. None of the above

3036. What is the particle size range of psuedometer..?

A. 0.8 B. 0.5

C. 0.6 D. 0.4

3037. What is the size of human hair ....?

A. 30 B. 80

C. 60 D. 70

3038. Which of the following bacteria causes ropiness in milk..?

A. Alcaligenes viscolactis

B. Alcaligenes viscolactis

C, subtiles

D. tetani

3039. Who derived the general equation for average particle size..?

A. Edmundson B. Cmein

C. Sefton D. Horbett

3040. In equation of average particle size what is the midpoint..............?

A. Equivalent radius

B. Equivalent diameter

C. Length

D. None of them

3041. Which of the following term means when the no on what of particle lying within a certain size range is plotted against size range.....................?

A. Particle size distribution

B. Frequency distribution

C. Fluidity

D. Viscocity

3042. What is the average size of red blood cell............?

A. 8.5 B. 7

C. 6 D. 10

3043. What is the AVERAGE particle size range of coase powder.................?

A. 100-200 B. 150-1000

C. 1000-3380 D. 10-50

3044. What is the shape of normal distribution curve............?

A. Bell shaped B. Sig moid

C. Straight line D. None of them

3045. In which type of curve positive $negative deviation from mean are uniform ....?

A. Frequency distribution curve

B. Long normal frequency distributio

C. Cumulative frequency distribution

D. All of them

3046. If the size distribution follows log normal pattern which equation is used for interconversion of size distribution..?

A. Admundson B. Chin

C. Sefton D. Hatch$ choate

3047. What is the normal size requirement if an aspirin tablet..?

A. Sieve no 180 B. Sieve no 32

C. Sieve no 18 D. None of them

3048. What is the requirement of particle of insulin zine camorphousinjection..?

A. 0.1-200 B. >2

C. 10>40D. D. 0.5-100

3049. Which of the following are methods of particle size determination..?

A. Optical microscopy

B. Sieving method

C. Sedimentation method

D. All of the above

3050. Which of the following equation is used for the conversion of number of distribution to? weight distribution?

A. Noyes Whitney equation

B. Higuchi Equation

C. Hatch Choate Equation

D. Henderson Hasselbalch

3051. What is the size range of particle in optical microscopy ..?

A. 0.2-100 B. 0.3-200
C. 100 D. None of them

3052. In this method the size is expressed in which terms..?

A. Dv B. Ds
C. Dp D. Dst

3053. Wat we can determine by optical microscopy method ....?

A. No distribution
B. Wt distribution
C. CONCENTRATION OF DRUG
D. Size of particle

3054. How lower limit of optical microscope could be brought down…?

A. By changing eye piece
B. By using electron microscope
C. BY changing resturing powder
D. None of them

3055. Which of the following terms defines it is the diameter if a circle with the same area as that of the particle observed the surface on which the particle resting..?

A. Projected area
B. Martin diameter
C. Ferit diameter
D. None of them

3056. The term rheology was suggested by which scientist...........?

A. Bingham j crawfond
B. Scott bliar
C. Eugene C. Bingham
D. Blake Lively

3057. Application of rheology in pharmacy was suggested by which scientist:

A. Newton B. Scott bliar
C. Robert Boyle D. Archimedes

3058. Which is the term used to define reciprocal of viscosity…?

A. Fluidity
B. Rate of shor
C. Velocity gradient
D. Force per unit ara

3059. What is the unit of absolute viscocity..?

A. Poise B. Antipoise
C. Stoke D. antistoke

3060. Which of the following scales are used to measure viscocity in industry..?

A. Saybott B. Redwood
C. Angler D. All of the above

3061. What is viscocity of castor oil..?

A. 0.363 B. 1000
C. 400 D. 1.19

3062. What is the dimension of relative viscosity..?

A. Gm/cm3 B. Stoke
C. Poise D. Dimensionless

3063. What are the compound exhibiting non Newtonian behaviour.............?

A. Cream B. Powder
C. Emulsion D. diluents

3064. Name the viscometer used to measure the Non-Newtonian viscosity?

A. Cup-Bob Viscometer
B. Brookfield rotating Viscometer
C. Falling Sphere
D. U Tube Viscometer

3065. What is the name of body exhibiting plastic flow..?

A. Black body B. Starting body
C. Bingham body D. Plastic body

3066. If the stress applied less than yield value the substance will acts as an ....?

A. Plastic B. Psuedoplastic
C. Dilatant D. Elastic

3067. What is termed as slope of rheogram..?

A. Fluidity B. Mobility
C. Viscosity D. None of the above

3068. What does yield value indicate in flocculated system ....?

A. Fluidity B. Mobility
C. Ploes no D. Force of flocculation

3069. The increase injected value depends on what..?

A. Forces of attraction between flocules
B. Flocules
C. Mobility
D. viscocity

3070. Psuedoplastic flow is shown by which type of solutions............?

A. Polymer dispersion
B. Suspension
C. Emulsion
D. All of the above

3071. Which of the following material in pseudoplastic ....?

A. Starch
B. Sodium alginate
C. Both A AND B
D. Sodium carboxy methyl cellulose

3072. What results to curved rheogram of pseudoplastic material..?

A. Viscocity of substance
B. Polymers
C. Shearing action n long chain molecules ex-polymer
D. Mobility of material

3073. What is caused of solvents associated to molecule of polymer is released..?

A. Decrease in viscocity
B. Decrease in size of dispersed molecule
C. Both a and b
D. All of the above

3074. Which of the following is material according to this definition materials which increases in resisitance to flow with increasing rate of shear..?

A. Plastic B. Pseudoplastic
C. Dilatant D. None of them

3075. Which of the following shear thickening system..?

A. Dilatant B. Plastic
C. Psuedoplastic D. None of them

3076. Which of the following is shear thining system..?

A. Dilatent B. Psuedoplastic
C. Plastic D. All of the above

3077. Which of the following statement is correct..?

A. Dilatant system returns to its original state of fluidity when stress is removed
B. Dilatant is a shear thiming system
C. FN=n1G-EQUATION describes dilator
D. All of the above

3078. In case of dilatant what is value of n..?

A. N=>1 B. N=<1
C. N=O D. N=0

3079. WHAT happens to value of n if degree of dilatancy increases..?

A. Decreases B. Increases
C. Constant D. None of them

3080. Which kind of behavior is exhibited by system if N=1..?

A. Dilatant B. Non –newtonian
C. Newtonian D. None of them

3081. Which of the following is example of dilatant flow.............?

A. Polymer dispersion
B. Emulsion
C. Suspension
D. All of the above

3082. Which type of flow is increase of psuedoplastic flow ....?

A. Plastic B. Dilatant
C. A and b both D. All of the above

3083. What kinds of equipments used for processing of dispersion ....?

A. Milling equipment
B. Blenders
C. High-speed mixiers
D. All of the above

3084. What are consistency curves on flow curves termed as ....?

A. Fluidity B. Viscocity
C. Rheogram D. None of them

3085. Which among the following system does not reform immediately when stress is removed ....?

A. Psuedoplastic B. Plastic
C. Dilatant D. thixotropic

3086. Which kind of particles do thixotropic substance have ....?

A. Symmetric

B. Asymmetric

C. Spherical

D. All of them

3087. Which kind of behaviour is shown by thirotropic substance ....?

A. Shear thining B. Shear thickening

C. Both A AND B D. None of them

3088. Which type of movement is exhibited by particle of thixotropic substance..?

A. Brownian motion B. No motion

C. Both a and b D. Thermal motion

3089. Which of the following system shows the formation of hysteresis loop..?

A. Plastic B. Psuedoplastic

C. Dilatant D. thixotropic

3090. Which area is has been proposed as a measure of thixotropic breakdown..?

A. Fluidity B. Mobility

C. Area of hysteresis D. Viscocity

3091. Which of the following equipments used in measuring thixotropic breakdown..?

A. Barometer

B. Monometer

C. Sphagomonometer

D. Planimeter

3092. The thixotropic coefficient depends upon what…?

A. Rate of shor B. Fluidity

C. Viscocity D. All of them

3093. Which of the following was scientist who observed negative thixotrophy.............?

A. Chong B. Bingham

C. Crowford D. None of them

3094. Which of the following solutions contain low solid content ....?

A. Thixotropic B. Dilatant

C. Plastic D. Anti-thixotropic

3095. Range of solid contant in anti-thixotropic substances ....?

A. 1-10% B. 0.1-100%

C. 10-19% D. 0.1-200%

3096. The statement that solid form gel more radily when gently shaken or otherwise shared than when allowed to formget while natural kept at rest describes which type of form............?

A. Rheopexy B. Thixotrophy

C. Pseudoplastic D. dilatant

3097. Which of the following substances shows negative thixotrophy ....?

A. Clay B. Bentonic

C. Nacmc D. Both a and b

3098. Which type of viscometer is used to determine viscosity of Newtonian liquid..?

A. Capillary B. Cup$bon

C. Falling sphere D. Cone $plate

3099. Which type of viscometer will be used to determine viscosity of methylcellulose solution ....?

A. Capillary B. Cup$bon

C. Falling sphere D. None of them

3100. Which of the low is used to calculate pressure difference in the arteries of capilliaries ....?

A. Poiseuill B. Manometer

C. Barometer D. None of them

3101. What is the average blood pressure at rest ....?

A. 120 mm/hg B. 100 mm/hg

C. 180 mm/hg D. 150 mm/hg

3102. Which of the following viscometer used to measure viscosity of Newtonian liquid..?

A. Hopper –falling ball

B. Capillary /ostward viscometer

C. Cup/bon

D. Bone of plate

3103. Which type of material is used to make up sphere of hoepphrsviscometer...........?

A. Glass B. Steel

C. Iron D. copper

3104. What is the example of cup/bon type of viscometer..?

A. Mac Michael B. Searle

C. Hoeppler D. Both a and b

3105. Which type of instrument should be used for system having viscocity below 20 up.?

A. Capillary B. Happhr

C. Stormer D. None of them

3106 Which of the following is example of ROTATIONAL plate viscometer...............?

A. Searle B. Mac Michael

C. Firranti-shirbey D. hoepphr

3107. Which of the following substances shows viscoclastic properties..?

A. Spectrum B. Curival fluid

C. Lotion D. All of them

3108. The compliance j, as a function of time is measured with an which instrument ....?

A. Creep viscometer

B. Cup/bon

C. Cone/plate

D. All of them

3109. What instrument is used to measure the viscoelasticity of dermatologic cosmetic material..?

A. Creep viscometer

B. Cup/bon

C. Cone/plate

D. ALL OF THEM

3110. Which of the following substances increases viscocity of H20..?

A. GLUCOSE

B. Hydrocolloids

C. Ploymers

D. None of them

3111. The intrinsic viscocity is used in determining which of the following factor..............?

A. Molecular weight of polymer

B. Analysis of drug

C. Concentration of drug

D. Both a and b

3112. A sample of Newtonian fluid is analyzed by applying s shear stress of 5000 dy/cm^2. the rate of shear is found to 100 sec-1 calculate the coefficient of viscosity /fluidity..?

A. 0.05 poise B. 0.01 poise

B. 0.02 poise D. 0.03 poise

3113. Which of the following is absolute viscosity of liquid paraffin ....?

A. <64 B. >30

C. 70/100 D. 410/9000

3114. The viscosities of water/chloroform at 250c are 0.8900/0.560 respectively .what is realative viscosity of chloroform ....?

A. 0.6323 B. 0.6292

C. 0.6121 D. 0.6494

3115. Which of the following is absolute viscosity of tween 80..?

A. 340/450 B. 1490.0

C. 1.2 D. 1.5

3116. Which of the following equation represents rate of sheer..?

A. F=F1/A B. F1/A *DV/DR

C. G=DV/DR D. F=NG

3117. IN GRAPH OF INTRISNIC VISCOSITY WHAT INTERSEPT VALUE REPRESENTS..?

A. FLUIDITY B. Mobility

C. Intrinsic viscosity D. Viscosity

3118. According to SI system one unit of poise is equal to..?

A. 0.2 nsm-2 B. 0.1nsm-2

C. 0.001 nsm-2 D. None of them

3119. Which of the following value is represents absolute viscosity of between 20..?

A. 340/450 B. 240/350

C. 410/9000 D. 76/100

3120. A plastic material has shown the yield value of 1800 dy/cm2 when the shear stress of 300 dy/cm2 is applied on the material the rate of shear was found 120 sec-1 .calculate the plastic viscosity..?

A. 9.98 poise B. 10 poise

C. 8.98 posie D. 11.34 poise

3121. Which of the following value represents intrinsic viscosity if dextrin 40 ....?

A. 0.16-0.20 B. 0.11-0.13

C. 0.27-0.32 D. 0.34-0.50

3122. Which of the following equation represents pseudoplastic flow rheogram..?

A. U=F-T/G B. FN=N1G

C. F=NG D. NONE OF THEM

3123. Which of the following represents intrinsic viscosity of dextron110..?

A. 0.27-0.32 B. 0.20-0.30

C. 0.01-0.10 D. 0.45-0.50

3124. Which of the following equation represents Reynolds no..?
A. Re=dvd/n
B. N=p1t1/p2t2/n2
C. N=kt/p
D. None of them

3125. On which principle falling sphere viscometer is based..?
A. Hoppler viscometer
B. Rotational viscometer
C. Capillary viscometer
D. None of them

3126. Which of the following value represents absolute viscositity of light liquid paraffin..?
A. >30 B. >64
C. 1.2 D. 5.816

3127. Cup/bob viscometer belongs to which category of viscometer..?
A. Rotational B. Hoppler
C. Capillary D. None of them

3128. Which of the following value represents viscosity of blood ....?
A. 4.0 B. 1.5
C. 1.01 D. 1.5

3129. What is the value of dynamic viscosity..?
A. 0.1 nsm2 B. 0.3 nsm2
C. Both a and b D. None of them

3130. Which of the following value represents kinematic viscosity of PEG 6000.?
A. 470/9000 B. 290
C. 450 D. 350

3131. WHICH OF THE FOLLOWING value h represents viscosity of blood plasma level..?
A. 1.5 B. 1.575
C. 2.0 D. 2.75

3132. What is the unit of kinematic viscosity..?
A. Poise B. Centipoise
C. Stokes D. None of them

3133. Which of the following properties are characterstic feature of particle..?
A. Size B. Shape
C. All of them D. Surface area

3134. Do flow of a particle affects the uniformity of particles..?
A. True B. False

3135. Particle size is normally denoted by which unit..?
A. Stokes B. Poise
C. Micrometers D. None of them

3136. One micrometers is equal to flow many millimetres ....?
A. 10-11mm B. 10-3mm
C. 10-7mm D. 10-9mm

3137. The term milimicrometer is presently called as what ....?
A. Nanometer B. Picometer
C. Decameter D. None of them

3138. The term nanometer is equal to which value ....?
A. 10-9 B. 10-11
C. 10-7 D. None of them

3139. Which of the following are applications of micromeritics in pharmacy ....?
A. Release /dissolution
B. Absorption /drug action
C. Physical stability
D. All of the above

3140. Do particle size of drug affect is release from its dosage forms..?
A. True B. False

3141. Which of the following property are important in collection of particles more than one size..?
A. Shape/surface area of individual particle
B. Size range /no or wt of particle
C. Physical stability
D. Both a and b

3142. The science of technology of small particles was given micromerities by whom..?
A. Seffon B. Horbitt
C. Chum/robinson D. Dalla valle

3143. Micrometer is also called as ....?

A. MICRON B. Nanometre
C. Picometer D. None of them

3144. Which of the following word symbolizes surface diameter ....?

A. Ds B. Dst
C. Dp D. Dv

3145. It is the definition of which of the following terms "the diameter of a sphere having the same surface area as the particles..?

A. Ds B. Dst
C. Dp D. Dv

3146. Which of the following would symbolizes volume diameter...........?

A. Ds B. Dst
C. Dp D. Dv

3147. It is definition of which of the following terms "the diameter of sphere having same volume as the particle..?

A. Dv B. Dst
C. Dp D. ds

3148. Which of the following terms symbolizes projected diameter.................?

A. Dp B. Dst
C. Ds D. Dv

3149. Which of the following terms symbolizes stokes diameter..................?

A. Dv B. Dst
C. Dp D. ds

3150. Particles of suspension ranges between what size..?

A. 0.5-10 micrometer
B. 50-100 micrometer
C. 150-1000 micrometer
D. 10-50 micrometer

3151. How stokes diameter is determined..?

A. Optical microscopy
B. Sedimentation
C. Sieving
D. None of them

3152. Particles of emulsion range between what sizes..?

A. 10-50 micrometer
B. 50-100 micrometer
C. 1000-3360 micrometer
D. 0.1-200 micrometer

3153. Which factor we can calculate an average particle size of sample..?

A. Particle size of distribution
B. Sedimentation
C. Sieving
D. All of them

3154. Which is the size range of average granule size..?

A. 1000-3360 B. 1500-3000
C. 2000-4000 D. 3000-7000

3155. What are the standard sizes of nanosphere?

A. 25 nm B. 50-100 nm
C. 21 nm D. 20 nm

3156. In how many standard sizes are nanosphere present..?

A. 60 B. 100-150
C. 22 D. 40

3157. Particle size is related to which 2 factors..?

A. Geometric shape
B. Surface regularity
C. Rugosity
D. All of the above

3158. Particle shape affects which of the following factors..?

A. Surface area
B. Flow of properties
C. All of them
D. Compaction of particles

3159. Which of the following parameter are important in studies of absorption /distribution..?

A. Surface area per unit /volume
B. Stability
C. Drug concentration
D. None of them

3160. Which of the following terms defines this "if the powder contains particles of one size..?

A. Monodisperse
B. Polydisperse
C. None of them
D. Both a and b

3161. How uniformly sized particles are obtained..?

A. By passing through sieves
B. By sedimentation
C. Both a and b
D. None of them

3162. Which of th following are applications of monosize particles in pharmacy ?

A. Standardization of instruments particle size analyzer
B. Occurate determination of pore size in caseof filters
C. For effective immunization normally antigens are made to assorbtion on uniform sized particles
D. All of the above

3163. Generally all of the pharmaceutical powders are...........?

A. Polydisperse
B. Monodisperse
C. Both a and b
D. None of them

3164. It is diffusion of which of the following terms "equipment sphere undergoing sedimentation at the same rate as the asymmetric particle ....?

A. Dst B DV
C. DS D. DP

3165. THE OPERATION In which oil ic determined into the pores of a powder metallurgy product is known as..?

A. Mixing B. Sintering
C. Impregnation D. infiltartion

3166. What is the mixture of potassium nitrate powedered charcoal and sulphur called..?

A. Paint B. Aluminium
C. Brass D. Gun powder

3167. THE TERMS pvc used in the plastic industry stands for.............?

A. Polyvinyl chloride
B. Polyvinyl carbonate
C. Phosphor vanadiu chloride
D. Phosphavinyl chloride

3168. In tablet formulation polyvinylpyrrolidone is commonly used as..?

A. Glidant B. Diluent
C. Lubricant D. binder

3169. Which one of the following is not an advantage of using the layering technique to produce pellets.?

A. Relative good yield
B. Highly reproductive final product
C. Not to east to scale up
D. Narrow particle size distribution

3170. Which of the following materials is not commonly found in a pellet formulation manufactured? by extrusion /speronisation...?

A. Drug substance B. Filler
C. Liquid binder D. surfactant

3171. Which of the following quality control test is not required for coating tablet

A. Dissolution test
B. Friability
C. Disintergration test
D. Uniformility of weight

3172. Magnetic filed intensity is a quantity```

A. Scalar B. Phasor
C. Vector D. variable

3173. Whichn of the following has the highest permability..?

A. Soft iron B. Steel
C. Air D. Per malkry

3174. Which of the following terms symbolizers stokes diameter..?

A. Dv B. Dst
C. Dp D. ds

3175. Paricles of suspension ranges between what size ....?

A. 0.5-10 micrometer
B. 50-100 micrometer
C. 150-1000 micrometer
D. 10-50 micrometer

3176. How stokes diameter is determined..?

A. Optical microscopy
B. Sedimentation
C. Sieving
D. None of them

3177. Change of state from solid to liquid is called

A. Vapourization
B. Condensation
C. Fusion
D. None of them

3178. The process in which solid directly changes to gas is called

A. Evaporation B. Melting
C. Sublimation D. None of them

3179. Define volume but no definite shpes is the property of..?

A. Solid B. Gas
C. Liquid D. None of them

3180. Dosage forms can be designed for administration of drug by all possible routes to achieve

A. Minimum therapeutic response
B. Maximum therapeutic response
C. Low therapeutic response
D. None of the above

3181. Liquid dosage forms are prepared by dissolving.

A. Preservative B. Surfactants
C. Active ingredients D. Supposotories

3182. Supposotories dosage forms can be admitted routes.

A. Oral B. Vaginal
C. Topical D. Rectal

3183. Liquid dosage forms are.

A. Monophasic and biphasic
B. Poultices or cataplasm
C. Lotions
D. None of the above

3184. Monophasic liquid dosage forms contain.

A. Two phase
B. One phase
C. Less than two phase
D. All of the above

3185. Drug is a..... . absorbed by liquid dosage forms.

A. Minimum B. Low
C. Rapidly D. None

3186. Simple syrup I. P. contain .... of sucrose

A. 33.3% w/w B. 66.7% w/w
C. 40.4% w/ w D. 87.7% w/ w

3187. Medicaments susceptible to.... are not suitable for liquid dosage forms.

A. Osmosis B. Hemolysis
C. Hydrolysis D. None

3188. Concentrates are required to be........... for use.

A. Solute B. Solvent
C. Dilute D. Distilled

3189. .... are sweetened concentrated solution of sucrose in viscous water or any other suitable aqueous vehicles.

A. Elixirs B. Tincture s
C. Drops D. Syrups

3190. Which of the following sweetened hydroalcoholic liquid preparations for oral administration.

A. Drops B. Syrups
C. Elixirs D. Tinctures

3191. The percentage of alcohol varies from.

A. 66.4% B. 20%
C. 4 - 40% D. 0.1 - 0.3%

3192. Elixirs are clear flavored sweetened...... liquid preparations.

A. Hydroscopic
B. Alcoholic
C. Hydroalcoholic
D. Hygroscopic

3193. Which one of the following medicated elixirs usually contain potent and nauseous drug like.

A. Antiviral
B. Antiulcer
C. Antibacterial
D. Antibiotic and anti tussives

3194. Elixirs do not need of adding preservatives If alcohol quantity is more than.....

A. 20% B. 30%
C. 50% D. 60 %

3195. Non - medicated elixirs are supplied in......

A. Small volume B. Bulk volume
C. Less volume D. None of the above

3196. Medicated elixirs are supplied in...

A. Small volume B. Bulk volume
C. Less volume D. All of the above

3197. Medicaments ate given in the form deteriorate rapidly.

A. Drops B. Syrups
C. Elixirs D. Droughts

3198. Drop are liquid preparations means for.
A. Young age B. Old age
C. Pediatric D. Children

3199. Drops are supplied in small volume containers e. g.
A. 5ml or 10ml B. 10 or 20ml
C. 20ml or 25ml D. 25ml or 50 ml

3200. Linctuses are viscous, oral liquid preparation for relief of...
A. Fever B. Pain
C. Cough D. Vomiting

3201. Linctuses are.... oral liquid preparations.
A. Rough B. Viscous
C. Soft D. Hard

3202. .... are liquid preparations intended for external applications without friction.
A. Liniments' B. Lotions
C. Elixirs D. Linctuses

3203. Collisions contain..... vehicle.
A. Evaporation B. Flexible
C. Volatile D. None

3204 ...... are aqueous solution used for the treatment of throat infection.
A. Elixirs B. Gargles
C. Cool water D. Throat paints

3205. Mouthwashes are aqueous liquid preparations used for?
A. Rinsing B. Deodorant
C. Both a and b D. None

3206. .... is the most commonly employed vehicle because of its viscous nature and sweet agreeable test use in throat paints.
A. Sucrose B. Dextrose
C. Sorbitol D. Glycerine

3207. .... are aqueous solution used to cleanse, deodorize, sooth, or medicated wounds after applying them with low pressure.
A. Nasal drops B. Mouthwashes
C. Sprays D. Douches

3208. The word 'douch' is commonly used for...
A. Oral solutions B. Nasal solutions
C. Vaginal solutions D. Eye solutions

3209. Douches are also supplied in the form of.
A. Gas from B. Liquid
C. Semisolid D. Poweders or tablets

3210. Eye drops should be....
A. Sterile B. None sterile
C. Pyrogen free D. None

3211. Micromoleculare solution consist of....
A. Micro partical B. Micro units
C. Micro polymer D. Nano partical

3212. The extent to which the solute dissolve at a particular temperature is known as.....
A. Viscosity B. Solubility
C. Sterility D. Tonicity

3213. The Solubilization technique was introduced by.
A. Hildebrand B. Scoft
C. Mc. Bain D. Hippocrate

3214. In which years Solubilization technique was Steblished.
A. 1920 B. 1946
C. 1937 D. 1980

3215. PH is helpful in enhancing the.
A. Sterility B. Solubility
C. Viscosity D. Stability

3216. When the solubility of drug is enhanced owing to the presence of large amount of addives the technique is refered as.
A. Cosolvancy B. Complexions
C. Hydrotrophy D. Preservation

3217. The number of moles of solids present in.
A. Viscosity B. Tonicity
C. Solubility D. None

3218. Which one of the following isotonic solution have the same number of.
A. Moles B. Litre
C. Gram D. K. G

3219. Saccharine is ..... times sweeter than sucrose.
A. 100 B. 350
C. 450 D. 550

3220. Biphasic liquid dosage forms preparations, the distributed phase is called dispersed phase and the vehicle is called.
A. Dispersion phase
B. Dispersion medium
C. Dispersion system
D. None

3221. Solid liquid dispersions are..
A. Suspension B. Emulsion
C. Capsules D. None

3222. Which one of the commonest vehicle for the liquid preparations.
A. Water B. Elixirs
C. Syrups D. Decoction

3223. Coloring agents are added to the liquid preparations to improve their.
A. Physical properties
B. Chemical properties
C. Biological properties
D. Organoleptic properties

3224. How many phases contain biphasic liquid dosage forms.
A. One phases B. None
C. Two phases D. Both a and c

3225. The rate of sedimentation are explained by.
A. Fric's first law B. Stock's law
C. Einstein's D. Newton 's law

3226. What is Einstein's Equation?
A. Dv/dt=dack/h' B. $E=mc^2$
C. F=ma D. pH=pka +log$[A/HA]$

3227. The flow property of suspensions explained by.
A. Stocke s B. Einstein
C. Newton D. Fric ' s

3228. As the shearing stress is increases the rate of shear is also.
A. Minimum B. Increase
C. Decrease D. None

3229. Newtonian flow is found in .... suspension.
A. Floculated
B. Defloculated
C. Viscosity
D. Flow property

3230. The rate of sedimentation of a floculated suspension is.
A. High B. Low
C. Uncontrolled D. None

3231. The sediment of a floculated suspensions is formed.
A. Slowly B. Rapidly
C. Medium D. None

3232. The process of dissociation of poorly soluble solutes in water in the presence of surfactant is called.
A. Sedimentation
B. Co solvency
C. Solubilization
D. Hydrotrophy

3233. Hyligher zeta potential gives defloculated type of suspension and results in.
A. Sedimentation B. Transparent form
C. Cake form D. Brittle form

3234. A synthetic sweetening agent which is nearly 200 times sweeter than sucrose and has no after tasts is.
A. Sorbitol B. Saccharine
C. Aspartame D. Cyclamate

3235. What is HLB value of tween 80 . ?
A. 10 B. 15
C. 20 D. 25

3236. Sodium oleate is a..... type of emulsifier..
A. Anionic B. Catatonic
C. Nonionic D. Ionic

3237. Emulsions are referedas .....
A. Solid - liquid dispersion s
B. Liquid - liquid dissociation s
C. Solid - liquid dispersion
D. None of the above

3238. Which one of the following btype of emulsifying agent s.
A. Anionic B. Cationic
C. Nonionic D. All of the above

3239. In which type of Emulsifying agent's contain both hydro phobic and hydrophilic portions.
A. Ionic B. Cationic
C. Nonionic D. Anionic

3240. Which of the following example of fatty alcohol polyethylene glycole ethers?
A. Poloxyl 40 stearate
B. Cetomacrogol 1000
C. Sodium lauryl sulphate
D. Sorbitan Monooleate

3241. In which years HLB system was founded.
A. 1945 B. 1949
C. 1950 D. 1955

3242. Who is defined HLB system.
A. Newton B. Griffin
C. Mc bain D. None

3243. Saponins are naturally occurring emulgents.
A. O/w B. W/o
C. Both a and b D. None of the above

3244. In which the following preparations of ointments.
A. Solid preparations
B. Liquid preparations
C. Semisolid preparations
D. All of the above

3245. What are the type of ointment bases.
A. Hydrocarbon B. Absorption
C. Water miscible D. All of the above

3246. Which of the following ointment base does not absorbed by the skin?
A. Hydrocarbon bases
B. Absorption bases
C. Water bases
D. Water bases

3247. What is non Emulsified bases or water - in - oil emulsions.
A. Water miscible bases
B. Water soluble bases
C. Absorption bases
D. Hydrocarbon bases

3248. What are the method of preparation of ointments.
A. Titration B. Fusion.
C. Sedimentation D. None of the above

3249. Which of the following example of an ointment prepared by fusion and containing a partically soluble solid.
A. White bees wax B. Paraffin
C. Benzoic acid D. Salicylic acid

3250. What is syrups. ?
A. None aqueous preparation
B. Aqueous preparation
C. Semisolid preparation
D. None

3251. Which one of the following method of preparation of syrups.
A. Solution with heat
B. Agitation without heat
C. Percolation
D. All of the above

3252. What is the formula of sucrose.. ?
A. C13 H22 o12 B. C12 H22 O11
C. C11 H22 O12 D. C10 H22 O10

3253. Which is the primary solvents for elixirs. ?
A. Water and alcohol
B. Glycerine and sorbitol
C. Propylene glycol
D. Flavoring agent

3254. What should be the alcohol percentage in elixirs.
A. 1 to 5 % B. 5 to 40%
C. 40 to 50% D. None

3255. What is the UEs of piperazine citrate.?
A. Anti inflammatory
B. Anti ulcer
C. Anthelmintic
D. Antibacterial

3256. In which condition linctuse is prescribed.
A. Dry cough B. Fever
C. Pain D. None

3257. Which one of the following semisolid dosage forms.
A. Ointments B. Creams
C. Jellies D. All of the above

3258. Which is following dosage form for infants, children, geriatric and mentally disturbed patients.?
A. Solid dosage form
B. Liquid dosage form
C. Semisolid dosage form
D. None

3259. Which is the monophasic liquid dosage form used in oral.?
A. Draought s B. Linctuse
C. Syrups D. All of the above

3260. What is usual dose of linctuses. ?
A. 5 ml B. 15 ml
C. 25ml D. 60ml

3261. Liniments are usually alcoholic and........ preparation.
A. Oral liquid B. Oily liquid
C. Fluid preparation D. Aqueous liquid

3262. Which is the fluid preparation for external use.

A. Collodions B. Lotions
C. Liniments D. Linctuse

3263. None polar solvents are are unable to reduce the attraction between the long of bstrong and weak electrolytes because of the solvents low.

A. Electric conso
B. High dielectric constant
C. Dielectric constant
D. Dipole interaction

3264. What is the CMC.?

A. Colloidal miscelle concentration
B. Critical miscelle concentration
C. Co solvancymiscelle concentration
D. None of the above

3265. The function of surfactant start only at. .

A. Miscelle B. CMC
C. HLB D. Shops

3266. Which solvents is used in combination to increase to solubility of drug solute are known as.

A. Solubilization
B. Complexation
C. Co solvents
D. Hydrotrophy

3267. Powder are the..... dosage forms.

A. Solid B. Liquid
C. Semisolid D. None

3268. What is effervescent granules.

A. Cresm B. Lotions
C. Powder D. Pastse

3269. Divided powder can be used in ....

A. Internal B. External
C. Both a and b D. None

3270. Which powder contain only one ingredient either in crystalline orbamorphous form is.

A. Divided powder
B. Compound powder
C. Simple powder
D. Bulk powder

3271. When the powders are supplied individually as a singal dose in separate packets they are called.

A. Bulk powder
B. Simpal powder
C. Comppund powder
D. Divided powder

3272. Which is the two example of the compound powders?

A. Aspirin
B. Paracetamol
C. Both a and b
D. Sodium bicarbonate

3273. Which of the following largest size of capsules?

A. 00 B. 0
C. 000 D. 5

3274. Which method can be done of filling of powder is.

A. Heat method
B. Dry method
C. Heap method
D. Wet method

3275. Which is the smallest size of the capsule?

A. 00 B. 000
C. 5 D. None

3276. Which of the following powders usually contain antibacterial agent like chlorhexidine and hexchlorophene?

A. Dentifrices
B. Surgical dusting powder
C. Both a and b
D. Effervescent powder

3277. Which types of powders are dispensed which required special techniques to dispense the ingredients show their peculiar properties.

A. Eutectic mixture
B. Effervescent powder
C. Powder to be reconstituted
D. All of the above

3278. In which condition the mixtures of powder when mixed turn to liquid.

A. Granules B. Eutectic
C. Dusting D. Dentifrices

3279. Which is not following effervescent granules?
A. Sodium bicarbonate
B. Citric acid
C. Acetylsalicylic acid
D. Tartaric acid

3280. Which gas is released as a results of acid - base reaction.
A. Oxigen B. Nitrogen
C. Helium D. Carbon dioxide

3281. Which stimulates the flow of gastric juice and accelerate absorption of medicament is.
A. Carbon dioxide
B. Nitrogen
C. Oxigen
D. None

3282. Which of the following substance is absorbe the moisture contain from the atmosphere.
A. Hydroscopic
B. Hygroscopic
C. Homogeneous
D. None of the above

3283. In which quantities for make the weight of ingredient or triturate for each powder upto 2 grains with lactose.
A. Imperial B. Metric
C. Both a and b D. None of the above

3284. Calibration of the moulds is done by using........ pastic in.
A. Lactose paste B. Gelatin
C. Fructose D. Maltose

3285. What is two method of effervescent granules.
A. Heat method B. Wet method
C. Dry method D. Both a and b

3286. In which method the powder mixture is moistened with a suitable liquid to form a coherent mass.
A. Heat method B. Dry method
C. Heap method D. Wet method

3287. In which all ingredients are melted together and stirred until cold.
A. Fusion B. Trituration
C. Dilution D. Diffusion

3288. Which one of the following layers of skin.
A. Hypodermis
B. Sebaceous
C. Sweat
D. Capillary loop in papilla

3289. Which is the innermost layer of skin?
A. Subcutaneous
B. Dermis
C. Epidermis
D. Hypodermis

3290. Stratum corner also called is.
A. Granules layer B. Horny layer
C. Basal layer D. Prickle cell layer

3291. Which is the one method of release rate of medicament from base?
A. Agar cup plate B. Diffusion
B. Heat D. Heap

3292. Which jelly is used as a vehicle for allergens in allergy test.
A. Electrocardiography
B. Patch
C. TDDS
D. None

3293. Which is the 1.2 to 2 percent jelly is used as lubricant and 5 to 10 % jelly as dermatological vehicle.
A. Tragacanth B. Sodium alginate
C. Pectin D. Starch

3294. Which jelly is feasible for acid products along with glycerol as dispersing and humectants?
A. Pectin B. Gelatin
C. Clays D. Tragacanth

3295. Which is the 7 to 20% bentonite forms a jelly used as dermatological bases.
A. Clays B. Polyvinyl alcohol
C. Gelatin D. Tragacanth

3296. Which method is employed to determine the release rate of antibacterial agents from the ointment bases.
A. Agar cup plate method
B. Diffusion
C. Heap
D. None

3297. What is lanoline.?
A. Hydrous wool fat
B. Jelly es
C. Hydrocarbon
D. Liquid paraffin

3298. PEG bases are highly...... In nature.
A. Hydrophilic B. Hygroscopic
C. Immiscible D. Water miscible

3299. What is the uppermost layer of skin.
A. Dermis B. Horny layer
C. Episermis D. Subcutaneous

3300. Which ointment bases are suitable for dry skin?
A. Absorption bases
B. Hydrocarbon bases
C. Water miscible bases
D. Water soluble bases

3301. Which is the nature of keratin?
A. Hydro philic
B. Lipophilic
C. Hygroscopic
D. Hydroscopic

3302. Which is the following buses are water soluble
A. Polyethylene Gylcore
B. MpsmEthyleneparbene sodium
C. PDS
D. EDTA

3303. Which are easily removable from the skin.
A. Water soluble bases
B. Water miscible base
C. Absorption bases
D. Hydrocarbon bases

3304. In which conditions are useful for acute lesion that has a tendency for oozing?
A. Jelly bases B. Pastes bases
C. Patch bases D. None

3305. ...... Are also called cataplasms.
A. Poultices B. Pastes
C. Jellies D. Starch

3306. What are cream?
A. Semisolid B. Liquid
C. Solid D. Pastes

3307. In which the drug or mixture of drugs with or without diluents are enclosed in a gelatin she'll.
A. Tablets B. Capsule
C. Injection D. None

3308. Which are preparations containing very fine powder of drugs that are taken up into the nose?
A. Snuffs B. Deodorant
C. Talcum D. Douch

3309. Which powder is mainly used to remove or neutralize foul smell of the skin.
A. Talcum powder B. Douch powder
C. Deodorant powder
D. Snuffs

3310. Which preparation is used for the cleaning of the surfaces of the teeth.
A. Insufflations B. Dentifrices
C. Deodorant D. Douches

3311. What are solid unit dosage forms intended for introduction into body cavities.
A. Supposotories B. Lozenges
C. Pastilles D. Pill

3312. Which one of the following sweetening agents for liquid dosage forms. ?
A. Cyclamate sodium
B. Sodium sulfite
C. Ascorbic acid
D. Glycerine

3313. Which agens are added to the liquid preparations to improve their organoleptic properties.
A. Flavoring agent
B. Coloring agents
C. Sweetening agents
D. Vehicles

3314. Which is the first synthetic color discovered accidentally was 'Mauveine' known as.
A. Violate to purple
B. Yellow to orange
C. Brown
D. Perkin's purple

3315. I'm which the range of benzoic acid and it's salts are used as preservatives.
A. 0.1 - 0.3% B. 0.1 - 0.2%
C. 0.1 - 0.4% D. None

3316. Which of the following mixture the provid uniform dosage.?

A. Simple mixture B. Syrups
C. Elixirs D. None

3317. Which monophasic liquid are suitable for any water soluble stable drugs.

A. Syrup B. Elixirs
C. Jellies D. Pastes

3318. Which one of the following monophasic liquid dosage from is promote healing of the wound.

A. Throat paints B. Douches
C. Gargles D. Mouthwashes

3319. Which the ratio is called sedimentation ratio.

A. Hu/Ho B. Ho/Hu
C. Both a and b D. None

3320. Why does this syrup turn to yellow?

A. Effect of heat
B. Effect of water
C. Effect of sugar
D. None

3321. What is the alcoholic content in the preparation of elixirs?

A. 0.3%v/v B. 0.4% w/v
C. 0.4 % v/v D. 0.5 % V/v

3322. Which of the following emulsions are.. Unstable system.

A. Dynamically
B. Chemically
C. Thermodynamically
D. None

3323. Which is nature of type of emulsions is cream white in appearance regardless of the oil used.

A. O/w B. W/o
C. Both a and b D. None

3324. .... nearly always form o/w types of emulsions di or trivalent actions soaps always will form W/o type of emulsions.

A. Tragacanth B. Starch
C. Acacia D. Sodium alginate

3325. Which dosage forms used in rectal vaginal or urethral cavities.

A. Supposotories B. Liquid
C. Syrups D. Elixirs

3326. In which dosage forms are used to treat local condition such as hemorrhoids in rectum and infections in vaginal.

A. Emulsions B. Suspension
C. Powder D. Supposotories

3327. Which are unit dosage forms hence there is no dose variations?

A. Supposotories B. Tablets
C. Capsules D. Cream

3328. The weight of one pessary varies from.. . . As the case may be.

A. 6 to 8 B. 4 to 8
C. 8 to 5 D. None

3329. Which one of the following types of supposotories.

A. Oleaginous bases
B. Hydrocarbon bases
C. Absorption bases
D. Water miscible bases

3330. In which years oleaginous bases introduced.

A. 1852 B. 1850
C. 1865 D. 1952

331. Which one of the following aqueous bases.

A. Glycero - gelatin
B. Macrogol bases
C. Soap glycerine bases
D. All of the above

3332. Which is dissolves in body secretion.

A. Aqueous bases
B. Glycerogelatin base
C. Macrogol bases
D. None of the above

3333. Which is also called carbowaxes.

A. Macrogol base
B. Glycerogelatin
C. Aqueous bases
D. None

3334. Which one of the following very hygroscopic in nature.

A. Oleaginous bases
B. Synthetic fat bases
C. Emulsions
D. Shoap glycerine bases

3335. Which is one popular brands in u. k.?
A. Witepsol B. Massa Estarinum
C. Massuppol D. All of the above

3336. Which moulds is not required in case of synthetic fate or macrogols bases.
A. Lubrication of moulds
B. Suppository moulds
C. Coca butter supposotories of mould
D. None of the y

3337. Which is technique supposotories can also be prepared by.
A. Compression B. Wet
C. Dry D. Granulation

3338. Which types of drug action by supposotories.
A. Local action
B. Inflammatory action
C. Both a and b
D. None

3339. Which one of the following length of human rectum is.
A. 5 to 10 cm B. 15 to 20 cm
C. 10 to 15 cm D. None

3340. Which one of the following factors affecting drug absorption from the rectum.
A. Coloniccontens B. Circulation routes
C. Ph D. All of the above

3341. What is the PH of rectal fluids.
A. 2 to 5 B. 5 to 7
C. 7 to 8 D. None

3342. Coca butter melts between.
A. 34 to 36 °c B. 25 to 30 °c
C. 44 to 46 c° D. 15 to 20 °c

3343. Which is recommended as a suppository base.
A. Hydrogenated palm kernel oil
B. Hydrogenated theobroma oil
C. Fractionated palm kernel oil
D. None of the above

3344. Which is used as lubricant for coca butter suppository.
A. Soaps
B. Glycerine
C. Alcohol
D. all LP of the above

3345. Eye drops should be prepared as.
A. Isotonic B. Hypotonic
C. Hypertonic D. Non sterile

3346. Theories of emulaification are characterized by one of the following Elixirs.
A. Film formulation
B. Phase inversion
C. Monomolecular adsoption
D. Solid particle adsoption

3347. Paediatric kaolin contain.
A. light kaolin
B. light magnesium oxide
C. heavy kaolin
D. Water

3348. Tweens are used in suspension as .
A. suspending agents
B. antioxidant
C. Flocculating agents
D. None

3349. The health insurance portability and accountability Act of.
A. 1946 B. 1992
C. 1990 D. 1996

3350. .... is the practice of pharmacy in private and government owned hospital.
A. Community pharmacy
B. Health system pharmacy
C. Nuclear pharmacy
D. Government service

3351. Nuclear pharmacy can be used in.
A. Radioactive drug
B. Synthetic drugs
C. Plants drug
D. None

3352. The offers opportunities to pharmacists of all educational levels.
A. Industrial pharmacy
B. Community pharmacy
C. Health system pharmacy
D. Nuclear pharmacy

3353. The job opportunities for pharmacists are expected to.
A. Community pharmacy
B. Health system pharmacy
C. Industrial pharmacy
D. All of the above

3354. Offers opportunities to pharmacists in various capacities.
A. Government service
B. Pharmaceutical education
C. Pharmaceutical journalism.
D. Organizational management

3355. The American pharmacists association (APHA) founding.
A. 1986 B. 1957
C. 1852 D. 1857

3356. The mission of ASAP is to represent it's more than ...... members includes
A. 25,000 B. 30,000
C. 24,000 D. 20,000

3357. The first half of this millennium was once refered to as.
A. Middle ages B. Dark ages
C. Modern ages D. None

3358. Who is defined the middle Ages?
A. Greco – roman
D. Hippocrates
C. Diocles
D. Galen

3359. The magical potions for curing were part of the duty of.
A. Doctor B. Pharmacists
C. Shaman D. none

3360. As western Europe struggled a new civilization crose among those who followed the teachings of.
A. Roman B. Muhammed
C. Galen D. Rhazes

3361. The Islamic nations Greek writing including those dealing with medicine were tranlated into.
A. Indian B. American
C. Arabic D. Europian

3362. Arabic culture had returned classical scientific and medical knowledge to.
A. Islamic B. American
C. Indian D. Europe

3363. Who is licensed to prepare and dispense medication counsel patients.
A. Doctor B. Shaman
C. Pharmacists D. None

3364. Who is responsible for the preparations of the dosage forms of drugs such as tablets, capsules, and sterile solution for injection.
A. Pharmacists B. doctors
C. Both a and b D. None

3365. Community pharmacist may be.
A. Independently owned small businesses
B. Part of large retail chains
C. Franchise operation
D. All of the above

3366. A chain pharmacy is.
A. Community pharmacy
B. Nuclear pharmacy
C. Health system pharmacy
D. Industrial pharmacy

3367. The examples of places where institutional pharmacies can be found.
A. Home health care
B. Long term care facilities
C. Managed care organization
D. All of the above

3368. Which country is top the world in exporting generic drugs worth us $ 15 billion in 2014.
A. India B. America
C. Japan D. Rush

3369. The pharma D curriculum usually required....... years to complete the degree requirements.
A. 2 academic B. 4 academic
C. 6 academic D. None

3370. What is the ACPE.?
- A. Accreditation council for pharmaceutical education
- B. American council for pharmaceutical education
- C. Pharmacy council for pharmaceutical education
- D. None

3371. A list of the govermental agencies that license pharmacists in the various states is available from.
- A. National Association of boards of pharmacy
- B. National community pharmacists association
- C. National professional organization of pharmacists
- D. None of the above

3372. Which committee recommends the action of central government and pharmaceuticals legislation?
- A. Chopra committee
- B. Mudaliar committee
- C. Bhore committee
- D. Bhatia committee

3373. Which of the following one professional degree in pharmacy.
- A. Pharma D
- B. B. Pharma
- C. M.Pharma
- D. PhD

3374. What is AACP.?
- A. Accreditation association of college of pharmacy
- B. American Association of college of pharmacy
- C. Australian association of college of pharmacy
- D. Auburn association of college of pharmacy

3375. Which of the following dermal preparations
- A. Film
- B. Paste
- C. Cream
- D. All of the above

3376. What is the type of oral dosage forms.?
- A. Aerosol
- B. Nebulizer
- C. Both a and b
- D. Tablet

3377. Which of the following dosage form for the drug to be administered under the skin.
- A. Subcutaneous
- B. Transdermal
- C. Topical
- D. None

3378. If 1 ml of av 0.1 N Hcl solution is added to 100 ml of pure water the PH is required from.
- A. 7 to 4
- B. 7 to 3
- C. 7 to 2
- D. 7 to 1

3379. The PH is change only ...... PH units.
- A. 0.09 PH
- B. 0.05 PH
- C. 0.08 PH
- D. 0.06 PH

3380. What is Henderson - hasselbalch equipment for a weak acid and it's salt.
- A. PH = PKa - PKb+ log [base/salt]
- B. [H3O+] = Ka [salt/acid]
- C. PH = PKa + log [salt/acid]
- D. None

3381. Kolthoff and Tekelenburg determined the...... of PH.
- A. temperature constant
- B. temperature coefficient
- C. temperature change
- D. temperature decrease

3382. What is PH indicatore of weak acid or weak bases
- A. thmol blue
- B. Methyl violet
- C. Methyl red
- D. Phenol red

3383. The PH rang of Bromocresol green.
- A. 3.7 to 5.4
- B. 5.2 - 6.8
- C. 4.2 - 6.2
- D. 3.1 - 4.4

3384. What is the PH rang of Alizarin yellow.
- A. 6.8- 8.4
- B. 8.0 - 9.6
- C. 10.0 - 12.0
- D. None

3385. An indicator......... is present in its ionic form.
- A. Methyl orange
- B. methyl violet
- C. Phenol red
- D. Methyl red

3386. What is the molar ratio, [salt/ acid], required to prepare an acetate buffer of PH 5.0?
- A. 1.74
- B. 1.74/1
- C. 1.74/2
- D. 1.75/1

3387. Who is the suggests universal indicatore.
A. Henderson - hasselbalch
B. Koppel and spiro
C. Van slyke
D. Merck index.

3388. .... Introduced the concept of buffer capacity.
A. Bower and bates
B. Palitzsch
C. Clark and lubs
D. Koppel and spiro and van slyke

3389. The buffer capacity of the blood in the physiological range PH..... is obtained as follows..
A. 4.76 to 6.86
B. 5.03 to 5.13
C. 7.0 to 7.8
D. None of the above

3390. What is PH of tears?
A. 6.5 to 7.6 B. 6.3 to 7.4
C. 7.4 to 7.8 D. All of the above

3391. The 24 hour urine collection of a normal adult has a PH averaging about 6.0 unit it may be as low as....... or high as.......
A. 4.6 or 7.4 B. 4.5 or 7.8
C. 7.8 or 4.5 D. None

3392. The PH scale was introduced by as.....
A. Sorensen B. Gifford
C. Both a and b D. Mellen and seltzer

3393. The plot of PH versus Mililiter of NAOH added produce the.....
A. Equivalonce point
B. titration curve
C. both a and b
D. None

3394. What is the chemical formulation of phosphoric acid.
A. H2Po4 B. H3Po4
C. HPo4 D. None

3395. What is the PBS.?
A. Phosphate buffered solution
B. Phosphate buffered saline
C. Phosphate buffered substance
D. Phosphate buffered system

3396. It is used for ophthalmic solution in the PH range of.
A. 5 to 6 B. 6 to 7
C. 7 to 9 D. None

3397. What is the PH of blood.
A. 7 . 3 B. 7.4
C. 7.6 D. 7.5

3398. What is the formula of molarity.?
A. Liter/moles B. Mililiter/ liter
C. Moles/ liter D. None

3399. What is the molecular weight of sodium bicarbonate.
A. 85.007 g/mol
B. 84.007g/mol
C. 84.008g/mol
D. None

3400. A 2.0% boric acid solution serves as an isotonic....... preparation
A. Dermatology
B. Orthopaedic
C. Ophthalmic
D. All of the above

3401. Which is the following solution the red blood cell are suspend.
A. 2.0% kcl B. 2.0% Naoh
C. 3.0% Nacl D. 2.0% Nacl

3402. The weak salt solution or water is salt to be.
A. Hypertonic B. hypotonic
C. Isotonic D. Hygroscopic

3403. What is the method of measurement of tonicity.
A. Hemolytic B. Freezing point
C. Hemolysis D. Isotonic

3404. The PH of a buffer solution and the change in PH upon the addition of an acid or base may be calculated by uses of the equation.
A. Buffer capacity
B. Buffer solution
C. Buffer equation
D. Buffer action

3405. Which is the following example of common ion effect.

A. In- B. OH-
C. Ac D. ΔTf

3406. The negative logarithm of Ka is called.

A. Dissociation exponent
B. Dissociation constant
C. Both a and b
D. None of the above

3407. The buffer solutions are not ordinarily prepared from..

A. Weak acid B. Weak bases
C. Strong bases D. Strong acid

3408. The PKa formic acid is.

A. 4.76 B. 3.75
C. 3.76 D. 3.93

3409. What is the PH of solution containing 0.1 mole of ephedrine and 0.1 mole of ephedrine hydrochloride per liter of solution.

A. PH =10.36 B. PH = 7.14
C. PH = 10.34 D. PH = 8.15

3410. How much is the PH increased by addition to the solubility of 0.1% physostigmine base, m.w 275.34?

A. An decrease of 1.93 PH units
B. An increase of 1.93 PH units
C. Both a and b
D. None

3411. what is the buffer capacity of a solution containing 0.20 m acetic acid and 0.10m sodium acetate.

A. beta 0.14 B. alfa 0.15
C. beta 0.15 D. beta 0.10

3412. The PH of the acetit acid solution has been.

A. Decreased B. Increased
C. equal D. None

3413. Calomel electrode is used for.

A. Mercury chloride
B. Sulphate mercury
C. Silver chloride
D. None

3414. An increase in the concentration of the buffer components resuls in a........ buffer capacity or efficiency.

A. Greater B. Reduce
C. Both a and b D. None

3415. The PH of the bicarbonate buffer in the blood.

A. PH = 7.4 B. PH = 7.3
C. PH = 7.5 D. PH =7.6

3416. When the PH of the blood gose....... life is in serious banger.

A. Below 6.9 or above 7.8
B. Below 6.8 or above 7.7
C. Both a and b
D. None

3417. Lacrimal fluid or tears have been found to have a great degree of buffer....

A. Buffer capacity B. Buffer solution
C. Buffer equation D. Buffer action

3418. When the sample is removed for analysis because of the loss of .... from the tear.

A. O2 B. Co2
C. No2 D. None

3419. If the strong acid is added to a..... solution containing equal quantities of acetic acid and sodium acetate.

A. 0.01 -m B. 0.1 N
C. 0.001-m D. 0.1m

3420. The PKa of pilocarpine is.

A. 7.15 B. 8.73
C. 7.14 D. None

3421. When sodium acetate is added to acetic acid the dissociation constant for the.

A. Weak base B. Strong base
C. Weak acid D. Strong acid

3422. Which of the following solution for tonicity.

A. Hypotonic B. Isotonic
C. Hypertonic D. All of the above

3423. The temperature corresponds to the freezing point of a .... solution?

A. 0.95 Nacl B. 0.85% Nacl
C. 0.60% Nacl D. 0.90% Nacl

3424. The PKb of ephedrine is?

A. 10.36 Pkb B. 4.76 pkb
C. 4.64 Pkb D. None

3425. How many isotonic solution of........... g of Nacl per 100 ml.

A. 0.9g of Nacl B. 0.8g of Nacl
C. 0.7g of Nacl D. 0.5g of Nacl

3426. If the red blood cells are suspended in a......... % Nacl solution.

A. 3.0% Nacl B. 2.0 % Nacl
C. 0.2 % Nacl D. 0.1 % Nacl

3427. How much sodium chloride is required to render 100ml of a 1% solution of apomorphine hydrochloride isotonic with blood serum.

A. 0.78 g B. 0.75 g
C. 0.76 g D. 0.71 g

3428. A 2.0 % solution of boric acid has the same osmotic pressure as the blood cell contents when determined by the.

A. Isotonicity value
B. Freezing point
C. Tonicity
D. PH concentration

3429. What is class 1st method of adjusting tonicity and PH

A. Cryoscopic method
B. White vicent method
C. Sodium chloride
D. Freezing point

3430. Sodium chloride equivalent method is used.

A. Isotonicity adjusting
B. Adjust the tonicity
C. Adjusting the freezing point
D. Adjusting the stability

3431. A second method for adjusting the tonicity of pharmaceutical solution was developed by.

A. Mellen and seltzer
B. white vincent
C. Husa and Adams
D. Roos and borm

3432. .... Suggested that the term isotonic.

A. Husa B. Mellen
C. Seltzer D. White vincent

3433. The presence in solution, result change in PH upon the addition of small quantities of.

A. Buffer solution C. Acid or alkali
B. Nacl solution D. Salt solution

3434. According to roos and borm published the first paper on buffer action in.

A. 1915 B. 1914
C. 1918 D. 1919

3435. The replacement of concentration by activities in the equilibrium of a.....

A. Weak bases B. Weak acid
C. Strong acid D. Strong bases

3436. The activity coefficient multiplied by the..

A. Mole concentration
B. Molar concentration
C. Equal concentration
D. Molar fraction

3437. An ionic strength no greater than about.

A. 0.1 or 0.2 B. 0.3 or 0.4
C. 0.2 or 0.5 D. None

3438. The addition of natural salts to buffers the PH of the solution by altering the.....

A. Ionic strength not altering
B. Activities equilibrium
C. Ionic strength
D. Alters activity coefficient s

3439. A positive dilution value singnifies that the PH...... With dilution of the buffer.

A. PH c onstant B. PH rises
C. PH decrease D. PH equilibrium

3440. A negative value singnifies that PH..... with dilution of the buffer.

A. PH decreases B. PH increases
C. PH constant D. pH equilibrium

3441. The change in PH with temperature for a large number of.

A. Water B. Buffer
C. salt solution D. None

3442. The temperature coefficients for the calomel electrode are given in the study by.

A. Deby – huckel B. Bates
C. Roots and borm D. Koppel and spiro

3443. Which is the following solution in a soft glass bottle is influenced by the alkalinity of the glass.

A. Boric acid B. Sodium chloride
C. Salicylic acid D. Ascorbic acid

3444. Indicators may be considered as.......

A. Strong acid or strong base
B. Weak acid and weak base
C. Weak acid and strong acid
D. Strong acid

3445. Methyl red show it's full alkaline color.......... at PH of about 6

A. Blue B. Green
C. Purple D. Yellow

3446. King is refered to as the.

A. Indicatore change
B. Indicatore altered
C. Indicatore constant
D. Indicatore equilibrium

3447. The ionization is represed by the.

A. Common ion effect
B. Common ion equilibrium
C. Common ion constant
D. Common ion change

3448. The indicatore is then predominantly in the form of Hin the..

A. Basic color B. Acid color
C. Weak color D. Strong color

3449. Indicatores can be combined to yield so called.

A. Only indicatores
B. Universal indicatore
C. Constant indicatore
D. None

3450. A universal indicatore is a PH indicatore that displays different colors as the PH transitions from PH.

A. 1 to 12 B. 13 to 14
C. 1.2 to 1.8 D. None

3451. The buffer capy changes as the ratio log ([salt] /[acid] increase with added..

A. Acid B. Base
C. Buffer D. salt

3452. When 0.01 mole of base is added to a 0.1 molar acetate buffer the PH increase from.

A. 6.8 - 8.4 B. 4.76 - 4.85
C. 5.2 - 6.8 D. None

3453. The reaction of an equivalent of an acid with an equivalent of a base is called.

A. Buffer capacity B. Buffer equation
C. Neutralization D. End point

3454. The plot of PH versus mililiter of..... added produces the titration curve.

A. Hcl B. NaoH
C. H_2O D. HCO_3

3455. A strong base has a high buffer capacity above a PH of.

A. 12 B. 10
C. 9 D. 6

3456. The buffer capacity of a solution of a strong acid was shown by ...... to be directly proportional to the hydrogen ion concentration.

A. Bates B. Gifford
C. Mason D. Van slyke

3457. The slope of the curve is a minimum and the buffer capacity is.

A. Decrease B. Constant
C. Greater D. Equilibrium

3458. The curves can be plotted by using the.

A. Buffer equation
B. Buffer capacity
C. Buffer solution
D. Buffer index

3459. The neutralization curve for the universal buffer mixture is lineare between PH.

A. 4 and 8 B. 8 and 12
C. 2 and 4 D. None

3460. The salt solution in this instance is said to be.

A. Hypertonic B. Hemolysis
C. Hypotonic D. Isotonic

3461. At a low pH a base is predominantly in the .... form

A. Gases B. Ionic
C. Acid D. Solid

3462. When the amount of base exceeds the limited .... of this form

A. Water solubility B. Solute
C. Solvent D. None

3463. The same salt concentration and same osmotic pressure as the red blood cell content and is said to be.

A. Hypertonic B. Hypotonic
C. Isotonic D. Hemolysis

3465. The salt solution in this instance is said to be.

A. Hypertonic B. Isotonic
C. Hypotonic D. Hemolysis

3466. A 2.0% solution of boric acid has the same .... as the blood cell contents.

A. Osmotic pressure
B. Isosmotic
C. Hemolysis
D. Hemolytic

3467. Which of the following example of uni - divalent electrolytes.

A. Sodium sulphate
B. Atropine sulphate
C. Both a and b
D. Calcium bromide

3468. What is the freezing point of both human blood and lacrimalfluid.

A. - 0.80°c B. -0. 52°c
C. - 0.90 °c D. None

3469. Which of the following ephedrine sulphate is

A. g × 0.23 = 0.23g
B. 0.3g × 0.21 = 0.063 g
C. 3.4 × 0.104 = 0.35 g
D. None

3470. We replace Nacl with....... as the isotonic agents.

A. Ephedrine sulphate
B. Propylene glycol
C. Sodium chloride
D. Procaine hydrochloride

3471. At a hydrogen ion concentration 1.75 × 10-5 what is the capacity of a buffer containing 0.10 moles each of acetic acid and sodium acetate per liter of solution.

A. 0.115 B. 0.113
C. 0.118 D. 0.112

3472. The buffer capacity depends on the value of the ratio.

A. [base]/[acid] B. [Salt] / [acid]
C. [Base]/ [Base] D. None

3473. The hydrogen ion concentration of such a solution is 10-12 and the total buffer capacity is.

A. Beta 0.020 B. Beta 0.023
C. 0.012 D. 0.028

3474. Which requires 20 times the amount of tears to restore the normal PH of the eye as compared with the result following two drops of? .....

A. Atropine sulphate
B. Sodium chloride
C. Epinephrine hydrochloride
D. Potassium chloride

3475. To reestablished the constant Ka at.

A. 3.75 × 10-2 B. 1.75 × 10-5
C. 3.20 × 10 -3 D. None

3476. The resistance to a change in PH is known as.

A. Buffer solution B. Buffer equation
C. Buffer action D. Buffer capacity

3477. Which is not universal indicatore.?

A. Methyl yellow
B. Phenolphthalein
C. Bromthylmol blue
D. Alizarin yellow

3478. Which method of granulation is suitable in case of poorly soluble drug?

A. Dry granulation
B. Moisture activated
C. dry granulation
D. Both A and C

3479. Which of the following example is correct to demonstrate dissolution or solubility Limited adsorption?

A. Penicillin B. Ibuprofen
C. Rifampin D. Galantamine

3480. Poorly water soluble drugs will be________ .

A. Slowly adsorp and show variable bioavailability
B. Slowly adsorpamd show maximum availability
C. Fastly adsorb and show good availability
D. Both A and C

3481. Which of the following equation can be used to determine release of active drug agent from dosage form?

A. Noyes-whitney
B. Hopfenberg
C. Baker- lansdale
D. None of above

3482. Critical step which play an important role in adsorption of drug from Tablet?

A. Dissolution
B. First pass metabolism
C. Disintegration
D. Enzymatic reaction and barriers

3483. Why milk is not taken along with antibiotic tablet?

A. Inhibit dissolution
B. Prevent adsorption
C. Inhibit disintegration
D. Prevent absorption

3484. Which of the following property make drug difficult to formulate?

A. Poor wetting and slow dissolution
B. Good wetting and fast dissolution
C. Both A and B
D. None of the above

3485. Which of the following is not used as a diluent?

A. Lactose anhydrate and spray dried lactose
B. Celutab
C. Dibetic calcium phosphate dehydrate
D. Sodium carboxymethyl cellulose

3486. Which of the following used as a dilutent, disintegrant , Binder as well as glidant?

A. Cellulose derivatives
B. Starch and its derivatives
C. Sorbitol
D. Both A and B

3487. In moisture activated drug granulation agglomerate size is between which of following range?

A. 150 to 160 um B. 100-450 um
C. 200-300um D. 150-500um

3488. What is the reason for lamination of tablet in storage period and compression?

A. Low level of glidant and binding agent
B. Air Entrapment between layers
C. High concentration of lubricant
D. Both A and C

3489. How can we inhibit the problem of capping and lamination while compressing tablet?

A. By improving granules size
B. By improving ratio of Binder agent
C. Why improving lubricant concentration
D. None of the above

3490. Super disintegrants swell up and disintegrate tablets within time_____.

A. 30 second B. 1 minute
C. 2 minute D. None of the above

3491. Which of the following used as a super disintegrant.

A. Veegum HV
B. Sodium starch glycolate
C. PVP
D. Sodium carboxymethylcellulose

3492. In liyophilized foam method, which of the following mixture is used to form tablet?

A. Mixture of gelatin, sugar ,drug
B. Mixture of gelatin ,starch, drug
C. Mixture of gelatin, PVP, drug
D. Mixture of gelatin, sugar or sugar drug and other component

3493. Zydin technology used in manufacturing of which type of tablet?

A. Dispensing tablet
B. Orally disintegrating tablet
C. Effervescent tablet
D. Hypodermic tablet

3494. While checking friability of tablets, loss should not more than______.

A. 1% B. 25%
C. 10% D. 8%

3495. In compression coated tablet, core coated by_________.

A. Sugar B. Both A and B
C. Polymer D. None of the above

3496. In compression coated tablet, coating material can be in the form of_________.

A. Liquid B. Granules
C. Powder D. Both B and C

3497. Compression coating is used for which type of a drug?
A. Anhydrous drug
B. Unstable drug
C. Moisture and heat labile
D. None of above

3498. In multi tablet system, tablet diameter is about_________.
A. 1-5 mm B. 1-10mm
C. 2.5-6mm D. 3-4mm

3499. In modified release Drug Delivery System repeat action tablet coating of layers is done by_______.
A. Slowly permeable barrier coating
B. Polymer Matrix barrier coating
C. Fast permeable barrier coating
D. None of above

3500. Which of the following drug is given in delayed release tablet form?
A. Erythromycin
B. Thalidomide
C. Venlafaxine hydrochloride
D. Oxtriphylline

3501. Which of the following is main disadvantage of immediate release tablet?
A. No drug release control
B. Disintegrate immediately
C. No special rate controlling feature
D. None of above

3502. Tablet triturates are generally contain ___________.
A. Two or more drugs
B. High amount of Potent drug
C. Small amount of potent drug
D. Complex form of drug

3503. How many tablets taken to check the friability of large number of tablet?
A. 10 B. 15
C. 20 D. 25

3504. What is the weight loss acceptance criteria for tablet friability?
A. Not more than 2%
B. Not more than 5%
C. Less than 1%
D. Less than 3%

3505. At which RPM, Roche friabilator is regulated to evaluate tablet friability?
A. 25 RPM B. 100 RPM
C. 50 RPM D. 10 RPM

3506. How many times tablet should taken in friability testing?
A. For 4 minutes at 25 RPM
B. For 5 minute at 25 RPM
C. For 3 minutes at 10 RPM
D. For 5 minute at 10 RPM

3507. Which of the following is rate cycle for Tablets in the tablet disintegration apparatus.
A. 30-40 cycle pe minute
B. 20-40 cycle per minute
C. 29-32 cycle per minute
D. Both A and B

3508. Which of the following solution used in testing of delayed release tablet?
A. N Hcl, 0.2 M phosphate buffer
B. 1%NaOH,0.2M phosphate buffer
C. 0.2N H2SO4, 0.3M phosphate buffer
D. 0.1N NaOH,0.3 M phosphate buffer

3509. Croscarmellose function as excipient in tablet.
A. Disintegrant B. Glidant
C. Binder D. None of above

3510. At which concentration, Colloidal Silicon oxide works as a glidant, antiadherent?
A. 2-5% B. 0.1-1%
C. 12-10% D. 1-3%

3511. Mean particle size, at which corn starch act as a excipient?
A. 15 um B. 20 um
C. 30 um D. 13 um

3512. Croscarmellose not used in which type of granulation?
A. Wet granulation
B. Dry granulation
C. Direct compression
D. All of above

3513. Which of the following used as a slow release controlling agent?
A. Ammonio methacrylate copolymer type A
B. Calcium phosphate dihydrate
C. Compactrol
D. Ammoniomethacrylate copolymer type B

3514. Which of the following is used as a direct compressible diluent?
A. Silicon dioxide
B. Dibasic calcium phosphate
C. Lactose
D. Both B and C

3515. Use of which type of diluent prevent risk of maillard reaction?
A. Cornstarch
B. 10 to 15% lactose
C. 10 to 90 % mannitol 60
D. None of above

3516. Hypromellose is which type of agent?
A. Immediate release control agent
B. Slow release control agent
C. Rate controlling agent
D. Sustained release control agent

3517. Mannitol is which type of diluent?
A. Soluble sugar alcohol diluent
B. Inorganic alcohol diluent
C. Soluble sugar Aqueous diluent
D. All of above

3518. The Crown thickness of individual tablet can be measured in_______.
A. NM B. Centimetre
C. Millimetre D. Micrometre

3519. Which of the following is a rapid method to measure the Crown thickness of tablet?
A. Micrometre scale method
B. Both A and B
C. Sliding Caliper scale method
D. None of above

3520. Acceptance variable range of tablet thickness with respect to standard value?
A. ±3% B. ±8%
C. ±5% D. ± 10%

3521. Which type of punches require for proper shape of a tablet?
A. Compression punch
B. Slotted punch
C. Revolving punch
D. None of above

3522. Conventional punches should run at which speed for proper shape of tablet?
A. High speed
B. Intermediate speed
C. Slow speed
D. None of above

3523. Convex surface of tablet increase risk of which type of tablet defect?
A. Capping B. Mottling
C. Lamination D. Cracking

3524. Which Instrument used to measure the uniformity of colour and gloss on a tablet surface?
A. Flame photometer
B. Both A and B
C. Micro reflectance photometer
D. None of above

3525. Which is the earliest tester used to evaluate tablet hardness?
A. Pfizer hardness tester
B. Monsanto hardness tester
C. Strong cobb tester
D. Schleunger tester

3526. When deep concave punches use in tablet punching, increased risk of which type of tablet defect?
A. Lamination B. Cracking
C. Whiskering D. Capping

3527. Which of the following is the cycle of tablet disintegration apparatus?
A. 15 to 30 cycle per minute
B. 20 to 40 cycle per minute
C. 40 to 56 cycle per minute
D. 28 to 32 cycle per minute

3528. Which of the following is also known as laboratory friabilator?
A. Roche friabilator
B. PTF 200 double drum friabilator
C. PTF 10 single drum friabilator
D. PTF 300 triple drum friabilator

3529. Which type of tablets undergo high friability weight losses comparative to conventional tablets?
A. Chewable tablet
B. Effervescent tablet
C. Multi compressed tablet
D. Both A and B

3530. To avoid the friability problem of tablet, granulation should contain atleast how much percentage of moisture?
A. 1 to 10% B. 10 to 30%
C. 2 to 4% D. None of above

3531. Which type of test used to evaluate rough handling friability of tablets?
A. Vibrational test B. Drop test
C. Plane impact test D. All of above

3532. Number of tablet taken to evaluate weight variation test according to IP?
A. 10 B. 15
C. 20 D. 25

3533. Formula used to determine the weight variation of tablet?
A. Composite weight / 10
B. Weight of tablet /number of tablet
C. Number of tablet / weight of tablet
D. None of above

3534. According to USB, number of tablets taken for weight variation test?
A. 10 B. 15
C. 20 D. 25

3535. Factor which directly contribute to content uniformity problem in tablet?
A. Excipient ratio
B. Compressed amount
C. Tablet weight variation
D. Both A and B

3536. Weight of tablet cannot be used as a potential and indicatore unless is it does not contain how much amount of active ingredient?
A. 20-50% B. 90-95%
C. 80-95 % D. Both B and C

3537. How many tablets are taken for content uniformity testing of low doses drug tablet?
A. 20 B. 30
C. 10 D. 15

3538. What is the mess size of basket use in USP disintegration apparatus?
A. 20 B. 15
C. 10 D. 25

3539. Indus disintegration Apparatus, tablet should remain at which distance from the bottom of beaker?
A. 2.5 cm B. 3.5 cm
C. 5 cm D. 4.5 cm

3540. How many glass tubes used in USB disintegration apparatus?
A. 10 B. 6
C. 3 D. 5

3541. What is the maximum degradation time for uncoated USP tablets?
A. 50 minute B. 20 minute
C. 30 minute D. 40 minute

3542. What is the minimum disintegration time of uncoated USB tablets?
A. 10 minute B. 5 minute
C. 15 minute D. 20 minute

3543. Direct and correct method for assessment of released drug from Tablet formulation?
A. In Vivo bioavailability
B. Both A and B
C. In vitro bioavailability
D. None of above

3544. Which of the following is USB Type II dissolution apparatus?
A. Basket type
B. Peddle type
C. Flow through cell type
D. Reciprocating cylinder type

3545. Which of the following test is restricted for the evaluation of tablet?
A. Dissolution
B. In vivo bioavailability test
C. In vitro bioavailability test
D. None of above

3546. Excessive dry granulation can lead to which type of tablet defect?
A. Lamination B. Whiskering
C. Capping D. Both A and B

3547. In compression coating, coating material found in_______________ form.

A. Powder B. Granules
C. Liquid D. Both A and B

3548. At which rotating speed, USP type-II apparatus is regulated for dissolution testing?

A. 25-30 RPM B. 25-40 RPM
C. 10-25 rpm D. 35-45 RPM

3549. Which of the following coating material used in compression coating?

A. Sugar B. Both A and B
C. Polymers D. None of above

3550. Waterproofing and Seal coat of tablet done by which material?

A. Shillacor polymer B. Sugar
C. Both A and B D. None of above

3551. Which solution is considered as waterproofing solution in seal coating?

A. Organic solution
B. Non aqueous solution
C. Alcoholic solution
D. All of above

3552. In seal coating, how many layers of coating can be applied?

A. 2-4 B. 3-5
C. 1-3 D. None of above

3553. Which of the following instrument used to measure the coated tablet?

A. Scale B. Gauge
C. Caliper D. Both A and C

3554. In supporting, how many layers of coating can be applied?

A. 2-6 B. 1-5
C. 3-8 D. 5-10

3555. In smothing, which type of coating material is applied for coating?

A. Thick sucrose solution
B. Thin sucrose solution
C. Powder sucrose
D. Both B and C

3556. For polishing of tablet, which of the following is generally use?

A. Carnauba wax B. Beeswax
C. Acacia D. Both A and

3557. Which of the following is the function of Fluid bed coating machine?

A. Spray coating of tablet
B. Coating of granules
C. Granulation
D. All of above

3558. What is the acceptable percentage range of film forming polymer in Aqua film coating solution?

A. 2%-8% B. 15%- 20%
C. 20%- 35% D. 7%-18%

3559. Which of the following is not film forming polymer?

A. Methyl cellulose
B. Poly ethylene
C. Cellulose acetate succinate
D. Hydroxy methyl cellulose

3560. Which spraying technique used in enteric coating of tablet by Rotatory Fluid bed coater?

A. Top spray technique
B. Bottom spray technique
C. Tangential spray technique
D. Both A and B

3561. Which of the following is not example of plasticizer used in film coating?

A. Propylene glycol
B. Dibutyl subacetate
C. Diethylphthalate
D. PVP

3562. In Fluid bed granulation, which type of spray technique can be use?

A. Top spray technique
B. Bottom spray technique
C. Tangential spray
D. Both A and B

3563. Which of the following Polymer is not use in enteric coating?

A. Carboxy cellulose
B. Eudragit L
C. Eudragit S
D. Acrylate polymer

3564. Separation of tablet in different layers lead to which type of tablet defect?

A. Capping B. Lamination
C. Whiskering D. All of above

3565. Tablet capping and lamination problem can be often removed by which process?

A. Precompression
B. Slowing tableting rate
C. Reducing final compression pressure
D. All of above

3566. Tablet produced by Deep concave punches show capping defect due to generation of__________.

A. Shear stress
B. Compression pressure
C. Die wall pressure
D. All of above

3567. Capping and lamination generally occurs due to which reason?

A. Lake of Cohesion
B. Low melting point substances
C. Air Entrapment
D. All of above

3568. Shear stress produced during tablet punching can be eliminate by using which type of punch?

A. Convex punch B. Flat punch
C. Both a and b D. None of above

3569. In some cases colloidal silica added in tablet formula to eliminate which tablet defect?

A. Picking and sticking
B. Capping and lamination
C. Mottling
D. All of above

3570. Which of the following is the reason for the motlling of tablet?

A. Use of colorant in direct compression
B. Particle size is too large
C. Colour differences of excipient
D. All of above

3571. Poor flow property of feed through Hopper can lead to which defect?

A. Arching B. Bridging
C. Rate holding D. All of above

3572. Method use to determine surface area of agglomerates?

A. Air permission
B. Gas adsorption
C. Both a and b
D. None of above

3573. What is the Angle of repose of free flowing material?

A. ≥30° B. ≤30°
C. ≥40° D. ≤40°

3574. Method generally use to determine angle of repose?

A. Tilting box method
B. Freestanding cone method
C. Revolving cylinder method
D. All of above

3575. Roller compactor used in which type of granulation method?

A. Wet granulation
B. Compression granulation
C. Dry granulation
D. Both B and C

3576. Roller compactor Exerts which type of pressure on compaction rolls?

A. Hydraulic pressure
B. Absolute pressure
C. Binding pressure
D. Vacuum pressure

3577. Which of the following is the first high shear powder blender?

A. Diosna mixer
B. Little Ford MGT mixer
C. Little Ford lodige mixer
D. Gral mixer

3578. Which of the following is the size range of round tablet

A. 4 /10-1 /2 inch B. 1/12 -1/15 inch
C. 3 /16 - 1/2 inch D. 4/5-1/3inch

3579. Which of the following diluent cannot be used in the water sensitive drug tablet formulation?

A. Debasic calcium phosphate
B. Anhydrous lactose
C. Calcium sulphate
D. None of above

3580. Diluent sorbitol show hydroscopic property at which humidity percentage?

A. 65% B. 75%
C. 70% D. 55%

3581. Which of the following sugar concentration solution can be used in wet granulation?

A. 80% dextrose
B. 50% glucose
C. 50-70 percent sucrose
D. Both B and C

3582. Which of the following Lubricant having low melting point?

A. Stearic acid
B. Polyethylene glycol
C. Talc
D. None of above

3583. In which range start of USB grade contain moisture?

A. 5-12 percent B. 12-20 percent
C. 11-14 percent D. 10-25 percent

3584. Which of the following step not involve in the dry granulation?

A. Screening B. Slugging
C. Milling D. None of above

3585. Differences between dug particle size and diluent bulk density can be late to __________ in the granulation.

A. Stratification
B. defects
C. Lump formation
D. None of above

3586. Single substance compressing can produce tablet which do not_______________.

A. Compact
B. Disintegrate
C. Dissolve
D. All of above

3587. What is the Angle of repose of poorly flowing material?

A. ≤30° B. ≥30°
C. ≤40° D. ≥40°

3588. Which of the following substance can be compress directly?

A. Sodium chloride
B. Sodium Bromide
C. Potassium chloride
D. All of above

3589. Direct compression of amine compound and spray dried lectose cause interaction by showing____________.

A. Yellow discoloration
B. Orange discoloration
C. Redis discoloration
D. None of above

3590. Which of the following granulation build up charge due to dry nature?

A. Dry granulation
B. Direct compression
C. Both a and b
D. None of above

3591. Compression granulation techniques used for____________.

A. Hydrophilic substances
B. Thermolabile substances
C. Hydrophobic substances
D. Both A and B

3592. Formulation of many Aspirin and vitamins are prepared by_____________.

A. Compression granulation
B. Wet granulation
C. Dry granulation
D. Both A and C

3593. Compaction pressure in compression granulation not result into______________.

A. Strengthening of Bond
B. Increase fluidity of mixture
C. Uniformity of the mixture
D. Both A and B

3594. Which of the following Mixture used for dry mixing of powder

A. Sigma blende B. Planetary mixture
C. Both a and b D. None of above

3595. Which of the following disadvantage of wet granulation?

A. Time consuming
B. Expensive
C. Labour intensive
D. All of above

3596. Equipment used in wet granulation is not useful for______________.

A. Dry mixing C. Aggregation
B. Dry milling D. Both A and C

3597. Which of the following equipment can be use for both powder blending and wet massing?

A. Sigma blender
B. Little Lodige mixer
C. Diosna mixer
D. Plow mixture

3598. Little lodige mixer is capable of doing powder mixing in______________.

A. 30-60 second B. 1 minute
C. 2 minute D. 20-40 second

3599. Gral mixture is modified version of ___________mixture.

A. Plow mixture B. Diosna mixture
C. Planetary mixer D. None of above

3600. Which of the following starch can be used in direct compression?

A. Sta-Rx 1500 B. Celutab
C. Emdex D. All of above

3601. At which percentage level veegum and bentonite act as a disintegrant?

A. About 10% B. About 20%
C. About 5% D. None of above

3602. At which concentration free gelatinized starches are work as a disintegrants?

A. 2% B. 5%
C. 10% D. 12%

3603. which of the following reduce friction between walls of die cavity and tablets surface?

A. Antiadherents B. Glidants
C. Lubricants D. All of above

3604. Which of following is not lubricant?

A. Steric acid B. Waxes
C. Cornstarch D. Polyethylene glycol

3605. Which of following act as a lubricant and glidant?

A. Talc B. Waxes
C. Cornstarch D. Celica derivative

3606. Which of the following act as a diluant Binder and disintegrates?

A. Glucose
B. PVP
C. Cellulose derivatives
D. All of above

3607. Roller compact capable of producing _________compact Ribbon like material.

A. 500kg B. 350 kg
C. 200 kg D. 800 kg

3608. Which of the following second most using lubricant?

A. Talc
B. Waxes
C. Polyethylene glycols
D. All of above

3609. Which of the following is the Most widely using lubricant?

A. Stearic acid derivatives
B. Stearic acid
C. Stearic acid salt
D. All of above

3610. Lactose EFK have faster disintegration time as compared to______.

A. Lactose anhydrous
B. Dextrose monohydrate
C. Celutab
D. All of above

3611. Which of the following have faster disintegration time?

A. Dipac
B. Celutab
C. Lactose anhydrous
D. Dextrose monohydrate

3612. Which of the following is the class of multiple compressed tablet?

A. Layered tablet
B. Compression coated tablet
C. Both a and b
D. None of above

3613. Which of the following is the reason for preparing multi compressed tablet?

A. Inhibit physical incompatibility
B. For repeat and prolonged action
C. Inhibit chemical incompatibility
D. All of above

3614. Delayed release action tablet release drug in which part of GI tract?
A. Stomach
B. Lower intestine
C. Upper intestine
D. None of above

3615. What is the function of aerosil as excipient?
A. Glidant
B. Lubricant
C. Anti adherent
D. All of above

3616. Which of the following substance used in enteric coating?
A. HPMC B. CMC
C. CAP D. PVP

3617. Sugar coated tablet disintegration time is_________.
A. 15 minut B. 60 minute
C. 30 minut D. 20 minute

3618. Sub coating is done in order to_________.
A. Build up size of tablet
B. Form uniform edges
C. To increase the bulkiness
D. All of above

3619. Which of the following is the type of perforated Pan system?
A. Accela cota B. Glatt coater
C. Hi coater D. All of above

3620. Chilsonator is used for___________.
A. Tablet granulation
B. Milling of powder
C. Tablet coating
D. None of above

3621. Eudragit used in which type of coating?
A. Sugar coating
B. Enteric coating
C. Film coating
D. All of above

3622. Which of the following substance used for film coating?
A. Shellac B. Gelatin
C. Zein D. Both A and C

3623. The wurster method is applicable in_________.
A. Tablet coating
B. Tablet compression
C. Tablet defects
D. Granulation

3624. Which of the following is step is important for release of drug from Tablet?
A. Ionization
B. Disintegration
C. Complexation
D. Dissolution

3625. Drug dissolution rate of tablet is given by which of following equation?
A. Maxwell's equation
B. Noyes Whitney equation
C. Acoustic equation
D. Michalis menten equation

3626. Sodium CMC is which type of adhesive?
A. Synthetic adhesive
B. Semi synthetic adhesive
C. Mucoadhesive
D. None of above

3627. Shellac is used to achieve which type of coating?
A. Hydrophilic Matrix coating
B. Lipophilic Matrix coating
C. Hydrophobic Matrix coating
D. None of above

3628. What is the mesh aperture diameter of IP disintegration apparatus?
A. 5 mm B. 1 mm
C. 2 mm D. 2.5 mm

3629. During tablet coating, improper distribution of coating solution before drying can cause which tablet defect?
A. Orange peel effect
B. Blistering
C. Cracking
D. None of above

3630. In matrix tablet formulation, which of following substances form hydrophilic matrix?
A. Aerosil B. HPMC
C. PVP D. Sodium CMC

3631. In Dissolution testing apparatus, flask maintained at which temperature?

A. 37° ± 4.9 °C B. 38° ± 0.9°C
C. 39° ± 0.5°C D. 37°± 0.5°C

3632. Tablet punch faces are plate by__________.

A. Aluminium B. Chromium
C. Zinc D. All of above

3633. Percentage of moisture present in Sta-Rx1500?

A. 10% B. 25%
C. 20% D. 30%

3634. Which of the following solution is called as Aqua coal ECD solution?

A. 25% w/v of ethyl cellulose dispersion
B. 10% w/v of ethyl cellulose dispersion
C. 30 % w/v of ethyl cellulose dispersion
D. 40% w/v of ethyl cellulose dispersion

3635. CAP dissolves at which part of GIT?

A. Stomach B. Intestine
C. Mouth D. None of above

3636. Which of following substance not use in polishing of tablet?

A. Carnauba wax B. Beeswax
C. Paraffin D. Acacia

3637. Kaolin use in _________.

A. Sealcoating B. Polishing
C. Subcoating D. None of above

3638. Oliec acid used as_______ in tablet coating.

A. Sealant B. Colouring agent
C. Polishing agent D. All of above

3639. How many coat of sugar syrup is applied for polishing of tablet?

A. 3-4coat B. 5-8 coat
C. 2-8coat D. 1-5 coat

3640. For polishing of tablet, what should be the speed of coating pan?

A. 20 RPM B. 12 RPM
C. 10 RPM D. 28 RPM

3641. Canvas lined Pan used for________.

A. Seal coating B. Smoothing
C. Subcoating D. Polishing

3642. Panpour method is used for which type of coating?

A. Sugar coating
B. Compression coating
C. Film coating
D. Chocolate coating

3643. How many Coats of grossing sugar syrup is applied for smoothening and colour coat?

A. 5-15 coat B. 10-30 coat
C. 20 coat D. 1-10 coat

3644. For smoothening of tablet, what should be the speed of coating pan?

A. 18 RPM B. 20 RPM
C. 12 RPM D. 25 RPM

3645. How many coats of gelatin / Acacia solution can be applied for sub coating?

A. 1-5 B. 5-10
C. 2 - 7 D. 3-9

3646. Which of the following route does not avoid first pass metabolism?

A. Buccal route B. Sublingual route
C. Parenteral route D. Oral route

3647. Which of the following method used in determination of tablet strength?

A. Friability B. Hardness testing
C. Both a and b D. None of above

3648. Tablet material adherence towards the die walls called as__________.

A. Sticking B. Mottling
C. Picking D. None of above

3649. Mannitol mostly used as sweetening agent in which type of tablet?

A. Sugar coated tablet
B. Chewable tablet
C. Both a and b
D. None of above

3650. According to IP, what is dissolution time of the enteric coated tablet in point 1 N Hcl?

A. 80 minute B. 190 minute
C. 120 minute D. 30 minute

3651. PVP is which type of adhesive?
A. Semi synthetic adhesive
B. Mucoadhesive
C. Synthetic adhesive
D. None of above

3652. Which of the following is not non enteric polymer?
A. Povidone
B. Eudragit E
C. Methyl hydroxyethyl cellulose
D. Eudragit L

3653. Which of the following is not soluble in intestinal fluid at pH 6 - 7?
A. Eudragit E B. Eudragit S
C. Eudragit L D. All of above

3654. What is the pH at which cellulose Acetate phthalate dissolve?
A. Above 6 B. At 7
C. Below 6 D. None of above

3655. Polymer which is completely insoluble in GIT fluid and water?
A. Ethyl cellulose
B. Eudragit E
C. Eudragit L
D. Hydroxypropyl methylcellulose

3656. Non enteric polymer which having solubility in aqueous as well as non aqueous fluid?
A. CAP B. PVAP
C. HPMC D. Ethyl cellulose

3657. Which of the following polymer can improve colorants dispersion in the coating solution?
A. Povidone B. HPMC
C. HPC D. All of above

3658. Which of following is non enteric Eudragit?
A. Eudragit L B. Eudragit S
C. Eudragit E D. Eudragit RL

3659. Which of the following polymer is used for enteric coating?
A. Eudragit E B. Eudragit RL
C. Eudragit L D. Eudragit RS

3660. Which of the following polymer is pH independent?
A. Eudragit S B. Eudragit RS
C. Eudragit E D. Eudragit L

3661. Which of the following polymer is pH dependent?
A. Eudragit S B. Eudragit E
C. Eudragit L D. Both A and B

3662. HPMC is soluble below________ temperature.
A. 40°C B. 48°C
C. 37°C D. 30°C

3663. Drugs sensitive to acid should be protected from acid in the pH range__________.
A. 1-3 B. 2-4
C. 1.5-3 D. 1-5

3664. Which of following is not plasticizer?
A. Low molecular weight polyethylene glycol
B. High molecular weight polyethylene glycol
C. Glycerine
D. Propylene glycol

3665. Polymer which is soluble in water?
A. Polyethylene glycol
B. Span
C. Propylene glycol
D. Both A and C

3666. Plasticizer which is used in coating solution of organic solvent?
A. Tween
B. Span
C. Polyethylene glycol
D. None of above

3667. For achieve proper distribution of colorant, In film coating solution particle size of colourant and should be_________________.
A. <10 B. <15
C. >10 D. >15

3668. Colour concentrate of Opalux-Opaquant used in which type of coating?
A. Sugar coating B. Chocolate coating
C. Film coating D. All of above

3669. Which type of colour concentrate used in film coating?
A. Opalux- Opaquant
B. Opaspray-Opaquant
C. Opadry
D. Both B and C

3670. Opadry used in which type of coating?
A. Film coating
B. Chocolate coating
C. Sugar coating
D. All of above

3671. Which of the following is example of Opaquant-extender?
A. Titanium dioxide
B. Talc
C. Silicate
D. All of above

3672. Miscellaneous component of film coating solution is ____________.
A. Surfactant
B. Antioxidants
C. Flavours
D. All of above

3673. Roughness in film coated tablet is generally observed when coating solution is applied by ________ method.
A. Spraying method
B. Both A and B
C. Panpour method
D. None of above

3674. Which method need additional step of drying for removal of latent solvent in film coating?
A. Panpour method
B. Pan spray method
C. Pan lading method
D. None of above

3675. Which method not need Spraying and automatic operator system for proper coating of tablet?
A. Pan pour method
B. Pan lading method
C. Pan spray method
D. All of above

3676. Sugar coating of tablet generally done by_______ method.
A. Pan spray method
B. Pan lading method
C. Pan pour method
D. All of above

3677. Coating solution is pumped at which pressure in airless spray system?
A. 250-3000psig B. 300-2500psig
C. n100-150psig D. 500-800psig

3678. Small orifice is used in which type of spray application system?
A. Airless spray system
B. Air atomized system
C. Pan spray system
D. None of above

3679. Coating solution is formed at which pressure in air atomized system?
A. 10-30psig B. 5-50psig
C. 15-40psig D. 50-100psig

3680. Which method is not used in sugar coating of tablet?
A. Pan spray method
B. Air atomized method
C. Airless spray method
D. All of above

3681. Adhesion test for film coated tablet is done by _______.
A. Hardness tester
B. Tensile strength tester
C. Friability tester
D. None of above

3682. Film coated tablets, diametral crushing strength is determined by __________.
A. Hardness tester
B. Friability tester
C. Tensile strength tester
D. All of above

3683. Lakes generally available contain how much amount of pure dye content?
A. 10-80 percent
B. 20-40 percent
C. 10-30 percent
D. 25-30 percent

3684. Which of the following lakes obtained from precipitation?

A. Dye B. Opaquant

C. Colorant D. None of above

3685. Hazing is term used for________.

A. Dull film B. Rough film

B. Removal of film D. All of above

3686. Thickness of film Coat of tablet is generally between which of the following range?

A. 30-150um B. 20-100 um

C. 10-90 um D. None of above

3687. Film Coat structure, under close examination can be _________ in appearance.

A. Non homogeneous

B. Distinct

C. Homogeneous

D. Both A and C

3688. Which of the following is a reason for non homogeneous appearance of film coat structure?

A. Insoluble ingredients

B. Crystalline ingredient

C. Non crystalline ingredients

D. All of above

3689. Which of the following polymer is mostly used in film coating?

A. Cellulose derivatives

B. Povidone

C. Eudragit E

D. All of above

3690. Particle size range of true latexes used in film coating?

A. 200-300 nm B. 20-80 nm

C. 10-100 nm D. 80-150 nm

3691. Which of the following equation used to determine particle diameter at which particle do not show the sedimentation in system?

A. Noyes Whitney equation

B. Hopfenberg equation

C. Stokes equation

D. None of above

3692. Which of the following polymer is produced by emulsion polymerization process?

A. Eudragit L100-55

B. Povidone

C. Eudragit NE30D

D. Both A and C

3693. Latex dispersion for film coating can be prepared by which method?

A. Emulsion polymerization

B. Emulsion trituration

C. Both A and B

D. None of above

3694 Which of the following polymer rarely used in film coating?

A. Methylcellulose

B. Hydroxyethyl cellulose

C. Hydroxypropyl cellulose

D. Hydroxypropyl methylcellulose

3695. Minimum film forming temperature of polymer determined by which method?

A. Emulsion polymerization

B. Both A and B

C. Glass transition

D. None of above

3696. Which of the following is the summarised equation of relationship between molecular weight and Apparent viscosity?

A. MWT=K(naap)k

B. naap=K×1/MWT

C. K=MWT/naap

D. None of above

3697. Which of the following used to lower the transition temperature?

A. Polymer B. Plasticizer

C. Opacifier D. All of above

3698. What is the function of plasticizer?

A. Increase strain

B. Increase film elongation

C. Decrease elastic modulus

D. All of above

3699. Which of the following is used for decreasing tensile strength?
A. Plasticizer
B. Disintegrate
C. Binder
D. Opacifying agents

3700. Presence of pigment generally reduce_______________ in formulation.
A. Elastic modulus
B. Tensile strength
C. Both A and B
D. None of above

3701. Stearic acid cause which tablet defect?
A. Sticking B. Lamination
C. Picking D. All of above

3702. Which of the following is not considered as tablet?
A. Tablet triturate
B. Troches and Lozenges
C. Pessaries
D. Both A and B

3703. Which of the following lubricant not used in the drug breakdown catalyzed by iron?
A. Talc B. Starch
C. Stearic acid D. All of above

3704. In Indian Pharmacopoeia, which test is not considered as official test for tablet?
A. friability B. Hardness
C. Disintegration D. Dissolution

3705. Which of the following tablet defect is due to high compression force?
A. Capping B. Picking
C. Sticking D. All of above

3706. Colorant added in which step of coating in spray coating?
A. Sealing B. Syruping
C. Polishing D. Sub coating

3707. Propyl gallate act as a ________.
A. Antioxidant
B. Preservative
C. Both A and B
D. None of above

3708. Peeling is term related with which type of coating?
A. Film coating B. Sugar coating
C. Both A and B D. None of above

3709. Non uniform colouring on tablet is called__________.
A. Mottling B. Orange peel effect
C. Both A and B D. None of above

3710. Which of the following instrument used to determine colour uniformity?
A. Reflectanespectro photometer
B. Tristimulus calorimetry
C. Micro reflectance
D. All of above

3711. Which of the following tooling is used for large tablet?
A. B tooling B. D tooling
C. BB2 link D. DD tooling

3712. In rotatory tablet press, what is the length of D and BB tooling punches?
A. 3 inch B. 7.5 inch
C. 5.25 inch D. 9 inch

3713. In rotatory tablet press, what is the diameter of barrel in BB tools?
A. 3 inch B. 0.45 inch
C. 9 inch D. 0. 75 inch

3714. In rotatory tablet press, what is the head diameter of BB tool?
A. 2 inch B. 5 inch
C. 1 inch D. 7 inch

3715. BB tooling and B tooling is different from each other in____________.
A. The length of lower punch
B. Diameter of head
C. The length of upper punch
D. All of above

3716. In D tooling, what is the diameter of nominal barrel?
A. 1 inch B. 2.5 inch
C. 5 inch D. None of above

3717. In rotatory tablet press, what is the D tools head diameter?
A. 1 inch B. 1.75 inch
C. 1.25 inch D. 2 inch

3718. What is the lower punch length in BB tooling?
A. 20 /40 inch B. 57 / 16 inch
C. 37 / 72 inch D. 90 /20 inch

3719. Glass transition method is used to determine the surface area of__________.
A. Granules B. Aggregates
C. Tablet D. Both A and B

3720. What is the formula for car's compressibility index?
A. Tap density - bulk density×100/tap density
B. Bulk density- tap density×100/tap density
C. Bulk density-Tab density×100/bulk density
D. None of the above

3721. To determine the true density of granules, which instrument is use?
A. Pycnometer
B. Refractometer
C. Hydrometer
D. All of above

3722. Which of the defect is caused by poor condition deep concave surface punches?
A. Lamination B. Whiskering
C. Capping D. All of above

3723. Which of the following defect is not tablet defect?
A. Orange peel effect
B. Rat holding
C. Whiskering
D. All of above

3724. Which of the following statement is not correct?
A. Subcoating build up the size of tablet
B. Stearic acid cause sticking
C. Whiskering is due to Deep convex punches
D. All of above

3725. Which of the following type of drug resistance compression for tablet formation?
A. Amorphous drug
B. Low density drug
C. Both A and B
D. None of above

3726. Tablet is __________form.
A. Unit dose form
B. Temper proof dosage form
C. Both A and B
D. None of above

3727. Which type of drug resist compression to form compact dose?
A. Amorphous nature
B. Low-density nature
C. Focculent nature
D. All of above

3728. Which type of drug need Entrapment and encapsulation before compression?
A. Drug sensitive to oxygen
B. Drug sensitive to light
C. Drug sensitive to moisture
D. Both A and C

3729. Nonuniform in organoleptic property like colour of tablet is considered as___________.
A. Orange peel effect
B. Mottling
C. Both A and B
D. None of above

3730. Orange peel effect term related with______coating.
A. Sugar coating B. Film coating
C. Both A and B D. None of above

3731. Along with orange peel effect which type of coating defect also take place?
A. Blistering B. Hazing
C. Roughness D. Bloom

3732. Dull film also called as________.
A. Hazing B. Bloom
C. Both A and B D. None of above

3733. Blooming of film coated tablet can occur When__________
A. When formulation processing temperature is too high
B. When tablet are exposed to high humidity
C. When formulation processing pressure is too high
D. Both A and B

3734. Blistering of coated tablet is due to______.
A. Solvent Rapid evaporation from Core
B. High temperature effect on elasticity
C. High temperature effect on strength
D. All of above

3735. Twinning of tablets occur when________.
A. Coating solution is thin
B. Low amount of coating solution use
C. Inefficient drying
D. All of above

3736. Which of the following processing step is not required for wet granulation?
A. Slugging B. Screening
C. Mixing D. Drying

3737. Removal of film of tablet from sharp corner of bisect is referred as________.
A. Lamination B. Cracking
C. Bridging D. All of above

3738. Which of the following is not reason for bridging of coated tablet?
A. High coating solution viscosity
B. Solvent Rapid evaporation from Core
C. Pressure improper atomization
D. Percentage of solid high in solution

3739. Bridging is term related with______________.
A. Film coated tablet
B. Tablet
C. Granules
D. Both A and C

3740. Drug intended to form tablets should must have________.
A. Fluidity
B. Compatibility with excipient
C. Compressibility
D. All of above

741. _____________ can be affected by granule density.
A. Compressibility B. Dissolution
C. Tablet porosity D. All of above

3742. What is the instrusion fluid pycnometer to determine granule density?
A. Benzene B. Mercury
C. Alcohol D. Both A and B

3743. Implantation tablet intended for implanta in __________ layer of skin.
A. Epidermis
B. Subcutaneous
C. Dermis
D. All of above

3744. Which of the following is the main purpose of implantable tablet?
A. Provide prolong drug action
B. Constant drug delivery
C. Both A and B
D. None of above

3745. What is the general length of implantable tablet?
A. 1 mm B. 8 mm
C. 10 mm D. 17 mm

3746. Which type of injector can be used to administer rod shaped in implantable tablet?
A. Sequent injector
B. Port injector
C. Kern injector
D. All of above

3747. What is the disadvantage of implantable tablet?
A. Tissue toxicity
B. Hypersensitivity can aoccur
C. Required surgical technique
D. All of above

3748. Granulation and drying process done in Fluid bed strength granulator within___________.
A. 60 to 90 minute or less
B. 60 to 90 minute or more
C. 20 to 25 minutes or less
D. 30 to 60 minute or less

3749. What is main objective of enteric coating?
A. Mask order
B. Target site drug release for absorption
C. Mast test
D. All of above

3750. Which of the following is a reason for millard reaction?
A. Reaction of reducing sugar with amino group

B. Reaction of reducing sugar with alkane group
C. Reaction of reducing sugar with benzene ring
D. Reaction of reducing sugar with alkyl group.

3751. Maillard reaction is______________.
A. Enzymatic reaction
B. Non enzymatic reaction
C. Catalysing reaction
D. None of above

3752. Which of the following model used for study of mechanism of dissolution?
A. Diffusion layer model
B. Danckwert's model
C. Interfacial barrier model
D. All of above

3753. Diffusion layer model also known as____________.
A. Film theory
B. Surface renewal theory
C. Fluid penetration theory
D. Both A and B

3754. Danckwert's model of dissolution also known as___________.
A. Penetration theory
B. Surface renewal theory
C. Film theory
D. Both A and B

3755. Which of the following law is applicable for dissolution testing of uniform size powder?
A. The Hixson- crowell cube root law
B. Maxwell's law
C. Danckwert's law
D. All of above

3756. Which of the following is USB Type -V apparatus?
A. Flow through cell
B. Paddle over disc
C. Cylinder type
D. Reciprocating holder

3757. According to USB rapidly dissolving drug do not dissolve less than 85% in ________ minute.
A. 80 minute B. 10 minute
C. 30 minute D. 50 minute

3758. Millard reaction also called as____________.
A. Browning reaction
B. Flavour reaction
C. Enzymatic reaction
D. Both A and B

3759. Which of the following USP type IV apparatus?
A. Flow through cell
B. Paddle over disc
C. Cylinder type
D. Reciprocating holder

3760. Which of the following factor generally not contribute in Millard reaction?
A. Temperature
B. Storage time
C. Moisture
D. Pressure

3761. Which of the following spray system can consume in fluid bed granulator?
A. Top spaying system
B. Tangential spring system
C. Side sprying system
D. All of above

3762. Maillard reaction is generally take place when temperature is above ______________.
A. 140°C B. 40°C
C. 100°C D. 85°C

3763. Which of the following is usually the diameter of aggregates (granules)?
A. 0. 2-4 mm B. 0.1-8mm
C. 4-8mm D. 5-9mm

3764. Which of the following is not the advantage of granules?
A. Prevent segregation
B. Reduce caking
C. Improve the flow property
D. None of above

3765. Which of the following is major factor affect the tablet stability?

A. Molecular binding
B. Light
C. Temperature
D. Humidity

3766. Colour stability studies of tablet is done by____________.

A. Colorimeter
B. Reflectometer with heat
C. Intense artificial light
D. All of above

3767. Which of the following is hardness measuring test?

A. Static indentation test
B. Scratch file test
C. Rebound test
D. All of above

3768. Which of the following formula used to calculate friability of tablet?

A. Friability= Initial weight - Final weight× 100
B. Initial weight
C. Friability= Initial weight ×100
D. Initial weight
E. Friability= Final weight-initial weight× 100
F. Initial weight
G. None of above

3769. Which of the following is not a type of porosity?

A. Microporosity
B. Miso porosity
C. Macroporosity e e
D. None of above

3770. Which of the following formula used for determination of pore volume in water evaporation method?

A. Pore = weight of saturated sample-weight of dried sample/density of water
B. Pore=Total volume - material volume
C. Both a and b
D. None of above

3771. Which of the following method not used in coating solution droplet size analysis?

A. Captive method
B. Browning method
C. Photographic method
D. Laser light skating

3772. Pore volume = total volume - material volume, formula comes under which method.

A. Direct method of porosity assessment
B. Water evaporation method
C. Indirect method of porosity assessment
D. All of above

3773. Which of the following is not a considerable method for atomization of film coating solution?

A. Ultrasonic atomization
B. Pneumatic atomization
C. Hydraulic atomisation
D. Counter atomisation

3774. Captive method used for__________ size analysis

A. Granule B. Droplet
C. Particle D. All of above

3775. In which of the following coating step of sugar coating, sugar in not use?

A. Seal coating B. Syruping
C. Sub coating D. Both A and B

3776. Which of the following is not used in polishing of tablet?

A. Beeswax B. Syrup
C. Paraffin wax D. Naphtha

3777. Which of the following is not a basic function of packaging of tablet?

A. Barrier protection
B. Agglomeration
C. Dost control
D. None of the above

3778. Who invent the single piece of gelatine capsules:

A. Mothes And Dublanc
B. Knull And Ruska
C. Hippocrates
D. Galen

3779 Green Bone is source of :-

A. Type A Gelatin
B. Type B Gelatin
C. Both
D. None

3780. Raw material testing of Gelatin:-
A. Solubility B. Particle size
C. Loss on drying D. All of the above

3781. Empty hard shells moisture content:-
A. 60% B. 50-70%
C. 12-15% D. 30%

3782. Gelatin capsule shells are:
A. Non-vegetarian B. Vegetarian
C. Both D. None

3783. What is the Form of HPMC:-
A. Hydroxypropyl Methyl cellulose
B. Hypromellose
C. Both
D. None

3784. Gelatin is soluble in:
A. Hot water B. Cold water
C. Oil D. HCL

3785. Isoelectric pH of gelatine A:
A. 0.1 B. 9
C. 6 D. 5

3786. Isoelectric PH of Gelatin B:
A. 5.2 B. 4.7
C. 2.9 D. 3.2

3787. Largest capsule size:
A. 0 B. 7
C. 4 D. 000

3788. Smallest capsule size:-
A. 5 B. 4
C. 8 D. 00

3789. In capsule size 1 fill the drug in ml :-
A. 1.50 B. 0.75
C. 0.90 D. 0.55

3790. How much quantity of quinine sulphate filled in capsule size 4 in Mg-
A. 0.75 B. 0.1
C. 0.21 D. 0.4

3791. How much amount of Iron present in Gelatin:-
A. Less than 15 ppm
B. More than 15 ppm
C. 0.3 ppm
D. None of the above

3792. What equipment are used in hard capsule shells manufacturing:-
A. Elli Lilly and company
B. Zanasinigris
C. Both a & b
D. Diosna Mixer

3793. Which Steps is not involved in filling capsule shells:-
A. Rectification & separate Body and cap
B. Dosing fill material
C. Joining and ejection
D. Centrifugation

3794. Dosing of fill material in capsules filled by which method:-
A. Direct filling method
B. Indirect Filling Method
C. Both
D. None

3795. Finishing machines For capsules:-
A. Pan polishing B. Ereweka kea
C. Cloth dusti ng D. All

3796. Optimum bloom strength of Gelatinis:-
A. 260 B. 90
C. 340 D. 150-250

3797. Rotofill use in :-
A. Fill Pellet in hard Gelatin capsule
B. Fill Powder in soft Gelatin capsule
C. Fill Powder in hard Gelatin capsule
D. None

3798. Hard capsules shells contain:-
A. Cap B. Body
C. Both D. Only A

3799. Who invented Rotary die process:-
A. Funker B. Michael
C. R.P.Scherer D. None

3800. Shape of Soft gelatin capsules are in these:
A. Oval B. Round
C. Oblong D. All

3801. Composition of soft capsules shells:-
A. Gelatin B. Water
C. Plasticizer D. All

3802. What temperature is best for determination of bloom strength:-

A. 10° for 17 hours B. 5° for 7 hours
C. 12 °for 6 hours D. 15° for 15 hours

3803. Following are example Of Plasticizers:-

A. Glycerin USP B. Sorbitol USP
C. Both D. None

3804. Hardness Ratios for soft capsules:-

A. 0.4/1 B. 0.8/1
C. 0.6/1 D. All

3805. Moisture content in soft capsules:-

A. 6-10% B. 7-9%
C. 3-9% D. 4-6%

3806. Preservatives used in soft capsules:-

A. Methyl paraben B. Propylparaben
C. Both D. None

3807. Which flavoring Agents used For soft Capsules:-

A. Ethyl vanillin B. Essential oil
C. Both D. None

3808. Area required for filling hard Gelatin capsules is:-

A. 20M2+10M2 ancillary
B. 200 ft2
C. 100 ft2
D. None

3809. Area requirement for Manufacturing of Ayurvedic Capsules:-

A. 100ft2 B. 300ft2
C. 160ft2 D. 800ft2

3810. What is the synonym for pearls:-

A. Spherical capsules
B. Oval capsules
C. Round capsules
D. None of the above

3811. Evaluation parameter for capsules:-

A. Uniformity of weight
B. Content of active ingredients
C. Disintegration
D. All of the above

3812. Drying of soft gelatin capsules are done at:-

A. 8-10°c B. 21-25°c
C. 15-20°c D. 35-37°c

3813. Moisture content is determine by:-

A. Toluene distillation
B. Azeotropic distillation
C. Both
D. None

3814. Disintegration time for soft gelatin:-

A. 60 minutes B. 30 minutes
C. 20 minutes D. 50 minutes

3815. Disintegration time for hard 3848. Green Bone is source of :-

A. Type A Gelatin B. Type B Gelatin
C. Both D. None

3816. Raw material testing of Gelatin:-

A. Solubility B. Particle size
C. Loss on drying D. All of the above

3817. Empty hard shells moisture content:-

A. 60% B. 50-70%
C. 12-15% D. 30%

3818. Gelatin capsule shells are:-

A. Non-vegetarian B. Vegetarian
C. Both D. None

3819. What is the Form of HPMC:-

A. Hydroxypropyl Methyl cellulose
B. Hypromellose
C. Both
D. None

3820. Gelatin is soluble in :-

A. Hot water B. Cold water
C. Oil D. HCL

3821. Isoelectric pH of gelatine A:-

A. 0.1 B. 9
C. 6 D. 5

3822. Isoelectric PH of GelatinB:-

A. 5.2 B. 4.7
C. 2.9 D. 3.2

3823. Largest capsule size:-

A. 0 B. 7
C. 4 D. 000

3824. Smallest capsule size:-

A. 5 B. 4
C. 8 D. 00

3825. In capsule size 1 fill the drug in ml :-
A. 1.50 B. 0.75
C. 0.90 D. 0.55

3826. How much quantity of quinine sulphate filled in capsule size 4 in Mg-
A. 0.75 B. 0.1
C. 0.21 D. 0.4

3827. How much amount of Iron present in Gelatin:-
A. Less than 15 ppm B. More than 15 ppm
C. 0.3 ppm D. None of the above

3828. What equipment are used in hard capsule shells manufacturing:-
A. Elli Lilly and company
B. Zanasinigris
C. Both a & b
D. Diosna Mixer

3829. Which Steps is not involved in filling capsule shells:-
A. Rectification & separate Body and cap
B. Dosing fill material
C. Joining and ejection
D. Centrifugation

3830. Dosing of fill material in capsules filled by which method:-
A. Direct filling method
B. Indirect Filling Method
C. Both
D. None

3831. Finishing machines For capsules:-
A. Pan polishing B. Ereweka kea
C. Cloth dusting D. All

3832. Optimum bloom strength of Gelatinis:-
A. 260 B. 90
C. 340 D. 150-250

3833. Rotofill use in :-
A. Fill Pellet in hard Gelatin capsule
B. Fill Powder in soft Gelatin capsule
C. Fill Powder in hard Gelatin capsule
D. None

3834. Hard capsules shells contain:-
A. Cap B. Body
C. Both D. Only A

3835. Who invented Rotary die process:-
A. Funker B. Michael
C. R.P.Scherer D. None

3836. Shape of Soft gelatin capsules are in these :-
A. Oval B. Round
C. Oblong D. All

3837. Composition of soft capsules shells:-
A. Gelatin B. Water
C. Plasticizer D. All

3838. What temperature is best for determination of bloom strength:-
A. 10° for 17 hours B. 5° for 7 hours
C. 12 °for 6 hours D. 15° for 15 hours

3839. Following are example Of Plasticizers:-
A. Glycerin USP B. Sorbitol USP
C. Both D. None

3840. Hardness Ratios for soft capsules:-
A. 0.4/1 B. 0.8/1
C. 0.6/1 D. All

3841. Moisture content in soft capsules:-
A. 6-10% B. 7-9%
C. 3-9% D. 4-6%

3842. Preservatives used in soft capsules:-
A. Methyl paraben
B. Propylparaben
C. Both
D. None

3843. Which flavoring Agents used For soft Capsules:-
A. Ethyl vanillin B. Essential oil
C. Both D. None

3844. Area required for filling hard Gelatin capsules is:-
A. 20M2+10M2 ancillary
B. 200 ft2
C. 100 ft2 D. None

3845. Area requirement for Manufacturing of Ayurvedic Capsules :-
A. 100ft2 B. 300ft2
C. 160ft2 D. 800ft2

3846. What is the synonym for pearls :-
A. Spherical capsules
B. Oval capsules
C. Round capsules
D. None of the above

3847. Evaluation parameter for capsules:-
A. Uniformity of weight
B. Content of active ingredients
C. Disintegration
D. All of the above

3848. Drying of soft gelatin capsules are done at:-
A. 8-10°c B. 21-25°c
C. 15-20°c D. 35-37°c

3849. Moisture content is determine by:-
A. Toluene distillation
B. Azeotropic distillation
C. Both
D. None

3850. Disintegration time for soft gelatin:-
A. 60 minutes B. 30 minutes
C. 20 minutes D. 50 minutes

3851. Disintegration time for hard gelatin:-
A. 40 minutes B. 30 minutes
C. 44 minutes D. 10 minutes

3852. How much Weight variation present in less than 300 mg capsules
A. 10% B. 15%
C. 20% D. None

3853. How much weight variation present in more than 300 mg capsules :-
A. 7.5% B. 8.7%
C. 9.8% D. 1.3%

3854. What are the Method of microencapsulation:-
A. Air suspension B. Phase separation
B. C. Both D. All of the above

3855. What is the reasons of micro encapsulation:- gelatin:-
A. 40 minutes B. 30 minutes
C. 44 minutes D. 10 minutes

3856. How much Weight variation present in less than 300 mg capsules
A. 10% B. 15%
C. 20% D. None

3857. How much weight variation present in more than 300 mg capsules:-
A. 7.5% B. 8.7%
C. 9.8% D. 1.3%

3858. What are the methods of microencapsulation?
A. Interfacial Polymerization
B. C-precipitation
C. Pulse laser ablation
D. Sonochemica

3859. What is the reasons for microencapsulation:-
A. Isolation of core from surrounding
B. Retarding evaporation
C. Pan coating
D. All

3860. Water soluble resin for microencapsulation :-
A. Gelatin B. Silicones
C. Zein D. Wax

3861. Ethyl cellulose is:-
A. Water soluble resin
B. Lipid
C. Water insoluble resin
D. Enteric coated

3862. Example of wax and lipid are :-
A. Paraffin B. Stearic acid
C. Bees wax D. All of the above

3863. Carnauba is:-
A. Wax /lipid B. Fat
C. Carbohydrate D. None

3864. Example of enteric resins:-
A. Zein B. Shellac
C. Both D. None

3865. Air suspension Method is used for :-
A. Solid B. Liquid
C. Gas D. All

3866. Particle size(microgram) for pan coating :-
A. 500-800 B. 100-300
C. 600-5000 D. None

3867. Advantage of microencapsulation:-
A. Mask bitter taste
B. Protect from environment
C. Reduction of hygroscopicity
D. All of the above

3868. Disadvantages of microencapsulation :-
A. Shelf life reduce
B. Cost production increase
C. Both
D. None

3869. Iron content in soft gelatin:-
A. 12 ppm B. 5 ppm
C. 15 ppm D. 10 ppm

3870. Which vehicle used in soft gelatin capsules :-
A. PEG B. Glycerol
C. Sorbitol D. None

3871. Water insoluble coating material for microencapsulation include :-
A. Ethyl cellulose B. Gelatin
C. Polyacrylate D. Both A&B

3872. Fumaric acid used in gelatin capsules shell is as:-
A. Plasticizer B. Antioxidant
C. Solubiliser D. Opacifier

3873. What concentration is required of plasticiser in soft gelatincapsule in %W/W:-
A. 5-8 B. 20-30
C. 10-20 D. 30-40

3874. When capsule stored at high temperature it becomes unacceptable because of :-
A. Soft spotted capsules
B. Bloated capsules
C. Both A & B
D. None of the above

3875. What is the sequence for capsules shells manufacturing in an autonomic process is:-
A. Dip,spin,dry,strip,trim,join the capsules
B. Spin,dry,strip,join
C. Dry,strip,join,dip,
D. None of the above

3876. Which water soluble substance used as coating material in microencapsulation process is:-
A. Polyethylene
B. Silicone
C. Hydroxyl ethyl cellulose
D. Paraffin

3877. Shells of soft gelatin capsules may be elastic or plastic like, by the addition of:-
A. Sorbitol B. Providone
C. PEG D. None

3878. Which part of capsules have more diameter :-
A. Cap B. Body
C. Shell D. None

3879. Which type of capsules present whole body:-
A. Hard gelatin
B. Soft gelatin
C. Semi solid capsules
D. Granules capsules

3880. Which material use in hard Gelatin capsules are:-
A. Solid B. Granules
C. Powder D. All

3881. Rotoweigh is used for :-
A. High speed capsules weigh machine
B. Capsule polishing machine
C. Fill powder in soft gelatine
D. Tablet punching machine

3882. Seidinader is used as:-
A. Capsule polishing
B. Capsules manufacturing
C. Capsules testing
D. Capsules weigh

3883. Which machine is used for fill powder in hard gelatine capsules:-
A. Rotofill B. Accogel
C. Accofill D. Rotofill

3884. What are the machine used for weight measurement :-
A. Vericap 1200 B. Rotoweigh
C. Dosator D. Both A & B

3885. Which Colours used in capsules:-
A. Sunset yellow B. Quinoline yellow
C. Red 30 D. All

3886. 90mg of material fill in which capsules size:-
A. 1 B. 6
C. 2 D. 5

3887. Which capsules size is used for veterinary :-
A. 000 B. 00
C. Both D. None

3888. Work of spinning in manufacturing:-
A. Remove excess gelatin
B. Join capsules
C. Remove moisture
D. For proper shape

3889. Printing and polishing of capsules are done at:-
A. Empty capsules
B. Filled capsules
C. Both
D. None

3890. Which of the following are Polishing machines:-
A. Erweka B. Rotosort
C. Both D. None

3891. Which excipient used in capsules:-
A. Colouring agent
B. Flow promoter
C. Binder
D. Both A&B

3892. Disadvantage of capsules :-
A. Not use hygroscopic material
B. Not used deliquescent
C. Both
D. None

3893. Which of the following material is not hygroscopic in nature:-
A. Nacl B. Sucrose
C. Urea D. Naoh

3894. Bloom strength for soft gelatin
A. 190gm B. 150gm
C. 210gm D. 90gm

3895. Vericap 1200 is used as:-
A. Capsule weigh machine
B. Capsule polishing machine
C. Both
D. None

3896. Bloom strength for hard gelatine capsule:-
A. 60gm B. 300gm
C. 250gm D. 432gm

3897. Viscosity of gelatin:-
A. 25-45 milipoise B. 3-6 milipoise
C. 4-5 milipoise D. 50-70 milipoise

3898. In capsules size 4 fill the drug in ml :-
A. 1.50 B. 1.37
C. 0.33 D. 0.23

3899. In capsule size 2 fill the drug in mg :-
A. 970 B. 300
C. 650 D. 400

3900. Which of the following capsules size is not in human use:-
A. 000 B. 00
C. Both D. None of these

3901. Macofar equipment consist which models :-
A. MT12 B. MT13/2
C. MT13/1 D. All of the above

3902. Methyl Paraben is used in capsules as :-
A. Preservatives B. Colorants
C. Binder D. Diluents

3903. Concentration of titanium dioxide is use in capsules :-
A. 0.2% B. 0.3%
C. 0.5% D. 0.1%

3904. Ethyl vanillin is used as:-
A. Flavouring agent B. Binding agent
C. Both D. None of the above

3905. Which material is used to prevent decomposition :-
A. So2 B. No2
C. Nh2 D. None

3906. Which of the following is not slug filling machine :-
A. Zanasi B. MG2
C. Lilly D. Macofar

3907. Base adsorption formula is:-
A. Wt of liquid base/wt of solid
B. (BA+S)X V/W=M/g
C. Both
D. None

3908. Who invented two piece telescopic capsules:-

A. Mothes B. Murdock
C. Dublan D. A &C

3909. What are the common source of collagen which are used in capsules manufacturing:-

A. Animal bone B. Hide portions
C. Frozen bone skin D. All

3910. Which material control the thickness of capsules wall:-

A. Viscosity B. Gelatin solutions
C. Both D. None

3911. Which type of soft gelatin capsules is discarded :-

A. Overfills B. Under fills
C. Foreign D. All

3912. Which machine operate at 73,000 capsules per hour :-

A. Rotoweigh B. Zanasi
C. Macofer D. Elli Lilly

3913. 0.2 gm of acetyl salicylic acid filled in which capsules :-

A. 9 B. 2
C. 00 D. 3

3914. Hartnett model is used as :-

A. Capsule imprinting machine
B. Capsule polishing machine
C. Capsule filling machine
D. Capsule weigh machine

3915. Methyl paraben and propylparaben are used in capsule in which concentration :-

A. 0.1% B. 0.2%
C. 0.3% D. 0.8%

3916. Concentration of essential oil used in capsules:-

A. 1% B. 2.0%
C. 5% D. 3%

3917. Which of the following is used as flavouring agent :-

A. Ethyl vanillin B. Essential oils
C. Both D. None

3918. What is the Purpose of acetaminophen in microencapsulation :-

A. Absorption base B. Flavour
C. Colour D. None

3919. Which kind of base is ascorbic acid:

A. Vegetable oil B. Water soluble base
C. Both D. None

3920. Preparations of encapsulation should have a PH range from......

A. 3.3-5.4 B. 8.3-9.5
C. 6-7 D. 2.5-7.5

3921. Hydrolysis and leakage are caused due to:-

A. High acidity B. High basicity
C. Alkaline pH D. None

3922. Water and alcohol are used in micro encapsulation as:-

A. Co solvent B. Hydrate
C. Solution D. None

3923. The number of gm of liquid base required to produce capsulable mixture, add with 1 gm solid...

A. Base absorption
B. Base adsorption
C. Both
D. None

3924. Base adsorption is the ratio of weight of the base .....

A. Weight of solid B. Weight in mg
C. Weight of liquid D. All of these

3925. Sealed soft capsules are measured under:-

A. Microscope B. IR
C. Scanner D. UV

3926. Which Mixer used in the formulation of soft gelatin capsules is :-

A. Ribbon blender B. V cone blender
C. Pony mixer D. All of the above

3927. Gelatin is weight on which instrument :-

A. Printomatic B. Milligram
C. Nanometer D. None of these

3928. Loss of water of soft gelatin capsule is prevented by:-

A. Proper packaging B. Sealing
C. Both D. None

3929. Size 00 capsules may occasionally used for:-

A. Humans B. Animals
C. Both D. None

3930. Gel strength is also known as :-
A. Bloom B. Viscosity
C. Hardness D. All of these

3931. The sealing temperature of soft gelatine is:-
A. 35-400 C B. 15-200
C. 40-800 C D. 60-670

3932. The thickness of wet shell of soft gelatin capsule is:-
A. 0.025-0.032 B. 0.2-0.5
C. 0.25-1.3 D. 0.123-0.125

3933. The product cost of capsules is directly proportional to:-
A. Shell thickness B. Polishing
C. Drug content D. None

3934. Particle size multiorifice centrifugal :-
A. 1-5000 B. 1-100
C. 5-5000 D. None

3935. Which property show charcoal in microencapsulation:-
A. Base B. Adsorbent
C. Both D. None of these

3936. Function of gelatin :-
A. Render the shell
B. Protection against light
C. Conceal the content
D. All of these

3937. Which material is used as suspending agent for oily base:-
A. Wax mixture B. Lipids
C. Oil D. All

3938. Which material is used as suspending agent form on oily base :-
A. PEG 4000 B. PEG 6000
C. Both D. None

3939. Which of the following dosage form is suitable for moisture sensitive :-
A. Tablet B. Suppository
C. Capsules D. Ointment

3940. Which of the following work on principle of dielectric constant &removes unfill capsules :-
A. Rotoweigh B. Rotofil
C. Vericap D. Accofil

3941. Which is responsible for reduced solubility of gelatin molecule by cross linking:-
A. -C-O-C- B. -COOH
C. -CHO D. -C-X-C-

3942. What is the % Relative humidity of empty capsules shells:-
A. 1-5 B. 15-30
C. 15-30 D. 45-60

3943. In multi orifice centrifugation method particle size are:-
A. 1-1500micrometer
B. 1-5000micrometer
C. 40-5000micrometer
D. 3-50micrometer

3944. Which of the following is not used in microencapsulation as cross linking agent :-
A. Tripolyphosphate Formaldehyde
B. Phase separation
C. Both
D. All of the above

3945. Which of the following is not used in microencapsulation as cross linking agent:-
A. Tripolyphosphate
B. Formaldehyde
C. Alcohol
D. Gluteraldehyde

3946. Which of the following is physicochemical evaluation parameter of micro encapsulation :-
A. Sieve analysis B. PH
C. Temperature D. Viscosity

3947. Purpose of the isosorbidedinitrate in microencapsulation :-
A. Sustained release
B. Solubility
C. Delay release
D. Viscosity enhancer

3948. Co solvent used in microencapsulation process:-
A. Glycerol B. Sorbitol
C. Both D. None

3949. Composition of the core material in microencapsulating processes :-
A. Drug or active constituent
B. Additives like diluents
C. Stabilizer
D. All of these

3950. Composition of coating material in microencapsulation processes:-
A. Inert polymer B. Plasticizer
C. Colouring agent D. All

3951. Wurster's processes is also known as:-
A. Rotary plate processes
B. Air suspension coating
C. Coacervation processes
D. Pan coating

3952. Dipping processes is done for :-
A. To remove moisture
B. To remove excess gelatin
C. Both
D. None

3953. Gelatin is used as a/an
A. Encapsulating agent
B. Viscosity agent
C. Antimicrobial agent
D. Tablet glidant

3954. Application of soft gelatin capsules:-
A. As an oral dosage form
B. As a suppository dosage form
C. Both
D. None

3955. In soft gelatin capsule the plasticizer used and gelatin ratio is.........
A. 0.8:1 B. 0.4:2
C. 0.3:1 D. 0.5:2

3956. 3 size of capsule will have ....ml capacity
A. 1.3 B. 0.56
C. 0.33 D. 0.95

3957. 490 mg of drug filled in which capsule :-
A. 3 B. 8
C. 0 D. 5

3958. 0.67 ml of drug filled in which capsule :-
A. 3 B. 0
C. 2 D. 00

3959. Dip coating means :-
A. Repeated coating and drying
B. Conduct charge
C. Air in coating pan is replaced by nitrogen
D. Acid insoluble coating

3960. Moisture content of empty capsule shell should be between......
A. 12-15% B. 20-25%
C. 5-8% D. 2-6%

3961. Bloom is measurement for.........of gelatine molecules:-
A. Dissolution B. Adhesiveness
C. Elasticity D. Cohesiveness

3962. Most alkaline product in soft gelatine capsule can cause:-
A. Tanning B. Leakage
C. Roughness D. None of these

3963. Pick false statement for the step of microencapsulation:-
A. Formation of three immiscible phase
B. Dissolution of coating
C. Deposition of coating
D. Rigidization of coating

3964. Which of the following is only applicable to solid core :-
A. Air suspension
B. Solvent evaporation
C. Spray drying
D. None of these

3965. Which of the following packaging commonly used in capsules packaging:-
A. Blister pack B. Strip pack
C. Both D. None

3966. Find correct one:-
A. 000 largest capsule size
B. 5 smallest capsule size
C. Both
D. None

3967. Vegetable capsules shells are made up of:
A. HPMC B. Chitosan
C. Gelatin D. None of these

3968. Gelatin is :-
A. Protein B. Fat
C. Carbohydrate D. Lipid

3969. Clindamycin capsules I.P.is used as :-
A. Allergy reaction B. Severe pain
B. Angina C. Headche

3970. DALACIN C 300 Mg brand name of :-
A. Clindamycin capsules I.P.
B. Isotretinoin capsules
C. Ivermectin tablet
D. None of these

3971. What are the example of I.P. capsules:-
A. Clindamycin capsules
B. Pregabalin capsules
C. Gapapentin capsules
D. Both a & b

3972. Which of the following is not I.P. capsules :-
A. Simethicone capsules
B. Cyclosporine capsules
C. Losium plus
D. None of these

3973. Which following step are involved in coacervation phase separation method :-
A. Formation of three immiscible phase
B. Deposition of coating in core
C. Rigidization
D. All of these

3974. Rotofill is manufactured by:-
A. Farmatic SNC
B. Parke Devis and company
C. Elli Lilly and company
D. Osaka Japan

3975. which formula used for soft gelatin capsule formulation for practical consideration :-
A. (BA+S) V/D=M/G B. (BA+V)
C. Both of these D. None

3976. In these equation (BA+S)V/D=M/G , BA stand for :-
A. Weight of liquid base
B. Solid
C. Volume
D. Mixture

3977. What are the grades for gelatin :-
A. Pharmagel A B. Pharmagel B
C. Both D. None

3978. Ph for the Pharmacogel A :-
A. 4.8-5.2 B. 3-5
C. 1-6 D. 9.7

3979. What is the ph for the Pharmacogel :-
A. 6.5 -7 B. 6..6-3.9
C. 6.5-9.5 D. 1.4-4.3

3980. Which of the following are not used as plasticizer in capsules:-
A. Sorbitol B. Glycerine
C. Mannitol D. None

3981. What type of material cause filling problems in capsules :-
A. Deliquescent or hygroscopic material
B. Inert powder
C. Granular powder
D. All of these

3982. Capsule shell are made with:-
A. Gelatin B. Pectin
C. Starch D. Shellac

3983. Gelatin and glycerin are used for the preparation of lamellae in a specified ratio Identify the correct one :-
A. 1:1 B. 9:1
C. 5:1 D. 10:1

3984. The shells of soft Gelatin capsules may be made elastic or plastic-like the addition of :-
A. Sorbitol
B. Hydroxypropyl Methyl cellulose
C. Polyethylene glycol
D. Providone

3985. High bloom Gelatin is used in the manufacture of :-
A. Soft Gelatin capsules
B. Hard Gelatin capsules
C. A& B
D. None of the above

3986. Which capsules contain less amount of plasticizer:-
A. Soft gelatine B. Tablet
C. Hard gelatin D. Pills

3987. Hard gelatin capsule having more bioavailability than these tablet this sentences state that:-

A. True B. Wrong
C. Both D. None

3988. Amoxicillin I.P. is used as :-

A. Antifungal
B. Antibacterial
C. Antimalerial
D. Anticancer

3989. The rate limiting step in the bioavailability of a capsule is :-

A. Disintegration B. Dissolution
C. Physical stability D. PH

3990. Gelatin is used as a binding agent in the following concentration:-

A. 2-10% B. 50-70%
C. 5-20% D. 100%

3991. Which of the following is used as plasticizer in capsule formulation:-

A. Glycerol B. Sorbitol
C. Propylene glycol D. All of the above

3992. Which of the following water insoluble material in microencapsulation :-

A. Ethyl cellulose
B. Polyethylene
C. Polyamide
D. All of the above

3993. Which particle size is used in air suspension :-

A. 1-1500 B. 5-5000
C. 35-5000 D. 600 mm

3994. The technique coacervation phase separation include :-

A. 2 steps B. 4 steps
C. 3 steps D. 9 steps

3995. Which of the following capsule filling machine is based upon Auger fill principle:-

A. Hoflizerkarg B. Osaka
C. Zanasi D. Capsugel type 8

3996. Particle size for spray drying and congealing method :-

A. 6000 B. 60
C. 600 D. 6

3997. Who is developed Multiforce centrifugal process:-

A. Southwest research institute
B. Northeast institute
C. Both
D. East institute

3998. Full form of SWRI:-

A. Southwest research institute
B. Southwest raw ingredient
C. Both
D. None

3999. Which of the following are major defects of Capsules shells during manufacturing:-

A. Double cap B. Black body
C. Loose piece D. Alll

4000. Which of the following are not minor defect of capsule:-

A. Trimming B. Wrinkles
C. Bubbles D. Scar end

4001. What are the critical defect of capsule shells:-

A. Cracky B. Hole on capsule
C. Short body D. All

4002. What is the rate limiting step in bioavailability of capsules:-

A. Dissolution
B. Disintegration
C. Physical stability
D. Ph

4003. What step not involved in capsule manufacturing:-

A. Stripping B. Slugging
C. Joining D. Spinning

4004. Which of the following enteric material used in manufacturing process of capsules:-

A. Zein
B. Shellac
C. Cellulose acetate Pthlate
D. None

4005. Which mill is used for particle size reduction of capsules:-

A. Ball mill B. Fluidized mill
C. Roller mill D. Cutter mill

4006. How much percentage is used of HCL in dry bone treatment

A. 6% B. 8%
C. 5% D. 7%

4007. The maximum capacity of capsule is represented by the number:-

A. 000 B. 00
C. 9 D. 5

4008. Plate processes method is used for :-

A. Soft gelatine
B. Hard gelatin
C. Both
D. None of the above

4009. Which material is used for manufacturing of gelatin:-

A. Dry bone B. Dry bone
C. Calf skin D. All of these

4010. Capsule is :-

A. Solid dosage form
B. Liquid form
C. Semi-solid dosage form
D. None

4011. Capsule is not given:-

A. Conscious patients
B. Unconscious patients
C. Coma
D. Both a&b

4012. Which Material fill in Capsules shell:-

A. Quinine sulphate
B. Granules
C. Powder
D. All of these

4013. Which of the following is not used as opasifying agent:-

A. Titanium dioxide
B. Carageenen
C. Both
D. None

4014. Which of the following test is performed after capsule shell mfg:-

A. Weight variations
B. Loss on drying
C. Disintegration
D. All of these

4015. Smudge on capsule is :-

A. Major defects
B. Minor defect
C. Critical defect
D. All of these

4016. Which dryer is used for drying soft Gelatin capsule:-

A. Tumbling dryer
B. Roller dryer
C. Drum dryer
D. None

4017. Which of the following are machine used for soft Gelatin Capsules manufacturing:-

A. Rotary die process
B. Reciprocating die
C. Plate process
D. All

4018. During QC stage which of the points are focused by Analysist:-

A. Eliminate damage particles
B. Conduct microbial testing
C. Thickness, appearance
D. All of the above

4019. What is the following is Latin term for powder:-

A. Pulvis B. Alibi
C. Luctor D. Magnum opus

4020. Powders are....

A. Solid dosage form
B. Liquid dosage form
C. Semisolid dosage form
D. Parental

4021. Dentifrices are used in formulation of :-

A. Bulk powder
B. Dusting powder
C. Enclosed powder
D. None of these

4022. Which of the following method is used for potent powder preparation:-

A. Granulation B. Trituration
C. Mortar and pestle D. Geometric dilution

4023. Fundamental law's of powders:

A. Kick's law B. Bond 's law
C. Rittinger's law D. All of these

4024. Gantt chart provide information about the

A. Closing schedule
B. Processing schedule
C. Production schedule
D. Labour schedule

4025. Stoke's law is used in

A. sedimentation B. Diffusion
C. Osmotic pressure D. Brownian motion

4026. Eye drops should be with ...... lachrymal secretion.

A. Hypertonic B. Isotonic
C. Hypotonic D. Hemolysis

4027. In which shapes of misclles.

A. Spherical
B. Sausage
C. Rod and lamellar
D. All of the above

4028. Bates expressed this quantitative in terms of a ....

A. Dilution factor
B. Dilution value
C. Dilution equilibrium
D. None

CHAPTER 2

Pharmaceutical Chemistry and Pharmacology

1. **The equilibrium constant k in this case is called?**
   A. Solut constant B. Solvent constant
   C. Indicater constant D. All the above
2. **The curve obtained is called?**
   A. pH - neutralization curve
   B. pH - titration curve
   C. Both (a) & (b)
   D. None
3. **The neutralization curve point include in?**
   A. Turning point B. Point of infection
   C. Both (a) & (b) D. None
4. **The pH interval between those two point is called?**
   A. Turning B. Infection
   C. Titration D. All the above
5. **The infection on the pH - neutralization curve depend upon?**
   A. Titration B. Concentration
   C. Indicater D. Acetic acid
6. **The titration of HCl with NaoH in the following repects in (caseCH3cooh)**
   A. The initial pH is higher
   B. The rate increase of pH during the titration is greter
   C. The pH at the equivalence point is higher
   D. All the above
7. **The disadvantage in such titration is that the infection on the pH - neutralization curve is very Small near the?**
   A. Very weak point
   B. Equivalence point
   C. Strong point
   D. Nutrition point
8. **The infection on the titration curve provide in?**
   A. The values of k1& k2 are not very Small
   B. The ratio k1 &k2 more then 10,000
   C. Both (a) & (b)
   D. None
9. **Titration of a polybasic acid with a strong base in the example in?**
   A. Sulphurous acid B. Nitric acid
   C. Calcium D. Chloride
10. **The case is quit similar to stepwise titration of a?**
    A. Diprotic acid B. Nitric acid
    C. Acetic acid D. Aprotic acid
11. **The contain substance absorb radiant energy & then emit if form of light the substance are called?**
    A. Fluorescent substance
    B. Chiropractic substance
    C. Intensity substance
    D. All the above
12. **The fluorescent substance & the phenomenon is?**
    A. Fluorecelence B. Fluorescence
    C. Fluorecarbon D. Fluorocomplex
13. **The neutralimetry which include all acid - base or neutralisation titration can be?**
    A. Alkalimetry B. Acidimetry
    C. Both (a) & (b) D. None
14. **The determination of the amount of an acid in a sample by titration with standard alkali called?**
    A. Alkane B. Alaklimetry
    C. Alkalifated D. Acidimetry

15. The determination of the amount of a base in sample by titration with standard solution in?

A. Alaklimetry B. Basemetry

C. Acidmetry D. All the above

16. The alaklimetry, the following substance can be used as primary standard in?

A. Sodium carbonate

B. Thallous carbonate

C. Sodium tetraborate decahydrate

D. All the above

17. The substance are generally used in acidimetry in?

A. Potassium acid phthalate

B. Oxalic acid dihydrate

C. Benzoic acid or sulphonic acid

D. All the above

18. The determination of the normality of the given acid solution by?

A. Alaklimetry

B. Thiosulphate solution

C. Isometrically

D. Iodometry

19. The liberated iodine is titrated with standard solution known as?

A. Chloride B. Magnesium

C. Thiosulphate D. All the above

20. The acid- base titrimetry in act?

A. Aqueous solution B. Non - aqueous

C. Both (a) & (b) D. None

21. The difficulties encountered in the titration of diluted solution of weak acid with alkali solution can be summarised as?

A. The infection on the pH - neutralisation curve small

B. The phenolphthalein colour coded away at the end point

C. Interference due to atmospheric co2

D. All the above

22. The solution of HCl gas in water called us?

A. Nitric acid B. Hydrochloric

C. Titration D. Solvent

23. The acidic or basic behaviour of solut dissolve in given solvent depend properties upon in?

A. Acid - base property of the solvent

B. Atoprulytic constant of the solvent

C. Dielectric constant of the solvent

D. All the above

24. The certain do not donate or accept protons hence do not show acidic or basic properties, these are called?

A. Aprotic B. Inert solvents

C. Both (a) & (b) D. None

25. Write are photogenic solvent in exampleknown as?

A. Amines B. Liquid ammonia

C. Alcohol or water D. All the above

26. Titration in basic solvent in?

A. Butylamine

B. Ethylenediamine

C. Dimethylformamide & liquid amonia

D. All the above

27. The problem of end point detection in non - aqueous titrimetry is not ?

A. Very simple B. Difficult

C. Strong titration D. Weak titration

28. The Fe3+ ion is reduced, hence it is the

A. Reductant B. Oxidant

C. Reduce D. All the above

29. Sn2+ ion is oxidised, hence it is the?

A. Oxidant B. Increase

C. Decrease D. Reductant

30. The pure water contain known as?

A. Water molecule B. Hydronium ions

C. Hydroxide ions D. All the above

31. The carminic acid give purple colour in?

A. Alkalis (oH-) B. Weak acid

C. Strong acid D. All the above

32. The litmus is used to test ether substance is?

A. Aqueous or non- aqueous

B. Acidic or alkaline

C. Solid or semisolid

D. All the above

33. **The addition of acid to indicater will shift equilibrium towards in?**

A. Right B. Left

C. Upper D. Lover

34. **The phenolphthalein change colour in?**

A. Distil water B. Solvent

C. Alkalis D. Alkenamine

35. **Which of the following is not an example weak acid ?**

A. Carbonic acid B. Sulfuric acid

C. Acetic acid D. Pyruvic acid

36. **The strong acid a large ka value in?**

A. True B. False

C. D.

37. **An amino. Acid act as acid & base known as?**

A. True B. False

C. D.

38. **The titration curve for precipitate reaction is similar to those obtain for?**

A. Acid - base B. Redox reaction

C. Both (a) & (b) D. None

39. **The concept of covalent bond was given by ?**

A. Lewis B. Kossel

C. Both (a) & (b) D. None

40. **The mean residence time of methane in atmosphere in years is?**

A. One to seven B. Two to seven

C. Three to seven D. Four to seven

41. **The major drawback of Mohr criterion is?**

A. Shape of the envelop

B. Shape of the weak

C. Shape of the small

D. Shape of the simple

42. **The principal of virtual work was developed by Mohr state weather the above substance is?**

A. True B. False

43. **Volhar,s method volume of given chloride solution in presenceof dilute is?**

A. NaoH B. HNo3

C. AgcN D. Both b & c

44. **The method is quite similar to one used to titrating silver by?**

A. Mohr method

B. Volhard method

C. Titration method

D. Redox method

45. **The volhard titration method can also used for determining by?**

A. Bromides B. Iodines

C. Both a & b D. None

46. **The metal ion is the complex is called?**

A. Central atom B. Central ion

C. Ionisation D. Atomic

47. **The several indicater are used in?**

A. Precipitation titration

B. Complexometric titration

C. Redox titration

D. Acid - base titration

48. **The volhard method for the determination of chlorine, bromine & iodine in the form of halides by?**

A. Complexometric

B. Precipitating

C. Equivaliting

D. All the above

49. **Why is EDTA titration called in?**

A. Rodox titration

B. Complexometric titration

C. Conductometry titration

D. Potentiometry titration

50. **The volhard,s was first described in?**

A. German chemist

B. Beer lomber law

C. Divyan chemist

D. None of this

51. **The is an indirect titration procedure used for determining the anions that precipitate with**

A. Nitric acid B. Chloride

C. Silver D. Sulphate

52. **The volhard method end point ferric alum distributed in colour by?**

A. Red colour B. Yellow

C. Pink colour D. Green colour

53. Write are precipitation type in the?

A. Direct B. Indirect
C. Both (a) & (b) D. Back titration

54. The EDTA titration technique in the?

A. Direct titration or indirect titration
B. Back titration method
C. Displacement titration
D. All the above

55. In certain metal like zinc, the ion - formation process is predominate hence it will have a?

A. Possative potential
B. Negative potential
C. Potential depend
D. All the above

56. The potential it acquired under such condition is referred to as it's?

A. Negative potential
B. Possative potential
C. Reversible potential
D. All the above

57. The magnitude of the electron potential is indicative of the metal ion concentration of the solution in which the electron is placed hence the electrode is ?

A. Indicator electrode
B. Ions
C. Indicator potential
D. Concentration

58. The solution in which it is placed such an electrode is called?

A. Electrode potential
B. Reference electrode
C. Active electrode
D. Concentration

59. Write are indicator electrode in the?

A. Metal electrode
B. Hydrogen electrode
C. Quinhydrone electrode
D. All the above

60. The (AgNo3)as a precipitating agent then it called?

A. Argentimetric B. Imargentimetric
C. Solventmetric D. Biomimetic

61. We have a conductor in in the form of an electrolyte solution,a special cell in?

A. Potential cell B. Conductivity cell
C. Oxidation cell D. Reduction cell

62. Electric conductivity of an electrolyte solution depend in?

A. Ions or mobility ions
B. Concentration ions
C. Temperature
D. All the above

63. Write are ion type in ?

A. Cation
B. Anions
C. Single or double charged
D. All the above

64. Write are conductivity cell type include in?

A. Wide mout hed cell
B. Cell for reactios producing precipitation
C. Dip type cell
D. All the above

65. Write are strong acid & strong base formula in?

A. HCl & NaoH B. NH4oH & HCl
C. HCl & NH4Oh D. NaoH &HCl

66. The pH of titration mixture for strong acid & strong base at equivalence point in?

A. 2 B. 2.7
C. 7 D. 6.2

67. The neutralization titration acid react with a base a form?

A. Salt & water B. Salt & acid
C. Salt & solution D. Salt & solvent

68. The ratio of number of gm - moles of a components to total number of gm mol in mixture or solution known as?

A. Molarity B. Molality
C. Mole fraction D. Normality

69. The number of gm - equivalent of solute per liter of solution in?

A. Molarity B. Molality
C. Mole function D. Normality

70. **The chemical regent form, which solution of required concentration can be prepared known as?**
A. Primary standard
B. Secondary standard
C. Diluted solution
D. All the above

71. **The number of gms of solute or 100 ml of solvent in?**
A. Molarity B. Molality
C. Normality D. Friability

72. **The redox potential depend up the?**
A. Ratio (ox) red B. Potential (ox) red
C. Indicator (ox) red D. None of this

73. **The potential of a platinum electrode can act as?**
A. Indicator potential B. Indicator electrode
C. Inductor solvent D. All the above

74. **The such as a piece of cu or ag in these conductor electrons carry electric current in?**
A. Metallic or electronic conductors
B. Electrolytic or ion conductors
C. Mixconductors
D. All the above

75. **The such as an aqeou8 solution of Nacl or cuso4here ions act carries in?**
A. Electrolytic conductor's
B. Ionic conductor's
C. Both (a) & (b)
D. None

76. **Which current is partly carried by ion & partly by electrons us is the case with a solution of an alkali metal in liquid ammonia known?**
A. Metallic conductor's
B. Electronic conductor's
C. Mixed conductor's
D. All the above

77. **Where R is constant for a given conductor & is called?**
A. Reductase B. Resistance
C. Reduce D. Reversible

78. **The titrant solution in small portions is add in the?**
A. Conductor B.Microburate
C. Beaker D. Indicator

79. **The minimum external voltage that must be applied in order to bring about continuous electrolysis is called?**
A. Decomposition B. Incompatible
C. Tetracomposition D. Distribution

80. **One gradually increasing the applied voltage there is only slight increase in current as show by the?**
A. Miniameter B. Milliammeter
C. Dichloremmeter D. Sudenlymmeter

81. **An amperometric titration can performed in?**
A. Polarographic cell
B. Precipitated cell
C. Redid cell
D. Conductors cell

82. **The dropping mercury cathode (DMC) is used in?**
A. Carmel electrode
B. Indicated electrode
C. Reference electrode
D. All the above

83. **The libreting 1 g eq of substance at electrone 96,487 Coulomb's are required, this quantity of electricity is called?**
A. Titration B. Faraday
C. Beer law D. Feja's

84. **The Coulomb is quantity of electricity given by the flow of one Ampere of current for?**
A. 3 second B. 5 second
C. 7 second D. 10 second

85. **The cerimetric titration also known as?**
A. Cerate oximetry B. Create reduction
C. Cerate developed D. Cerate crimetry

86. **Write are oxidizing agent in?**
A. Oxygen B. Antiseptic
C. Disinfectants D. All the above

87. **Write are standard oxidant in?**
A. Potassium permanganate
B. Potassium bromate
C. Potassium dichromate & iodine
D. All the above

88. The method of volumetric chemical analysis developed by?

A. Ion Athanasius B. Solvent

C. Formation D. Shape

89. The irreversible specific indicator In?

A. Methyl orange in oromatometry

B. Visual indicator

C. Nitridometry

D. Iodostarchy

90. Write external indicator in?

A. Bromatometry B. Nitritometry

C. Visual indicator D. All the above

91. The bromatometty is a titration process in which the?

A. Bromination B. Bromimetry

C. Brominated D. Brominivity

92. Bromatometry process is a?

A. Acetate process

B. Titration process

C. Non titration process

D. Chemical process

93. The bromination of a indicator in?

A. Strong indicator

B. Weak indictor

C. Chemical indicator

D. Stable indicator

94. The point when the reactants are done reacting in?

A. Equivalence point

B. End point

C. Both a & b

D. Non depend end point

95. The dichrometry a most significant techniques used in?

A. Quantitative analysis

B. Quality analysis

C. Precipitatate analysis

D. Protogenic analysis

96. Type of titration classifieds into type based reaction involved in?

A. Acid - base titration

B. Complexometric titration

C. Redox titration &precipitation titration

D. All the above

97. The titration widely used in the ?

A. Food industry

B. Packing industry

C. Concentration industry

D. Product colour industry

98. Potentiometric cell has following part in?

A. Electrode & sult bridge

B. Analyticall solution

C. Galvanometers

D. All the above

99. Write are indicator electrode in?

A. Metal electrode

B. Hydrogen electrode

C. Both a & b

D. Catomel electrode

100. Write are reference electrode in?

A. Catomel B. Metal electrode

C. Quinhydron D. Hydrogen electrode

101. Which one of the following is a weak acid?

A. HNO3 B. HI

C. HF D. HBr

102. Which of the following is not an example of weak acid?

A. Lactic acid B. Carbonic acid

C. Sulfuric acid D. Pyruvic acid

103. The process of adding known concentration until complete the reaction with volume is called as?

A. Titrant B. Titration

C. Tirrent D. Titrend

104. The Titration end point determined by change in colour by?

A. Indicater B. Burette

C. Instrument D. Measuring cylinder

105. In standard solution which of the following is accurately known as ?

A. Volume

B. Pressure

C. Temperature

D. Normality, strength or %chemicals

106. The ability of chenille in each liter of solution is known as?

A. Normality

B. Strength

C. Molecule weight

D. Equivalent weight

107. The required concentration can be prepared from chemical regant is called as?
A. Titration B. Indicator
C. Primary standard D. Secondary standard

108. Acid-base titration in invalve as?
A. Single reaction
B. Proced to completion
C. Neutralisation reaction
D. Stoichiometric reaction

109. The standard always contain known as?
A. Acid
B. Base
C. Primary standard
D. Concentration solute

110. Acid-base titration equivalent quantities hydronium ions and hydroxide ion are present?
A. At beginning point
B. At end point
C. At middle point
D. Titration

111. Strength of acid and base equivalence hclparts by weight?
A. 36.5 B. 40.0
C. 58.5 D. 18.0

112. The Titration strongacid and strong base the equivalence point know as?
A. Wlll be below pH 7.0
B. Above pH of 7.0
C. At of pH 7.0
D. With above pH of 7.0

113. Acid whose molecule contains only one replaceable (or ionisable) hydro in called?
A. Acetic acid B. Monobasic acid
C. Nitric acid D. All the above

114. Write in molarity formula known as?
A. Molarity-distance travelled solute/distance travelled solvent
B. Kilogram per liter / mol wt
C. Wt present per liter / mol wt
D. None of this

115. Primary standard in acid-base titrametry substance commonly used are ?
A. Sodium bicarbonate
B. Borax
C. Benzoic acid
D. All the above

116. Displacement titration notice acid act asvery weak at?
A. Nitric acid B. Monopretic acid
C. Monoprotic acid D. None of this

117. The phenomenon is known as?
A. Titration B. Rosin
C. Naphthal D. Fluorescence

118. Acidic primary standard as following substance generally used in ?
A. Potassium acid phtahalate
B. Benzoic acid
C. Oxalic acid
D. All the above

119. Alkaline primary standard as following substance can be use?
A. Sodium carbonate
B. Thallium carbonate
C. Potassium iodate
D. All the Above

120. Write the potassium acid phtahalate formula known as?
A. Khc8h4o4 B. H2c2o42h2o
C. C6h5cooh D. None

121. Write the sodium carbonate formula known as?
A. Khco3 B. Na2co3
C. Ti2co3 D. Nene of this

122. Write the benzoic acid formula known as?
A. H2c2o42h2o B. C2h5oh
C. C6h5cooh D. Agno3

123. Write the potassium iodate formula known as?
A. Agno3 B. Ki
C. Kio3 D. None of this

124. Write the sulfuric acid formula known as?
A. Nh4so4 B. Nh2so3h
C. Khco3 D. Nahco3

125. The aqueous solution of electrolytes contain ad?
A. Metal B. Lactose
C. Ion D. Acid

126. Non aqueous titration carried out by?
A. Water insoluble. Drug
B. Alkaline drug
C. Water soluble drug
D. All the above

127. Write non aqueous titration one useful as?
A. Leveling point
B. Differentiating solvent
C. Both (a) & (b)
D. None

128. The acidic or basic behaviour of a solute dissolved in a given solvent depend upon?
A. Acid-base properties of the solvent relative the solute
B. Autoprotolysis constant of the solvent
C. Dielectric constant of the solvent
D. All the above

129. Write is one used of non aqueous titration known as?
A. Solvent B. Acid
C. Base D. Thymol blue

130. The autoprotolysis constant formula given by ?
A. Ks= bhsh× b5- / b2sh
B. Ks= hsh×as- / a2sh
C. Both (a) &(b)
D. None

131. In problems the alkalimetric determination of weak acid in?
A. Aqueous solvent
B. Aqueous solute
C. Aqueous medium
D. None of this

132. The term antoprotolysis mean that no other substance is heated in the proton transfer process as?
A. Inert or aprotic solvent
B. Protophilic solvent
C. Photogenic solvent
D. All the above

133. In aqueous medium dissociate practically completely provided the solution is not very concentration as?
A. Hcio4 B. Hcl
C. Both (a) &(b) D. None

134. Non aqueous is very weak acid such as?
A. Amino acid B. Ethylenediamine
C. Per chloric acid D. Phenols

135. Write non aqueous acid-base concept in?
A. Bronsted &Lowery
B. Shortcomings
C. Hydrated
D. None of this

136. Write oxidation addition of such as?
A. Hydrogen B. Sulphate
C. Oxygen D. Reduct

137. Write oxidation involve as ?
A. Loss oxygen B. Loss sulphate
C. Loss carban D. Loss hydrogen

138. Oxidation - reduction titration in substance to be determined is either?
A. Oxidant or oxygen
B. Reduct or oxygen
C. Oxidised or reduced
D. Oxidation or range

139. The oxidation - reduction reation are most widely used method in?
A. Quality analysis
B. Quantitative analysis
C. Both a & b
D. None

140. Write are oxidation equation known as?
A. Mol. Wt of the oxidat / change in oxidation number per mol. Of the oxidant
B. Mol. Wt of the oxidation / change in oxidant no. Per molecule of the oxidation
C. Both a & b
D. None

141. Write are in general eq. Wt of a reductant as?
A. Mol.wt of reductant / change in oxidation no. Per molecule of reductant
B. Mol. Wt of reduction no. Per molecule of reductant
C. Both (a) & (b)
D. None

142. Write in this method invalves redox reation as?
A. Finding out the product of the reation
B. Setting up a partial equation for oxidation
C. Setting up a partial equation for reductio
D. All the above

143. Write iodine are two types known as?
A. Ido & oxide
B. Iodimetry& iodometry
C. Sodium & chloride
D. None of this

144. The titrimetric method very useful reation involving known as?
A. Iodine B. Either
C. Sulphate D. Acid

145. Write are iodimetric determination of iodine oxidant in?
A. Strong oxidant B. Weak oxidant
C. Both (a) &(b) D. None of this

146. Write are iodometry iodine oxidant determination in?
A. Weak oxidant B. Strong oxidant
C. Bath (a) &(b) D. None

147. Write are weak oxidant which can be reduce by reductants ?
A. Sodium thiosulphate
B. Salphurous acid
C. Arsenious oxide
D. All the above

148. Write are strong oxidant , which can be reduce by reductants as?
A. Cuso4 B. Klo3
C. Kmno4 D. All the above

149. Write are standard solution of an oxidant used in as ?(oxidimetric method)
A. Reduction B. Titration
C. Oxidation D. None of this

150. Write are oxidimetric method procedure is called as?
A. Oxidant B. Reduct
C. Oxidimetric D. Oxidiometric

151. Write are at in typevisual indicator used in redox titrimetry
A. 1 B. 2
C. 3 D. 4

152. Write are visual indicators used in redid titrimetry?
A. Reagentserving as its own indicator (self indicater)
B. External indicator
C. Internal indicator
D. All the above

153. Write are self indicators one example known as?
A. Kmno4 B. Agno3
C. H2so4 D. None of this

154. Write are external indicator in standard solution at known ?
A. Mgso4 B. Kmno4
C. K2cr2o7 D. Agno3

155. The titration involving precipitation reation in?
A. Much smaller in no.
B. Strong smaller in no.
C. Weak smaller in no.
D. All the above

156. Write in requirement for precipitation titration at in standard solution as?
A. Ph
B. Sodium chloride
C. Potassium thiocyanate
D. Magnesium thiocyanate

157. Write a gravimetric determination the rate of precipitation can be?
A. Increase B. Decrease
C. Weak D. Strong

158. Write are precipitant reaction in the substance can be?
A. Must be slow B. Must be fast
C. Both (a) & (b) D. None

159. The most important precipitation reaction in?
A. Reduct analysis
B. Oxidant analysis
C. Titrimetric analysis
D. All the above

160. The most important precipitation reaction in titrimetric analysis are those which involve the use of silver nitrate this are called?

A. Nargentimetric determination

B. Argentimeyric determination

C. Both (a) &(b)

D. None of this

161. Write precipitation in laboratory exercises method known as?

A. Mohr method B. Volhard method

C. Both (a) & (b) D. None

162. Write are determination of normality of the given chloride solution by?

A. Silver titration B. Mohr titration

C. EDTA titration D. Fejan titration

163. Write are volhard method for determination by

A. Magnesium B. Chloride

C. Silver D. All the above

164. Write in potassium thiocyanate formul

A. KHNS B. kCNS

C. KCLS D. KcNL

165. Which are strongly absorbed by precipitates known as?

A. Solvent precipitate

B. Colloidal precipitate

C. Sodium precipitate

D. Equivalence precipitate

166. Write in several metal ion can be determined by using a standard solution of?

A. Calcium B. EDTA

C. Buffer D. Acid

167. Write are main type of precipitate titration are

A. Volhard method B. Fajans method

C. Mohr method D. All the above

168. Write are volumetric analysis titration used known as

A. Pipette B. Burette

C. Beaker D. Stand

169. The EDTA form with several matels these are called as?

A. Metal chelonates

B. Either chelonates

C. Solvent chelonates

D. None of this

170. The complexing agent EDTA is called as?

A. Cholen B. Chelon

C. Chilen D. Chelonrate

171. These indicater from stable, brightly coloured complexes with most ions these are called?

A. Metalechloride indicater

B. Melallochromic indicater

C. Metalloidate indicater

D. None of this

172. Volhard method, which of the following salt should be cogulated during the titration known?

A. Silver sodium B. Silver cyanide

C. Silver bromide D. Silver chloride

173. The above is due to formulation of as

A. Silver chromate B. Silver cynide

C. Silver thiocyanateD. Silver chloride

174. Write are following is a back titration in?

A. Mohr method B. Volhard method

C. Fajan's method D. All the above

175. Write complexing agent known as?

A. Water soluble complexes

B. Water insoluble complexs

C. Both (a) & (b)

D. None

176. Write are EDTA agent known as?

A. Chelating agent B. Sequestering agent

C. Both (a) & (b) D. None

177. Write are replacement titration solution used known as?

A. Chloride B. Sulphur

C. Calcium D. Magnesium

178. The stability of the sparingly soluble salt is decrease by?

A. Inorganic solvent B. Organic solvent

C. Both (a) & (b) D. None

179. Electrometric titration method include are?

A. Potentiometric titration

B. Conductometric titration

C. Coulometry titration

D. All the above

180. When a metal electrode is depend in a solution containing it's?

A. Ions B. Solvent

C. Either D. Standard

181. Write in a reaction between cuso4&Zn (s)?

A. Zinc undergo oxidation

B. Zinc experiences an increase in the oxidation

C. Undergos oxidation

D. All the above

182. Write old painting can be restore oxidizing agent known as?

A. H2so4 B. H2o

C. H2o2 D. H2po4

183. Write are oxidizing agent known ?

A. Are mostly ether

B. Are mostly metal

C. Are mostly non either

D.Are mostly non metal

184. Write hydrogen act as a reducing agent known?

A. By taking oxygen

B. By giving electron

C. Both (a) & (b)

D. None

185. Write oxidizing agent does not include ?

A. Potassium chloride

B. Potassium iodide

C. Potassium bromine

D. Potassium chlorine

186. Write are oxidation also referred known as?

A. Combustion B. Respiration

C. Both (a) & (b) D. None

187. Write are activation energy can lowered use known?

A. Solvent B. Enzyme

C. Catalysts D. All the above

188. It's reversible potential which is show by E is given by?

A. E=E + RT/nF in = amn+

B. E=E - RT/nF in mn+

C. E=E+ RT/nF In = ms+

D. Nene of this

189. Potential of a single electrode can not be measured it is therefore coupled with another electrode where potential known this called?

A. Reverce electrode

B. Reference electrode

C. Active electrode

D. Inactive electrode

190. The potential assumed by the electrode is known?

A. Reversible evident

B. Reversible electrone

C. Reversible potential

D. All the above

191. The metal ion concentration of the solution in which the electrode is placed , hence this electrode is known as?

A. Indicater solvent B. Indicater electrode

C. Indicater electron D. Indicater starch

192. Write are quantitative analysis can be divided known as?

A. One major categories

B. Two major categories

C. Three majorcategories

D. Four majorcategories

193. The method of quantitative analysis known as?

A. Classlal method

B. Instrument method

C. Physiochemical method

D. All the above

194. An instrument method requires calibration which is done with the help of solution known as?

A. Weak solution

B. Strong solution

C. Concentration solution

D. None of this

195. The method of quantitative analysis based on the measurementof electrical property are briefly called?

A. Electron method

B. Electrical method

C. Electrode method

D. None of this

196. The visual titrimetry potentiometric titration types chemical reaction known ?
A. Two chemical reaction
B. Four chemical reaction
C. Three chemical reaction
D. None of this

197. Write are type potentiometric titration chemical reaction include known as?
A. Acid-base potentiometric
B. Redox potentiometric
C. Potentiometric titration based on precipitation & complexation reaction
D. All the above

198. The potentiometric titration of given HCl solution with alkali solution using known?
A. Liquidhydrone - catomel electrode system
B. Quinhydrone - catomel electrode system
C. Both (a) & (b)
D. None

199. Write are potentiometric titration can be used to known as?
A. Coloured solution
B. Non coloured solution
C. Colour indicater
D. Indicater allow

200. The colour change of indicater cannot be located by usingknown?
A. Titrametric technique
B. Equivalent technique
C. Potentiometric technique
D. None of this

201. The equivalence point of the titration can be?
A. Accurately determined
B. Non accurately determined
C. Both (a) & (b)
D. None

202. In acid- base titration hydron quinhydrone atimory & glass electrode can act as?
A. Indicater suitable
B. Indicater electrode
C. Indicater electron
D. Indicater potassium

203. The view point of electricalconduction substance can be divided into?
A. Two categories B. Four categories
C. Six categories D. Seven categories

204. Those substance which permit the passage of current through them (conduct electric current) are called?
A. Indicator B. Conducters
C. Condrant D. Conducting

205. While substance which do not conduct electricity are known as?
A. Indicator B. Insulators
C. Electrode D. None of this

206. The nature of charged particles present in conductors the can be divided into?
A. Two conductors B. Three conductors
C. Four conductors D. Five conductors

207. Write are conductors they can be following type known as?
A. Metallic or electronic conductors
B. Electrolytic or ionic conductors
C. Mixed conductors
D. All the above

208. We have a conductors in the form of an electrolytes solution a spaicel cell known ?
A. Counductility B. Conductivity
C. Condract D. None of this

209. Write are are conductivity cell used in a?
A. Conductometric titration
B. Conductlitiy titration
C. Conductvelant titration
D. Conductvelence titration

210. Write are application of conductometric titration known as?
A. Titration of a strong acid with a strong base
B. Titration of a strong acid withweak base
C. Titration of a weak acid with weak acid
D. All the above

211. Write are titration strong acid with a strong base formula known as?
A. HCl - NaoH B. HCl - NaoH
C. Na+ - NH4oH D. None of this

212. Write are titration strong acid with a weak base known as?
A. HCl - NaoH
B. CH3 COOH - NH4OH
C. HCl - NH4OH
D. None of this

213. Write are titration weak acid with a weak base known as?
A. CH3COOH - NH4OH
B. HCl - NaOH
C. CH3COOH - HCl
D. None of this

214. The potential acquired by the electrode under such a condition is called?
A. Reversible B. Unreversible
C. Both (a) & (b) D. None

215. This distrabance of equipment associated with the flow of current is called?
A. Electrolytic polarization
B. Equilibrium
C. Electron dipping
D. None of this

216. These Three type of titration are bassed on the measurement of electrical properties these are called ?
A. Oxidation titration
B. Reduction titration
C. Electrimetric titration
D. Electrical titration

217. The non-aqueous titration solvent includesknown as?
A. Aprotic solvents
B. Photogenic solvents or protophilic solvents
C. Amphiprotic solvents
D. All the above

218. Interference due to water in titration know as?
A. Aqueous titration
B. None aqueous titration
C. Both (a) & (b)
D. None

219. Non aqueous titrations of weakBase with?
A. Nitric acid B. Acetic acid
C. Perchloric acid D. None of this

220. The Non aqueous titration of weak acid with?
A. Alkoinxide B. Alkoxides
C. Alkenxide D. None of this

221. The non aqueous titration are- those in which acidic or basic substance are carried out using?
A. Aqueous solvent
B. Non aqueous solvent
C. Methanol solvent
D. Aprotic solvent

222. Those Non - aqueous solvent can be explained by using Lowery bronsted according know as?
A. Acid is a proton donor
B. Base is a proton donor
C. Both (a) & (b)
D. None

223. Write aprotic solvent known as?
A. Chloroform B. Benzene
C. Both (a) & (b) D. None

224. Write are protogenic solvent example known as?
A. Sulphuric acid B. Hydrochloride acid
C. Nitric acid D. All the above

225. Write are strong basic solvent is called as?
A. Label solvent B. Levelling solvent
C. Weak solvents D. Strong solvents

226. The other hand a weakly basic solvent has weak tendency to accept proton, hence this solvent called?
A. Aceptentiating solvent
B. Differentiating solvent
C. Leveling solvent
D. All the above

227. Write in defferentiating solvent are not useful in?
A. Aqueous titration
B. Non aqueous titration
C. Precipitation titration
D. Acid titration

228. The both protogenic & protophilic properties example known as?
A. Acetic acid B. Alcohol
C. Both (a) & (b) D. None

229. The non-aqueous titration of weak base with?
A. Alkoxides B. Perchloric acid
C. Arctic acid D. All the above

230. When weak base like pyridine are dissolve in?
A. Acetylene acid B. Acetate acid
C. Acetic acid D. None of this

231. When weak bases like pyridine in acetic acid equivalent amount of acetate ions are?
A. Reduced B. Produced
C. Precipitation D. Oxidized

232. The indicater method several indicater are available and are used to in the end opinion?
A. Retect B. Reduct
C. Oxidant D. Detect

233. The application of redox titration using?
A. Cerric ammonium sulphate
B. Cerric potassium sulphate
C. Cedric methacholine chloride
D. All the above

234. Write are type method redox titration known as?
A. Direct titration B. Back titration
C. Both (a) & (b) D. None

235. The redox titration can be explained with equation in the oxidation is?
A. Loss of protons B. Loss of electrons
C. Loss of chlorides D. None of this

236. The redox titration can be explained with the reduction is?
A. Loss of electrons
B. Gain electrons
C. Loss of proton
D. Loss of reduction

237. Write are back titration example known?
A. Drug like chloramphenicol
B. Metronidazole
C. Nitrosa
D. All the above

238. The diazotisation titration are carried out for the drug estimation of drug containing in?
A. Primary aromatic amines group
B. Secondary aromatic amines group
C. Standard aromatic amines group
D. All the above

239. Write are diazotisation example known as?
A. Hydrolysis B. Chloride
C. Ions D. Acids

240. The diazotisation titration although procedure for individual drug are?
A. One drug B. Two drag
C. Indifferent drugs D. Different drugs

241. Write are diazotisation titration type method include in?
A. Direct method B. Reverse method
C. Special method D. All the above

242. The direct titration with nitric solution act in?
A. Benzocaine B. Dapsone
C. Procaine D. All the above

243. Conversion to amino group by chemical reaction by reduction in?
A. Metronidazole B. Secnidazole
C. Chloramphenicol D. All the above

244. The primary aromatic amino group can be diazotised by using?
A. Methyl B. Diazepam
C. Nitrite solution D. All the above

245. The diazotisation titration lonversion to amino group by chemical reaction by hydrolysis known as?
A. Paracetamol (acetyl derivative)
B. Pathalyl sulphathiazole (pthayl derivative)
C. Succinyl salphathiazole (saccinyl derivative)
D. All the above

246. The acid solution of the drug liberate benzylhydryzine which can be diazotised to give?
A. Acetylhide B. Benzylazide
C. Methylazide D. None of this

247. The complexometric titration are those in which complexing agent is used to?
A. Ions B. Divalent
C. Polyvalent D. All the above

248. The complexing agent is an electron?
A. Accepting ion B. Donating ion
C. Both (a) & (b) D. None

249. If a single bond is formed between a complexing agent & metal it's called?
A. Divalent B. Ligand
C. Lebling D. Poyvelnt

250. If a complexing can from more then one bond with polyvalence ion then it is considered a polydentate called as?

A. Achelating agent B. Chelating agent
C. Conduct agent D. Sequestring agent

251. The complex form is soluble in water, thenit is called?

A. Accurately agent
B. Sequestering agent
C. Chelating agent
D. All the above

252. The such complexing agent is unidenetate in nature called as?

A. Aco-ordination compound
B. Co-ordination compound
C. Organic compound
D. Inorganic compound

253. Write are full form (WCN) known in complexometric titration in?

A. Weak weak co-ordination number
B. Wold co- ordination number
C. Wernen co-ordination numbers
D. Attached co-ordination number

254. Dimethylglyoxime & salicylaldoxime are example for?

A. Sequestering agent
B. Chelating agent
C. Lingand agent
D. None of this

255. The ethylene diamine tetraacetic acid is example in?

A. Chelating agent
B. Ligand agent
C. Sequestrum agent
D. All the above

256. The EDTA full form in ?

A. Ethylene diether tetra acetic acid
B. Ethylene dichloro tetra acetic acid
C. Ethylene diamine tetra acetic acid
D. Ethylene dinitro tetra acetic acid

257. The stability of the complex in acidic pH in?

A. Increase B. Decrease
C. Both (a) &(b) D. None

258. The stability of the complex in temperature is?

A. Increased B. Decreased
C. Ionisation D. All the above

259. The complexometric titration is type of method determining end point in?

A. Potentiometric method
B. Amperometric method
C. Conductometric method
D. All the above

260. In indicater used in complexmetric titration are called?

A. Am indicater B. Pm indicater
C. Sm indicater D. Lm indicater

261. Indicater used in complexometric titration known as?

A. Mordan black II or eriochrome blackT
B. Xylenol orange
C. Murexide
D. All the above

262. The complexmetric titration type include in?

A. Direct titration
B. Replacement of one complex by another
C. Alkalimetric titration of metal
D. All the above

263. The direct titration a weight amount of the substance to be

A. Estilated B. Estimated
C. Estibride D. Estiacute

264. Estimated example include in?

A. Bismuth - nitrate , carbonate, oxynitrate, subnitrate
B. Calcium - chloride gluconate lactate
C. Zin - sulphate oxide undecenoate
D. All the above

265. The complexation is favoured by?

A. Chelating B. Heating
C. Decrease D. Increase

266. When sharp end point is not obtain by?

A. Direct titration or back titration
B. Alkalimetric titration
C. Indirect titration
D. All the above

267. Masking and demasking agent are those wich?
A. Precipitate or conductometric
B. Precipitate or complex ions selectively
C. Precipitate or acid or base
D. None of this

268. The end point of the titration in soap titration with?
A. Formulation salt
B. Formulation lathar
C. Formulation sodium
D. Formulation chloride

269. The end point of the titration in the soap titration method is at formulation lather that stand for about time known as?
A. 2 minutes B. 4 minutes
C. 6 minutes D. 8 minutes

270. The estimation of hardness can be determine by type known as?
A. 4 B. 2
C. 6 D. 8

271. Write are estimation can be determine method known?
A. Soap titration method
B. EDTA method
C. Redox titration method
D. All the above

272. The water which form lather directly with the soap called?
A. Soft water B. Distil water
C. Hard water D. All the above

273. The EDTA method is called?
A. Precipitation titration
B. Complexion titration
C. Complexometric
D. Complement titration

274. The water wich forms precipitates when with saop is called?
A. Soft water B. Hard water
C. Purified water D. Distil water

275. the EDTA method used indicater in?
A. Methyl B. Benzene
C. Strach D. Crichrom blacky

276. The EDTA in the ability to form with metal ion is?
A. Acetate form B. Basic form
C. Suitable complex D. Unsuitable complex

277. The colour of dye metal complex & dye are in
A. Same B. Different
C. Both (a) &(b) D. None

278. The EDTA method is used drops of indicater in?
A. 1 to 2 drops B. 3 to 4 drops
C. 5 to 6 drops D. 7 to 8 drops

279. The buffer used in the EDTA solution must have in pH?
A. 5 B. 10
C. 15 D. 20

280. All of the following act us masking agent known ?
A. Ammonium chloride B. Iodine
C. Iron D. Floride

281. The alkalimetric titration is?
A. Iodine B. NaoH
C. Calcium D. EDTA

282. The silver & gold are titrated by?
A. Chlorotetracynonickate
B. Tetracyanonicketate
C. Both (a) &(b)
D. None

283. All the following can produce selective complexometric titration in?
A. Direct titration B. Back titration
C. Choice indicter D. Indirect titration

284. The solubility of the sparingly soluble salt decrece by?
A. Inorganic solvent
B. Organic solvent
C. Increase solvent
D. All the above

285. Which of the following is a back titration method in?
A. Mohr method
B. Volhard method
C. Distribution method
D.Absorption method

286. The effect of increase in temperature on stability complex is?
A. Decrease B. Increase
C. Effect D. No effect

287. Write are complexing agent in?
A. Water soluble complex
B. Water insoluble complex
C. Both (a) & (b)
D. Water complex not include

288. Write are disodium salt of EDTA is ?
A. Hexadenate B. Fexadenate
C. Tetradenate D. Mondenate

289. Write are ethylene diamine is?
A. Dibenate B. Bidenate
C. Tetradenate D. Chlorodenate

290. The complex formation with act metals,ligand may be act in?
A. Natural B. Electron donor
C. Both (a) & (b) D. None

291. The water act in?
A. Monodentate B. Hexacyandenate
C. Bidenate D. Ethredinated

292. The equipuvalent weight of a substance is defined as the part by?
A. Number of that substance
B. Hemically
C. Weight of that substance
D. None of this

293. The neutralisation or acid - base reaction are very suitable for?
A. Titrimetric analysis
B. Redox titration
C. Precipitation titration
D. All the above

294. Write are magnesium oxide formula in?
A. Mgso B. Mgo
C. Mo D. Mao

295. The eq. At of an acid is that weight of it which contain one replaceable in?
A. Sodium B. Hydrogen
C. Calcium D. Bromide

296. An acid whose molecule contain only one replaceable (or ionisable) hydrogen is called?
A. Monobasic acid B. Nitric acid
C. Phosphoric acid D. Sulphuric acid

297. If a contain 1g eq. Of a substance per liter, it is called?
A. Weak solution B. Strong solution
C. Normal solution D. Difficult solution

298. The selecting a suitable regent & preparing it's?
A. Test solution B. Standard solution
C. Both (a) & (b) D. None

299. The substance commonly used as primary standard in acid Base titration are known as?
A. Faroic acid B. Adipic acid
C. Benzoic acid D. All the above

300. There is a small difference between, the equipment point and end point this difference is known as?
A. Titration error B. End point error
C. Both (a) & (b) D. None

301. high performance liquid chromatography is technique are used
A. separation B. purification
C. identification D. all of the above

302. which one of the following is the full form of HPLC
A. high performance liquid chromatography
B. high profile liquid chromosomes
C. high profile liquid chromatography
D. none of the above

303. how many phases in HPLC
A. one B. two
C. three D. four

304. which one of the following is the phase of HPLC
A. stationary & mobile phase
B. transparent phase
C. semi transparent
D. automobile phase

305. mobile phase are
A. polar B. non polar
C. both A&b D. none of the above

306. stationary phase are
A. non polar B. polar
C. both A&b D. none of the above

307. one which of the following full form of MPLC
A. medium pressure liquid chromatography
B. medium pressure liquid chromosomes
C. medium profile liquid chromatography
D. medium performance liquid chromatography

308. which solvent used in HPLC
A. helium B. nitrogen
C. oxygen D. carbondioxide

309. -------------- is generates an electrical signal that can be amplified and presented in the form of a chromatography of solute concentration as a function of time
A. detector B. amplified
C. capacitor D. none of tha above

310. based on principle of separation which type of HPLC technique is performe
A. adsorption chromatography
B. ion change chromatography
C. gel chromatography
D. all of them

311. what is the particle size of stationary phase
A. 5-10 u B. 7-10 u
C. 4-19 D. 8-13

312. the column used for HPLC are generally made by
A. copper B. iron ore
C. stainless steel D. graphites

313. --------------are used for supporting the liquid phase
A. microporous B. pellicular
C. both A&b D. none of the above

314. porous pluges of stainless steel or teflon are used in
A. ends of the column
B. packing of the column
C. both A&b
D. none of the above

315. most commonly the detector is a variable wavelength
A. ultravoilet visible spectrophotometer
B. flurемeter
C. refractive index monitor
D. all of them

316. porous material used in HPLC
A. silica B. alumina
C. both A&b D. none of the above

317. pellicular column material used of HPLC
A. inactive silica B. active silica
C. active alumina D. all of them

318. when was HPLC invented
A. 1970 B. 1987
C. 1965 D. 1945

319. the resolving power of a chromatography column increase with column
A. number of theoretical plates
B. number of resolving power
C. both A&B
D. none of the above

320. in which system the stationary phase may be coated into the insert support
A. liquid - liquid partition system
B. liquid - solid partition system
C. liquid - semi solid partition system
D. solid - solid partition system

321. for a typical adsorbent such as silica gel the most popular pore diameters are
A. 10 and 50 A0 B. 60 and 100 A0
C. 100 and. 150 A0 D. 236 and 250 A0

322. in reversed phase HPLC there is a
A. non polar solvent / polar column
B. polar solvent / non polar column
C. non polar solvent / non polar column
D. none of the above

323. which of the following (s) is /are the advantages of HPLC over traditional LPLC (lowpressure liquid chromatography
A. sample recovery
B. molecules
C. ideal for ionic species and large molecules
D. all of them

324. which of the following statements is true for a refractive index detector in HPLC
A. it is more sensitive than a uv detector
B. it can only be used for isocratic elutions
C. it does not respond to many solutes
D. none of the above

325. the eluent strenght is a measure of
A. solvent adsorption energy
B. solvent absorption energy
C. solvent diffusivity
D. solvent mixing index

326. An isocratic elution in HPLC is one in which the composition of the solvent
A. remains constant

B. change continuously
C. change in a series of steps
D. none of the above

327. high pressure liquid chromatography can be performed only in column
A. column B. row
C. stationary D. none of the above

328. A gradient elution in HPLC is one in which the composition of the solvent
A. remain constant
B. is change continuously or in a series of steps
C. both A&B
D. none of the above

329. Dwell volume is defined as
A. the volume of solvent contained in a liquid chromatography column
B. the time required for the gradient to reach the column
C. the volume of the column between the point at which solvent are mixed and beginning of the column
D. none of the above

330. gravity feed method for solvent delivery is not used with narrow column packed with
A. fine mesh particles
B. large mesh particles
C. mesh product
D. none of the above

331. when was chromatography invented
A. 1906 B. 1980
C. 1954 D. 1974

332. which column acted as an sdsorbent and the different substance got adsorbed to different extent and this gave rise to coloured bands at different position on the column
A. calcium carbonate
B. sodium carbonate
C. calcium sulphate
D. none of the above

333. chromatography may be regarded as a method for
A. detection B. purity
C. separation D. identification

334. when was introduce in partition and paper chromatography technique
A. 1956 N.k jain B. 1941 martin
C. 1978 khandelwal D. none of the above

335. which one of the following is the full form of TLC
A. thin layer chromatography
B. thin layer chromosomes
C. thin layer conlusion
D. none of the above

336. chromatography are two phases
A. distribution & dissolution
B. equilibrium & distribution
C. equilibrium & equivalent
D. none of the above

337. the chromatography method separation in general involes are following step are--
A. adsorption or retention of a substance or substance on the stationary phase
B. separation of the adsorbent substance by mobile phase
C. both A&B
D. none of the above

338. chromatography is physical method used to separate and analyse
A. simple mixture B. complex mixture
C. viscous mixture D. metals

339. in which type of chromatography the stationary phase held in a narrow tube and the mobile phase is forced throught is under pressure
A. column chromatography
B. planer chromatography
C. liquid chromatography
D. gas chromatography

340. in chromatography the stationary phase can be supported on a ......
A. solid or liquid B. liquid or gas
C. solid only D. liquid only

341. in chromatography which of the following can be mobile phase made of...
A. solid or liquid B. liquid or gas
C. gas only D. liquid only

342. which of the following cannot be used as an adsorbent in column adsorption chromatography

A. magnesium oxide
B. silica gel
C. activated alumina
D. potassium permanganate

343. which of the following types of chromatography involes the separation of substance in a mixture over a 0.2 mm thick layer of a adsorbent ....

A. gas liquid B. column
C. thin layer D. paper

344. in chromatography cannot used to purity ....

A. non volatile B. volatile substance
C. water D. none of the above

345. the size of a thin layer of adsorbent is about

A. 0.1mm B. 0.2mm
C. 0.3 mm D. 0.4mm

346. the chromaplates or thin layer chromatography plate is made up of.........

A. wood B. glass
C. fibre D. Metal

347. the eluant filled in the closed is......

A. mixture of gases
B. mixture of a liquid or gas
C. mixture of solid
D. mixture of liquid

348. chromatography technique are based on diffirent absortion mechanism ....

A. surface adsorption
B. partition
C. ion exchange
D. all of them

349. which is third absorption phenomena is that.......

A. ion exchange B. partition
C. exchange D. none of the above

350. which is the four mechanism of chromatography technique are.........

A. pre dominates B. dominates
C. no exchange D. none of the above

351. which of the following of the full form of Rf value

A. retardation factor B. ratio factor
C. resonance factor D. none of the above

352. which phase the retardation factor the fraction of an analyte are .....

A. mobile phase B. stationary phase
C. column D. none of the above

353. which coating material used for TLC ......

A. silica gel B. alumina
C. both A&B D. none of the above

354. which the plate is placed in a development chamber at an angle are .....

A. 450C B. 600C
C. 670C D. 780C

355. thickness for thin layer chromatography are ....

A. 0.0 to 2.0mm B. 0.3 to 4.6 mm
C. 0.4 to 5.6 mm D. 0.1 to 0.6 mm

356. stationary phase material for used for adsorption chromatography

A. starch B. lactose
C. sodium D. none of the above

357. adsorption chromatography has been extensively used for......

A. separation B. purification
C. assay D. none of the above

358. chromatography involves two naturally ....

A. immiscible phase B. miscible
C. soluble phase D. none of the above

359. the gas -solid chromatography is chromatography as per basic principle involved ...

A. exclusion B. ion exchange
C. Adsorption D. absorption

360. if the mobile phases in gas movement of solute in determind by.........

A. boiling point B. melting point
C. solubility D. volatility

361. an adsorbent may be described as.....

A. solid B. liquid
C. voletile oil D. emulsion

362. an adsorbent is porous may be ......

A. finelly divided B. partially divided
C. divided D. none of the above

363. adsorption chromatography can be carried out .....
A. column B. thin layer modes
C. both A&B D. none of the above

364. langmuir adsorption isotherm is know as......
A. M. k1k2C/1+k2 C
B. K. K1K2M/1+K2C
C. m. K2K3C/1+K2
D. k. K1K5C/1+K2C

365. when compound used as the stationary phase in adsorbents ..
.A. silica acid
B. calcium oxide
C. magnesium oxide
D. all of them

366. hydroxyapatitve (calcium phosphate) is widely used for .....
A. separation of protein
B. nucleic acid
C. Both A&B
D. none of the above

367. the stronger adsorbents naturally have more ......
A. polar structure
B. non polar structure
C. polar and non polar
D. none of the above

368. commonly used low polarity solvent are .....
A. hexane B. heptane
C. toluene D. all of them

369. commonly highly polar solvent include are ...
A. propan-1-ol B. butan-1-ol
C. acetone D. all of them

370. they also decrease the resolving power of the ..
A. column B. mobile phase
C. stationary phase D. none of the above

371. the disadvantage with adsortion chromatography howere less in the fact tha is .....
A. empirical B. non reproducible
C. both A&B D. none of the above

372. the column chromatography is matrix may be .....
A. cellulose starch B. silica gel
C. both A&B D. none of the above

373. The mobile solvent phase is generally are ...
A. organic solvent immiscible
B. water
C. both A&B D. none of the above

374. liquid - liquid chromatography especally in the HPLC is used for
A. separation of a very range biological compound
B. purification
C. identification
D. none of the above

375. the separation of compound that are readily soluble in...
A. organic liquid
B. sparingly soluble in water
C. both A&B
D. none of the above

376. partition chromatography is intermediate between ....
A. adsorption
B. ion exchange chromatography
C. both A&B
D. none of the above

377. The ratio of the concentration of the compound in two solvent is constant and is know as......
A. partition coefficient
B. partition size
C. partition reduction
D. none of the above

378. silica gel is used for ....
A. fine white powder
B. granules
C. fine powder
D. none of the above

379. gel filtration or gel exclusion chromatography is technique is variously know.....
A. gel filtration
B. molecules sieve filtration
C. exclusion chromatography
D. all of them

380. gel chromatography is are.....
A. simple chromatography
B. reliable method
C. both A&B
D. none of the above

381. porous glass granules have been used as.....
A. molecular sieves
B. molecular size
C. molecular shape
D. none of the above

382. haemoglobin can be separated from.....
A. sodium chloride
B. sodium potassium
C. benzen
D. sodium hydroxide

383. Fractionation of mixture of biopolymers is the most wide spread application of gel chromatography can also used ..
A. preparative purposes
B. identification
C. assay
D. none of the above

384. The main application of the gel chromatography are...
A. Purification
B. molecular weight determination
C. solution concentration
D. all of them

385. The effluent volume of globular protein are largely determind by......
A. molecular weight
B. molecular formula
C. molecular mass
D. none of the above

386. The main application of exclusion chromatography is the purification macromolecules ...
A. viruses
B. protein
C. enzyme
D. all of them

387. The amino acid can be separated from.....
A. peptides
B. hormones
C. granules
D. none of the above

388. solution of high molecular weight substance can be concentration by the addition of...
A. dry sephadex G-25
B. dry sephadexG-28
C. dry sephadex G-29
D. none of the above

389. water and low molecular weight substance are absorbed by....
A. swelling gel
B. foming gel
C. both A&B
D. none of the above

390. The use of column of sephadex G-25 solution
A. high molecular weight
B. low molecular weight
C. both A&B
D. none of the above

391. the low molecular weight components are distributed between ....
A. mobile phase
B. stationary phase
C. both A&B
D. none of the above

392. Exclusion chromatography is one of a number of method commonly used for.....
A. reversible binding of a ligand to a micromolecules
B. Irreversible binding of a ligand to a micromolecules
C. both A&B
D. none of the above

393. when was column chromatography developed ....
A. 1900
B. 1930
C. 1902
D. 1903

394. column chromatography was developed by the american petroleum chemist in...
A. D.T day in 1900
B. D.S day in 1900
C. both A&B
D. none of the above

395. column chromatography is also known as...
A. adsorption chromatography
B. gel chromatography
C. gas chromatography
D. paper chromatography

396. The principle of selective adsorption is used in...

A. column chromatography

B. gel chromatography

C. both A&B

D. none of the above

397. The banded column of adsorbent is termed as.....

A. chromatogram B. chromatograph

C. Both A&B D. none of the above

398. The portion of a column which is occupied by a particular substance is called its.....

A. Zones B. adsorbence

C. Both A&B D. none of the above

399. This process of recovery of constituent from the chromatogram is known as...

A. elution B. adsorbence

C. zones D. none of the above

400. Long and narrow tubes are used for....

A. difficult separation

B. simple separation

C. both A&B

D. none of the above

401. separating column are used in .....

A. detachable adapters

B. change adapters

C. both A&B

D. none of the above

402. The adsorbents is packed between two sintered....

A. glass discs

B. small bore taflon tube

C. both A&B

D. none of the above

403. Aluminium oxide activated by heating about....

A. 200-3000C B. 400- 6000C

C. 400-5000C D. 100-300OC

404. carbone dioxide is most widely used for.....

A. adsorbent B. purity

C. Assay D. none of the above

405. polyacrye amide particle size are......

A. Ca 0.04 mm B. Ca. 0.06 mm

C. Ca. 0.09 mm D. Ca. 0.07 mm

406. polycrye amide are suitable for the separation of.....

A. lower fatty acid

B. higher fatty acid

C. fatty acid

D. none of the above

407. The column chromatography solvent used for this purpose are called ..,

A. eluants B. zones

C. both A&B D. none of the above

408. optical detector old type of flow analyser which are small cell made from

A. glass B. quarts

C. both A&B D. none of the above

409. Detectors based on.....

A. heat of adsorption

B. cold of adsorption

C. adsorption

D. none of the above

410. These detector are known as.....

A. micro adsorption detector

B. micro molecules detector

C. micro grame detector

D. none of the above

411. conductivity detector are suitable for lonsed substance in......

A Aqueous solution D. water solution

C. both A&B D. none of the above

412. The rate of the flow of solvent throught the column is controlled by.......

A. suction pump B. pump inhibitor

C. both A&B D. none of the above

413. The analysis is adsorbent may be pushed out completely with the ....

A. wooden pestle B. pluger

C. both A&B D. none of the above

414. The volume of solvent is known as.....

A. retention volume B. Rf value

C. both A&B D. none of the above

415. Peak resolution is determined by ....

A. selectivity B. efficacy

C. enfluence D. none of the above

416. **The plate number can be increased by....**
A. simply increasing the column length
B. simply decreasing the column length
C. both A&B
D. none of the above

417. **The maximum number of peaks that can be separated by a specific chromatographic system is called the ....**
A. peak capacity B. peak capablity
C. both A& B D. none of the above

418. **Peak capacity is determined by....**
A. acceptable separation
B. separation
C. both A&B
D. none of the above

419. **Nature of solvent of low viscosities are generally used for ....**
A. high efficiency separation
B. low efficiency separation
C. both A&B
D. none of the above

420. **The common preparative separation .sample /column packing ratio have range found to be .....**
A. 1:20 to 1:100 B. 1:30 to 1:200
C. 1:21 to 1:300 D. 1:19 to 1:400

421. **The usual particles size ranges from…**
A. 100 to 200 mesh B. 100 to 150 mesh
C. 100 to 160 mesh D. 100 to 190 mesh

422. **Difficult soluble samples are generally separated at….**
A. Higher temperature
B. Low temperature
C. Medium temperature
D. None of the above

423. **Column chromatography analysis capillaries made of….**
A. glass B. Copper
C. Both A&B D. Sulphate

424. **Capillaries internal diameter are …**
A. 0.05-2 mm B. 0.06-2 mm
C. 0.07-3 mm D. 0.07-4 mm

425. **An optical detector is used for the analysis of steroids by.**
A. Gradient elution B. Elution
C. Efficacy D. None of the above

426. **The separation of cis/trans isomer is based on.**
A. Steric factor B. Influence factor
C. Both A&B D. None of the above

427. **Separation of tautomeric mixtures these could be done by.**
A. Column chromatography
B. Gas chromatography
C. Paper chromatography
D. None of the above

428. **Pyruvic acid and indolyl pyruvic acid could be separated in the ..**
A. Liquid phase B. Solid phase
C. Semi solid phase D. None of the above

429. **Affinity chromatography is technique are**
A. Electrophoresis B. Centrifugation
C. Both A&B D. None of the above

430. **Group specific ligands commonly used in affinity chromatography**
A. Lysine B. sucrose
C. Mannitol D. Starch

431. **A wide range of enzyme and other protein, including receptor protein and immino globulins has been purified by**
A. Affinity chromatography
B. Column chromatography
C. Paper chromatography
D. Gas chromatography

432. **Immobilised single stranded DNA can be used to.**
A. Isolate complementary RNA and DNA
B. Complementary DNA and RNA
C. Both A&B
D. None of the above

433. **Whist this separation can be archived on**
A. Gas B. Column
C. Paper D. None of the above

434. **affinity chromatography can be exploited to**
A. Concentrate dilute solution
B. Separate native and denatured micromoles

C. Both A&B
D. None of the above

435. Cibacron blue is one of the numbers of triazines dyer can be used in
A. Ligand to purity protein
B. Ligand to purity enzyme
C. Both A&B
D. None of the above

436. The interaction is not genuinely specific the term sometimes technique are
A. Hot ligand chromatography
B. dye ligand chromatography
C. Cold ligand chromatography
D. None of the above

437. The most commonly used in chelating ligands for the metal ions
A. Ethyl
B. Tris ethylenediamine
C. Chloramine
D. None of the above

438. Protein purified technique include by
A. Monoxide B. Superoxide
C. Aminoxide D. None of the above

439. The affinity chromatography is use for the separation of a mixture of the cell into
A. Homogeneous
B. Homogeneous population
C. both A&B
D . None of the above

440. Covalent chromatography from other form of
A. Column chromatography
B. Gas chromatography
C. Affinity chromatography
D. None of the above

441. The sample components can be sensed by a detector and monitored by
A. Data B. Recorder
C. Both A&B D. None of the above

442. It is possible to measure the inlet pressure of the column with a
A. manometer B. Nanometer
C. Minimeter D. Momometer

443. Which of the following is not used for detection in gas chromatography
A. Infrared spectroscopy
B. NMR
C. Flame ionization
D. Electrical conduction

444. which of these effect result from slow injection of a large sample volume
A. Increased resolution
B. Decreased resolution
C. Nonlinear detector response
D. Constant resolution

445. the gas chromatography trace obtained after an experiment is called as
A. chromatograph B. Chromatogram
C. Chromatophore D. None of the above

446. Which of the following detector give a concentration depends signal
A. Electron capture detector
B. thermal conductivity
C. Infra-red detector
D. All of them

447. What useful information can be found from a diameter plot
A. The selectivity factor
B. Optimum mobile phase flow rate
C. Optimum column temperature
D. Optimum column length

448. Resolution is proportional to the
A. Number of theoretical plates in a column
B. Square root of the number of a theoretical plate in a number
C. Square of the number of the theoretical plates in a number
D. None of the above

449. Derivation of a sample is carried out to
A. Reduce polarity of the analytes
B. Increase the detector response
C. Increase volatility rof the analytes
D. All of them

450. Which pf the statement is correct
A. Gas chromatography is used to analyse solid
B. gas chromatography is used to analyse gases

C. Gas chromatography is used to analyse gases solution and solid
D. All of them

451. Which of the following detector give mass flow depend signals
A. Electron capture detector
B. Field ionization detector
C. Thermal conductivity detector
D. All of them

452. Helium is generally preferred as carries gas over nitrogen and hydrogen because -
A. It is inert
B. It has a lower viscosity
C. It doubles up as a party gas for balloon and funny voices
D. All of them

453. the column is heated to
A. Prevent analyte condensation within the column
B. Control elution of the efferent analyte
C. Reduce band broadening to get sharper peak
D. all of them

454. sample retention in the column is measured by
A. Retention time B. Retention factor
C. Retention index D. All of them

455. Which is the following are not used as stationary phase in a gas chromatography
A. Polysloxanes
B. silica
C. Cyclohexene
D. None are used as stationary phase

456. Doubling the column length increase resolution by a factor of
A. (2) 0.5 B. 2
C. 3 D. 4

457. Which of the following gases in a unsuitable for are as a gas chromatography carrier gas
A. nitrogen B. Helium
C. Oxygen D. All of them

458. Which of the following is not an ideal characteristic of a detector used a gas chromatography
A. Linear response to the solution
B. Short response time
C. High reliability
D. Sensitive to the change in the flow rate of carrier gas

459. Filter photometer detector is primarily responsive to which of the following compound /elements
A. Volatile sulphur or phosphorous compound
B. Nitrogen
C. Potassium
D. Helium

460. Flame ionization detector in also know a
A. Calorimetry B. katharometer
C. Polarimetry D. None of the above

461. Gas – solid chromatography is based upon
A. Selective adsorption on liquid
B. Selective adsorption on solid
C. Both A&B
D. None of the above

462. Gas liquid chromatography is based upon the partition between the
A. Gas an immobile liquid phase
B. Gas an immobile solid phase
C. Both A&B
D. none of the above

463. Gas solid chromatography was developed by
A. G.D kohler B. G.K kohler
C. G.C kohler D. None of the above

464. The gas liquid chromatography is more popular than
A. Gas liquid chromatography
B. Gas solid chromatography
C. Gas semi solid chromatography
D. None of the above

465. Gas liquid chromatography was originated by
A. A.T.P martin in 1951
B. A.T.K martin in 1952
C. A.J.D martin in 1954
D. None of the above

466. The analysis is completed in a

A. Long time B. Short time
C. Both A&B D. None of the above

467. Gas chromatography is a present one of the most widely used for

A. Assay B. purification
C. separation D. None of the above

468. Gas chromatography can be further subdivided into

A. Gas -liquid chromatography
B. Gas -solid chromatography
C. Both A&B
D. None of the above

469. When a gas or vapour comes in contact with

A. Adsorbent B. adsorption
C. Purification D. None of the above

470. Gas – liquid chromatography is consists of a

A. Mobile phase B. Stationary phase
C. Both A&B D. None of the above

471. The gas chromatographic separation is carried out in

A. Tubular column B. column
C. Both A&B D. none of the above

472. The gas chromatography is a tubular column made of

A. glass B. Teflon
C. Both A&B D. None pf the above

473. The adsorbent are packed in the form of

A. Granules
B. Fine size graded powder
C. Mixer
D. None of the above

474. The most widely used carrier Glaser are

A. Hydrogen B. Helium
C. Nitrogen D. All of the above

475. Hydrogen gas that may react with

A. Saturated compound
B. Unsaturated compound
C. Both A&B
D. None of the above

476. Liquid sample are generally introduce by

A. Hypodermic syringe
B. hyper dermic syringe
C. Hex dermic syringe
D. None of the above

477. Packed column are prepared by

A. Packing metal
B. Glass tubing
C. Granules stationary phase
D. All of the above

478. The porous polymer are stableup to

A. 3000 C B. 2500C
C. 5600C D. 350OC

479. Porous polymer beads are mechanically strong and can be easily packed on

A. Column B. glass
C. Tubing D. None of the above

480. Open tubular column are made of

A. Long capillary tubing
B. Short capillary tubing
C. Both A&B
D. None of the above

481. Open tubular column uniform and narrow internal diameter is

A. 0.026-0.076cm B. 0.025-0.075cm
C. 0.064-0.086cm D. 0.026-0.089 cm

482. The ionization detector are based on the

A. Conductivity of gases
B. Electrical conductivity of gases
C. Both A&B
D. None of the above

483. The detector responds to all organic compound except

A. Sodium B. Formic acid
C. Folic acid D. Amino acid

484. Electron capture detector can be used as the bases for an ionization detector know as

A. Electron capture detector
B. Electron avoid detector
C. Both A&B
D. None of the above

485. Chlorinated pesticides can be determined down to

A. Sub pictogram
B. Sub equivalent gram

C. Both A&B
D. None of the above

486. The ECD is most frequently used for detection and measurement can be
A. Environment
B. Environment pollutants
C. Pollution
D. None of the above

487. The general requirement for the liquid phase
A. Good solvent property of the compound
B. High thermal stability
C. Low vapour pressure
D. All of the above

488. The temperature programming may be carried in
A. Linear B. Natural or ballistic
C. Both A&B D. None of the above

489. The evaluation efficiency of a column is expressed by ....
A. Number of numerous plates in the column
B. Number of theoretical plates in the column
C. Both A&B
D. None of the above

490. The uncorrected or experimental retention volume chromatography is given by
A. VR =TRF2 B. VR=trfc
C. Both A&B D. None of the above

491. In which of the following method are liquid samples injected into in the column in chromatography
A. Gas – tight syringe
B. Micro syringe
C. Rotary sample valved
D. Solid injection syringe

492. Which of the following is the commonly used support material for the packed column an gas chromatography
A. Glass
B. Metal
C. Diatomaceous earth
D. Stainless steel

493. Which of the following is the advantages of straight packed column
A. It can be packed uniformly
B. it can be repacked easily
C. It can compact
D. None of the above

494. Sample injection port must be maintained at a temperature at which rapid vaporization occur but ....does not occur
A. Thermal degradation
B. thermal production
C. Both A&B
D. None of the above

495. Capillary column are open tubular column constructed from which of the following material
A. Glass B. Metal
C. Stainless steel D. Fused silica

496. Slow injection of large samples leads to band broadening and loss of ....
A. Dissolution B. Diffusion
C. Resolution D. None of the above

497. Which of the following is the disadvantages of hydrogen which can be used as carrier gas in gas chromatography
A. Dangerous to use
B. Expensive
C. Reduced sensitivity
D. High density

498. Chromatography is a physical method that is used to separate and analyse
A. Simple mixture B. Complex mixture
C. Viscous mixture D. Metal

499. In chromatography the stationary phase can be supported on a..
A. Solid or liquid B. Liquid or gas
C. Solid only D. Liquid only

500. Chromatography can not be used to ....
A. Purify substance B. Impurify substance
C. Both A&B

501. A large number of applications have been achieved by
A. GLC
B. Liquid chromatography
C. Gas chromatography
D. None of the above

502. The detection of steroid drug used by
A. Athletes in international sports
B. Administered to animal races
C. Both A&B
D. None of the above

503. Hazardous pollutants such as Carbone monoxide can be monitored by
A. Paper chromatography
B. Gas chromatography
C. Both A&B
D. None of the above

504. Analysis of volatile fatty acid produced by
A. Fungus B. Bacteria
C. Microbus D. Noe of the above

505. Most of the compound are non-volatile HPLC is used for
A. Separation B. Food analysis
C. Both A&B D. None of the above

506. It is known that inorganic compound are mostly are
A. Volatile B. Non volatile
C. Ointment D. None of the above

507. A number of metals chelates have been separated by
A. GC B. GLC
C. HPLC D. None of the above

508. Infrared spectrometry is a very
A Weak B. Strong
C. Powerful D. None of the above

509. Infrared spectrometry is usually carried out at
A. Pressure
B. Atmospheric pressure
C. Positive pressure
D. Negative pressure

510. A condensed sample gives the spectrum normally obtained by
A. Conformational IR
B. Conventional IR
C. Both A&B
D. None of the above

511. The pyrolysis of polymer followed by
A. Identification B. Separation
C. Assay D. None of the above

512. The pyrolysis of polymer separation by
A. Liquid -liquid chromatography
B. Gas chromatography
C. Paper chromatography
D. None of the above

513. The pyrolysis of polymer are identification by
A. IR spectroscopy
B. Spectrometry
C. Mass spectrometry
D. None of the above

514. Ion exchange was first reported by two British agricultural chemists by
A. 1960 B. 1850
C. 1260 D. 1976

515. Natural and synthetic inorganic cation exchange were used for
A. Harding hard work
B. Softening hard work
C. Both A&B
D. None of the above

516. Modern ion exchange resin were first used in
A. 1936 by Adams and holms
B. 1935 by Adams and holms
C. Both A&B
D. none of the above

517. Ion exchange may be defined as a
A. Irreversible reaction
B. Reversible reaction
C. Both A&B
D. None of the above

518. ion exchange separation is mainly carried out in
A. Column packed B. Packed
C. Both A&B D. None of the above

519. These exchanges are also called
A. Acidic ion exchange material
B. Alkali ion exchange material
C. Both A&B
D. None of the above

520. Cation exchange posses are
A. Positive B. negative
C. Both A&B D. None of the above

521. Anion exchanger have possess are -
A. Positive change B. Negative change
C. Both A&B D. None of the above

522. The selective desorption of the bound molecularis achieved by -
A. PH B. Ionic concentration
C. Both A&B D. None of the above

523. A cation exchanger is -
A. Low molecular weight
B. High molecular weight
C. Both A&B
D. None of the above

524.Anion exchanger are generally supplied in the form of -
A. Salts B. Organic compound
C. Solvent D. None of the above

525. The practical use of the dissolved material must be present also in the dissociated from it is to be retained by
A. Protein B. Resin
C. Amino acid D. Folic acid

526. An ion exchange resin may be characterised by
A. The number of ion active
B. The number of cation group
C. The group of alcohol group
D. None of the above

527. The exchange capacity of an anion exchange is determined by
A. Sodium chloride B. Sodium nitrate
C. Sodium sulphate D. Potassium

528. The technique are generally used to bring solution in contact with ion exchange resin
A. Batch method B. Column method
C. Both A&B D. Capillary method

529. The batch method is used for
A. Softening of water
B. Production of deionised
C. Both A&B
D. None of the above

530. Deionised water can be used in
A. Conduction experiment
B. Preparing solution silver nitrate
C. Biological studies
D. All of them

531. The resin to be used should have a
A. Small particle size
B. Large particle size
C. Medium particle size
D. None of the above

532. The ion exchange chromatography technique has played a unique role in the discovery of the elements in the
A. Actinide series
B. Citric acid
C. Potassium chloride
D. None of the above

533. Separation of sugars method was developed by
A. Kym and zill 1951 B. Kym and zill 1645
C. Both A&B D. None of the above

534. Ion exchange chromatography has been used to
A. Separation of complex mixture
B. Separation of granules
C. Both A&B
D. None of the above

535. Ion exchange chromatography has been used to separated the complex mixture 18 amino acid obtained by
A. Acid hydrolysis of protein
B. Acid hydrolysis of enzyme
C. Both A&B
D. None of the above

536. Carbonate is invariably present in solution of sodium hydroxide used for
A. Volumetric determination
B. Colorimetric derivation
C. Both A&B
D. None of the above

537. Ion exchange is especially used for treatment of
A. Low grade uranium deposits
B. High grade uranium deposits
C. Both A&B
D. None of the above

538. Capillary electro chromatography is packed with a

A. HPLC stationary phase

B. Gas chromatography

C. Both A&B

D. None of the above

539. The column packing can be

A. Porous B. Round

C. Both A&B D. None of the above

540. Micellar electro kinetic chromatography is a more versatile made the

A. Capillary zone electrophoresis

B. Tube zone electrophoresis

C. Both A&B

D. None of the above

541. Separation of sample component is archived by the

A. First or separator column

B. Second or separator column

C. Both A&B

D. None of the above

542. Ion chromatography has been used mainly for the

A. Separation of inorganic unions

B. Separation of organic

C. Separation of inorganic cation

D. None of the above

543. The pump used in ion chromatography is usually

A. Metallic B. Non metallic

C. Silver D. Gold

544. The injection valve must introduce a reproducible sample volume into the

A. Gas chromatography

B. Ion chromatography

C. Paper chromatography

D. None of the above

545. Analyte quantities can be determined

A. Semi automatically

B. Automatically

C. Both A&B

D. None of the above

546. Ion chromatography is first and for most a

A. Qualitative B. Quantitative

C. Identification D. Assay

547. The determination of carbohydrates is one of the most common application of IC with-

A. amperometry detection

B. Amplifier detection

C. Both A&B

D. None of the above

548. Amperometry is also used with more

A. Ions B. Traditional ions

C. Both A&B D. None of the above

549. The determination of amino acid was first widely used for

A. Paper chromatography

B. ion chromatography

C. Both A&B

D. None of the above

550. Mass spectrometer technique has been applied to

A. Oligosaccharides B. Sulfonic acid

C. Both A&B D. None of the above

551. Components which have small value of k have affinity for

A. Mobile phase B. Stationary phase

C. No phase D. Solution

552. Supercritical fluid chromatography recently developed technique that is hybrid between -

A. Liquid and solid

B. Gas and liquid

C. Semi solid volatile oil

D.None of the above

553. which the critical temperature is

A. 32.10 C B. 31.10 C

C. 40.10C D. None

554. Which the critical pressure is

A. 74.9 bar B. 72.10 bar

C. 72.9 bar D. none

555. The supercritical fluid is delivered to the column by a
A. Modified HPLC pump
B. HPLC pump
C. None modified HPLC pump
D. None of the above

556. The application of SFC include the analysis of mixture of
A. Triglycerides B. Hydrocarbon
C. Both A&B D. None of the above

557. HPLC has been a very popular technique for the analysis of
A. Polar non volatile B. Non polar
C. Efficacy D. None of the above

558. Various classes of polar compound have been analysed by
A. Packed B. Capillary column
C. Both A&B D. None of the above

559. Flash chromatography technique was developed by professor Clark still in the late of
A. 1980s B. 1970s
C. 1990s D. 1986s

560. The pressure of the solid usually cause the mixture to
A. Bump B. Pump
C. Bulk D. Taped

561. The separated components can be located bye
A. Thin layer chromatography
B. Smooth layer chromatography
C. Both A&B
D. None of the above

562. Dry column flash chromatography is one of the most valuable technique for
A. Separating compound in the synthetic laboratory
B. Unfortunately,
C. Both A&B
D. None of the above

563. The eluting solvent need to be a mixture of
A. Non polar B. Polar
C. Both A&B D. None of the above

564. The column can be protected by covering it with a piece of
A. Filter paper
B. Whatman filter paper
C. Simple paper
D. None of the above

565. The column is eluted using a series of hexane ethyl acetate mixture of increasing
A. Ability B. Molarity
C. Polarity D. Normality

566. If the simple components are coloured the progress of the separation can be
A. Monitored visually
B. Monitored capacity
C. Both A&B
D. none of the above

567. Chiral chromatography involves the separation of
A. Stereoisomer B. isomer
C. Both A&B D. None of the above

568. Chiral chromatography HPLC column are commercially available are
A. Normal B. Reversed phase
C. Both A&B D. none of the above

569. The diastereomers were subsequently separated in the normal or revers phase made of
A. Chromatography
B. Stereoisomer
C. Steroid
D. None of the above

570. Analytical chromatography system can be adapted to preparative separation which ....enantiomer can be collected
A. Impure B. Miscellaneous
C. Pure D. None of the above

571. Chiral stationary phases can uniquely contribute to studies of the -
A. Nature molecular recognition
B. Molecular recognition
C. Both A&B
D. None of the above

572. it has been show that chromatography parameter obtained by-
A. Chiral stationary phase
B. Chiral mobile phase
C. Chiral autonomic
D. None of the above

573. Chiral affinity by-
A. Protein B. Ovomucoid
C. Chymotrypsin D. All of then

574. Valuable information of drug protein intact ion can be deduced from
A. Chromatographic parameter
B. Chromatographic apparatus
C. Both A&B
D. None of the above

575. 2- aryl propionic acid the widely used for -
A. Anti –diabetic
B. Anti -cancer
C. Anti –inflammatory
D. Anti-hypertension

576. Chromatography parameter with shed light on the mechanism of chiral recognition by the
A. Enzyme B. Protein
C. Hormones D. None of the above

577. Efficient separation was obtained on the
A. Alpha 1-acid glycoprotein
B. beta 1-amino acid glycoprotein
C. Gamma 1- amino protein
D. None of the above

578. The a-chymotrypsin stationary phase was developed mainly by
A. Weiner B. Co-workers
C. Both A&B D. None of the above

579. The three hydroxyls on each glucose unit can be derivatized to from stands around the
A. Chiral sucrose B. Chiral glucose
C. Chiral mannitol D. Chiral benzene

580. The exterior surface is hydrophilic surrounded by
A. Hydroxyls B. Carbone
C. Hydrogen D. Hexane

581. The structure of these type of stationary phase is based is single stands of
A. Chiral selector B. Chiral projector
C. Both A&B D. None of the above

582. Displacement chromatography can be attributed to Tiselius who in
A. 1940 B. 1943
C. 1969 D. 1976

583. The technique was discovered by
A. Horvath B. wrath
C. Thomson D. None of the above

584. Displacement chromatography process can be broken down into the distinct phases
A. Loading B. Displacement
C. Regeneration D. all of them

585. Antigenic vaccine protein and antisense...... has also been demonstrated
A. Oligonucleotides B. Nucleosides
C. Nucleotide D. None of the above

586. Mobile phase is a ....
A. Polar B. non polar
C. Semi synthetic D. None of the above

587. The aqueous components of the mobile phase usually contain for
A. 0.1 to 0.5% formic or acetic acid
B. 0.1 to 0.5 % amino acid
C. 0.1 to 0.5 % folic acid
D. None of the above

588. Chromatography technique have been used in blood processing and purification since the ......
A. 1982s B. 1980s
C. 1994s D. 1992s

589. Blood plasma is the liquid components of ....
A. Water B. Blood
C. Virtus fluid D. None of the above

590. In whole blood red blood cell are suspended within the plasma ...
A. Leukocytes B. Platelets
C. Both A&B D. None of the above

591. The goal of extract specific material that are present in blood
A. Plasma B. Purification
C. Processing D. All of them

592. Albumin is a soluble protein with considerable structure stability
A. Highly water soluble
B. Highly water insoluble
C. Water
D. none of the above

593. The Cohn process incorporating cold ethanol /fractional has been used for

A. Globulin purification
B. Albumin purification
C. Both A&B
D. None of the above

594. When Cohn fractionation started being used in

A. 1946 B. 1962
C. 1972 D. 1999

595. Chromatographic method for separation started being adopted in the early

A. 1980 s B. 1999 s
C. 1992 s D. 1996 s

596. Fast protein liquid chromatography commonly used in

A. Biochemistry B. Enzymology
C. Both A&B D. None of the above

597. The column used in fast protein liquid chromatography are

A. Large tube (mm ID)
B. Medium tube
C. Small tube
D. None of the above

598. Reversed phase chromatography has a historical background in

A. 1980s B. 1970s
C. 1996s D. 1972s

599. Size exclusion chromatography is used for

A. Polymer characterization
B. Polymer
C. Polymer identification
D. None of the above

600. New forms of chromatography are developed in the .

A. 1930s and 1940s
B. 1950s and 1970s
C. 1999s and 1997s
D. 1960s and 1980s

601. Which of the following wavelength range is associated with uv spectroscopy?

A. 0.8 - 500um B. 400 - 100nm
C. 380 - 750nm D. 0.01 - 10 nm

602. Which of the following compounds does not absorb light in the uv/visible spectrum.

A. Aspirin B. Paracetamol
C. Chloralhydrate D. Phenobarbitone

603. What is the wavelength range for uv spectrum of light.

A. 400nm- 700nm B. 700nm to 1mm
C. 0.01nm to 400nm D. 10nm to 400nm

604. Beer Lambert's low given the relation between which of the following.

A. Reflected radiation and concentration
B. Scattered radiation and concentration
C. Energy absorption and concentration
D. Energy absorption and reflected radiation

605. Which of the following is not a limitation of beer lamberts low which give's the relation between absorption thickness and concentration.

A. concentration must be lower
B. Radiation must have higher bandwidth
C. Radiation source must be monochromatic
D. Dose not consider factors other then thickness and concentration that affect absorbance.

606. Beer's low states that the intensity of light decrease with respect to............

A. concentration B. Distance
C. composition D. volume

607. which of the following is not true about absorption spectroscopy?

A. It involves transmission.
B. scattering is kept minimum
C. Reflection is kept maximum
D. Intensity is an indication of concentration.

608. what is the unit of absorbance which can be derived from beer lamber's low?

A. Cm B. 1 unit
C. 2 unit D. No unit

609. In infrared spectroscopy which frequently range is known as the fingerprint region.

A. 400 -1400cm-1 B. 400 - 1400 cm-1
C. 900 - 600 cm-1 D. 600 - 250 cm -1

610. In which of the following ways absorption is related to transmitted?

A. Absorption is the lagarthm of transmittance.

B. Absorption is the reciprocal of transmittance.

C. Absorption is the negative

D. Absorption is a multiple of transmittance.

611. Lambert's low states that the intensity of light decrease with respect to...........

A. Concentration B. Distance

C. Composition D. Volum

612. Transmittance is given as T=P/P0. If P0 is the power incident on the sample what does. P represent?

A. Radiant power transmitted by the sample

B. Radiant powder absorbed by the sample

C. Sun of powers absorbed and scattered

D. Sun of power's transmitted and reflected

613. The represenration of beer lambert's low is given as A= abc if 'b'represent's distance c'represents concentration and A respresents absorption. What does a' represent?

A. Intensity B. Transmittance

C. Absorptivity D. Admittance

614. What is the unit of absorbance which can be derived from beer lambert's low?

A. L mol-1 B. L gm-1cm-1

C, Cm D. No unit

615. which of the following is not a source used in mid infrared spectrophotometer?

A. Nernst glower

B. High pressure mercury are lamp

C. Globar

D. Nichrome wire

616. which of the following is the wave number of near infrared spectrometer?

A. 400 - 200cm-1 B. 200 - 10 cm-1

C. 12500 - 4000cm -1

D. 50 - 1000 cm -1

617. which of the following options are correct in terms of wavelength for the different type of IR spectrometer.

A. Near IR: 0.8. -2.5mm

B. Mid IR: 0.8 - 2.5 mm

C. Far IR: 50-100mm

D. Mid IR: 50-100 mm

618. which of the following is not a composition of nemst glower or nernst filament?

A. Oxides of zirconium

B. Oxides of Barium

C. Oxides of thorium

D. Oxides of thorium

619. what is the composition of Globar rod which is used as a source in mid IR spectroscopy?

A. silicon carbide B. Silver chioride

C. Silicon dioxide D. Silver carbide

620. which of the following is not used as pyroelectric material used in pyroelectric transducer in infrared spectroscopy?

A. Triglycine sulphate

B. Deutrated triglycine sulphate

C. Some polymers

D. Tetraglycine sulphate

621. which of the following is the principle of golay cell which is used as a detector in IR Spectroscopy.

A. Expansion of gas upon heating

B. Increase in resistance due to increase in temp. And vice versa.

C. Decrease in resistance due to increase in temperature.

D. Temperature difference gives rise to a potential difference in the material

622. what is the name of this solid sample treatment technique?

A. pressed pellet B. Mull technique

C. Solid films D. solid run in solution

623. spectroscopy deals with interaction of electromagnetic radiation with matter. What is the speed of this radiation in vacuum in m/s?

A. 6×10 B. 5×10

C. 7×10 D. 3×10

624. which type of Qwantwm transition take place in ultra violet and visible spectroscopy?

A. Rotation of molecules

B. Nuclear

C. Bonding electrons

D. spin of nuclei in magnetic field

625. which of the following is not a property or parameter of electromagnetic radiation?

A. wavelength B. voltage
C. wave number D. Amplitude

626. Which of the following is not a type of spectroscopy?

A. Gammaray
B. XRay
C. Nuclear magnetic resononce
D. sound

627. Electromagnetic radiation can travel through vacuum.

A. true B. High
C. false D. low

628. which of the following is false about wavelengths of electromagnetic radiation?

A. Radiation with short wavelength have high energies.
B. radiation with long wavelengths have low energies
C. Energy does not depend on wavelength
D. Energy depends on wavelength

629. which of the following is the wavelength of microwave radiation.

A. 10 -780 nm B. 0.78 - 30um
C. 0.6 - 10 m D. 0.75-3.75nm

630. How is wave number of electromagnetic radiation related to wavelength?

A. It is the reciprocal of wavelength
B. It is directly proportional to wavelength
C. It is not related to wavelength
D. it is equal to wavelength

631. Velocity of electromagnetic radiation is more in vacum than in any medium.

A. True B. high
C. False D. low

632. what is the correct seque for the processes occurring in a mass spectrometer?

A. Lonization vaporization deflection acceleration
B. Vaporization acceleration ionization
C. Vaporization ionization acceleration deflection
D. Lonization vaporization acceleration deflection.

633. which compound would be expected to show intense IR absorption at 2250 cm-1

A. CH3 CH2 CH2 CO2H
B. (CH3)2 CHCN
C. CH3 CH2 CH2 CONH2
D. (CH3)2 CHCH2 OH

634. which compound gives two distinct peoks in it's proton NMR

A. C6H6 B. CH3OCH3
C. C6H5OH D. CH2 CH4 OH

635. which of the following wavelength range is associated with uv spectroscopy.

A. 0.8 - 500um B. 400 - 100nm
C. 380 - 750nm D. 0.01- 10nm

636. which of the following compounds does not absorb light in the uv/ visible spectrum.

A. Aspirin B. paracetmol
C. Chloral hydrate D. Phenobarbitone

637. In which region of the electromagnetic spectrum does an Absorption at 800nm come.

A. visible B. vacuum - uv
C. Infrared D. Near - uv

638. According to the beer Lambert low on which of the following does absorbance not depend.

A. Distance that the light has travelled throught the sample.
B. solution concentration
C. Extinction coefficient of the sample.
D. Colour of the solution.

639. Which of the following statements is correct.

A. Infrared radiation has a lower wave number than visible.
B. Microwave radiation possesses more energy than infrared radiation.
C. Uv radiation a longer wavelength than infrared radiation.
D. IR radiation has a shorter wavelength than visible light.

640. In uv spectrophotometer sample cell is made up of.

A. Glass B. Quartsz
C. Both D. None

641. In a uv visible spectrophotometer the path length is normally.
A. 10mm B. 10cm
C. 10um D. 100nm

642. Which of the following is not true about fourier transform infrared spectrophotometer.
A. It is of non dispersive type.
B. It is useful ulnere repetitive analysis is required
C. size has been reduced over the years
D. Size has increased over the years.

643. What is the main reason for other types of thermal detectors are not being used in FTIR spectrophotometer?
A. Less accuracy B. Less precision
C. Slower response D. Less sensitivity

644. Which of the following is the reference that is generally used in FTIR interometer?
A. Air B. Nacl solution
C. Alcohal D. Base solution

645. In michelson's interometer the frequency of the detector out put can be determined by translating the............ Of movable mirror and the......... Of monochromatic radiation.
A. Velocity, Wavelength
B. Thickness, intensity
C. Length, velocity
D. Angle, Intensity

646. why is the computer necessary in fourier transform spectrometer?
A. To display the detector out put
B. To process the detector output
C. To determine the amplitude.
D. To determine the frequency

647. In NMR spectrophotometer the homogenous magnetic field varied continuously by.
A. Magnet B. Rf - transmitter
C. Sweep generator D. Rf - receiver

648. Deuterated solvent in an NMR sample is used to.
A. Stabilizer the magnetic field
B. set the chemical shift reference
C. Obtain good field homogeneity across the sample
D. Both {a} and {c}

649. wave number is number of wave per
A. Millimeter B. Inch
C. Centimeter D. Meter

650. Which of the following is the fundamental NMR equation.
A. Y=2π u/h1 B. Wo= YHo
C. V=YHO/2π D. V =YHo/2π

651. Which type of energy transition is shown by IR Spectroscopy.
A. Rotational B. Bond - breaking
C. Vibration D. Electronic

652. As wave no. Increases wave energy-
A. Decreases B. Remains
C. Increase D. No relation

653. Which of the following is bending vibration.
A. Scissoring B. Rocking
C. Wagging D. all of these

654. when a fundamental vibration couples with an overtone or combination band the coupled vibration is called.
A. Differential Band
B. Combination Bond
C. Dipole moment
D. Fermi Resonance

655. Fermi resonance is often observed with.
A. Carbonyl Compounds
B. I hydrocorban Compounds
C. Amino Compounds
D. Nitro Compounds

656. In IR - Spectroscopy sample can be prepared by using.
A. Sodium chloride (Nacl)
B. Nijal mull
C. Potassium Bromide
D. All of these

657. 2250 cm-1 is base value for the absorption What of bands (IR-spectroscopy)
A. O -H B. C - H
C. N - H D. C= N

658. what is the base value for absorption of c=o bond (in IR Spectroscopy)
A. 1100 cm-1 B. 1650 cm-1
C. 1715 cm-1 D. 2150cm-1

659. Interfere gram is essentially a plot of intensity versus.

A. Time B. Frequency

C. Both of these D. None of these

660. Which of the following main component of mass spectroscopy deal with resolving the ions into their characteristics mass components according to their mass to charge ratio?

A. Ion source B. Detector system

C. Analyzer D. Analyzer tube

661. what are the main criterial on which mass spectrometer used for?

A. Composition in sample

B. Relative mass of atoms

C. Concentration of elements in the sample

D. Properties of sample

662. Which species of the following is used to bombard with the sample for which mass spectroscopy has been performad?

A. Alpha particles B. Electrons

C. Neutrons D. Protons

663. Separation of ions in mass spectrometer take place on the basic of which of the following.

A. Mass

B. Charge

C. Molecular weights

D. Mass to charge ratio

664. Which type of ionic species are allowed to pass through the slit and reach the collecting plate?

A. Negative ions of all masses

B. Positives ions of the specific mass

C. Negative ion of the specific mass

D. Positives ions of all masses.

665. Which of the following statements is not true about mass spectometry?

A. Impurities of masses different from the one being analysed interferes with the result.

B. It has great sensitivity.

C. It is suitable for data storage.

D. It is suitable for library retrieval.

666. In mass spectrometer the ion currents are measured using which of the following?

A. Scintillation counter

B. Electrometer tube

C. Ion counter

D. Electric fields

667. The procedure for mass spectroscopy starts with which of the following processes?

A. The sample is bombarded by electron beam

B. The ions are separated by passing them into electric.

C. The sample is converted into gaseous state

D. The ion are detected

668. In mass spectrometer the ions are sorted out in which of the following ways?

A. By accelerating them through electric field B. By accelerating them through magnetic field

C. By accelerating them through electric and magnetic filed

D. By applying a high voltage

669. Which of the following detectors are used in mass spectroscopy.

A. photomultiplier tube

B. Photo tube

C. Photo voltanic cell

D. Thermopille

670. How is the wavelength controlled in an FTIR Spectrometer

A. By a michelson interferometer

B. By a computer

C. By a laser

D. By calibration with a standard sample

671. what type of technique is FTIR spectroscopy?

A. A dispensine technique

B. An absorbance technique

C. An emission technique

D. A uv vistechniqe

672. What does the spectrum of nitrogen (N2) look like?

A. The same as that of air

B. It has only p-and r-branches

C. The same as that of corbon monoxide

D. It does not have one

673. What are the selection rules for FTIR absorption?

A. absorprion only occurs for symmetrical molecules

B. Absorption only occurs with dipole change.

C. Abdorption requires an add vibration quantum number

D. Absorption requires promotion to a new quantum level

674. What occurs when the moving mirror in an FTUR spectrometer is the same distance from the beamsplitter as the static mirror.

A. Constructive intefrence

B. Radio interference

C. Destructive inter ference

D. The spectrum is measured

675. Which infred technique can measure two spectra at once.

A. FTIR Spectroscopy

B. Dispensive infrared Spectroscopy

C. FTIR ATR Spectroscopy

D. FTIR microscopy.

676. Which spectrometer is the more complicated dispersive or FTIR.

A. diapersive B. Neither

C. FTIR D. FTIR Spectroscopy

677. In what Regina of the spectrum does infrared radiation occur?

A. At the low energy

B. Between the visible and uv regions.

C. Between the visible and microwave region

D. Between the visible and x-ray region's

678. What occurs when a molecule absorbs infrared radiation.

A. It warms up B. It fliearound

C. It spins faster D. It vibrates faster

679. Bolometer a type of detector is also known as.......

A. Resistance temperature detector

B. Thermistor

C. Thermocouple

D. Golay cell

680. Which of the following is not a technique for preparing solid samples in IR spectroscopy?

A. Solid run in solution

B. Mull technique

C. Solid films

D. Thin films

681. Which of the following is not used as pyroelectric material used in pyroelectric transducers in infrared Spectroscopy.

A. Triglycine sulphate

B. Deutrated Triglycine sulphate

C. Somepolymers

D. Tetraglycine sulphate

682. Ultraviolet light is used in.

A. low enforcement

B. Rador

C. Nuclear medicine

D. Fluorese scence microscopy

683. Corn smut is particularly.

A. Useful B. meaningful

C. harmful D. damaging

684. Fluoresence microscopy is an excellent for materials made of.

A. Chlorine B. Fluorine

C. Fluoresce D. Copper

685. Cygnus loop is an example of.

A. gamma rays B. visible spectrum

C. x-rays D. uv rays

686. Lithography uses.

A. ultraviolet B. x-rays

C. gamma D. visible rays

687. Vibration spectroscopy involves the transition filling in the spectral range of.

A. 100-1000cm-1 B. 300-3000cm-1

C. 400-4000cm-1 D. 500-5000cm-1

688. Which of the region of IR spectra appears between (1400- 600) cm-1

A. Functional groupregion

B. Fingerprint region

C. Low - frequency region

D. None of the mentioned

689. select the correct statement from the following option.

A. IR spectra can identify the unknown material's

B. It can determine the amount of component's in a mixture

C. It can also determine the quality of a sample.

D. All of the mentioned

690. Which of the following molecule have infrared active vibration

A. NO B. H_2

C. CH_4 D. All of the mentioned

691. which of the following can't show a vibrational absorption spectrum?

A. OCS B. H_2O

C. CO_2 D. $CH_2=CH_2$

692. Which of the following is not a type of bending molecular vibration?

A. Twisting B. Stretching

C. Wagging D. Rocking

693. What is the absorption frequency (cm-1) of - C=N functional group.

A. 3610- 3640 B. 1690-1769

C. 1180-1360 D. 2850-2960

694. presence of a functional group in a compound can be established by using.

A. Chromatograph

B. IR Spectroscopy

C. mass spectrometer

D. x-ray diffraction

695. Select the incorrect option from the following option.

A. IR spectroscopy helps in determination of purity.

B. IR spectroscopy helps in determination of force constant from vibrational spectrum.

C. IR spectroscopy helps in identifying an unknown an unknown compound

D. None of the mentioned

696. IR spectroscopy helps in detecting the presence of hydrogen bonding.

A. high contiontration

B. true

C. low contiontration

D. false

697. All bodies behave as source of.......

A. Electromagnetic radiation

B. IR radiation

C. Uv radiation

D. None of the mentioned

698. which of the following represent a spectrum of frequency emission?

A. Absorption spectra

B. Emission spectra

C. Em spectra

D. None of the mentioned

699. spectrography doesn't computer the energy of frequency spectrum.

A. True B. False

C. low D. high

700. Which of the following source is used for exciting bodies electrically?

A. DC are B. AC arc

C. Spark D. All of the mentioned

701. which of the following is more used core in spectrometer?

A. Graphite B. Aluminium

C. Carbon D. Fullerie

702. Which of the following represent emission specta?

A. Continuous spectra

B. Line spectra

C. Band spectra

D. all of the mentioned

703. Every spectrograph requires dispersion.

A. true B. false

C. high D. low

704. Dispersion of radiation is carrid out by........

A. Prism

B. Grating

C. Diamand

D. Both prism and grating

705. IR absorption patten in absorption spectrograph is known as........

A. Finger print B. Absorption

C. signature D. graph

706. identify the type of instrument calibration error (s) shown in this graph.

A. Hysteresis error
B. Linearity error
C. Both zero and span error
D. Zero error

707. Identify the type of instrument calibration error.

A. Span error B. Zero error
C. Hysteresis error D. Linearity error

708. When calibrating an instrument you may detect the presence of hysteresis error by.

A. Comparing the instrument against a knoun standard that is free from any hysteresis.
B. Comparing accuracy at certain points both going up and down the calibration scale.
C. Deadband
D. Both a and c

709. Which of the following adjustment is usually adjusted first in an instrument rewiring calibrat

A. Deadband B. Span
C. Hystersis D. Linearity

710. A pressure transmitter has a calibrated measurement range of 200 to 300 PSIG and an out put range of 4-20 MA what is the expected out if the input pressure medication is 235 PSIG?

A. 1.6MA B. 5.6MA
C. 16.5MA D. 12.5MA

711. A PH transmitter has a calibrated range of 5to 9 ph with a 4 -20 MA out put what is the phmeasurement if the transmitter's out put is equal to 17.3 MA?

A. 4.156 PH B. 6.599 PH
C. 8.325 PH D. 8.460 PH

712. The purpose of documenting an As found calibration in addition to documenting the As left calibration for an instrument is to.

A. Ensure perfect accuracy
B. Help other's locate the instrument
C. Eliminator instrument hysteresis
D. Measure calibration drift.

713. A smart transmitter is one that.

A. communicate using foundation fieldbus
B. Has a micro processor built inside
C. Transmiter without inbuilt sensor
D. none of these

714. Which one of the following techniques can be used for the detection chromotograph?

A. UV absorbance or refracting index measurement.
B. Increase in tempratus
C. Ionization in flame
D. Tharmal conductivity

715. Considering high performance liquid chromatography which one of the following statemeis FALSE.

A. HPLC B. TLC
C. Columns longer than 50 meters have been used here to increase the efficiency of separation
D. none of these

716. According to beer's low for a colored solution which one of the following statements is false.

A. The present transmission is not directly proportioal to the concentration
B. The absorbance is directly proportional to the concentration.
C. The absorbance does not change when the cell path length increase.
D. both a and c

717 Deutorium and tungsten lamps are used as a light source in one of the following techniques.

A. Nuclear magnetic resonance spetrophotometers
B. X-rays diffractometers
C. Gas chromatograph
D. uv / visival spectrophotometer's

718. Which one of the following arrangements for the sequence of the main components of a UV/ visible spectrophotometer is correct.

A. Light source-monochromator-sample cell - Detector-Readout
B. light source-sample cell-detector - monochoromator- readout.
C. Light source-detector-sample cell - monochomater - readout
D. none of these

719. Which one of the following radiation has the longer wavelength.

A. infra red B. visible

C. x-ray D. Uvtraviolet

720. The energy associated with infra red is enough to make.

A. Electronic transitions

B. vibration and ratatinal transitians

C. A full separation of the electron in the outer shell

D. X-rays fluorescence

721. The moisture in an organic substance is determined by.

A. Potentiometric titration

B. x-ray fluorescence

C. x-ray absorption

D. karl fisher titration

722. The technique used used to identify a functional group in an organic molecule is

A. Coulometry

B. X-ray fluorescence

C. Infrared spectrometer

D. Conductometry

723. One part per million is the same as

A. 1ug /g B. 1mg /kg

C. 1mg /mg D. all of the above

724. Narrow line spectra are emitted by

A. hot solids

B. Excited poyatomic molecules

C. Molecule in the ground molecular state

D. Excited atoms

725. What are the demonstration of the molar absorptivity in the beer'slow expectation?

A. Mol per liter

B. Gram permol

C. Liters per mol. Centimeter

D. Microgram per square centimeter

726. The region of the electromagnetic spectrum in wwhich the highest energy photons are observed is the.

A. Uv B. Microwave

C. Infrared D. X-ray

727. Grating is a device used in the spectrophotometer to function as.

A. A light source

B. A detector

C. A monochromator

D. A nibulizer

728. An important advantage of a double -beam spectrometer over a single - beam specphotometer is that.

A. It permits cancelation of slow variation of the source powder.

B. micowave

C. infared

D. none of these

729. Helium rather than argon after is used as the carrier gas in GLC when TCD isused as the detector becouse

A. He has a higher ionization potential

B. He is more inert

C. He has stable isotopes which separate and cause a change in column behavior

D. He has a higher thermal conductivity.

730. Reversed phase HPLC is the technique in which.

A. Statioanary phase is solid and mobile phase is liquid

B. The stationary phase is made of very fine particles

C. The stationary phase or is non polar and the mobile phase isrelatively polar

D. None of these

731. How should the concentration of a colorless sample be determined.

A. using a UV spectrophotometer

B. Using a VIS spectrophotometer

C. Either a UV or VIS spectrophotometer

D. Using an indicator solutionand ph paper

732. In mass spectrometry the atomic mass unit amuis defined as

A. 1/2 of the mass of one neutral c-12 atom

B. The mass of any individual atom expressed in grams

C. The mass of a deuterium atom

D. The mass of male of hydrogen atoms expressed in daltons.

733. What happens to the molecules in the ion source of the mass spectrometer

A. They are ionized and split in fragments
B. They lose hydrogen atoms only
C. They are ionized only
D. They are excited and emit radiation at vsarious wavegths

734. How many equivalent NMR protons are in butonoic acid?

A. 8 B. 2
C. 6 D. 4

735. The wave number of a transition is 2000 cm-1 in what part of the electromagnetic spectrum does this come?

A. infrared B. Radiowave
C. Microwave D. Uv - visible

736. The frequency of a transition is 5.4×10 HZ what are is the corresponding wavelength?

A. 5.6×10-6m B. 560nm
C. 5.6×10-8m D. 180 000cm

737. According to the beer lamber low on which of the following does absorbance not depend?

A. Extinction coefficient of the sample
B. Colour of the solution
C. sample solution
D. solution concentrate

738. The dichromate ion absorbs light of wavelength close to 500 nm based on this information what can you concluded?

A. solution of the dichromate ion arecolorless.
B. The dichromate ion absorb within the visible region
C. The dichromate ion absorb in the UV region
D. The dichromate ion absorb outside the visible region

739. Which of following statemnt is correct?

A. solution concentration
B. Infrared radiation has shorter
C. infrared radiayion
D. microwave radiation

740. Which statement is correct?

A. wavelength is directly proportional to energy
B. Wavenumber is directly proportional to wavelength
C. wavelengh is directly proportional of frequency.
D. wavenumber is directly proportional to energy

741. A shift to lower Wavenumber for an absorption in a spectrum corresponds to-

A. A lose of intensity
B. A shift to lower wavelength
C. A shift to higher energy
D. A shift to lower frequency

742. The UV /VIS spectroscopy

A. Generates colored spectrum
B. can determine the concetratio
C. can be used to make light visible
D. can determine to sample

743. The unit an spectrometer on the x-axis is

A. Meter B. Centimeter
C. Per centimeter D. all of these

744. The unit of NMR spectrum on the x-axis is

A. Herts B. Cm-1
C. PPM D. Cm-3

745. In a mass spectrometry

A. The analyzed substance remains intact
B. Large quantities
C. the analyzed substance is ionized
D. large quantity of the substances is required.

746. A mass spectrometry delivers the evidence about.

A. The color of a substance
B. The reactivity of a substance
C. The molecular mass of a substance
D. None of these

747. Following group has the IR range of 2100-2200 cm-1

A. C=C - Stretching B. C-C- Stretching
C. C=C, -Stretching D. C=O-Stretching

748. Homoannular diene base valve.

A. 2.15nm B. 235nm
C. 253nm D. 245nm

749. K band is seen is which of the flowing transition.

A. π -π* B. n - π*

C. 2/π D. π = 2/27

750. Electron donating group cause's.

A. Increse Deshiclding

B. Increase shielding

C. Decrease shielding

D. decrease shielding

751. Refarence standard of NMR in aqucous solvents.

A. Tetra methyl silane

B. Trimethylsilane

C. a and b

D. Trimethylsilyl pranesulphonic acids.

752. IR radiation source

A. Deuterium discharge lamp

B. Mercury are lamp.

C. Incandescent lamp

D. none

753. following are UV -ViS and IR detectors respectively.

A. Bolometer and PMT

B. PMT and bolometry

C. Thermalconductivity and PMT

D. None

754. The unit's of coupling constant

A. Hertz B. Angstroms

C. PPM D. All the above

755. Nujol is a........

A. Vegetable B. Mineral oil

C. Fixed oil D. Edible oil

756. What is the condition for mclafferty raarragement of to occur.

A. Presence of hydrogen

B. Presence of a s. drogen

C. presence of unsturation

D. presence of beta hydrogen

757. The beer Lambert low given a linear correlation with positive grandient b/w.

A. molar extinction coefficient and concentration

B. Absorbance and concentration

C. wavelength and absorbance

D. Molar extinction coefficient and absorbance.

758. Which of the following is not a absorption spectroscopy

A. Pand S B. P and Q

C. Q and R D. Qand S

759. The base value of unsaturated ketone is taken as

A. 235 B. 215

C. 280 D. 250

760. Thickness of the sample medium in UV - visible spectroscopy is related to.

A. Beer's low

B. Lambert's low

C. Beer's Lambert's low

D. None

761. sigma* and n-sigma*electronic transition are possible in.

A. Benzene B. Toluene

C. Bromine D. Naphthalene

762. Absoption bound originator's due ton -π transition of a single chromophoric group is.

A. R-bond B. k - bond

C. B - bond D. E - bond

763. Electrum withdrawing group cause.

A. Increase Deshieldiding

B. Increase shielding

C. decrease shielding

D. Decrease

764. The IR absorption occurs when.

A. Vibration frequency equal to IR frequency.

B. Processional frequency equal to IR frequency.

C. vibration equal's to processional frequency.

D. None of the above.

765. minimum energy required for the fragmentation to occur in mass spectroscopy

A. 70 Kev B. 70Mev

C. 70Ev D. 70Mev

766. If the absorption of electromagnetic radiation by matter result in the emission of radiation of the same or large wavelengh for a long or short time.

A. Lyminescence
B. Fluorescence
C. Phosphorescence
D. Spontoanrous

767. if the absorption of electromegnetic radiation by matter result in the same or longer wavelengths for a short time.

A. Luminescence
B. Fluorescence
C. Phosphorescence
D. Spontaneus emission

768. Prompt emission of x-ray by an atom ionized by a higher energy x-ray is a type of which of the following phenomena?

A. Luminescence
B. Fluorescence
C. Phosphoreson
D. Spontaneous emission

769. The measurement of intensity of Fluorescence x-rays provide a simple and........ Way to...... Anlydis.

A. Destructive guantative
B. Non - Destructive quantative
C. Destructive qualitative
D. Non - destructive qualitative

770. The energy of emitted x-ray depends upon the....... Of the atom and their intensity depends upon the.

A. Atomic number amount of sample
B. Mass number amount of same
C. Mass number concentration or atoms
D. Atomic number concentration of atom's

771. The problem of spectral interference is not severe in x-ray spectroscopy.

A. True B. high
C. low D. false

772. In x-ray Fluorescence spectrometer the relationship between the excitation intensity and the intensity of Fluorescence does not depend on which of the following.

A. Spectrum of the incident radiation
B. Incident engle
C. Moleculer wight
D. molecular weight

773. Which of the following is the principle of flame Emission photo meter's

A. Radiation is absorbed by non- excited atomes in vapour state and are excited to higher state.
B. Medium absorbs radiation and transmitted radiation is measured
C. Colour and wavelength of the flame is measured.
D. Only wavelength of the flame is measured.

774. In flame emission photo meters the measurement of..... Is used for qualitative analysis

A. Colour B. Intensity
C. Velocity D. Frequency

775. In flame emission photo meter the measurement of........ Is used for quantitative analysis.

A. colour B. colour
C. velocity D. frequency

776. Which of the following is not an advantage of lamiar flow burner used in flame photometry?

A. Noiseless
B. Efficient atomization of sample
C. Stable flame for analysis
D. Sample containing two or none solvents can be buaned efficienty

777. Laminar flow burner used in flamephotometer's is also known as.....

A. Turbulent burner
B. Tatol consumption burner
C. premix burner
D. Nozzle mix burner

778. which of the following is the advantage of prism monochromator's

A. Dispersion is non -overlapping
B. Dispersion is over
C. Dispersion occurs in non- linear manner
D. Dispersion occurs. In a linear

779. which of the following is the advantage of grating monochromator?

A. Dispersion is non -/overlapping
B. Dispersion occurs in non - linear mannar.
C. Dispersion is overlapping
D. Dispersion occurs in a linear manner.

780. Which of the following is not a detector used in flame emission photometer's.

A. Photonic cell
B. Phoyovoltaic cell
C. Photoemissive tube
D. Chromatogram

781. Which of the following is not an application of flame emission photometer's.

A. Analysis of biological fluids
B. Determination of sodium potassium in soil
C. Determination of metals such as mn cu
D. Analysis of complex mixture

782. The flame emission Photometer's identify the unmarked component.

A. Filter B. Atomiser
C. Pressure regulator
D. Burner

783. The glass tube of photo emissive tube identify the part which is indicate.

A. Anade B. Grid
C. Cathode D. Dynode

784. Which of the following is not an advantage of a photovoltaic cell which is used as a detector in flame emission photometer's

A. portable
B. No external supply
C. Robust in construction
D. Does not show fatigue

785. The main advantage of Fluorescence over UV - VIS spectrophotometer is -

A. It's sensitivity
B. It's compatibility with separation techniques
C. It's compatibility with most analytes
D. None of the above

786. Select the true statement about Fluorescence spectroscopy of molecules in the UV -visible region.

A. Emission usually occurs at energies that are greater than the energies of excitation.
B. Emission usually occurs at energies that are less than the energies of excitation
C. a and b
D. None of the above is accurate.

787. Accuracy is defined as-

A. The closeness of a measured value to the real value
B. The measure of how often an experimental value can repeated
C. both a and b
D. None of these

788. Which of the following is an application of molecular spectroscopy.

A. Structure investigation
B. Study of energetically reaction
C. Basis of understanding of color's
D. All of the mentioned.

789. Reversed phase HPLC is the technique in which.

A. Stationary phase is solid and mobile phase is liquid.
B. The stationary phase is non polar and the mobile phase is relatively
C. The stationary phase is made of very fine particales
D. The stationary phase has been silinized withdimethyldichlorosilane.

790. Uv spectroscopy is the best example for-

A. Absorption spectroscopy
B. Absorption and Emission
C. Emission spectroscopy
D. None of the above

791. flamphotometerry fluorimetry are examples for.

A. Emission Spectroscopy
B. Absorption Spectroscopy
C. Molecular spectroscopy
D. Molecular Spectromiter

792. The study of Absorption of visible radiation whose wavelength ranger's from 400nm - 800nm is know as.

A. Uv Spectroscopy
B. Visible spectroscopy
C. IR Spectroscopy
D. NMR Spectroscopy

793. In visible spectroscopy if the colour of the solution is red them which colour filter is preferred.

A. Violet B. Orange
C. Yellow D. Green

794. The detectors used in uv/visible spectrophotometers are called as -
A. Photometric detectors
B. Photo voltaic cell
C. Photo emissive cell's
D. Photo multiplier tubes

795. In spectrophotometers the wavelength accuracy is given as.
A. +, - 0.01nm B. +, -10nm
C. +, -1nm D. +, - 0.1nm

796. A system is said to obey Beer's low when a plot of concentration vs absorbance gives a -
A. Curved line
B. Straight light
C. Perpendicularline
D. Horizontal line

797. Factors which are responsible for the deviation of Bee's low are -
A. Assciation
B. Disciation
C. Faculty development of colour
D. All of the above

798. Uv Spectroscopy the absorption of uvradiation ranges from.
A. 800 - 1000nm B. 200- 400nm
C. 400 - 600nm D. 600 - 800nm

799. Anti-hypertensive to be avoids during pregnancy :
A. Diuretics B. Ace inhibiter
C. Nonreactive D. All of these

800. Beer's low is related to.
A. Concentration B. Both a and b
C. Path length D. None of the above

801. Lamber's low is related to
A. Concentration B. Both a and b
C. path length D. None of the above

802. The sample cell in a UV spectrophotometers is made up of.
A. Colour corrected glass
B. polystyrene
C. Quartz
D. Polymers

803. In a flourimeter is primary filter is used to
A. Absorb uv and transmit visible Radiation
B. Transmit uv and absorb visible radiation
C. Transmit uv and absorb visible radiation
D. None of the above

804. The source of light in flouri meter is
A. Tungsten lame
B. Mercury vapour lamp
C. Corbon are
D. Hydrogen discharge lamp.

805. The sample cell commonly used in flourimeter is made up of.
A. Quartz B. Fused silica
C. Polystyrene D. Glass

806. At higher tempture flourescence intensity.
A. Increases B. Decreases
C. Is un altered D. None of the above

807. Flame phetometry involves excitation of
A. Lons B. Neutral atoms
C. Solid partides D. Neutral Toms

808. The grating in uv spectrophotometers is made up of
A. Glass B. Polystyrene
C. Quartz D. potassium bromide

809. In uv spectra of a pair of qeometrical isomers when compared to the Cis isomer. Trans isomer.
A. Absorbs at lower wavelength
B. Has no. Absopption
C. Absorbs a higher wavelength
D. None of the above

810. Saturated aliphatic hydrocarbons given uv peak in the following region.
A. Above 400nm B. 200 - 300nm
C. 300 - 400nm D. less then 200nm

811. Non aqueous titration equation can be expressed by.
A. Arrhenius
B. Beer's low
C. Lewis concept
D. Lowery Bronsted theory

812. In IR Spectroscopy a region in which the number of bending and is usually more than the number of stretching vibration is called as

A. Absorption region
B. Aromatic region
C. Functional group region
D. finger print region

813. The device used in spectrophotometet to disperse the polychromatic light constituent wave length.

A. Collimating device
B. Monochromator
C. Facussing ans
D. All the above

814. The important dispersion devices used in Spectrophotometers are.

A. Prism B. Gratinges
C. Lences D. Both a and b

815. The sample containers in spectrophotometers or colorimeters are called.

A. Test tabes B. Capillary tubes
C. Cuvettes D. None of the above

816. Cuvettes meant for uv region are mode of.

A. Glass B. Silica
C. Quartz D. Both a and b

817. Infrared gas cell are made up of

A. Glass B. Silica
C. Quarts D. Both a and c

818. In uv / visible Spectrophotometers the main detectors that are used are-

A. photocells
B. Photomultiplier tubes
C. phototubes
D. all of the above

819. In flame photometry the absorbance is due to

A. Color of the solution
B. Luminous flame
C. The colour imparted to the non luminaus by the elements
D. Absorption spectrum.

820. The forIR detector are.

A. Themocouples B. phototubes
C. Golay cells D. all of the above

821. The important application of spectrometry are -

A. Qualitative analysis
B. Quantative analysis
C. Enzume assay
D. All of the above

822. Wave number is measured in

A. Cm B. nm
C. Cm-1 D. fresnd

823. The wave number and energy of EMR are.

A. Directtly prortional
B. Inversely propartional
C. Not related
D. None of the above

824. The sample cell in a UV spectrophotometer is made up of

A. Colour corrected glass
B. Polystyrene
C. Quartz
D. Polymers

825. The ratio of electronic energy tovibrational energy in a molecule is.

A. 1:100 B. 1:10
C. 10:1 D. 100:1

826. π - π* triplet transition result's in

A. UV absorption B. Phosphorescence
C. Flourescence D. Excitation

827. π -π* single transition result in

A. Uv absorption
B. Exitation
C. phosphorescence
D. Flourescence

828. In a flourimeter the primary filter is used to

A. Absorb UV and transmit visible radiation
B. Transmit UV and absorb visible
C. Transmit UV and visible readiation
D. None of the above

829. In a flourimeter the secondary filter is used to -

A. AbsorbUV and transmit visible raditio

B. Transmit UV and absorb visible

C. Transmit UV and visible radiation

D. None of the above.

830. In most of the flourimeter the angle between the incident beam and emission beam is

A. 45° B. 135°

C. 90° D. 180°

831. The source of light in a flourimeter is

A. Tungsten lamp

B. Mercury vapour lamp

C. Carbon are

D. Hydrogen discharge lamp.

832. The sample cell commonly used in a flourimeter is made up of

A. Quartz B. Fused silica

C. polystyrene D. Glass

833. At higher temperature Flourescence intensity

A. Increases B. Decreases

C. Is unaltered D. None of the above

834. If viscosity of a solution is increased, fluoresence intensity

A. increases B. is unalted

C. Decreases D. None

835. The presence of the following group increases Flourescence intensity.

A. Amino group B. Nitro group

C. Both a and b D. None of the above

836. The presence of the following group decreased the Flourescence intensity.

A. Amino group B. Carboxylic group

C. both a and b D. None of the above

837. The main advantage of Fluorescence over UV-VIS Spectroscopy is

A. Its Sensitivity

B. It's compatibility with separation

C. It's compatibility with most analytes

D. All of the above

838. Select the true statement about Flourescence spectroscopy of molecules inthe UVvisible regiin

A. Emission usually occurs at energy that are greater than the energies of excitat.

B. Emission usually occurs at energies of exicitationh

C. bith a and b

D. none of these

839. How manyequivalent NMR protons are in butanoic acid?

A. 8 B. 2

C. 6 D. 4

840. The wave number of a transition is 2000 cm-1 in what part of the electromagnetic spectrum does this come.

A. IR B. Microwave

C. Radiowave D. Ultraviolet

841. In a prism monochromtor the principle is

A. Reflection B. Scattering

C. Re - inforcent D. Dispersion

842. In an interference filter the wavelength of the light which is transmitted depends.

A. Incident light - wavelength

B. Dielectric constant of the medium used

C. Order of light

D. both b and c

843. In a spectrophotometric titration then % transmission.

A. Increases

B. Decrerease

C. No change

D. Can not be predicted.

844. In a spectrophotometeric titration volume of titrant is plotted against.

A. % transmission B. Either a or b

C. Absorbance D. Wavelength

845. The following solution can be estimated by dpectrophotometric titration

A. Coloured solution

B. Colourless solution

C. Turbid suspension

D. All of the above

846. We can not UV spectra less than 200nm because
A. Of lack of source of light
B. No compound absorbs less than 200nm
C. both a and b
D. Oxygen interferes

847. A non - fluorescent organic molecule after absorption of UV energy loose energy by
A. Reemission of radiation
B. Reflection
C. Refraction
D. Heat

848. A fluorescent molecule after absorption of UV flucreesant losses part of the energy by means of
A. Collisian
B. Vibration transition
C. Deactivatian
D. Ratatianal transition

849. A flourimeter can be converted into a nephtometer by inserting
A. UV filter B. IR filter
C. Visible D. Can not be done

850. The absorben activity of an adsorbent can be increased by
A. Decreasing the surface area
B. Decreasing the particles size
C. Increasing the temperature
D. all of the above methed

851. Non aqueous titration can be carried out by
A. Potentiometry B. Amperometry
C. conductometry D. spectrophotometry

852. Standard hydrogen electrode can be used as
A. primary reference electrode
B. secondary reference electride
C. both a and b
D. Indicator electrode only

853. The finger print region in IR spectrum range from
A. 4000 - 3000 cm-1B.Less than 1500cm-1
C. 3000 - 2000 cm-1D. above 600 cm-1

854. The largest peak in the mass spectra is called as-
A. mass peak B. base peak
C. metastable peak D. m+ 2 peak

855. mass spectra is usually a
A. Band spectra
B. positive ion spectra
C. Absorption spectra
D. emission spectra

856. IR spectra is concerned with
A. vibration
B. Electronic transitions
C. Rotations
D. spin of protons

857. UV spectra is abtained as a result of
A. Emission of UV radiation
B. Absorption and remission of UV
C. Absorption of UV rays
D. Change in spin of electrons

858. Which of the following is not a source used in mid infrared spectrophotometer.
A. Nernst glower
B. Globar
C. High pressure mercury are lamp
D. Nichrome wire

859. The vibration without a center of symmetry are active in which of the following region?
A. IR but inactive in raman
B. Raman but inactive in raman
C. Raman and IR
D. Inactive in both Raman and IR

860. Compelling indications for use of antihypertensive drugs :
A. Heart failure
B. Diabetes
C. Chronic seal disease
D. All of these

861. The frequency of vibration of a bond is a function of which factor?
A. Bond order
B. Force constant of the bond
C. masses of the atoms involved in bonding
D. Force constant of the bond and masses of the atoms

862. The vibration without a center of symmetry are active in which of the following region.

A. IR but inactive in raman

B. Raman and IR

C. Raman but inactive in raman

D. Inactive in both Raman and IR

863. Which of the following is the wave number of near Infrared spectrometer

A. 4000 -200cm-1 B. 200 -10cm-1

C. 12500 -10cm D. 60 -1000 cm-1

864. Which of the following options are correct in terms of Wavelength for the different types of IR spectrometer.

A. Near IR 0.8 - 2.5mm

B. Mid IR 0.8 - 2.5mm

C. Far IR 2.5 -50mm

D. Mid IR 50 - 100 mm

865. what is the composition of yelobar rod which is used as a source in mid IR spectroscopy

A. silicon corbide B. silver chloride

C. Silicon dioxide D. siliver carbide

866. Which of the following is not used as pyroelectricmaterial in pyroelectric transducens in infrared spectroscopy.

A. Triglycine sulphate

B. Some polymers

C. Deutrated triglycine sulphate

D. Tetraglycine sulphate

867. What is vibration spectroscopy.

A. IR in an earthquakes

B. A class of spectroscopy techniques which analyzer molecular motion

C. When you shine a flashlight through a prism and shake it

D. The study of epileptic ghosts infrared spectroscopy.

868. The picture to the right is a representation of.

A. A spring with two balls attached to it

B. A short carbon chain with large endgroup

C. A circuit diagram of two point charges connected by a resistor

D. A simple harmanic ascilatot

869. Which of the following will oscillate the fastest?

A. A large mass on a weak spring

B. A large mass on a stiff spring

C. A small mass on a stiff spring

D. A small mass on a weak spring.

870. A simple harmanic ascilator may absorb energy............?

A. Any time

B. When the freqvencics match excthy

C. When the amplitudes are the same

D. At no time

871. In the past IR spectra he'd to be acquired one wave length at a time which took a look can we collect spectra so quickly today?

A. We are smarter than the people.

B. some guy figured out a better.

C. The courier transfer Algorithm allows us to scan all frequencies at once.

D. Light is faster today that is used to be.

872. Which of the following is not an IR vibrational mode.

A. Stertching B. Scissoring

C. Rocking D. Rolling

873. When does n carbonyl (C=0) stretch appear in an IR spectrum?

A. 720 -720 B. 1870 - 1650

C. 3640 -3250 D. 650 – 000

874. When casting a film on water why is it important, why is it important to chase a solvent which is less water.

A. So that the solvent and water don't mix

B. So the water does not evaporate before the solvent

C. So you can from a film

D. So the solution will float on top of the water.

875. Why is it important to where gloves when handling solt plates?

A. There might be some toxic chemimcal left on the solt plate

B. There is moisture on your fingers which will damage the salt plate.

C. All of the above

D. The oils and dirt on your finger's will affect your spectrum.

876. why is it important to squire a background spectrum.

A. So you don't see carbon dioxide in your spectrum

B. So you don't have peaks characteristic of your substrate in your spectrum.

C. Because a picture always looks better on a nice background.

D. A and B only

877. What type of solar radiation is potentially damaging to the eyes

A. Visible light
B. Infrared rays
C. UV light
D. Un visible light

878. What type's of UV radiation are dangerous?

A. Only uv- A is dangerous

B. Only UV - B is dangerous

C. Only UV - A and B dangerous.

D. Both are dangerous.

879. The safest sunglasses are mode out of what material?

A. Ordinary plastic
B. Glass
C. Polycarbonate
D. All of these

880. What is the mast immediate danger to children's eyes from extreme overexpasure to the sun?

A. Glancoma
B. Photokeratitis
C. Skin cancer
D. Both A and

881. When buying sunglasses look for those that block what percentage of UV?

A. 90% UV - and UV - B

B. 100% UV - and 90% UV - A

C. 99 - 100% UV - A and UV -B

D. Only A and B

882. People who work in which of the following jobs are at increased risk of UV eye damage.

A. life guards

B. both of the above

C. Tollbooth operators

D. None of these

883. What else can I do to cut my exposure to UV rays?

A. Wear a brimmed hat

B. stay indoors during

C. both of the above

D. life gurds

884. Adding UV caotiong to prescription glasses is which of the following?

A. Expensive
B. Free
C. Inexpensive
D. None of these

885. Uv spectrascopy the absorption of UV radiation ranges from.

A. 800 - 1000nm
B. 200 - 400nm
C. 400 - 600nm
D. 600 - 800 nm

886. In a UV visible spectrophotometer the path length is normally

A. 10 mm
B. 10 cm
C. 10um
D. 100nm

887. The unit of NMR spectrum on the x -axis is-

A. Herts
B. cm-1
C. ppm
D. none of these

888. Bending vibration include following except

A. Rocking
B. Sterching
C. Twisting
D. Wagging

889. Radiafrequency radiation is associated with

A. NMR

B. IR

C. Mass spectroscopy

D. UV

890. Number of NMR signal generated by acetone is.

A. 2
B. 6
C. 3
D. 1

891. The unit of magnetic field strength in NMR is

A. Cycles second
B. pulse /second
C. Gaus
D. Debye

892. NMR signal is obtained in 14, dioxane.

A. 3pears
B. 2 peaks
C. 1 peak
D. 4 peaks

893. Basic principle underlying FT-IR is?

A. Polarization
B. Diffraction
C. Rafraction
D. IR

894. In IR spectroscopy the changes in electronic energy is always associated with charge in.
A. Rotationnal energy
B. vibrationnal
C. vibrational and ratatianal
D. all of these

895. A solvent used in NMR studies is.
A. Chloroform
B. Carbon tetrachloride
C. Acetone
D. ethanol

896. cyclo butane have NMR signal is.
A. 1 B. 2
C. 4 D. 3

897. IR spectra is concerned with.
A. vibration B. electronic tansitions
C. Rotation D. spin of protons.

898. For calibration of wave number scale in IR......... Is used.
A. Holmium filter
B. Polystyrene film
C. polystyrene film
D. Polyvinyl film

899. For obtaining IR radiation nernst filament should be healed to... C°
A. 500 - 1000 B. 1000 - 1500
C. 2000 - 2500 D. 1000 - 1800

900. Which of the following requires the most enerrgs in IR..
A. Wagging
B. Twisting
C. Asymmetric bend
D. Asymmetric stretch

901 Which is an example of colloid
A. Milk B. Butter
C. Blood D. All of the above

902. Which of the following step include gravimetric analysis
A. Sampling
B. precipitation
C. Disputation of sample
D. All of the above

903. In which process of precipitation progresses include
A. precipitation
B. Nucleation
C. Crystal growth
D. All of the above

904. The filtering media as in gravimetric analysic
A. Filterpaper
B. Filter pulp
C. Filter mats
D. All of the above

905. When the solubility of BaSO4 is greatest the precipitation of Baso4 is done in which media
A. Acidic B. Basic
C. Amphoteric D. All of the above

906. Due to common ion (so2) the poor dissociation of Baso2 the solubility of Baso4
A. Increases B. Not effect
C. Decreases D. None

907. The ppt of inorganic solid are more soluble in
A. Polar solvent B. Non polar
C. Semi polar D. None

908. Which of the following factor effect the rate of deposition in crystal growth
A. Natural of solvent
B. Natural of ion
C. Impurities
D. None of the above

909. Which of the following is impotent step in gravimetric analysis
A. Coup legation B. Semi precipitation
C. Precipitation D. None of above

910. Which of the following physical quantity effect supersaturated solution
A. Fixed pressure
B. Fixed agitation
C. Fixed temperature
D. All of the above

911. Which of the following step is not involved in precipitation
A. Nucleation B. Crystal growth
C. None of above D. Both a and c

912. The rate of diffusion in crystal growth depended on

A. Nature of ions B. Temperature
C. Rate of stirring D. All of the above

913. Gravimetric analysis covering the major factor of

A. Precipitation product
B. Solubility product
C. None of above
D. Insoluble product

914. The % aluminium in potassium alum can be determine by

A. Precipitation method
B. Copexometry
C. Gravimetric
D. All of the above

915. The pore pharmaceutical substance are quantiarlity converted free compound and the basic of gravimetric analysic

A. Progesterone suspension
B. Mephobarbital tablet
C. Both a and b
D. Phenacaine hydrochloride

916. Solubility of PPT increases by

A. Increases in pressure
B. Increases in solid concentration
C. Increases in temperature
D. None of above

917. The contamination of PPT by substance which are soluble are mother liquor called as

A. Precipitation
B. Nucleation
C. Co precipitation
D. None of above

918. When electrolyte is added to colloidal solution the colloidal particle joint together to form bigger particles the codes less

A. Precipitation B. Colligation
C. Deliration D. Post precipitate

919. The number of gram of the desired constituent in 1gm of the substance weighed generally employed as

A. Law mass action
B. Comom ion factor
C. Gravimetric factor
D. None

920. The substance which are estimated by gravimetric are

A. Free acid B. Free salt
C. Free base D. Both A and B

921. Which is not consider in the principle of grevemetry

A. Law of mass action
B. Solvent precipitation
C. Common ion effect
D. Principle of solubility product

922. Gravimetric analysis are based an

A. Precipitate B. Temperature
C. Weight D. None of above

923. Common ion effect absorbed in

A. No change in the equilibrium consent
B. The relative contrition of the reacting substance by change
C. The conisation of reacting component mass change
D. All of the above

924. Technique by which an elements or compound is obtained in its present form through insoluble subsequent weighing is

A. Precipitation titration
B. Gravimetric analysis
C. Complexes metric analysis
D. None of above

925. In actual gravimetric analysis final weight of product is usually accomplished by which standard method

A. Solvent extraction
B. Distillation
C. Ignition
D. A and B

926. Gravimetric analysis is based up on

A. Qualitative precipitation
B. Quantitative compilation
C. None
D. Quantitative precipitation

927. Which is not a violet step in succesple gravimetric method

A. Identify an insoluble form with definite composition

B. Convert the precipitate altimetry to reasonably memorable form
C. Wash the PPT free of co precipitation at and impurities as for as possible
D. None of above

928. The mass of HaBr2 precipitated when 15.00 ML of 0.337 MHG (NO3) solution is added to excess KBR solution is
A. 2.01 g B. 1.76 G
C. 1.82 G D. 1.65 g

929. Which of the following is not a property required as the substance chosen for use a precipitated in a gravimetric
A. Law solubility
B. Stable when heated to 110.c
C. Able to be stored for an extended time without deterioration
D. Has known formula

930. Potassium alum are
A. KAI (So)2.12 H2o
B. None of above
C. KAI (So)2.24.H2o
D. Caocl2.8H2o

931. How would you assay the following drug gravimetric
A. Sodium chloride
B. Barium sulphate
C. Potassium alum
D. Piperazine phosphate

932. 2.49 of carbon reacts with 0.80 g hydrogen to form a hydrocarbon the empirical formula of the hydrocarbon will be
A. C4H B. CH4
C. C3H D. C2H6

933. Magnesium chloride and silver nitrate solution are mixed given that precipitated reaction occurs the precipitated is likely to be
A. Mg(No3)2 B. AgNo3
C. Mgcl2 D. Agcl

934. What is washing of precipitates is generally not used for
A. Pure water B. NaoH
C. Ethanol D. None of above

935. Which added for the washing of precipitates are colloidal solution
A. Electrolyte B. None of above
C. Water D. NaoH

936. What is the thus pure water cannot be used as a
A. Wash liquid
B. None of above
C. Wash precipitate
D. Both A and B

937. What is adsorption of an ion on the concentration of the ion present in the solution
A. Particle depends
B. None of above
C. Charge depends
D. Both A and B

938. What is the size of the ion influence the process
A. Adsorption B. Heating
C. Particle D. None of above

939. What is the type of co precipitate can be understood by considering the process of growth
A. Crystal B. PPT
C. Liquid D. None of above

940. Precipitate in some cases on heating the PPT
A. 100-110.C B. None of above
C. 20-40 . C D. 200-350. C

941. What is the participated for example by heating the PPT
A. Agcl B. None of above
C. H2o D. Na++

942. Precipitate are this problem is solved by heating the PPT to a sufficiently are
A. High temperature
B. Nature temperature
C. Low temperature
D. None of above

943. What is the washed PPT may contain occluded are
A. Adsorbed water B. None of above
C. Heating water D. Solubility

944. What is the composition of the wash solution depended upon the properties of the PPT

A. Chemical B. Both A and B

C. Solubility D. Physically

945. What is the washing of precipitate the correct procedure is to a small volume of wash liquid each time of washing

A. 10 ml B. 45 ml

C. 23 ml D. 11 ml

946. What is the precipitate some are dried at ordinary

A. Temperature B. None of above

C. Cooling D. Heating

947. Thermo gravimetric analysis the temperature of a substance is gradually

A. Decreases B. Increases

C. Both D. Weight

948. What is the thermal decomposition are the substance that is weighed has a definitechemical composition

A. Caco3 alone B. Caso4

C. Caso2 D. None of above

949. In this section some gravimetric procures are described

A. Laboratory exercises

B. None of above

C. Chemical method

D. Nature exercises

950. What is the colloid particles are very small in size hence their surface to would be very high

A. Mass rati B. None of above

C. Particle size D. Adsorption

951. In the beginning these particles there exists several important in

A. No charge B. Positive

C. Both B and D D. Negative

952. What is the beginning these particle are of colloidal size and have a large number

A. Ag+ and Cl- ions B. Na+

C. Cl++ D. None of above

953. What is the Ag+ ions on the particle surface attract are

A. Ag+ and Cl B. Both A and B

C. Positive ions D. Negative ions

954. This is called preferences adsorption the above example

A. Ag+ and Cl B. NaoH

C. Na+ D. OH-

955. These Cl- ions now attract positively charge sodium ions thus forming

A. Primary layer B. Secondary layer

C. Electrical D. Both A an B

956. What is the Ions in solution particle size

A. 108 cm B. 58 cm

C. 99 cm D. 12 cm

957. What is the colloidal particles are charged

A. Electrically B. Chemical

C. Sun light D. None of above

958. Which are very small in size have a very high surface to mass ratio

A. Colloid particles B. None of above

C. Ions D. Adsorption

959. What is adsorption of ions on precipitates let us consider the process of precipitation

A. Salt B. None of above

C. Solution D. Solubility

960. Which now it has been found that only those particle settle at the bottom whose diameter is greater than

A. 10-4 cm B. 23 cm

C. 11-6 cm D. 12-9 cm

961. The adsorption are colloidal range particle of diameter

A. Diameter 10-7-10-4 cm

B. None of above

C. Diameter 11-8-17 cm

D. Demeter 10-14 cm

962. What is the gravimetric determination

A. Chloride B. None of above

C. Silver chloride D. A and C

963. Precipitation of chloride as silver chloride are the add solution

A. Distilled water B. Ethanol

C. HNo3 D. A and C

964. Precipitation are chloride silver chloride precaution are the glass ware

A. Wash bottles B. Polyethylene

C. Glass D. Filtration

965. Gravimetric determination of chloride of silver chloride are procreation method

A. Preparation of the sample solution

B. All of the above

C. Preparation of chloride as silver

D. Digestion of the precipitation

966. What is the digestion of the precipitate solution added

A. Agno3 B. H2o

C. HNo3 D. Cl

967. Which are filter crucibles porous percolation sintered glass are used to precipitate

A. Digestion precipitation

B. Sample precipitate

C. Weighing precipitate

D. None of above

968. What is the digestion of the precipitate process of digestion brings about

A. Coagulation B. Anti coagulation

C. Filtration D. None of above

969. What is the digestion in the upper clear liquid called supernatant solution droup

A. AgNo3 B. H2o

C. HNo3 D. Agcl

970. Washing the filtrate should be collected and few drops of dilute added

A. HCL B. H2o

C. None of above D. H2so4

971. Silver ions combine with to form insoluble Agcl

A. Cl B. Agcl

C. Ag+ D. None of above

972. What is the ionic reaction has been used for the determination

A. Gravimetric B. Precipitate

C. Chemical D. Physical

973. AgNo3 soln and weighing the resultant PPT of the after washing and drying

A. AgNo3 B. Hcl

C. H2o D. HaNo3

974. A slight excess of HCl is added so that are completely precipitates

A. Ag+ ions B. None of above

C. Hcl D. Silver ion

975. Gravimetric are solubility of Agcl due to the formation solution chloride complexes of silver

A. Increases B. equable

C. Decreases D. A and C

976. What is the barium as barium sulphate are use are determination

A. Gravimetric B. Silver nitric

C. Silver chloride D. None of above

977. The barium sulphate are formula

A. Baso4 B. Agso4

C. H2so4 D. None of above

978. It barium is to be determination in a given solution its definite is taken in a beaker

A. H2so4 B. None of above

C. H2o D. A and C

979. Precipitation form homogenous soln aro another method of precipitant is to add the given sol

A. Sulphuric acid B. Choride

C. Nitric acid D. A and C

980. The formula weight of Baso4 is

A. 233.42 B. 233.45

C. 244.30 D. 233.34

981. The formula weight of Bacl2.2H2ois

A. 244.32 B. 322.43

C. 243.54 D. 243.54

982. The gravimetric factor for the the conversion is

A. Baso4 B. A and C

C. Bacl2 D. None of above

983. What is the gravimetric determination of calcium as calcium oxalate the sample containing is dissolved in hot Hcl and added

A. Ammonium oxalate
B. None of above
C. Barium sulphate
D. Calcium carbonate

984. Calcium as calcium oxalate the mixture is heated with to dissolve the solid and solution is boiled for

A. HCL B. Cao
C. H2o D. None of above

985. There are several inorganic ions that be precipitated by adding

A. Organic reagent B. Organic precipitate
C. A and B D. None of above

986. What is the gravimetric method using have been developed for almost all the elements

A. Organic precipitants
B. None of above
C. Reagents
D. Solubility

987. What is the cheated compounds obtained by the reaction between metal

A. Metal ions B. A and D
C. Insoluble D. Organic precipitates

988. The precipitates obtained with organic precipitants are made of coarse particles which are easily

A. Filtered B. Dissolution
C. Precipices D. none of above

989. When Nickel metal determine what will be organic precipitants form

A. Diethyl glyoxime B. Quinaldic acid
C. Cupferron D. None of above

990. When aluminium metal determine what will be organic precipitant form

A. 8-hydroxy guinoline
B. None of above
C. Cupferron
D. 8- nitro so nathol

991. When cupferron organic precipitant what will be metal determined form

A. Iron B. Aluminium
C. Zinc D. Nickel

992. When cobalt metal determine what will be organic precipitins form

A. Copper B. Zinc
C. Iron D. None of above

993. When zinc metal determined what will be organic precipitant form

A. Quinaldic acid B. Nickel
C. Copper D. Iron

994. It is a white crystalline solid which is poorly soluble in water but fairly soluble in alcohol

A. Benzoinoxime B. Cupferron
C. Quinaldic acid D. None of above

995. This is an expensive reagents are

A. Quinaldic acid B. Iron
C. None of above D. Zinc

996. This reagent gives insoluble complexes with

A. Cu B. A and c
C. Cd D. Co

997. What is the precipitates so obtained are influenced by the PH of the solution for example

A. Zinc B. None of above
C. Iron D. H2o

998. What is A3 percent aqueous solution of sodium salt of the acid is used as regent

A. Anthranalic acid B.All of the above
C. Nitric acid D. Nickel

999. Anthanalic acid in neutral or waking acidic solution the reagent precipitants solution are

A. Zn B. A and C
C. Ni D. None of above

1000. What is the salicylaldoxime the reagent solution is prepared in water alcohol mixture are

A. Bl B. A and C
C. Pd D. Cu

1001. What is the electro gravimetric are the platinum electrodes are used for

A. Electrolysis B. None of above
C. Cathode D. A and c

1002. What is the electro gravimetric determination of copper are this method

A. Electro deposition B. None of above
C. Titrimetric analysis D. Battery

1003. What is the barium sulphate the digestion of precipitate increases ....and given same purification

A. Particle size B. A and C
C. Surface area D. None of above

1004. What is the aluminium as aluminium oxide the precipitation is usually carried the out in the presence of NH4cl add solid and drops

A. Methyl red indicator
B. None of above
C. Methyl yellow indicator
D. Alcohol

1005. What is the addition of ammonia is continued till the colour of the solution the indicator show the PH of the solution which should be maintained within the range

A. 6.5 to 7.5 B. 7.9 to 8.9
C. 8.2 to 7.8 D. 5.8 to 8.9

1006. What is the leade is precipitated as lead chromate by the addition of

A. Sodium chromate solution
B. None of above
C. Potassium chromate solution
D. A and C

1007. What is the precipitates of lead chromate is almost as

A. Insoluble in dilute acetic acid
B. All of the above
C. Soluble in dilute acetic acid
D. Soluble in dilute nitric acid

1008. Which are the if the substance is insoluble in water dissolve it in the minimum quantity

A. HNo3 B. NH4OH
C. H2so4 D. None of above

1009. What is the calcium as calcium carbonate or calcium oxide are added indicator

A. Methyl B. Phinophathline
C. H2so4 D. None of above

1010. What is the calcium will be precipitated as CaC2o4 .H2o

A. Cao B. C2o4
C. CaCo2 D. None of above

1011. What is the zinc is precipitated as zinc ammonium phosphate form a zinc salt solution solution by adding

A. Diammonium hydrogen phosphate
B. Sodium nitric
C. Ammonium sulphate
D. None of above

1012. Which is the zinc ammonium phosphate are procedure added to drops of methyl red indicator solution changes in colour form

A. Red to yellow B. None of above
C. Green D. Blue

1013. The precipitate of Mg(NH4) Po4.6H2o is usually contaminated with the impurities of

A. B and C
B. Ammonium phosphate
C. Magnesium phosphate
D. Sodium phosphate

1014. What is the oxine is almost

A. Colourless B. Crystalline
C. Insoluble water D. All of the above

1015. Which is the oxine added solution as

A. NH4cl B. None of above
C. H2so4 D. So4

1016. What is the purity and thermal stability of both the the can be determined

A. Primarily standards
B. A and C
C. Secondary standards
D. None of above

1017. What is the TGA involves the use of a

A. Thermal balance B. Potency
C. Pyrolysis curve D. None of above

1018. What is the organic precipitants usually have a
A. High molecular weight
B. None of above
C. High temperature
D. Low molecular weight

1019. Which are the some important organic percipients as
A. Diethyl glyoxime
B. Ammonium sulphate
C. 8-hydroxyquinoline
D. A and C

1020. The best procedure to use when filtering an aqueous solution of collect a precipitate is to
A. Use large volume of to ensure that all soluble matters separated from the precipitates
B. Wash the precipitate with a minimum amount of water
C. Warm the solution the before filtering
D. Not wash the precipitates at all

1021. A sample of an unknown substance was found to contain 0.24 g of carbon 0.040 g of hydrogen and 0.32 g of oxygen the empirical formula of the known was
A. Ch3o B. C2H2o
C. CH2o D. C2H4o2

1022. Sodium nitrate NaNo3 cannot be analysed gravimetric be Cory
A. The stability sodium nitrate is very low
B. All compound containing ions or nitrate ions are soluble
C. Sodium nitrate is insoluble
D. Sodium nitrate soluble

1023. Fe3+ metal ion form the precipitin with
A. 2N NH4oH B. (NH)2 Hpo4
C. 2NH2so4 D. None of above

1024. The strongly heated required in
A. Fe2o3 B. Cuo
C. Baso4 D. All of the above

1025. Zn2+ metal ion form the precipitins with
A. Zno B. Mg-(NH4)
C. Al2o3 D. None of above

1026. Cu2+ metal ion form the participate with
A. Cuo B. Zno
C. Al2+ D. None of above

1027. Mg2+metal ion form the precipitin with
A. Mg-(NH4) B. Zno
C. Agcl D. None of above

1028. Ag+ metal ion form the precipitates with
A. Agcl B. Zno
C. Zn D. Cuo

1029. Zn2+ metal ion form the precipitates with
A. 10% Na2Co3 soln
B. 20% Na2co3 soln
C. 11% H2so4 soln
D. None of above

1030. Cu2+ metal ions form
A. cuo B. Al
C. Zno D. None of above

1031. So42- metal ion form the precipitins with
A. 2% Bacl2 solution
B. 20% Na2co3 solution
C. 5% Aaso4 solution
D. None of above

1032. Cl –metal ion form the precipitates with
A. 1% AgNo3 solution
B. 10% Cl solution
C. 5% Agcl solution
D. None of above

1033. Agcl precipitate wash with
A. Cold water +few drops of conc. HNo3
B. Hot water
C. Water containing NH4oH
D. None of above

1034. Mg2+ precipitates ions washed with
A. So42- B. Cl
C. Cuo D. None of above

1035. Agcl precipitant ions washed with
A. Cl- B. Cu
C. So4- D. Zno

1036. So42- metal ion for the wash liquid with
A. Hot water
B. Water containing HNo3
C. Cool water
D. None of above

1037. Zn 2+metal ion are the treatment of ash with
A. Filtered i a sintered crucible
B. Conc. HNo3
C. Same as for Zn
D. None of above

1038. Cr2o3 precipitant was liquid with
A. Water+2% NH4NO3
B. Ammonia solution
C. Same as for Ag
D. None of above

1039. Ba2+ metal ion are the wash liquid with
A. 10% K2cr2o7 solution
B. 4% AgNO3sloution
C. Same as for solution
D. None of above

1040. Nickel dimethyl glyoxime cheated precipitate are the treatment of ash with
A. Filtered in a sintered glass crucible
B. Some as for Ag+
C. Conc. Hno3
D. None of above

1041. Mg oxidant precipitates was liquid with
A. 1: 40 ammonium solution
B. Water +2% NHNo3
C. Some as for Ag
D. None of above

1042. Pb2+ metal ions form the ions washed with
A. Cro42-
B. So42-
C. Cl
D. None of above

1043. Cu 2+ metal ions form the drying and ignition with
A. Dried at 110-120 C
B. None of above
C. 105-110 C
D. 134- 150 C

1044. Ni 2+metal ions form the precipitates with
A. 1% dimethyl glyoxime alcohol solution
B. 20% Cl solution
C. 10% Agno3 solution
D. None of above

1045. Baso4 precipitate form the treatment of ash with
A. Conc. H2so4
B. Conc. H203
C. Conk HNO3
D. None of above

1046. What is the zinc as zinc oxide the solution again added drops indicator as
A. Phenolphthalein
B. None of above
C. H2so4
D. NaoH

1047. What is the zinc as oxide the solution added drops indicators as colour as
A. Pink colour
B. Red
C. Blue
D. Yellow

1048. What is the zinc as zinc oxide the use of solution in sacking the filter paper
A. Ammonium nitrate
B. Nitric acid
C. Sulphuric acid
D. None of above

1049. What is the benzyl penicillin may be estimated gravimetrically of precipitation as the
A. 1- ethyl benzyl piperidinium salt
B. None of above
C. Sodium salt
D. Potassium salt

1050. What is the sodium or potassium salt of benzyl penicillin are
A. Nac16H17N2o4s
B. A and C
C. Kc16H16N2o4s
D. None of above

1051. What is the proguanil cupric oomplex the method is based upon the fact that when an
A. Ammoniac solution
B. Ammoniacal cupric
C. Sodium solution
D. None of above

1052. What is the quantitative precipitation of the in soluble proguanil complete taken place which is filtered and weighed to a constant weight
A. 130 C
B. 234 C
C. 150 C
D. 236 C

1053. What is the sodium lauryl sulphate it contains the equivalent of not less than of alcohol
A. 58% w/w
B. 12% w/w
C. 45% w/w
D. 23 %w/w

1054. What is organic precipitants formed are covalent in nature and hence are soluble in solvent

A. Non polar solvent
B. None of above
C. Polar solvent
D. Inorganic solvent

1055. What is the organic precipitate thus complex of cupferron is soluble in ether and hence facilitates its separation from other metal present in a

A. Large volume solution
B. Polar solution C. Non polar solution
D. None of above

1056. What is the urea reagent form metal precipitated with

A. Fe B. All of the above
C. Al D. Zn

1057. What is the dimethyl glyoxime DMG precipitant form metal precipitated with

A. Ni B. None of above
C. Cu D. Zn

1058. Precipitant H2s form the reagent with

A. H2s B. OH
C. Cu D. None of above

1059. What is the dimethyl sulphate reagent form the precipitant with

A. So42- B. H2s
C. OH D. None of above

1060. 8- acetoxy quinoline reagent form the metal precipitated with

A. Al B. All of the above
C. Mg D. Zn

1061. The KSP of caf2 is 4.2 *10-11 in pure water in acidic solution the solubility of Caf2 is expected to

A. Increases because Ca2+ ions is acidic
B. Increases because F ions is basic
C. Decreases because Ca2+ ions is acidic
D. None of above

1062. A solution is known to contain ions of Ag+ cu2+ what will happen when 1.0 m is added to the solution

A. No precipitate will form
B. Both Agcl and pbCl2 will precipitate
C. Only Agcl will precipitate
D. All of the above

1063. Which has the greatest molar solubility in water at 25 C

A. Ammonium nitrate
B. None of above
C. Barium sulphate
D. Copper phosphate

1064. When mixed which pair of aqueous solution will form precipitates

A. KNO3 and cabr2
B. CaCl2 and K2Co3
C. NaNo3 and NH4
D. None of above

1065. Which of the following substance does not form a precipitate with silver ions

A. Hydro chloric acid
B. Sodiumbromide
C. Sulphuric acid D. Potassium nitrate

1066. The solubility of the precipitate will with decreasing the temperature

A. Increases B. None of above
C. Decreases D. No effect

1067. What will be the effect an solubility of the precipitates it PH is decreased when anion of the salt is the conjugate of weak acid

A. Increase B. None of above
C. No effect D. Decrease

1068. What is precipitation titrations are those in which a result in the formation of a precipitate

A. Sparingly soluble salt
B. Sparingly insoluble salt
C. Chemical reaction
D. None of above

1069. One of the main reasons for the limited of such titration is the lack of suitable indicators to detect the

A. End point
B. None of above
C. Chemical reaction
D. No effect

1070. What is the furthermore thecomposition of the precipitate may not be exactly known owing to the as

A. Co precipitation effect
B. Chemical effect
C. precipitation
D. No effect

1071. Thus the main precipitation filtrations are the argentometric filtrations which employ a standard solution of

A. Silver nitrate B. None of above
C. Sodium nitrate D. Calcium carbonate

1072. What is decapitation titration are the complex formation reaction is involved rather than precipitation reaction

A. No change in oxidation states occurs
B. Other reaction
C. Change in oxidation states occurs
D. None of above

1073. When Ag NO3 is added to a solution of either

A. Nacl/ KCl B. NaNO3
C. Nao2 D. None of above

1074. What is the AgNO3 is added to solution of Nacl KCl a colour precipitation

A. White precipitate
B. Yellow precipitate
C. Blue precipitate
D. None of above

1075. Both these reaction may be employed for the titrimetric determination of

A. Ag+ B. Thiocyante
C. All of the above D. Halides

1076. What is the precipitation titration are the solution of Nacl and KSCN are

A. Colourless B. None of abov
C. Crystalline D. Odourless

1077. What is the equivalent mass of a salt in a precipitation reaction is

A. Molar mass of the salt
B. None of above
C. Mohr's method
D. Volhards method

1078. What is the precipitation filtration are the mass of in the filtration of ions is its molecular mass

A. AgNO3 B. Nacl
C. Cl- D. A and C

1079. It is the turbidity procedure for the determination of Ag+ with Cl- first introduced by gay Lussaa in

A. 1832 B. 1865
C. 1946 D. 1895

1080. What is the Gay lussac turbidity method is A standard solution of Nacl is treated with a solution

A. AgNO3 B. Ag+
C. Nacl D. None of above

1081. What is the turbidity methods are Nacl solution is added to the silver solution is the presence of free HNO3 and small quantity of pure precipitated

A. AR Ba(NO3)2 B. KSCN
C. K2cro4 D. None of above

1082. What is the in neutral solution of Nacl and AgNO3 this method are

A. Mohr's method
B. Turbidity method
C. Volhard method
D. None of above

1083. Potassium chromate K2cro4 solution is used as an indicators whereas in silver nitrate and KSCN an acidic solution of ferric alum is used an indicator are this method

A. Volhards method
B. None of above
C. Mohr's method
D. Fijians method

1084. Potassium chromate an only be used in neutral solution since

A. Ag2cro4 dissolves in acids
B. All of the above
C. Alkaline solution
D. Silver oxide

1085. What is the Fijians adsorption indicatotors are the consider the at the surface of precipitate

A. Electric charge B. A and D
C. No charge D. Negative charge

1086. Which is the indicators are some Cl is adsorbed on the precicipitated Agcl surface imparting a negative charge to the crystal are used indicator

A. Fijian's method B. None of above
C. phenolphthalein D. NaoH

1087. What is the adsorption of the negatively charge due anion on the positively charge surface change the colour of the due

A. Oichloro fluooe sceinate anion
B. Tetra bromo fluore senates anion
C. Fluoresceinate anion
D. All of the above

1088. Mohr's method is

A. Direct titration method
B. A and C
C. Indirect method
D. No t effect methods

1089. Mohr's method is direct titration methods used for determination

A. Cl- and Br-
B. AgNO3
C. Gall
D. None of above

1090. Mohr's methods is direct titration method used for determination of Cl and Br in natural PH and it is not used for

A. Iodine
B. Copper
C. Zinc
D. None of above

1091. Preparations of AgNo3 0.1 m this is method

A. Standardisation of AgNo3
B. None of above
C. Standerton of NaoH
D. A And C

1092. What is the precipitation are combination of two ionic species to form a

A. Insoluble product
B. None of above
C. Indirect product
D. Soluble product

1093. What is precipitation are the effect of ph increases of PH and decrees

A. Solubility
B. None of above
C. adsorption
D. Temperature

1094. Volhards method is

A. Indirect method
B. Colorimetric method
C. Direct method
D. None of above

1095. Formation of soluble cloured compounds method is

A. Volhards methods
B. Fijians' method
C. Molar's method
D. All of the above

1096. Mohr's method is direct titration of

A. AgNO3
B. HNO3
C. K2cr2o7
D. None of above

1097. Mohr's method are used for indicators

A. K2cr2o7
B. Phenolphthalein
C. NaoH
D. None of above

1098. Volhards methods are used for indicators

A. Fe2+
B. K2cro7
C. NaoH
D. None of above

1099. Mohr's method is end point

A. Red colour of Ag chromates
B. Blue colour
C. Yellow colour ppt
D. None of above

1100. Volhards method is end point

A. Red soluble compless of Fescn
B. Yellow insoluble complex
C. Blue soluble complex
D. None of above

1101. Titration is carried out at neutral or slightly alkaline PH are this method

A. Mohr's method
B. Fejjan method
C. Volhards method
D. None of above

1102. What is the determine of halides at acidic PH are method

A. Volhards method
B. Fejjan method
C. Mohr's method
D. All of the above

1103. Volhards method is colour of fescN fades aboves

A. 25.c
B. 20.c
C. 50. C
D. None of above

1104. What is the method determine of iodide not possible as it adsorb chromate ions so use will get false end point

A. Mohr's method
B. Volhards method
C. Fejjan method
D. None of above

1105. Volhards method is determination of halides is possible

A. Cl B. I
C. Br D. All of the above

1106. Fajjans method is

A. Direct method B. Simple method
C. Indirect method D. None of above

1107. Fajjans method are used the indictore

A. Fluorescain B. NaOH
C. HNO3 D. All of the above

1108. Precipitation Titration and preparation of their 0.IN standard solution are

A. Silver nitrate B. Ammonium oxide
C. Calcium oxide D. None of above

1110. What is AR AgNo3 molecular wt

A. 160.87 B. 169.8
C. 167.97 D. 195.56

1111. Fejjan method are the end point and colour

A. Pink colour B. Red colour
C. Blue colour D. Yellow

1112. Fejjan method are the reagent use

A. AgNo3 B. Cl
C. H2SO4 D. None of the above

1113. Fajjans method of use of is

A. Adsorption indicator
B. NaoH
C. Phenophthaline
D. None of the above

1114. Fluorescain indicator are colour for yellow to pink and what used with

A. Cl B. I
C. Br D. All of the above

1115. Tartrazine indicator are colourless for used

A. Ag+ B. Z-
C. Cl- D. All of the above

1116. Argentometry used for

A. Halides B. Turbidity
C. Fejjan D. None

1117. Argentometry are the use for indicator

A. Without indicator B. No indicator
C. With indicator D. A and c

1118. Which is the method are introduced indicator which adsorb on surface of PPT at equivalence are method

A. Kazimierz Fejjan B. Volhards method
C. Mohr's method D. None

1119. Kazimierz Fejjan are used of the indicator are acidic dyes is

A. Fluoresen B. Phenophthaline
C. Rhodamine D. None

1120. Kazimierz Fejjan are used of the basic dyes of indicators

A. Rhodamine B. NaoH
C. Fluorescain D. None

1121. Colloidal ppt are the adsorption of indicators use

A. Ions on ppt and colour change
B. No colour change
C. Ions anppt and blue colour
D. None

1122. What is the Argentometry are the without indicators used for

A. Turbidity method B. Volhards method
C. Mohr's method D. None

1123. Argentometry are the with indicators used for method

A. Mohr's method B. Volhards method
C. Fejjan method D. All of Adove

1124. What is the used for indicators arewithout indicator and with indicator

A. Argentometry B. Turbidity
C. Colourimery D. None of above

1125. What is the Titration curve based on

A. P-values B. C-values
C. S-values D. None of the above

1126. Mohr's method is

A. I.p dialysis fliuds B. AgNo3
C. Nacl dextross D. A and c

1127. Volhards method is based on

A. Ammino ghrlline B. Nacl
C. AgNo3 D. All of the above

1128. Phenyl mercuric acitic are based on method

A. Volhards method B. Fejjan method
C. Mohr's D. None

1129. Nacl are based on the this method
A. Volhards method B. Fejjan method
C. Mohr's D. None of the above

1130. Sodium chloride and dextross injection these are used as
A. Fluids B. Electrolute
C. Nutrient D. All of the above

1131. All these injection are the stored in a
A. Single dose container
B. No containers
C. Double dose container
D. None of the above

1132. What is the potassium chloride are molecular wt
A. 74.55 B. 57.87
C. 72.67 D. 86.97

1133. These is a potassium chloride are
A. Colourleess B. Crystalline
C. Odourless D. All of the above

1134. It should not contain less than 99% of KCl when determine by Titration with standard AgNo3 this method
A. Mohr's method B. Fajjans method
C. Volhards method D. None

1135. What is the potassium chloride are the stored in containers to prevent absorption of moisture
A. Closed container B. Open contains
C. Single container D. None of above

1136. Kbr is used as a
A. Sedative B. Convulsants
C. Anti convulsants D. A and c

1137. Dichloro fluorescein indicators dissolve 0.lg Dichloro Fluorescain of
A. 95% ethanol
B. 40%alcohol
C. 96% sodium nitrate
D. None

1138. Ferric alum2indicator this is a saturated solution of Ferric alum in the
A. 1m HNO3 acid B. A and c
C. 5m H2SO4 acid D. None of the above

1139. Which is a sodium or potassium chloride can be used as a
A. Primary standard
B. Thiocyante solution
C. Secondary standard
D. None

1140. What is the sodium or potassium chloride can be used as a primary standard for solution
A. AgNo3 B. H2SO4
C. HNO3 D. None of the above

1141. When the AgNo3 solution has been standard with any one of these methods thise solution can be used to standard
A. Potassium Thiocyante solution
B. Calcium nitrate solution
C. Silver nitrate solution
D. None of above

1142. In the Titration end point can be determined by change in colour by
A. Measuring cylinder
B. Burettle
C. Indicator
D. None of above

1143. What is the quantity of chemical in each liter of solutions is known as
A. Strength B. Molecular wt
C. Normality D. None of above

1144. When the exactly required concentration can be prepared form chemical reagent is called as
A. Primary standard
B. A and c
C. Secondary standards
D. None of above

1145. The process of adding known concentration until it complete the reaction with known volume is called as
A. Titrant B. Titration
C. Analysis D. Titrennd

1146. What main types of precipitation Titration ar
A. Volhards B. Fejjan
C. Mohr's D. All of the above

1147. The function ofd extrinsic a protective colloidal is to prevent coagulation of colloidal are

A. Silver chloride B. Calcium carbonate
C. Silver nitrate D. None of above

1148. What is the titrated two additional portions of AgNo3 solution with fix the title value

A. Thiocyante
B. Potassium carbonate
C. Silver nitrate
D. None of above

1149. What types of drugs are analysed by this method

A. Carbromal B. KCl infusion
C. Nacl infusion D. All of the above

1150. When the ionic products is less than the solubility products the solution is

A. Saturated B. Qvantative
C. Unsaturated D. None of above

1151. Dichloro Fluorescain are the it is a

A. Weakly acids solution
B. Simple solution
C. Stogly basic solution
D. None of above

1152. It is orange colour powder dye sparingly soluble in alcohol are

A. Eosin
B. Dichloro Fluorescain
C. Fluorescain
D. None of above

1153. When the diphenyl carbazone are the 0.2% alcohol solution of diphenyl carbazone is used as

A. Adsorption indicator
B. Effect of acid
C. Phenophthaline
D. None of above

1154. Factor affecting the solubility the precipitated

A. Effect of temperature
B. Effect of acid
C. Effect of solvent
D. All of the above

1155. What is the solubility of inorganic salt is reduced by addition of organic seventh such as

A. Ethanol B. Propanol
C. Methanol D. All of the above

1156. What is the absorption indicators are the easin for colors

A. Yellow green B. Orange to blue
C. Pink to red D. None of above

1157. Which is the Fluorescain indicators are the application of and PH

A. 7-10 B. 8-9
C. 6-11 D. None of above

1158. Nacl form is a

A. Colour less B. Crystal
C. Odourless D. All

1159. What is the Nacl intended for parenteral administration should not contain more than

A. 0.1% w/w B. 16% w/w
C. 0.2%w/w D. 0.7%w/w

1160. What is the sodium chloride and dextross injection these are used as

A. Neutrient B. Fluid
C. Electrolyte D. None of above

1161. Determination of the amount of Hcl and HNO3 acids present together solution the mixture is titrated standard alkali using indicators as

A. Phenophthaline B. NaoH
C. H2So4 D. None oak above

1162. Which of the following is responsible for the acidic PH of normal rain water as

A. Co2 B. So2
C. No2 D. Nh3

1163. Which of the following gases is a contributor to the formation of acid rain

A. H2 B. So2
C. O3 D. Nh3

1164. Which of the following is a general property of bases

A. Taste sour
B. Conduct electric current in solutions
C. Turn litmus
D. None

1165. The solution with the lowest PH is

A. 1.om Hf
B. 1.0m HcooH
C. 1.0m hcn
D. 1.om cH2 cooH

1166. As the (H3o)+ in a solution decrease the(oH)

A. Increase and the PH decrease
B. Increase and the PH increase
C. Decrease and the PH increase
D. None

1167. A solution of know concentration is the definition of a

A. Buffer solution
B. Natural solutions
C. Standard solutions
D. None

1168. Non metal oxide showings of reduction with acidic or alkaline are called as

A. Acidic oxide
B. Ammphoteric acid
C. Basic oxide
D. Neutral oxide

1169. Amphéteric oxides react with acidic to form

A. Salt
B. Acid and base
C. Water
D. A and c

1170.solvent as an acid on Titration with a base and act as a base on Titration with acid is known

A. Protogenic
B. Aprotic
C. Protopholic
D. Ammphoteric

1171. Which solvent can be used in non aqueous Titration

A. Acetic acid
B. Semi normal acetic
C. Glacial acetic acid
D. All of the above

1172. Which drug can be determination by acidic ethical non aqueous Titration

A. Nalidixic acid
B. Acyclovir
C. Fluorescain
D. All of the above

1173. None aqueous Titration as carried out for

A. Water insoluble drugs
B. Weekly base drugs
C. Weakly acidic drug
D. All of the above

1174. Which indicator is employed for determination of acetazolamide

A. Azo violent
B. Crystal violet
C. Thymol blue
D. Potentiometer ice determination

1175. Indicators used in alkaline metric non aqueous titration is

A. Thymol blue
B. Crystal Violet
C. Iron salt
D. All of the above

1176. What is the solvent amphiprotic are the example

A. H2o
B. C2H5OH
C. CH3OH
D. All of the above

1177. What is the oxyhalides solvent are the example

A. Pocl3
B. Scocl2
C. Nocl
D. All of the above

1178. Which forms the example c6H6. C6H6. CH3 are the this solvent ex

A. Aprotic
B. Acid
C. Basic
D. None of above

1179. The non aqueous titration used solvent

A. A question solvent
B. Acidic solvent
C. Non aqueous solvent
D. None of above

1180.Indicator used in acidimetric non aqueous titration is

A. Thymol blue
B. Iron salt
C. None of above
D. Crystal violet

1181. Which is the neutral solvent are

A. Methanol
B. Propanol
C. Ethanol
D. All of the above

1182.What is the type of solvent

A. Acidic
B. Oxyhalides
C. Basic
D. All of the above

1183.What is the acidic solvent are theexample as

A. CH3COOH
B. HF
C. HcooH
D. All of the above

1184. What is the basic solvent are characterised of

A. Tendency to release protons
B. A and c
C. Tendency to accept protons
D. None of above

1185. The titration in non aqueous solvent recently are being widely used in the analysis of drug
A. Pharmaceutical industry
B. Food industry
C. Chemical industry
D. None of above

1186. What is the solvent exerts a treatment influence on the solute
A. Acid properties B. A and c
C. Base properties D. None of above

1187. Which one is aprotic solvent
A. Chloroform B. Sodium
C. Benzene D. None of above

1188. Such titration can also be used for the titration of the substance
A. Not soluble water B. Aqueous
C. Soluble water D. None of above

1189. The non aqueous titration can be explained by the using they
A. Bronsted cowry B. Volhads method
C. Mohrs method D. None of above

1190. What is the non aqueous types
A. Aprotic solvent
B. Protophilic solvent
C. Photogenic solvent
D. All of the above

1191. Aprotic solvent are the example as
A. Chloroform
B. Sodium
C. Calcium carbonate
D. None of above

1192. What is theprotogenic solvent are
A. Acidic in nature B. A and B
C. Basic in nature D. None of above

1193. What is the non aqueous solvent are protogenic solvent are examples
A. Hcl B. A and C
C. H2so4 D. None of above

1194. Protophllic solvent are the
A. Basic in nature B. A and c
C. Acid in nature D. None of above

1195. Protophillic solvent are the the example
A. Liquid ammonia B. Ketone
C. Amine D. All

1196. What is the amphiprotic solvent
A. Water B. Weak organic acid
C. Alcohol D. All of the above

1197. Acidimetry in non aqueous titration is
A. Adrenline B. Amtriptyline
C. Albendazole D. All of the above

1198. Which is the Allkalimetry in non aqueous titration of acidic subtance
A. Phenobarbitone B. Acetazolamide
C. Ethosuximide D. All of the above

1199. Classification of non aqueous solvent are depending on the solvent
A. Ionisation of solvent
B. None of above
C. Organic solvent
D. Acidic solvent

1200. For example of ionisation solvent
A. NH3 B. So2
C. H2o D. All of the above

1201. The molecule that affords group for attachment to metal ion
A. Chelate B. Trivalent metal ion
C. Bivalent metal ion D. Ligand

1202. Which one is a bivalent metal ion
A. Calcium B. Aluminium
C. Iron D. Strontium

1203. The example of trivalent metal ion is :-
A. Calcium B. Iron
C. Strontium D. Aluminium

1204. Which one of these is a tetravalent metal ion :-
A. Strontium B. Aluminium
C. Iron D. Calcium

1205. What affects the complex formation & detection?
A. Effect of Ph
B. Stability
C. Usage of PM indicator
D. All of above

1206. In which solution cobalt-EDTA complex is fairly stable?
A. Concentrated sulphuric acid
B. Concentrated hydrochloric acid
C. Perchloric acid
D. All of above

1207. Which one enhance the ionization of complex & lowers the value of stability constant (k)

A. Pressure B. Temperature
C. Viscosity D. Density

1208. What decreases the value of stability constant (k)

A. Addition of electrolytes
B. Removal of electrolytes
C. Addition of indicators
D. None of above

1209. The solubility of salt of EDTA is .... times more than parent compound

A. 25 times B. 50 times
C. 75 times D. 100 times

1210. The equivalence point in complexometric titration is observed by the help of :-

A. Metallochromic indicators
B. Acid-base indicators
C. Redox indicators
D. All of the above

1211. At equilibrium attained a metal buffer solution is largely influenced by change in ......

A. PH B. Temperature
C. Viscosity D. Density

1212. Which is served as a chelating agent to yield a dye-metal complex?

A. Metal ion B. Buffer solution
C. PM indicators D. All of above

1213. What should be the pH of ammonia buffer to standardize 0.5M disodium edetate solution?

A. 07 B. 08
C. 10 D. 12

1214. Which indicators used to standardize 0.5M disodium edetate solution?

A. Eriochrome black-T
B. Mordant black 2
C. Solochrome black-T
D. All of the above

1215. The agent which form complex with one of the metal ion present in solution is called?

A. Masking agent B. Demasking agent
C. Chelating agent D. Ligand

1216. Which indicator is used to standardize calcium carbonate?

A. Eriochrome black-T
B. Hydroxy napthol blue
C. Calcon mixture
D. None of the above

1217. Which indicator is used to standardize magnesium chloride

A. Mordant black 2
B. Calcon mixture
C. Eriochrome black-T
D. Hydroxy napthol blue

1218. Which one is used as a complexing agent for cobalt copper & led?

A. Sodium sulphide
B. Thio glycerol
C. Ammonium chloride
D. Dimer caprol

1219. Ammonium fluoride used as a masking agent for?

A. Iron B. Zink
C. Copper D. Cobalt

1220. Which one can not assayed by residual titration method?

A. Cadmium B. Aluminium
C. Iron D. Led

1221. Bismuth forms a stable complex by reacting with EDTA at the pH of?

A. 1.0 B. 3.0
C. 4.0 D. None of the above

1222. Analysis of calcium containing compounds are done bye :-

A. Aqueous titration
B. Non aqueous titration
C. Complexometric titration
D. Potentiometric titration

1223. Metal indicators can be used in?

A. Complexometric titration
B. Potentiometric titration
C. Aqueous titration
D. Acid base titration

1224. Analysis done bye using mordant black Black 2 indicator is :-
A. Non aqueous titration
B. Precipitation titration
C. Acid-Base titration
D. Complexometric titration

1225. Indicators used in complexometric titration are :-
A. Methyl orange
B. Metal indicators
C. Mordant black 2
D. All of the above

1226. EDTA method can also be termed as :-
A. Precipitation titration
B. Acid-base titration
C. Complexometric titration
D. Potentiometric titration

1227. Magnesium oxide content in magnesium compound are determined by using :-
A. Precipitation titration
B. Aqueous titration
C. Acid-Base titration
D. Complexometric titration

1228. Complexometric titration helps in the determination of :-
A. Acidic drug B. Non metal ions
C. Metal ions D. All of the above

1229. Titration of bismuth is done in :-
A. Acidic solution B. Alcoholic solution
C. Neutral solution D. Neutral solution

1230. EDTA is a ligand :-
A. Tertadentate ligand
B. Octadentate ligand
C. Hexadentate ligand
D. Pentadentate ligand

1231. In the assay of lotions containing Copper & zink, which of the following is used to mask copper by precipitation
A. Glycerine B. Thioglycerol
C. Thyocynate D. 8hydroxy quinoline

1232. In complexometric titration, which are used as masking agents?
A. Ammonium fluoride
B. Dimercaprol
C. Pottasium iodide
D. All of the above

1233. The metal indicator complex in complexometric titration must carry the stability of
A. Sharp colour change
B. Resist dissociation
C. None of the above
D. Both A & B

1234. Murexide can also be termed as :-
A. Ammonium purpurate
B. Ammonium nitrate
C. Ammonium tartrate
D. Ammonium succinate

1235. Under complexometric titration, which is not correct statement for direct titration method?
A. Interference occurs due to presence of other ions
B. Slow complexation reaction
C. Both A & B
D. None of the above

1236. In which type of complexometric titration sodium alkali is used?
A. Back titration
B. Replacement titration
C. Direct titration
D. Indirect titration

1237. The process of adding known concentration till the completion of the reaction with known volume is termed as:-
A. Analysis B. Titrant
C. Titration D. Titrend

1238. In each litre of solution, the quantity of solution is defined as :-
A. Strength
B. Normality
C. Molecular weight
D. Equivalence weight

1239. Exact concentration required can be prepared from chemical reagent is :-
A. Secondary standard
B. Primary standard
C. Both A&B
D. None of the above

1240. Combination of metal cation with Lewis bases, results in the species called as?
A. Complex ion B. Non metal ion
C. Metal ion D. All of the above

1241. During ancient time, the method used for the analysis of polyvalent & bivalent metal ions is?
A. Precipitation titration
B. Gravimetry methods
C. Spectroscopy method
D. Redox methods

1242. In recent time, which reagent is used to detect metal ions?
A. HCl B. EDTA
C. Sodium bicarbonate
D. All of the above

1243. Which type of indicators are incorporated with EDTA to detect metal ions
A. HCL B. Sodium bicarbonate
C. EDTA D. All of the above

1244. A compound that is formed by the combination of a metal ion with a molecule that is capable of donating electron is :-
A. Complex B. Mixture
C. Chelate D. All of the above

1245. Combination of a polyvalent metal ion with a molecule containing donating group is called :-
A. Chelate B. Mixture
C. Ligand D. solution

1246. In complexometric titration, which are used as masking agents?
A. Ammonium fluoride
B. Dimercaprol
C. Pottasium iodide
D. All of the above

1247. The coordination number of silver is :-
A. 2 B. 6
C. 4 D. 8

1248. what is used as a solvent in the determination of fluoride by precipitation?
A. Dilute Hcl
B. Dilute nitric acid
C. Dilute sulphuric acid
D. All of the above

1249. The titration of cyanide with silver ion is known as :-
A. Leibig titration B. Volhard method
C. Mohr's method D. Iodimetry

1250. Km/Kn >_ 1000000 is the equation for aparant stability so what is the Km and Kn in equation:-
A. Apparent stability constant
B. Apparent solubility constant
C. Both
D. None

1251. Which one form complex with cyanide ion and form mask substance
A. Cadmium B. Zink
C. Copper D. All of the above

1252. Which one of these cannot masked by cyanide
A. Alkaline earth metals
B. Aluminium
C. Nickel
D. Silver

1253. What is used as a demasking agent for the complex of cyanide with zink & cadmium?
A. Acidic anhydride B. Borax
C. Chloral hydrate D. None of the above

1254. What can be taken as the end point in determination of concentration of cyanide?
A. When solution becomes turbid on addition of AGCN
B. When solution becomes transparent on addition of AGCN
C. When solution becomes turbid on addition of silver nitrate
D. When solution becomes transparent on addition of silver nitrate

1255. To make the end point more sharp, what should be added to cyanide solution?
A. Ammonium hydroxide
B. Potassium Iodide solution
C. Silver cyanide solution
D. Both A and B

1256. A molecule of Silver nitrate is chemically equivalent to how many molecules of KCN
A. 5 molecules B. 2 molecules
C. 3 molecules D. 4 molecules

1257. What is the use of ion exchange resins in complexometric titration
A. To remove cations
B. To remove non ionic compounds
C. To remove anions
D. None of the above

1258. What is the reason behind masking of metal ions by kinetic masking?
A. Kinetic inetrness
B. Kinetic activeness
C. Kinetic saperation
D. All of the above

1259. Which agent is also termed as versene?
A. Silver B. Copper
C. EDTA D. none of the above

1260. What colour is shown by solochrome black at the end point
A. Pink to blue B. Blue to yellow
C. Yellow to blue D. Red to blue

1261. Which titration is envolved for determining the proportions of individual cations in mixtures :-
A. Acid - Base titration
B. Redox titration
C. Complexometric titration
D. None of the above

1262. In EDTA titration, end point is generally detected by :-
A. PH sensitive indicators
B. Metal-ion sensitive indicators
C. Metal indicators
D. None of the above

1263. Replacement or substitution titration may be used for the metal ions that do not reactor r(react unsatisfactorily) with a metal indicator :-
A. True B. False

1264. Carbonic acid gives purple colour on reaction with :-
A. Acids B. Alkalis
C. Weak acids D. All of the above

1265. Addition of indicator to acid shifts the equilibrium towards :-
A. Right B. Left
C. Up D. Down

1266. Phenolphthalein shows the color changes in :-
A. Alkalis B. Water
C. Acids D. Salt solution

1267. Color of dyes changes over a specific pH range is :-
A. Acid-Base indicator B. Reactant
C. Catalyst D. Product

1268. The substances which can also act like acid or base are termed as :-
A. Base B. Amorphous
C. Amphoteric D. Alkalis

1269. Non aqueous titration can be done for :-
A. Water insoluble drugs
B. Weakly acidic drug
C. Weakly basic drug
D. All of the above

1270. Which is the aprotic solvent from the following :-
A. Chloroform B. Benzene
C. Both A & B D. None of the above

1271. Which one is protogenic solvent :-
A. Sulphuric acid B. Hydrochloric acid
C. Nitric acid D. All of the above

1272. Which one is protophillic solvent :-
A. Sodium hydroxide
B. Sodium methoxido
C. Lithium methoxide
D. All of the above

1273. Which one from the following is useful in non aqueous titration :-
A. Differentiating solvent
B. Levelling solvent
C. Both A & B
D. None of the above

1274. Water may intervension with non aqueous titration by :-
A. Acting as strong base than the weakly acidic drug
B. Acting as strong acid than the weakly acidic drug
C. Both A & B
D. None of the above

1275. Standardization of perchloric acid can be done by using :-

A. Oxalic acid

B. Tartaric acid

C. Benzoic acid

D. Pottasium hydrogen pthalate

1276. For the titration of halogen acid if salt of weak bases, which one from the following is added :-

A. Lead acetate B. Mercuric acetate

C. Bismuth iodide D. Copper sulphate

1277. From the following, Which is used as a non aqueous titration indicator

A. Crystal violet B. Thymol blue

C. Oracet blue B D. All of the above

1278. If both the acid and base are strong electrolytes, the solution at the end point will be neutral

A. True B. False

1279. The exact pH of solution at the equivalence point can be calculated from ionization constant of :-

A. Weak acid Or weak base

B. Concentration of solution

C. Both A & B

D. None of the above

1280. For any actual titration, the correct end point will be characterized by a definite value of the concentration of :-

A. Hydrogen ion B. Titrant

C. Titrand D. None of the above

1281. The first theory of indicator action was suggested by :-

A. Arrhenius B. Bonsted - Lowry

C. W. Ostwald D. Volhard

1282. The first theory of indicator action was based on the concept of :-

A. Very weak organic acid indicators

B. Very weak bases

C. Both A & B

D. Concentration of solution

1283. What will be the equivalence point of salt solution after hydrolysis :-

A. Slightly alkaline & acidic

B. Slightly acidic

C. Slightly basic

D. Strongly acidic

1284. The exact pH of the solution at the equivalence point can be calculated from:-

A. Ionization constant of weak acid

B. Ionization constant of weak base

C. Concentration of solution

D. All of the above

1285. For any actual titration the correct end point is characterized by a definite value of hydrogen ion concentration, which depends on the :-

A. Nature of acid

B. Nature of base

C. Concentration of solution

D. All of the above

1286. Benzalkonium chloride is categorise as

A. Acidic preservative

B. Mercurial preservative

C. Neutral preservative

D. Quaternary ammonium compound

1287. Pure water contains: -

A. Hydronium ions only

B. Water molecules only

C. Hydroxide ions only

D. All of the above

1288. What if (H30+) of a solution is less than (-OH) , the solution is :-

A. Always acidic

B. Always basic

C. Always neutral

D. Might be acidic basic or neutral

1289. The pH scale in general used ranges from:-

A. 0-1 B. 0-7

C. 0-14 D. 1-7

1290. KOH can be classified in the below equation as :-

KOH(aq.) -------→K+(aq.) + OH-(aq.)

A. Strong acid B. Weak acid

C. Strong base D. Weak base

1291. pH of buffer solution depends upon the concentration of :-

A. Acid B. Conjugate base

C. Salt D. Both A & B

1292. Carminic acid gives purple color with
A. Acid B. Alkali
C. Weak acid D. All of them

1293. pH can be kept constant with the help of :-
A. Buffer solution
B. Super saturated solution
C. Saturated solution
D. Unsaturated solution

1294. Addition of acid to indicator creates the equilibrium towards :-
A. Left B. Right
C. Up D. Down

1295. Phenolptheline shows the change of color in :-
A. Alkalis B. Water
C. Acid D. Salt solution

1296. The exact pH of the solution at theequivalence point can be calculated from :-
A. Ionization constant of weak base
B. Ionization constant of weak acid
C. Concentration of solution
D. All of the above

1297. If the Solute is in high concentration, then the solution is :-
A. Highly concentrated
B. Low concentrated
C. High temperature
D. Low temperature

1298. For any actual titration the correct end point will be characterized by definite value of H+ ion concentration of the solution, which depends upon the :-
A. Nature of acid & base
B. Concentration of solution
C. Indicators used
D. Both A & B

1299. Which substances changes colour according to hydrogen ion concentration of the solution :-
A. Redox indicators
B. Complexometric indicators
C. Acid-Base indicators
D. Aqueous indicators

1300. The observed colour of an indicator in solution is determined by the ratio of the concentration of the acidic & basic forms:-
A. True B. False

1301. The pH of solution will depends upon the :-
A. Indicator added to it
B. Acidity of solution
C. Nature of solution
D. Strength of solution

1302. The ionic strength of solution is related to:-
A. The activity coefficient
B. Nature of solution
C. Concentration of solution
D. partition coefficient

1303. When making colour comparison for the determination of pH of solution, the condition between two solutions will be :-
A. Indicator concentration should be same
B. Ionic strength should be equal
C. Both A & B
D. None of the above

1304. What should be the colour range of indicator (methyl orange)
A. 2.9 - 4.6 B. 3.0 - 5.0
C. 4.2 - 6.3 D. 1.2 - 2.8

1305. What should be the colour of phenolphthalein in acid solution :-
A. Red B. Yellow
C. Blue D. Colourless

1306. 1-carboxybenzeneazodimethylaniline is the chemical name of :-
A. Methyl red B. Ethyl red
C. Ethyl orange D. Phenolphthalein

1307. ethyl red shows which colour in alkaline solution :-
A. Red B. Orange
C. Yellow D. Blue

1308. Which indicator is available either as free acid or as the sodium salt :-
A. Methyl red
B. Quinaldine red
C. Phenolphthalein
D. Methyl orange

1309. Sulphonphthaleins are usually suplied in acid form :-

A. True B. False

1310. Quinaldine red indicator is prepared by dissolving 1g. in .... Of 80% ethanol

A. 100ml B. 10ml
C. 50ml D. 25ml

1311. Which type of indicator is used to have a sharp colour change over a narrow & selected range of pH :-

A. screened indicators
B. Natural indicators
C. Mixed indicators
D. pH indicators

1312. The colour change of a single indicator may also be imlroved by the addition of a pH sensitive dyestuff.

A. True B. False

1313. The neutralisation processes can be understood by studying the changes in the :-

A. Hydrogen ion concentration
B. Hydroxide ion concentration
C. Hydronium ion concentration
D. None of the above

1314. The neutralisation curve is obtained by plotting pH against the :-

A. Concentration of solution
B. Indicators added
C. Percentage of acid neutralized
D. Strength of solution

1315. Precipitation curve can be evaluated by determining the pH at various stages during the titration using :-

A. Potentiometric method
B. Redox method
C. Complexometric method
D. Neutralisation method

1316. In which type of titration the analyte displaces a reagent , usually from a complex, & the amount of displaced reagent is determined by appropriate titration :-

A. Potentiometric titration
B. Displacement titration
C. Redox titration
D. Complexometric titration

1317. Displacement titration of hydrolysed salts is the titration of :-

A. Weak base with strong acid
B. Weak acid with weak base
C. Strong acid with strong base
D. Strong acid with neutral solution

1318. Which acid behaves as monoprotic acid in titration :-

A. Hydrochloric acid B. Sulphuric acid
C. Boric acid D. Perchloric acid

1319. The solvents include those substances which may be considered chemically neutral & virtually unreactive under the conditions are :-

A. Aprotic solvents
B. Protogenic solvents
C. Protophillic solvents
D. Amphiprotic solvents

1320. Carbon tetrachloride & toluene are the examples of :-

A. Protophillic solvents
B. Amphiprotic solvents
C. Aprotic solvents
D. Protogenic solvents

1321. . ... Are the solvents include those substances which posseses high affinity for electrons :-

A. Aprotic solvents
B. Amphiprotic solvents
C. Protogenic solvents
D. Protophillic solvents

1322. Which of the following solvents are used for the non aqueous titration:-

A. Glacial ethanoic acid
B. Acetonitrile
C. Alcohols
D. All of the above

1323. Which of the following are the indicators used in non aqueous titration :-

A. Crystal violet B. Methyl red
C. Thymol blue D. All of the above

1324. In Precipitation titration which reagent is used as the reagent :-

A. Silver nitrate
B. Ammonium purpurate
C. Sulphuric acid
D. Hydrochloric acid

1325. Precipitation titration can also be termed as :-
A. Coulometry
B. Spectrophotometric titration
C. EDTA Titration
D. Argentimetric titration

1326. Determination of end point in precipitation titration is evaluated by
A. Mohrs procedure
B. Kjeldahls method
C. Volhards method
D. None of the above

1327. In precipitation titration, formation of a soluble coloured compound is examplified by :-
A. Kjeldahls method
B. Mohrs procedure
C. Volhards method
D. Both A & B

1328. Precipitation titration is carried out for the determination of :-
A. Chlorides B. Bromides
C. Iodides D. All of the above

1329. In which type of titration, adsorption indicators are used :-
A. Precipitation titration
B. Complexometric titration
C. Redox titration
D. Acid-Base titration

1330. Fluorescein is the .... Indicator
A. Metal-Ion
B. Mixed indicators
C. Adsorption indicators
D. Acid-Base indicators

1331. Which are the adsorption indicators from the above :-
A. Fluorescein
B. Tartrazine
C. Dichlorofluorescein
D.All of the above

1332. The Ksp of CaF2 is 4.2×10-^{11} in pure water. In acidic solution the solubility of CaF2 is expected to :-
A. Increase because Ca^{2+} ion is acidic
B. Decrease because Ca^{2+} ion is acidic
C. Increase because F- ion is basic
D. Decrease because F- ion is basic

1333. A solution is known to contain ions of Ag^+, Cu^{2+} & Pb^{2+}. What will happen when 1.0M HCL is added to the solution.
A. No precipitate will form
B. Only AgCl will precipitate
C. Both AgCl & $PbCl^2$ will precipitate
D. All 3 ions will form precipitate

1334. Which has the greater molar solubility in water at 25· C.
A. Ammonium nitrate
B. Barium sulphate
C. Copper(2) phosphate
D. Lead(2) carbonate

1335. When mixed, which pair of aqueous solution will form precipitate :-
A. KNO^3 & $CaBr^2$
B. $NaNO^3$ & (NH^4) ^{2}
C. K2SO^4& (NH^4) ^{2}S
D. $CaCl^2$ & K^2CO^3

1336. Which of the following statement about Mohr's method is incorrect:-
A. The pH of the reaction mixture should not be too high to prevent the formation of undesirable precipitates
B. The pH of the reaction mixture should not be too low to prevent the conversion of chromate ions to dichromate ions
C. This method is used to determine the concentration of chloride ions in a water sample
D. A bluish-green precipitate can be observed at the end point of the titration

1337. Which of the following substances does not form a precipitate with silver ions
A. Hydrochloric acid
B. Sulphuric acid
C. Pottasium nitrate
D. Sodium bromide

1338. Which of the following statements are correct :-
A. A specific volume of analyte is transferred into a conical flask for titration by a pipette
B. The titrant is run from the burette into the conical flask

C. Precipitation titration is a type of volumetric analysis.
D. All of the above

1339. The solubility of the precipitate will .... With decreasing the temperature.
A. Increase
B. Decrease
C. No effect
D. Initially decreases then increase

1340. What will be the effect on solubility of the precipitate if pH is decreased when anion of the salt is the conjugate of weak acid
A. Increase
B. Decrease
C. No effect
D. Initially decrease then increase

1341. In titration of chloride ions with silver nitrate solution, ... Is used to serve as indicator.
A. Methyl orange
B. Tartrazine
C. Pottasium chromate
D. Phenolphthalein

1342. At the end point in the titration of chloride ions with silver nitrate solution, the chromate ions combine with silver ions to form :-
A. Silver dichromate
B. Silver chromate
C. silver nitrite
D. None of the above

1343. The silver chromate , obtained from the titration of chloride ions with silver nitrate is :-
A. Insoluble
B. Partially soluble
C. Completely soluble
D. Sparingly soluble

1344. The solubility of product of silver chromate increases with :-
A. Decreasing temperature
B. Increasing temperature
C. Increasing acidity of solution
D. Decreasing acidity of solution

1345. The precipitation titration should be performed in the condition of :-
A. High temperature
B. Low temperature
C. Room temperature
D. All of the above

1346. In precipitation titration, By using a mixture of .... & .... such as to give a neutral solution, the danger of raising the pH of unbuffered solution beyond the limits is minimised
A. Pottasium chromate & pottasium dichromate
B. Silver chromate & silver nitrate
C. Silver hydroxide & pottasium chromate
D. Pottasium dichromate & silver nitrate

1347. In precipitation titration, the formation of a soluble coloured compound is examplified by the :-
A. Kjeldahls procedure
B. Mohr's method
C. Volhard's procedure
D. Arrhenius theory

1348. Volhard's method is used for the titration of :-
A. Silver B. Iron
C. Magnesium D. Gold

1349. Volhard's method for the titration of silver in the presence of :-
A. Free nitric acid
B. Standard pottasium thiocyanate
C. Ammonium thiocyanate
D. All of the above

1350. Volhard's method can be used in the determination of .... In acid solution:-
A. Bromides B. Iodides
C. Chlorides D. All of the above

1351. Fluorescein & dichlorofluorescein (adsorption indicators) are suitable for the titration of :-
A. Chlorides B. Nitrates
C. Iron D. Calcium

1352. Determination of chlorides are carried out in :-
A. Acidic Solution
B. Basic solution
C. Neutral solution
D. All of the above

1353. Determination of bromide can be done by using :-
A. Volhard's method
B. Mohr's titration
C. Kjeldahls method
D. Ostwald's method

1354. Most suitable adsorption indicator for the titration of bromide is :-
A. Phenolphthalein
B. Dichlorofluorescein
C. Fluorescein
D. Eosin

1355. Because of adsorption phenomena, the mohr's method cannot be applied to the titration of :-
A. Iodides B. Bromides
C. Chlorides D. Thiocyanates

1356. Because of distinguishing the colour change of pottasium chromate & adsorption phenomena, which is the suitable adsorption indicator:-
A. Fluorescein B. Dichlorofluorescein
C. Eosin D. All of the above

1357. Determination of silver in dil. Nitric acid solution by titration with std. Thiocyanate solution is done in the presnnce of :-
A. Iron(3) B. Nickel
C. Magnesium D. Sulphur

1358. What should be the temperature during the Determination of silver in dil. Nitric acid solution by titration with std. Thiocyanate solution
A. 25· C B. 35·C
C. 40·C D. 45·C

1359. Name the anions whose silver salts are slightly soluble in water but soluble in nitric acid :-
A. Phosphate B. Chromate
C. Arsenate D. All of the above

1360. In precipitation titration, theinstruments are used for determination purpose are :-
A. Potentiometry B. Amperometry
C. Coulometry D. All of the above

1361. Which methods are particularly useful for titrating mixtures of halides with silver nitrate.
A. Iodimetry B. Potentiometry
C. Amperometry D. None of the above

1362. OXIDATION-REDUCTION TITRATION

If acidified pottasium dichromate (K2Cr2O7) acts as an oxidizing agent, colour changes from:-
A. Orange to red B. Orange to green
C. Yellow to red D. Yellow to green

1363. In acidified solution of pottasium dichromate (K2Cr2O7), dichromate ion become reduced to :-
A. Chromate (5) ions
B. Chromium (3) ions
C. Chromium (2) ions
D. Chromium (4) ions

1364. Oxidation involves :-
A. Loss of hydrogen B. Loss of oxygen
C. Gain of electron D. Gain of hydrogen

1365. In a reaction between CuSo4(s) & Zn(s)
A. Zinc experiences an increase in the oxidation state
B. CuSo4 undergoes oxidation
C. Zn undergoes oxidation
D. All of the above

1366. Oxidizing agents are :-
A. Mostly non metals
B. Mostly metals
C. Decrease in transition state
D. Mostly transition metals

1367. In copper oxide (CuO) & carbon monoxide (CO) reaction, reducing agent is :-
A. CuO B. CO
C. CO2 D. Cu

1368. Upon oxidation of acidified pottasium magnet, purple colour of magnese :-
A. Stays B. Changes to pink
C. Changes to blue D. Become colourless

1369. Hydrogen acts as a reducing agent,

A. By taking oxygen
B. By giving electrons
C. By taking hydrogen
D. Both A & B

1370. Reduction involves :-

A. Loss of electrons
B. Gain in hydrogen
C. Gain in oxygen
D. Loss of oxygen

1371. Oxidizing agents does not include :-

A. Pottasium iodide
B. Pottasium chromate
C. Pottasium dichromate
D. Bromine solution

1372. An oxidant :-

A. Gives oxygen B. Accepts electrons
C. Gives hydrogen D. Both A & B

1373. While pottasium iodide (KI) is a powerful reducing agent:-

A. The iodide ion is oxidized to iodine
B. The iodide ion is reduced to iodine
C. The iodine ion is reduced to iodide
D. The iodine ion is oxidized to iodide

1374. While iodide ion (I-) oxidizes to iodine (I2) , a change in colour from colourless to :-

A. Brown B. Pink
C. Blue D. Violet

1375. Oxidation is reffered to as :-

A. Combustion B. Respiration
C. Transpiration D. Both A & B

1376. While passing hydrogen over heated CuO(s) black colour is oxidized to :-

A. Golden colour B. Pink colour
C. Blue colour D. Colourless

1377. What procedures should be carried out to determine the titration error in Oxidation-Reduction titration :-

A. Change in ionic charge
B. Change in Cationic charge
C. Change in electrodes
D. Change in solution

1378. Potassium permanganate is not :-

A. Secondary standard
B. Primary standard
C. Both A & B
D. None of the above

1379. Reducing substances (traces of organic matter) which will react with potassium permanganate to form :-

A. Hydrogen peroxide
B. Pottasium dichromate
C. Sodium oxalate
D. Manganese dioxide

1380. Permanganate is inherently unstable in :-

A. The presence of potassium
B. The absence of potassium ions
C. The absence of manganese ions
D. The presence of manganese ions

1381. The presence of manganese dioxide catalyses the .... Of the permanganate solution.

A. Auto decomposition
B. Preservation
C. Purity
D. None of the above

1382. Acidic & alkaline solutions are .... Than neutral solution :-

A. Less stable B. More stable
C. Unstable D. Concentrated

1383. Potassium permanganate can be stored in:-

A. Transparent polybags
B. Ampules
C. Dark coloured bottles
D. All of the above

1384. Hydrogen peroxide is usually available in the form of aqueous solution containing how much amount of hydrogen peroxide :-

A. 7%, 5%, 9%
B. 6%, 10%, 20%
C. 10%, 15%, 16%
D. 6%, 12%, 30%

1385. One of the good example of self indicating reagent is :-

A. Phenylanthranilic acid
B. Diphenylamine
C. Potassium permanganate
D. Methylene blue

1386. Standard solutions of exactly known concentration can be prepared by weighing out the pure dry salt by dissolving it in the proper volume of water.

A. True B. False

1387. Pottasium dichromate is powerful oxidizing agent as compared to potassium permanganate :-

A. True B. False

1388. Pottasium dichromate is used only in :-

A. Acidic solution B. Alkaline solution
C. Neutral Solution D. Both A & B

1389. Determination of iron in iron ores are followed by using :-

A. Pottasium chromate
B. Potassium permanganate
C. Potassium dichromate
D. Hydrogen peroxide

1390. Chemical oxygen demand (COD) is expressed in terms of :-

A. Mg. Of oxygen required per litre of water
B. Mg of oxygen required per gm. of water
C. Gm. of oxygen required per litre of solution
D. Mg. Of water required per litre of oxygen

1391. Cerium (4) sulphate is powerful .... agent :-

A. Oxidizing B. Reducing
C. Neutral D. None of the above

1392. Cerium sulhate can be used only in :-

A. Basic solution B. Neutral solution
C. Indicators D. Acidic solution

1393. Cerium (4) sulphate may be used to determine reducing agents in the presence of :-

A. High concentration of sulphuric acid
B. High concentration of hydrochloric acid
C. Low concentration of sulphuric acid
D. Low concentration of hydrochloric acid

1394. Cerium(4) sulphate is used to determine reducing agents in the presence of :-

A. High concentration of hydrochloric acid
B. High concentration of sulphuric acid
C. Low concentration of hydrochloric acid
D. Low concentration of sulphuric acid

1395. Direct titration with cerium(4) sulphate in a dilute HCl medium for iron(2) can accurately performed at :-

A. 70'C
B. 65'C
C. Room temperature
D. 58'C

1396. Solution of cerium(4) sulphate may be prepared by dissolving cerium(4) sulphate Or the more soluble ammonium cerium(4) sulphate in :-

A. Dilute (0.6-1.0M) hydrochloric acid
B. Dilute (0.5 - 1.0M) sulphuric acid
C. Conc. (0.5-1.0M) sulphuric acid
D. Conc. (0.5 - 1.0M)hydrochloric acid

1397. In oxidation-reduction titration, which indicators are used to determine copper in brass :-

A. Ferroin
B. N-phenylanthranilic acid
C. Both A & B
D. None of the above

1398. At which pH values, arsenite can be titrated with iodine solution:-

A. Between 4 & 9 B. Between 5 - 10
C. Below 5 D. Above 10

1399. In which type of solutions, arsenate is reduced to arsenite :-

A. Alkaline solution
B. Strongly acid solution
C. Neutral solution
D. Weak acidic solution

1400. The titration with standard solution of iodine can also be termed as :-

A. Potentiometry B. Redox titration
C. Iodimetry D. Complexometry

1401. The titration deals with the iodine liberated in chemical reactions can be termed as :-

A. Iodimetry B. Iodometry
C. Complexometry D. Potentiometry

1402. The titration deals with the standard solution of iodine can be termed as :-

A. Complexometry B. Iodometry
C. Potentiometry D. Iodimetry

1403. In iodometric titration, the tri-iodide ion is formed when :-

A. The excess of iodine ion is present
B. The excess of iodide ion is formed
C. The excess of potassium iodide is present
D. The iodine ion is absent

1404. Which are the stronger oxidizing agents than iodine or tri-iodide ions :-

A. Potassium permanganate
B. Potassium dichromate
C. Cerium (4) sulphate
D. All of the above

1405. In iodimetry, the solution for titration is used :-

A. Iodine in pottasium dichromate
B. Iodine in potassium permanganate
C. Iodine in potassium iodide
D. None of the above

1406. Which theory is not good for nonprotonic solvents

A. Lowery bronsted theory
B. Lewis's theory
C. Usanovich theory
D. Lux flood concept

1407. According to Lewis's theory acid is:-

A. Electron pair donor
B. Electron pair acceptor
C. Yield a proton
D. Accept a proton

1408. According to Lewis's theory when neutralization occurs which type of bond produces:-

A. Ionic bond
B. Non ionic bond
C. Coordinat covalent bond
D. All of above

1409. According to usanovich theory what is base

A. Which give anions
B. Which give electrons
C. Which combines with cation
D. All of above

1410. Which titration is done to obtain pure product

A. Gravimetry B. Acid base titration
C. Redox titration D. Complexometri

1411. which one is used to determine tha final weight of product in gravimetry

A. Solvent extraction
B. Ignition
C. Volatilization D. All of above

1412. Wahi is the theory of gravimetry analysis:-

A. Law of mass action
B. Solubility product
C. Common ion effect
D. All of above

1413. The rate of reaction of is directly proportional to the product of molecular Concentration is said by:-

A. Principal of Solubility product
B. Law of mass action
C. Common ion effect
D. All of above

1414. In gravimetry analysis the principal of Solubility product is applicable to:-

A. Occurrence of precipitation
B. Prevention of precipitation
C. Dissolution of a substance
D. All of above

1415. Which one is a solubility product of aluminium hydroxide:-

A. 1.1 × 10 -33 B. 1×10-33
C. 8.8×10-5 D. 1.1×10-5

1416. 1×10-50 is the solubility product of

A. Barium sulfate B. Lead sulfate
C. Mercuric sulfide D. Calcium oxalate

1417. The molar mass of a compound CH2O is 180 gm per mol -1 so what is the molecular formula of that particular compound:-

A. CH2O B. C6H12O6
C. C5H10O5 D. C3H6O3

1418. What will be precipitate obtain after the reaction of magnesium chloride and silver nitrate:-

A. Mgcl2 B. Agcl
C. Mgno3 D. AgNo3

1419. Which one is not able to react or form precipitate in gravimetry analysis because of low stability :-

A. S ilver nitrate B. Silver chloride
C. Sodium nitrate D. Sodium chloride

1420. What is the type of precipitate
A. Crystalline B. Curdy
C. Gelatinous D. All of above

1421. What is the reason of the formation of crystalline precipitate:-
A. Composition of salt
B. Aggregate of small porous particles
C. Jelly like consistancy
D. All of above

1422. Which type of precipitate is formed by the aggregates of small porous particles:-
A. Gelatinous B. Curdy
C. Crystalline D. All of above

1423. What is the characteristics of a precipitate form:-
A. Low Solubility
B. Form large precipitate
C. Easily convert into weighed form
D. All of above

1424. What should be characteristics of weighed form:-
A. Have adequate stability
B. Coincide with chemical formula
C. Error should be less
D. All of above

1425. The process used for converting the colloidal suspension into filterable mass is called:-
A. Agglomeration B. Acid base titration
C. Mohars titration D. None of above

1426. What is the particle size range of colloidal suspension:-
A. 0.1mue to 0.2mue
B. 0.1mue to 1 mue
C. 0.1 mue to 0.5 mue
D. 0.1 mue to 10mue

1427. The stability of colloidal suspension is because of:-
A. Adsorption or anion or cation on surface of particles
B. Absorption of cations or anion on the surface of particles
C. Both
D. None

1428. The ultra microscopy of colloidal suspension is based on:-
A. Particle size B. Tyndal effect
C. Temperature D. None of above

1429. The viscous jelly like colloids are called
A. Lyophobic colloids B. Lyophilic colloids
C. Emulsoids D. Both B and C

1430. Which one is an example of lyophobic colloids
A. Gold B. Silver
C. Iron D. Copper

1431. Coagulation of colloids is done by:-
A. Heating with stirring
B. Increase concentration of electrolyte added
C. Both
D. None

1432. Wich one is more difficult to coagulate:-
A. Emulsoids B. Suspensoids
C. Both D. None

1433. The production of large crystals from small crystal by mother liquor is called:-
A. Post precipitation B. Digestion
C. Occlusion D. None of above

1434. The precipitation should be carried out in
A. Hot solutions B. Cold solution
C. Normal solution D. All of above

1435. Which one is a fast speed filter paper
A. No. 31 B. No. 30
C. No. 32 D. No 40

1436. No 52 whatman filter paper is of type
A. Fast speed B. Medium speed
C. Slow speed D. All of above

1437. For the filtration of gelatinous precipitates which one is used:-
A. Normal filter paper
B. What man filter paper
C. Filter pulp
D. Filter mates

1438. Gooch crucible is made up of
A. Asbestos B. Silika
C. Porcelain D. All of above

1439. What is the pore size of G2 type sintered glass crucible:-

A. 100-120 microns
B. 40-50 microns
C. 5-10 microns
D. 20-30 microns

1440. Which one of sintered glass crucible have pore size 5-10 microns:

A. G1 B. G2
C. G3 D. G4

1441. If the drying of precipitate is done on temperature above 200•c than which one is used

A. Silica crucible
B. Glass fiber disk
C. Sintered glass crucible
D. Munroe crucible

1442. When lead sulfate precipitates washed by sulfuric acid than what is sulfuric acid

A. Electrolyte B. Precipitant
C. Both D. None

1443. In the precipitation titration of picric acid and piperazine phosphate which one is a analyte

A. Barium sulfate B. Picric acid
C. Piperazine phosphate D. All of above

1444. In the precipitation titration of barium sulfate and potassium dichromate which one is a precipitant

A. Picric acid
B. Potassium dichromate
C. Thiacetazone
D. Barium sulfate

1445. Which solution in iodometric titration is used to determine the acid content of solutions iodometrically Or in the standardisation of solutions of strong acid:-

A. Standard solution of iodine
B. Potassium iodate solution
C. Potassium iodide solution
D. Potassium dichromate solution

1446. Which solution is used as the source of known quantity of iodine in iodometric titration:-

A. Potassium dichromate solution
B. Potassium iodate solution
C. Potassium iodide y
D. Standard solution of iodine

1447. POTENTIOMETRIC TITRATI What is the potential of a substance :-

A. Redox potential
B. Reduction potential
C. Oxidation potential
D. Both A & B

1448. Which one have a tendency to accept electrons :-

A. Iron B. Copper(2) +
C. Nickel D. Cobalt

1449. What is used for electroanalytical chemistry

A. Amperometry B. Acid - base titration
C. Potentiometry D. None of the above

1450. Which one of these is used to make salt bridge in potentiometric titration:-

A. NaCl B. KCl
C. MgCl D. NaOH

1451. Which one of these is important part of potentiometry :-

A. Formation of salt bridge
B. Analytical solution
C. Electrodes
D. All of the above

1452. Which one has relationship between potential & .... Of solution :-

A. Electric current B. Charge
C. PH D. None of the above

1453. Which one is a reference elctrode as well as an indicator :-

A. Calomel electrode
B. Hydrogen electrode
C. Both A & B
D. None of the above

1454. Platinum is used with which type of electrode :-

A. Acid - Base electrode
B. Redox electrode
C. Calomel electrode
D. Antimony electrode

1455. What is the main aim to put silver - silver nitrate electrode :-
A. Contains less toxicity
B. Thermally stable
C. Both A & B
D. None of the above

1456. Laws of positive charge is called as :-
A. Anionic reaction B. Cathodic reaction
C. Both A & B D. None of the above

1457. What happens when titrate is added with electrode in potentiometric titration
A. Change in electrode potential
B. Change in reaction time
C. Change in temperature
D. All of the above

1458. Which one not affects the reference electrode :-
A. Temperature
B. Composition of solution
C. Electric current
D. pH

1459. Electronic instruments are resistant to :-
A. Glass B. Metal
C. Organic matter D. All of the above

1460. Which one is the type of differential titrator :-
A. Simple titrator B. Compound titrator
C. Atomic titrator D. None of the above

1461. What is used to determine the end point in potentiometry :-
A. HCl B. EDTA
C. Copper D. Cadmium

1462. Which one of these has the zero electrode potential :-
A. Calomel B. Hydrogen
C. Antimony D. All if the above

1463. Which one of these is the combination electrode :-
A. Glass electrode
B. Metal electrode
C. Organic matter electrode
D. None of the above

1464. In a laboratory scale the use of potentiometry is :-
A. Determination of concentration
B. Saperation of liquids
C. Identification of compounds
D. Flow of current

1465. For which purpose the potentiometric titration is used in the field of characterization :-
A. Anions B. Cations
C. Acids D. Bases

1466. Which one is the indication of completion of potentiometric titration:-
A. Colour change
B. Precipitation formation
C. Complex formation
D. None of the above

1467. What is the location of junction potential :-
A. Electrodes B. Salt bridge
C. Analyte D. Solution

1468. What is the use of aluminium trioxide in a glass membrane electrode :-
A. As an analyte B. As a membrane
C. Indicator D. None of the above

1469. Which solution is filled in glass bulb of glass membrane electrode :-
A. NaCl B. NaOH solution
C. HCl D. HBr

1470. Which one acts as a key compound for calomel electrode :-
A. KBr. B. NH^4OH
C. KCl D. NaCl

1471. What is the use of silver chloride electrode:-
A. Determination of silver
B. Determination of chloride
C. Determination of silver chloride
D. Both A & B

1472. What is the use of hot chrome in the world of electrodes :-
A. To wash platinum electrode
B. To wash hydrogen electrode
C. For better reaction
D. All of the above

1473. The presence of .... Acts as drawback for electrodes:-

A. Complexing agents
B. Cations C. Anions
D. Oxidizing agents

1474. What is used with half cell electrode of calomel :-

A. Iron B. Copper
C. Mercury D. Platinum

1475. What temperature is related to normal hydrogen electrode:-

A. 25 B. 50
C. 75 D. 100

1476. The pH range of 3 to 8 is of :-

A. Antimony electrode
B. Platinum electrode
C. Pcalomel electrode
D. Hydrogen electrode

1477. What is the use of thin glass bulb electrode

A. Indicator electrode
B. Reference electrode
C. Normal electrode
D. All of the above

1478. The concentration of calcium oxide is .... for manufacturing of glass electrode :-

A. 2 B. 4
C. 6 D. 8

1479. Which state is not permitted for glass electrode :-

A. Cold state B. Dry state
C. Moisture state D. All of the above

1480. Silver sulphide is used in .... :-

A. Hydrogen electrode
B. Antimony electrode
C. Platinum electrode
D. Crystalline membrane electrode

1481. Calomel electrode is also called as :-

A. Liquid membrane electrode
B. Liquid-liquid electrode
C. Membrane-membrane electrode
D. All of the above

1482. What is the use of urease enzyme used in urea electrode :-

A. Hydrolysis B. Oxidation
C. Rensidification D. Reduction

1483. Which one is not a type of enzyme based electrode :-

A. Urea electrode B. Penicillin electrode
C. Urease electrode D. Hydrogen electrode

1484. Which one of electrode used CO2 & No2 as analyte:-

A. Glass electrode
B. Calomel electrode
C. Platinum electrode
D. Gas sensing electrode

1485. Poggendoffs competition method is used to measure :-

A. Concentration of analyte
B. Concentration of solution
C. EMF of cell
D. All of the above

1486. The pH of glass electrode is depends on temperature, is said by :-

A. Dragondoff B. Nernst
C. Mohr D. Poggendoff

1487. In potentiometric titration, the initial concentration of test solution is determined by :-

A. Nernst equation
B. Grans plot
C. Oxidation number
D. Reduction number

1488. Two identical pure platinum wires is used for :-

A. Bi-metallic System
B. Tri-metallic system
C. Tetra-metallic system
D. None of the above

1489. Direct potentiometry used two electrodes to determine :-

A. Concentration gradiant
B. Endpoit
C. EMF
D. Al of the above

1490. Tungsten is not used in .... type of potentiometry

A. Redox titration
B. Acid-Base titration
C. Complexometric titration
D. Precipitation titration

1491. What happens when the change in EMF in polarized electrode :-
A. Increased current
B. Decreased current
C. Constant current
D. None of the above

1492. What is the resistance of glass membrane of glass electrode :-
A. High B. Low
C. Constant D. None of the above

1493. Which electrode has low divalent ions than hydrogen ions :-
A. Hydrogen electrode
B. Glass membrane electrode
C. Calomel electrode
D. Platinum electrode

1494. Nernst given the relation between .... :-
A. Concentration
B. Temperature
C. Potential of solution
D.All of the above

1495. When the rate of change of potential is maximum, it shows the end point of ....:-
A. Acid-Base titration
B. Potentiometry
C. Gravimetric titration
D. Complexometric titration

1496. Accuracy based titration is :-
A. Acid base titration
B. Redox titration
C. Complexometric titration
D. Potentiometry

1497. Calomel electrode is not a .... :-
A. Indicator electrode
B. Reference electrode
C. Both A & B
D. None of the above

1498. In potentiometric titration, the curve is plotted between potential & .... ?
A. Current B. Volume
C. Potential D. Temperature

1499. Nernst equation is related to :-
A. Potential B. Concentration
C. Current D. Voltage

1500. In Complexometric titration which type of electrode is used
A. Hydrogen B. Antimony
C. Platinum D. Mercury

1501. Mercurus sulfate electrode is used to determine the compounds like :-
A. Aromatic B. Hydrocarbons
C. Halides D. Volatiles

1502. Precipitation is the formation of ?
A. Crystals in solution
B. Solid in solution
C. Both a) & b)
D. None of them

1503. Which indicator is most commonly used in precipitationtitration ?
A. Silver nitrate B. Phenopthalin
C. methyl orange D. None of the above

1504.Precipitation is type of process -
A. Ionic B. Non-ionic
C. reduction D. Oxidation

1505. According to end point detection method , procedure are widely used in precipitation titration
A. Mohrs method B. Volhard method
C. Fajans method D. All of the above

1506. Indicator used in Mohrs method
A. Chromate B. Methyl blue
C. Both a) & b) D. None of the above

1507. Which method is used in water analysis ?
A. Fajan's method B. Mohr's method
C. Volhard's method D. None of these

1508. Which method is based on precipitaion of absorption indicator ?
A. Fajan's method B. Mohr's method
C. Volhard's method D. None of these

1509. Absorption indicator works best when :
A. They do not precipitate out silver ion when the indicators are at low temperature
B. They bind to the precipitate only when excess silver ion is present to produce colour
C. Both a) & b)
D. None of these

1510. Halides can be determined by titrating with AgNo3 using which indicator :

A. Na2CrO4 B. Saffranin
C. KmNo4 D. Phenolphthaelin

1511. Precipitation titration is also called :

A. Argentometric titration
B. Potentiometric
C. Redox titration
D. None of the above

1512. In precipitation titration :

A. The reaction is fast and stoichiometry is known
B. The reaction is slow and stoichometery is unknown
C. The reaction is fast but stoichiometry is unknown
D. None of these

1513. Diffrence between the titration curve of precipitation reaction and strong acid and bases reaction is :

A. We put solubility product of precipitate instead of the ionic product of water
B. The curve is same
C. None of them

1514. (NaCl + AgNO3 -› AgCl + NaNO3)in this reaction which one is precipitating agent and which one is analyte :

A. Ag+ is analyte and Cl- is precipitating agent
B. Ag+ and Cl- both are analyte
C. Ag+ and Cl- b oth are precipitating agent
D. Ag+ is precipitaing agent and Cl- is analyte

1515. What is neccessary to form precipitate :

A. Cation or anion B. Cation or cation
C. Anion or anion D. None of them

1516. What are basic requirment of a precipitation reaction useful in titrimetric analysis :

A. The precipitate must be practically insoluble
B. The reaction should be rapid
C. The equilance point or end point must be possible to detect during the titration
D. All of the above

1517. Which one is not the limtation in precipitation titration :

A. Only few number of ions such as halide ions can be titrated by the precipitation titration
B. Co-precipitated may be occured
C. Slow rate of reaction
D. None of them

1518. In any system in which a solid is in equiibrium with its solution , how will you determine the product of ion cocentration:

A. By Solubility product
B. By concentration of solid
C. Both A) & B)
D. None of them

1519. When a precipitating reagent is added to solution containing two aninons , both of which form slight soluble salts with the same cation e.g. when silver nitrate is added to a soution containing both chloride and iodide . Than which salt will precipitate first :

A. AgCl will be precipitate first
B. AgI will be precipitate first
C. Both will precipitate at the same time
D. Both will not precipitate

1520. When AgNo3 is added to the solution of either Nacl which colour precipitate will be form :

A. White
B. Blue
C. Greyish
D. No precipitate will form

1521. Why precipitation titration use is limited :

A. Lack of suitable indicators to detect endpoint
B. Slow rate of reaction
C. Both of them
D. None of the above

1522. Which drug is titrated by the precipitation titration :

A. Aminophylline B. Theophylline
C. Barbiturate D. Heloperidone

1523. Dimenhydrinate is determined by which titration :

A. Acid- base titration
B. Oxidation - reduction titration
C. Complexometric titration
D. Argentometric titration

1524. From following drug which is determind by Volhard's method :

A. Sodium chloride injection
B. Dextrose injection
C. Both of them
D. None of the above

1525. Phenylmercuric acetate is determined by :

A. Gay lussac method
B. Fajan's method
C. Volhard's method
D. Mohr's method

1526. Intraperitoneal dialysis fluid (for chloride) is determined by :

A. Gay lussac method
B. Fajan's method
C. Volhard's method
D. Mohr's method

1527. Which drug is not determined by precipitation titration :

A. Chlorpenothanne
B. Ethinamide
C. Aminophylline
D. Barbiturate

1528. Sodium chloride and Dextrose injection is determined by which method :

A. Mohr's method
B. Volhard's method
C. Gay lussac method
D. Fajan's method

1529. Chlorobutol is determined by which titration :

A. Precipitation titration
B. Acid base titration
C. redox titration
D. complexometric titration

1530. Dimenhydrinate is determied by which method :

A. Volhard's method
B. Fajan's method
C. Gay lussac method
D. Mohr's method

1531. Phenymercuric acetate is determined by which titration :

A. Argentometric titration
B. Complexometric titration
C. Acid-base titration
D. Redox titration

1532. In precipitation titration how end point is determined in Gay lussac method :

A. On the basis of turbidity
B. By addition of indicatior
C. Both a) & b)
D. None of the above

1533. Why potassium chromate is used as a indicator in precipitation titration :

A. Potassium chromate show turbidity in presence of excess silver ions
B. Postassium chromate turns red in the presence of excess silver ions
C. Potassium chromate show blue colour in presence of excess silver ions
D. None of the above

1534. Absorption indicator is used in titration :

A. Redox titration
B. Acid- base titration
C. Precipitation titration
D.None of them

1535. Which is the absorption indicator :

A. Fluorescein B. Eosin
C. Dichlorofluoresin D. All of the above

1536. What is the colur of potassium dichromate indicator :

A. Orage B. Red
C. Blue D. Green

1537. Determination of chlorides and bromides with standard mercurous perchlorate solution By using which indicator :

A. Bromophenol blue
B. Bromo cresol blue
C. Seffranin
D. Crystal green

1538. Titration of standardised AgNo3 Solution with potassium thiocynate solution . Name the method :

A. Mohr's method B. Volhard's method
C. Fajan's method D. Gay lussac method

1539. In ksp of CaF2 is 4.2 x 10-11 in pure water. In acidic solution the solubility of CaF2 is expected to :

A. Increase because the Ca2+ ion is acidic

B. Increase because the F+ ion is acidic
C. Decrease because the Ca2+ ion is acidic
D. Decrease beacuse the F+ ion is acidic

1540. A solution is known to contain Ag , Cu and Pb . What will when 0.1 M HCl is added to the solution :
A. No precipitate will form
B. Only AgCl will precipitate
C. Only AgCl and PbCl will precipitate
D. All ion will precipitate

1541. Which has a greatest solubility in water :
A. Ammonium Nitrate
B. Barium sulphate
C. Copper (II) phosphate
D. Lead (II) phosphate

1542. When mixed, Which pair of aqueous solutions will form precipitate :
A. KmNo3 and CaBr2
B. K2So4 and (NH4)2S
C. NaNO3 and (NH4)2 CO3
D. CaCl2 and K2Co3

1543. Which of the following statement about Mohr's method is incorrect :
A. The pH of the reaction mixture should not be too high to prevent the formation of undesirable precipitate
B. This method is used to determine the concentration of chloride ion in water sample
C. The pH of the reaction mixture should not be too low to prevent Conversion of chemistry ions into dichromate ions
D. The blueish-green colour is observed at the end-point

1544. Which of the following statemant is incorrect about Volhard's Method :
A. AIn this method AgNo3 is treated with potassium thiocynate solution
B. Bthe reddish -brown colour is obtain at the end point of titration
C. This method is carried out in HNO3 medium
D. None of them

1545. Which of the following statment about fajan's method is incorrect :
A. Fanjan's method uses adsobption indicator B. Fajan's method does not use Siver nitrate in its reaction
C. The end point is determined by the stoichiometric reaction of silver ion and chloride ion to form a colored adsorbed layer on the silver chloride precipitate
D. This method has helped in the quantitative determination of chloride ions in various sample solutions

1546. Which of the following substance does not form precipitate with Siver ion :
A. Hydrochrolic acid
B. Sulphuric acid
C. Potassium nitrate
D. Sodium bromide

1547. What reacts with silver nitrate to form white ppt :
A. Any chloride can react with the silver nitrate to form white ppt
B. Any bromide will reacts with silver nitrate to form white ppt
C. Both a & b
D. None of them

1548. What is the colour of silver bromide precipitate :
A. Yellow B. Green
C. Red D. Blue

1549. How do you pricipitate Silver silver nitrate:
A. By adding HCl in silver nitrate solution
B. By adding Nacl in silver nitrate solution
C. Both a & b
D. None of the above

1550. The solubility of the precipitate will ....with decreasing the temprature :
A. Increase
B. Intially increase and than decrease
C. Decrease
D. No effect

1551. What will be the effect on solubility of precipitate when pH is decreased when anion os the salt is the cojugate of weak acid :

A. Increase

B. Intially increase than decrease

C. Decrease

D. No effect

1552. Acid base titration is used for :

A. Determination of unknown concentration of acid

B. Determination of unknown concentaration of both

C. Detrmination of unknwon concentatration of Acid - base

D. To determine quality of acid - base

1553. Neutralization reaction in acid - base titration produce

A. Salt B. Neutralized base

C. Both a) & b) D. Sugar

1554. Who invented acid - base titration :

A. Karl fischer

B. Svante arrhnius

C. George Ernst Stahl

D. None of them

1555. In acid-base titration at equvilance point :

A. Numbers of moles of OH ions and numbers of moles of H ions are equal

B. Numbers of moles of OH ions are greator than H+ ions

C. Number of moles of OH ions are lesser than numbers of moles of H+ ions

D. Both a) & b)

1556. Gram equivalent of a substance is :

A. Number of grams of reagent which in reaction corresponds to a gram- atom or gram-ion (1.008) of hydrogen

B. Number of grams of reagent which in a given reaction corresponds to a gram-atom or gram-ion (1.1) of hydrogen

C. Number of grams of reagent which in a reaction corresponds to a gram-atom or gram-ion(2.0) of hydrogen

D. None of them

1557. An acid whose molecule contains only one replaceble hydrogen is called :

A. Dibasic acid B. Monobasic acid

C. Both of them D. none of them

1558. Acetic acid is :

A. Monobasic acid B. Dibasic acid

C. Tribasic acid D. None of them

1559. H2CO3 is :

A. Monobasic acid B. Dibasic acid

C. Tribasic acid D. None of the above

1560. HClO4 is :

A. Dibasic acid B. Tribasic acid

C. Monobasic acid D. None of the above

1561. The basicity of an acid is defined as :

A. Number of ionizable hydrogen atoms present in a molecule of an acid

B. Number of unionisable hydrogen atoms present in a molecule of an acid

C. Number of ionisable hydrogen atom presnt in base

D. Numbers of unionisable hydrogen atom present in base

1562. For the titrimetric calculations the concentration of the reagent soln must be:

A. Known

B. Unknown

C. In dosen't depend on concentration

D. None of the above

1563. In terms of molarity the gram molecula weight of substance means its mol wt expressed in:

A. Gram B. Miligram

C. Kilogram D. None of them

1564. 80 g of NaOH in 5 liter solution , calculate the molarity :

A. 2g B. 10g

C. 16g D. 15g

1565. The success of titrimetric procedure depends on :

A. Selecting a suitable reagent

B. Choosing a suitable indicator

C. Concentration of reagent solution must be known

D. All of the above

1566. A substance which contain water molecule, it is not good for :

A. Primary standards

B. Secondary standards

C. Both a) & b)

D. None

1567. In acid - base titration oxalic acid and copper sulphate are used as :

A. Primary standards

B. Secondary standards

C. Both a) & b)

D. Not used

1568. The indicator phenolphthalein is a :

A. Strong base B. Weak base

C. Strong acid D. Weak acid

1569. What is range in which methyl red genrally changes the colour :

A. 0.2-1.8 B. 2.9-4.0

C. 4.2-6.3 D. 10.8-13.0

1570. Pheolphthalein is with acid and base :

A. Acid is colurless and base Red

B. Acid is yellow and base is red

C. Acid is red and base is colurless

D. Acid and base both are colourless

1571. Why pheolphthalein is dangerous :

A. It may cause eye irritation

B. It cause skin irritation

C. Both a) & b)

D. None of them

1572. An acid whose basicity is more than one is called :

A. Monobasic acid B. Dibasic acid

C. Polybasic acid D. Both a & b

1573. Orthphosphoric acid (H3PO4) is a:

A. Monobasic acid B. Triprotic

C. Tribasic acid D. Both b & c

1574. What is florescent indicator :

A. That absorb radiant energy and emit it in the form of light

B. That absorb light

C. aromatic property

D. None of them

1575. When flourescent indicator is used in titration , the titration is performed in :

A. Silica flask B. Glass flask

C. Both a & b D. None of them

1576. When flourescent indicator is used ,Why titration is not performed in glass flask :

A. A flask made up glass will not permit ultravoilet light to enter

B. A flask made up of glass will break easily when flourescent indicator is used

C. A flask made up of glass react with flourescent indicator

D. All of the above

1577. Which is not a fluroscent indicator :

A. Rosin B. Chromotropic

C. Fluorescein D. Nitramine

1578. The determination of an amount of an acid in a sample , by titration with a standard alkali is called :

A. Alkalimetry B. Acidimetery

C. Both a & b D. None of them

1579. The determination of the amount of a base in a sample by titration with standard acid solution is called :

A. Alkalimetry B. Basicimetry

C. Acidimetry D. All of the above

1580. Which is the best indicator for detection of end point in the titration of weak acid and strong base :

A. Methyl orange (pH 3-4)

B. Bromothymol blue (pH 6-6.75)

C. Methyl red (pH 4-6)

D. Phenolphthalein (pH 8-9.6)

1581. Strongest base is :

A. HSO4– B. HSO3–

C. CH3COO– D. CH3O–

1582. Which dissociate Strongly :

A. HCL ->H+ + Cl-

B. NaOH -> Na+ + OH-

C. Both a & b D. None of them

1583. The number of moles of KMnO4 that are requried to react completely with one mole of ferrous oxalate in acid medium is :

A. 3/5 B. 2/5

C. 4/5 D. 1

1584. 10g of NaOH in 1 liter solution calculate the Molarities :

A. 2 B. 0.4
C. 0.25 D. 0.125

1585. 73.0 g of HCL in 1 liter solution , calculate the Normality :

A. 2 B. 1
C. 0.5 D. 0.01

1586. Bromocreasol green is yellow in acid and in Alkaline :

A. Blue in colour B. Green in colour
C. Red in colour D. Yellow in colour

1587. What is the colour of methyl yellow indicator in acid :

A. Red B. Brownish
C. Yellowish - green D. Colourless

1588. What is the pH range of Bromophenol red indicator :

A. (10.2 - 11.0) B. (6.9 - 7.0)
C. (10.6-12.) D. (5.2-6.8)

1589. What is the pH range of Phenolphthalein indicator :

A. (0.2-1.8) B. (6.0 - 8.1)
C. (8.3 - 10.0) D. Both a & b

1590. Which the best indicator in the titration of Strong acid with Strong base :

A. Neutral red (6.8 - 8.0)
B. Penolphthalein (8.3 - 10.0)
C. Nitramine (10.8- 13.0)
D. Cresol red (0.2 - 1.8)

1591. 35.46 g of HCl contains 1.008 g of replaceable hydrogen , the equvivalent weight of HCL is :

A. 55.0 B. 29.6
C. 35.46 D. 26.4

1592. CH3OH contain hydroxyl group then why it cannot regarded as a base

A. It dot contain hydroxyl group
B. It does not ionise
C. Both a & b
D. None of them

1593. The basicity of H2SO4 is 2 and its mol wt is 98.08. Calculate its equvivalent weight :

A. 49.04 B. 98.08
C. 60.2 D. 46.0

1594. In the quation PbO + HCl -> PbCl2 + H2O . How many moles of HCl is requried to balance the equation :

A. 1 B. 2
C. 3 D. 4

1595. Which one of the following is responsible for the acidic pH of normal rainwater :

A. CO2 B. SO2
C. NO2 D. NH3

1596. Which one of the following is the contributor to the formation of acid rain :

A. H2 B. SO2
C. O3 D. NH3

1597. Which one is the property of base :

A. Taste Sour
B. Conduct electric current in solution
C. Turn litmus red
D. Concentration of h3O is greator than oh

1598. Which solution has lowest pH :

A. 1.0M HF B. 1.0M HCOOH
C. 1.0M HCN D. 1.0 CH3COOH

1599. A solution of known Concentration is the defination of :

A. Buffer Solution
B. Saturated solution
C. Standard solution
D. Unsaturated Solution

1600. A solution which resist tge change in the pH when acid or alkali added to it :

A. Buffer Solution B. Neutral Solution
C. Standard Solution D. Saturated Solution

1601. A chemical species which produce hydrogen ion in solution is known as :

A. Arrehnius acid B. Lewis Acid
C. Arrehnius base D. Lewis base

1602. If 1.0 x 10-4 solution has pH of 10.0 , the solute is called as

A. Weak acid B. Strong acid
C. Weak base D. Strong base

1603. A substance that is non - metal oxides which show no reaction with acid or alkali is :

A. Amphoteric acid B. Acidic oxides
C. Neutral oxides D. basic oxides

1604. Acids or bases are form when acid react with :

A. Amphoteric oxide B. Water
C. Salts D. None of them

1605. What is the pH of lemon juice:

A. 2 B. 6
C. 10 D. 8

1606. Select an Alkali :

A. Strong acid B. Water soluble base
C. Weak acid D. None of them

1607. Any substance that increases the concentration of H3O+ ion in water are called as :

A. Bronsted Acid B. Arrehnius acid
C. Bronsted base D. Arrehinius base

1608. Any substance that decreases the concentrationof H3O+ ion in water are called as :

A. Bronsted Acid B. Lewis acid
C. Bronsted base D. Lewis base

1609. Select an Strongest Conjugate acid :

A. HClO4 B. CH3COOH
C. H2S D. H2O

1610. HSO4- is a :

A. Conjugate acid B. Conjugate base
C. Both a & b D. None of them

1611. The pka of an indicator is 4. . what is the ph range of an indicator :

A. 8-10 B. 6-7
C. 3-5 D. 1-2.5

1612. What does the pka of an indicator tells you:

A. Strength of acid
B. Strength of base
C. Both a & b
D. None of them

1613. What is the pka of acetic acid :

A. 4.76 B. 5.8
C. 8.0 D. 7.6

1614. What is the pka of weak acid :

A. 4.5 B. 1.2
C. 7.0 D. 8

1615. Th pH range of an indicator phenolphthalein is 8.0 - 10.0 . What its pka:

A. 10 B. 2.3
C. 5.6 D. 9.4

1616. The pka of an indicator is 1. Its pH range is:

A. 3.2-4.4 B. 0.2-1.8
C. 4.0-5.6 D. 5.3-7.6

1617. Why direct titration of boric acid with NaOH is not possible :

A. Because Boric acid form precipitate
B. Because Boric acid is very weak acid
C. Because boric acid is very strong acid
D. None of them

1618. In the assay of hydroxyzine dichloride which is a antihistaminic drug . Which indicator is used :

A. Cresol red
B. Methyl orange
C. Tymol blue
D. Phenolphthalein

1619. By which titration the assay of phenarmine maleate in pharmaceutical industry is perform :

A. Acid - Base titration
B. Complexometric titration
C. Both a & b
D. Precipitation

1620. In the titration of strong acid and weak base which indicator is choosen :

A. Cresol red B. Tymol blue
C. Methyl orange D. Phenolphthalein

1621. The moisture content in non-aqueous titration should not more than :

A. 10 % B. 0.05%
C. 15 % D. 5 %

1622. Which statement is not true about non-aqueous titration :

A. Titration of water insoluble drug is performed by this method
B. Titration of weak acid or weak basic drug is not possible
C. Solvents are expensive
D. Greater care in the control of temprature is needed

1623. In the assay of metronidazol which indicator is used :
A. Crystal voilet
B. Methyl red
C. Glacial acetic acid
D. All of the above

1624. The titration curve is the plot of the pH of the analyte solution versus :
A. pH of the titrant
B. Volume of titrant added
C. Volume of analyte
D. None of them

1625. 33 ml of 3M HCL is titrated with Naoh to form water and sodium chloride. How many moles of sodium hydroxide is consumed in this reaction :
A. 3 mol B. 10 mol
C. 33 mol D. 100 mol

1626. 50 ml of 0.5 M barium hydroxide is required to fully titrate a 100 ml solution of sulfuric acid . what is the intial concentration of acid :
A. 100 M B. 50 M
C. .25 M D. .5M

1627. In the titration of a weak acid with strong base . At equivalence point what is the pH of the solution :
A. > 7 B. 7
C. < 7 D. 0

1628. Titration curve exhibit asymptote at very large volume of added titrant . which of the following parameter determine asymptote :
A. The pH of the intial solution
B. The slope of the curve on the titration curve
C. The ka of the intial solution
D. The pH of the titrant

1629. Which of the following criteria accurately describes the primary diffrence between strong versus weak acid :
A. Negative versus positive pH
B. Complete versus partial ionization in solution
C. Proton donation versus electron acceptance
D. Presence versus absence of halogen ion in chemical structure

1630. In the following statement which perfectly describe the " Buffer " region in the titration curve :
A. The flat portion of the curve after the equivalance point
B. The flat portion of the curve just before the equivalence point
C. The steep portion of the curve after the equivalence point
D. The concave portion of the curve after the addition of titrant

1631. 10ml of 0.5M calcium hydroxide is required to titrate 50 ml of hydrochloric acid . what is the intial concentration of acid :
A. 1/5 M B. 5 M
C. 1/10 M D. 10 M

1632. Red litmus paper turn .... When put in alkaline soltution :
A. Yello B. green
C. Blue D. Orange

1633. Blue litmus paper turns red :
A. Acidic condition B. Alkaline condition
C. Both a & b D. None of them

1634. Which titrant is most widely used in Non-aqueous titration :
A. NaOH B. Acetic acid
C. Perchloric acid D. None of them

1635. According to IP which indicator is used in the analysis of Diazepam :
A. Methyl red B. Bromophenol red
C. Methyl orange D. Crystal violet

1636. In the titration of HCL with NaOH the , pH at equivalence point is 7 but if a weak acid like CH3COOH with NaOH at equivalence point the pH is more than 7. This is due to:
A. Hydrolysis of salt formed
B. Reduction of salt formed
C. Oxidation of salt formed
D. Nome of the above

1637. The pH at the equivalence depends on the relative values of :

A. Ka B. Kb

C. Both a & b D. None of them

1638. In sparingly soluble salt like siilver phosphate if HCL is added than the solubility will be :

A. Increase

B. decrease

C. No effect

D. Intially increase than decrease

1639. Each colour is associated with particular pH in

A. Litmus indicator

B. Universal indicator

C. Methyl blue indicator

D. Phenolphthalein indicator

1640. Diffrece between the weak acid and strong acid can be findout through :

A. Litmus indicator

B. Universal indicator

C. Crystal voilet indicator

D. Methylene blue indicator

1641. A buffer solution is consist of :

A. A weak acid in solution

B. A strong acid in solution

C. A weak base in solution

D. a weak acid and its conjugate base in solution

1642. Which one is not strong acid :

A. HCl B. H2SO4

C. HnO3 D. H2SO3

1643. In litmus paper the pH-7 show trough the colour of :

A. Red B. Blue

C. Green D. Yellow

1644. acid become colourless when :

A. Pholphthalein indicator is added

B. When litmus indicator is added

C. Universal indicator is added

D. All of the above

1645. when acid react with metal carbonate :

A. Carbon dioxide gas is released

B. Dihydrogen gas is released

C. Dioxygen gas is released

D. Dinitrogen gas is released

1646. When strong acid combine with strong base the nature of salt will be :

A. Neutral B. Basic

C. Acidic D. Slightly basic

1647. In neutralization reaction, instead pH meter :

A. Barometer is used

B. Gas syringe is used

C. Heat senson is used

D. None

1648. In which titration phenolphthalein indicator is used :

A. Acid - base titration

B. Precipitation titration

C. Potentiometric titration

D. All

1649. Common property that both acid and base have :

A. Both have sour taste

B. Both show red colour when litmus paper is used

C. Both conduct electricity

D. All of the above

1650. The acid neutralizing capacity of antacid tablet is determined by :

A. Acid - base titration

B. gravimetric

C. Precipitation titration

D. Counductometric titration

1651. In which titration coloured complex is used to indicate the end - point of titration:

A. Oxidation - reduction titration

B. precipitation titration

C. Complexometric titration

D. Acid - base titration

1652. Complexometric titration is also called :

A. Chelatometry titration

B. Argentometry titration

C. Non - aqueous titration

D. None of them

1653. How complex are formed in complexometric titration :

A. When metal ion react with anion
B. When cation react with anion
C. When a central atom react with positive ion
D. All of the above

1654. The groups (anion/neutra/positive) attached to the central (cation/metal ion) are called :

A. Ligands B. Neutral atom
C. Chelate D. None of them

1655. Which bond is usually formed between the central cation and the ligand :

A. Covalent bonds B. Hydrogen bonds
C. ionic bonds D. Polar bonds

1656. Ligands which posses only one electronegative donar atom and contain only one unshared pair of electron are called

A. Mondentate B. Bidentate
C. Tridentate D. Polydentate

1657. Polydentate contain :

A. Only one point of attachment with central cation
B. Two point of attachment with the central cation
C. Three points of attachemtn without central cation
D. Multiple point of attachment with central cation

1658. All polydenate ligands are also called as the chelating lingands because :

A. The complex formed by them involve the formation of 5 -6 membered hetrocyclic rings
B. The complexes formed by them involve the formation of homocyclic ring
C. Both a&b
D. None of them

1659. Which of the following Statement is not true about complexometric titration :

A. In Complexometric titration the complex form in the end point of titration os coloured
B. Metal ion is neecessary for the formation of complex
C. Complex only form when ligand posses only one electron pair to donate
D. Complexometric titration is a form of volumetric analysis

1660. Complexometric titration is useful in the determination of :

A. Non-metal ion B. Metal ion
C. Chelate D. Ligands

1661. Chelating agent form strong complex with metal ion in the ratio of :

A. 1:1 B. 1:4
C. 1:3 D. 2:1

1662. Molecule composed of metal and chelates are known as :

A. Coordination complexes
B. Non-coordination complex
C. Ligands
D. None of the above

1663. Most common chelating agent belong to the group of compound called :

A. Polyaminocarboxylic acid
B. Nitrogen containing compound
C. Halogen containing compound
D. Oxygen contaning compound

1664. The higher the valency of metal ion the more stable the :

A. Complex B. lingand
C. Metal ion D. None of the above

1665.Ethylene diamine is a type of ligand :

A. Mondentate B. bidenatate
C. Polydentate D. Hexadenatate

1666. What is the full form of EDTA :

A. Ethylenediamine tetraamino acid
B. Ethylenediamine triamino acid
C. Ethylenediamine triacetic acid
D. Ethylenediamine tetra acetic acid

1667. Which type of ligand EDTA is :

A. Polydenatate B. Hexdenatate
C. Both a&b D. Monodenatate

1668. What is the pH of EDTA :

A. 4-6 B. 10-12
C. 1-4 D. 8-10

1669. Which of the following statement is not true about EDTA :

A. EDTA forms 1:1 complexs with metal ion
B. EDTA is hexdenatate ligand
C. EDTA is dangerous chemical
D. None of them

1670. One of the most common chelating used for complexometric titration in analytical chemistry :

A. Acetylacetone B. Alizarin
C. EDTA D. Benzotriazole

1671. The ability of the polydentate ligands to form more stable metal complexes than thos formed by similar monodentate ligands is called :

A. Chelation
B. Chelate effect
C. Complex formation
D. None of them

1672. The solubility of metal chelates in water depends on :

A. Presence of hydrophillic groups in metal
B. ph of metal ion
C. Both a&b
D. None of them

1673. Which is used to mask Cu by precipitation in the assay of lotion containing Cu and Zn :

A. Thiocynate
B. Glycerines
C. 8-hydroxy quinoline
D. Thioglycerol

1674. Tiron is used for masking :

A. Al B. Ti
C. Botha&b D. None

1675. Which is used as a masking agent in complexometric titration :

A. Ammonium fluride
B. Dimercaprol
C. Potassium iodide
D. All of the above

1676. In complexometric titration , the process by which a substance is so transformed that it does not take part in any particular reaction :

A. Masking B. Demasking
C. Chelation D. Complex formation

1677. Which one is not a masking agent :

A. Acorbic acid B. Ammonium fluride
C. Triethanolamine D. None

1678. What is the use of masking agent in complexometric titration :

A. To decrease the pH of reaction
B. To increase the rate of reaction
C. To mask the unwanted content or impurities in reaction
D. None of them

1679. Which is used to mask copper in complexometric titration :

A. Thioglycerol B. Triethanolamine
C. Ascorbic acid D. All of the above

1680. Which masking agent is used to mask heavy metals in complexometric titration :

A. KCN/NaCN B. Thioglycerol
C. Hg2+ D. All of the above

1681. Complexometric titration curves are constructed between :

A. Negative logarithm of metal ion concentration (pM) versus milli-litres of titrant
B. Negative logarithm of metal ion concentration versus concentration of ligand
C. Concentration of metal ion versus concentration of complex
D. None

1682. In complexometric titration curve , the greator the value of apparent stability constant :

A. The sharper the end point (at constant pH)
B. The greator the ph of reaction at end point
C. The faster the reaction
D. None

1683. Find the incorrect statement for direct titration method under complexometric titration :

A. Slow complexation reaction
B. Interference occur due to the presence of other ion
C. Both a&b are correct
D. None

1684. Which statement is incorrect of Displacement titration under complexometric titration :
- A. This titration is used for metal ion which do not react with metal indicator
- B. Displacement titration is also called subsitution titration
- C. Reaction is very fast
- D. None of them

1685. In which type of complexometric titration sodium alkali is used :
- A. Direct titration
- B. Indirect titration
- C. Replacement titration
- D. Back titration

1686. Alkaloids like codeine can be determined by which type of complexometric titration:
- A. Direct titration
- B. Indirect titration
- C. displacement titration
- D. Back titratipn

1687. Barbiturate forms metal complex with :
- A. Zinc
- B. Mercury
- C. Both a&b
- D. None of the above

1688. Chlorpromazine forms metal ion complex with:
- A. Zinc
- B. Mercury
- C. Both a&b
- D. None of them

1689. Which one is the most stable complex :
- A. Fe(H2O)6]3+
- B. [Fe(NH3)6]3+
- C. [Fe(C2O4)3]3-
- D. [FeCl6]3

1690. From the complex of CO(NH3)6 Cl2 , How many ions are produced :
- A. 6
- B. 4
- C. 3
- D. 2

1691. On which factor the stability of complex depends :
- A. Charge on the central metal atom
- B. Basic nature of ligands
- C. Nature of metal ion
- D. All of the above

1692. Why erichrome black T is used in complexometric titration
- A. As an indicator
- B. To make complex
- C. As an reagent
- D. To maintain temprature

1693. Metellochromic indicator is used in which type of titration :
- A. Acid-base titration
- B. EDTA titration
- C. Precipitation titration
- D. Redox titration

1694. The metal indicator complex must have sufficient stability to :
- A. Resist dissociation
- B. Sharp colour change
- C. Both a&b
- D. None of the above

1695. Which indicator is used in chelatometery titration :
- A. Methyl red
- B. bromophenol blue
- C. Cresol blue
- D. Eriochrome black T

1696. The first metal ion indicator used in EDTA titration :
- A. Eriochrome Black T
- B. Calmagite
- C. Murexide
- D. Xylenol orange

1697. What is the colour of Calmagite indicator at pH10 in complexometric titration :
- A. Green
- B. Colourless
- C. Blue
- D. Red

1698. The colour change of metal ion indicator depends on :
- A. pH
- B. Temprature
- C. Viscosity
- D. Ligand

1699. In the assay of CaCo3 and CaCl2 which indicator is used :
- A. Solochrome dark blue or calcon
- B. Xyenol orange
- C. Murexide
- D. Patton and reeder's indicator

1700. In which titration mordant black II indicator is used :
- A. Conductometry titration
- B. acid-base titration
- C. Complexometric titration
- D. All of the above

1701. Which indicator is used in the direct titration procedure for Ca^{2+} :

A. Hydroxynaphthol blue
B. Cresol red
C. Methyl blue
D. Nitramine

1702. How many grams of EDTA is required to dissolve in 1 litre water . To prepare EDTA Solution :

A. 1 B. 2
C. 3 D. 4

1703. In complexometric titration , the colour change is sharper at which pH :

A. 15 B. 10
C. 4 D. 12

1704. The titration of cynide with silver ions is known as :

A. Liebig titration
B. Arrehenius titration
C. Karl fischer titraton
D. None of them

1705. The appearance of white turbidity of mercuric nitroprusside marks the end point in the titration of :

A. Mercuric nitrate with standard KCl solution
B. Ammonium nitrate with KCl solution
C. Silver nitrate with KCl solution
D. None of them

1706. For the titration of 25 ml of 0.1 M Nacl , How many ml of mercuric nitrate soln is required :

A. 5 ml B. 10 ml
C. 15 ml D. 20 ml

1707. EDTA is used in some food product as a :

A. Preservative B. Colouring agent
C. Taste enhancer D. None

1708. By which method the hardness of water is determined :

A. EDTA method
B. Precipitation method
C. Gravimetric metnod
D. All of the Above

1709. In Complexometric titration , bismuth is titrated in which solution :

A. Alkaline acidic B. Acidic solution
C. Neutral D. Alcoholic

1710. The indicator Murexide is also called as :

A. Ammonium purpurate
B. Ammonium tartrate
C. Ammonium succinate
D. Ammonium nitrate

1711. Indicate method for detecting the end point of mercurimetric titration :

A. Iron alum
B. Diphenyl Carbazone
C. Murexide
D. Sodium nitroprusside

1712. What condition is neccessary in order to carry out complexometric titration :

A. Strong acidic solution
B. Neutral solution
C. Presence of buffer solution
D. All of the above

1713. Which forms more stable complex with EDTA :

A. Ca^{2+} B. Mg^{2+}
C. Both a&b D. None

1714. Which is more stable complex :

A. Metal - EDTA complex
B. Metal EBT complex
C. Both a & b
D. None

1715. Find the inccorrect statment about complexometric titration :

A. Complex serve as a end point detection
B. Metallochromic indicator are used
C. Without EDTA titration cannot be possible
D. Buffer solution is used

1716. Which of the following is a titrant in Complexometric titration :

A. Na_2SO_4
B. Nacl
C. ethyldiamenetetra acetic aid
D. NaOH

1717. Which of the following statement are correct :

A. Metallochromic indicator forms complex with metal ion
B. EDTA is weak acid
C. EDTA is a strong acid
D. All of the above

1718. Which of the following analysis refers to the complextation titration :
A. Titration of barium salts with H2SO4
B. Titration of calcium chloride with EDTA
C. Titration of potassium cynide with AgNo3
D. All

1719. Which statment about dissodium salt of EDTA is correct :
A. Dissodium salt of EDTA is more stable than EDTA
B. Disodium salt of EDTA is less stable than EDTA
C. Disodium salt of EDTA is also used in acid base titration
D. Disodium salt of EDTA is also used in precipitation titration

1720. EDTA is :
A. Dibasic acid B. Tribasic acid
C. Tetrabasic acid D. None

1721. Which is more soluble in water :
A. EDTA
B. Disodium salt of EDTA
C. Both is soble at same level
D. Both are insoluble

1722. For the determination of calcium by EDTA titration which indicator is used :
A. Murexide B. Methyl blue
C. Both a&b D. Phenolphthalein

1723. Which of the following drug compound is determined by back complexometric titration :
A. PbSO4 B. CaC2O4
C. Both a & b D. None

1724. Which of the drug compound cannot be analysed by direct complexometric titration :
A. NaCl B. NH4Br
C. CaCL2 D. MgSO4

1725. In the titration of calcium by EDTA titration the end point is marked by change in colour from red to :
A. Green B. Blue
C. Purple D. Colourless

1726. Accorrding to IP, the assay of Dibasic calcium phosphate is performed by which titration :
A. Complexometric titration
B. Precipitation titration
C. Acid - base titration
D. Counductometry titratrion

1727. In the determination Ca in insoluble salt such as a phosphate which indicator is used :
A. Hydroxynaphthol blue
B. Murexide
C. Bromopyrogallol red
D. Fast sulphon black

1728. For the determination of calcium in calcium lactate tablets which titration is performed :
A. Precipitation titration
B. EDTA titration
C. Redox titration
D. All of the above

1729. Determination of calcium using Eriochrome black T as indicator :
A. Direct titration
B. Indirect titration
C. Displacement titration
D. Back titration

1730. According to IP , Magnesium hydroxide assay is performed by which titration :
A. Acid-base titration
B. Complexometric titration
C. Both a&b
D. Redox titration

1731. The magnesium carbonates are assayed by complexometric titration with :
A. EDTA B. NaOH
C. Mg2SO4 D. Na2CO4

1732. In the determination of magnesium by EDTA titration which indicator is used :
A. EBT B. Murexide
C. EDTA D. None

1733. Determination of Calcium and magnesium in sea water is performed by which titration :
A. EDTA titration
B. Complexometric titration
C. Chelatometery titration
D. All of the above

1734. In the determination of hardness of water by Complexometric titratiion which Indicator is used :

A. EBT
B. Methyl red
C. Murexide
D. Methyl blue

1735. In the determination of water which buffer solution is used :

A. NH4OH-NH4CL
B. HCL
C. Nacl
D. KCl

1736. What pH of buffer is required in determination of hardness of water by complexometric titration :

A. 5
B. 10
C. 15
D. 20

1737. Which is used as a demasking agent :

A. Ascrobic acid
B. Formaldehyde acetic acid
C. Magnesium
D. Triethanol amine

1738. Which shows kinetic masking :

A. CO2+
B. Cu2+
C. Cr3+
D. Fe3+

1739. Which one not produce selective complexometric titration :

A. Demasking
B. Control of pH
C. Choice of indicator
D. Back titration

1740. In what condition back titration of EDTA is not used :

A. Insoluble complexes
B. Titration that require heat
C. Analyte that form inert complex
D. When no pM indicator is available

1741. Disodium salt of EDTA is :

A. Monodentate
B. tridentate
C. Hexadentate
D. Tetradentate

1742. When a complex is formed with metal ion , ligand act as a :

A. Neutral
B. Electron donor
C. Both a&b
D. Cation

1743. Water is:

A. Monodentate
B. tridentate
C. Hexadentate
D. Tetradentate

1744. Which masking agent is use for mercury :

A. Ammonium fluride
B. Iodide
C. Ascrobic acid
D. Triethanolamine

1745. Complexing agent forms :

A. Water soluble complex
B. Water insoluble complex
C. Both a&b
D. Precipitate

1746. Which one serves as a masking agent :

A. Cu
B. Co
C. CN
D. Ni

1747. If the temprature increses , the stability of complex :

A. Increases
B. No effect
C. Intially increase than decrease
D. Decreases

1748. From following compound for which the replacement titration is perfomed :

A. Calcium
B. Magnesium
C. Zinc
D. All of the above

1749. Which one is not used as a masking agent:

A. Ammonium fluride
B. Iodide
C. Iron
D. All of the above

1750. In the oxidation reduction titration for the detection of end point :

A.Redox indicator is used
B. Potentiometer is used
C. Both a&b
D. Metallochromic indicator is used

1751. Redox titration involve :

A. Idometery
B. Bromometry
C. Cerimetry
D. All of the above

1752. In which titration the solution of iodine is treated with reducing agent :

A. Acid - base titration
B. Redox titration
C. Precipitation titration
D. Complexometric titration

1753. In which titration starch indicator is used :
A. Acid - base titration
B. Redox titration
C. Precipitation titration
D. Complexometric titration

1754. On which basis the titrant is selected in oxidation reduction titration
A. Its standard reduction potential E0
B. pH
C. Acidity
D. None

1755. Which titrant is used in Redox titration :
A. KMnO4 B. Iodine
C. AgNo3 D. All of the above

1756. Select non-oxidizing agent :
A. H2O2 B. HNO3
C. KMnO4 D. H2S

1757. Select Non - reducing agent :
A. H2O2 B. HNO3
C. KmNO4 D. All

1758. From following statment which one is true about Oxidizing agents :
A. They are non-metal
B. They are metals
C. Decrese in oxidation state
D. They are mostly transition metal

1759. Which one is the reducing agent in the reaction of CuO and CO :
A. CuO B. Cu
C. CO D. CO2

1760. In Redox titration whose molarity is considered :
A. Molarity of released proton in case of Oxidising agent
B. Molarity of released electron in case of reducing agent
C. Both a&b D. None

1761. When postassium permagnate is analyze against a colourless titrant which indicator is used :
A. Starch B. Iodine
C. Both a&b D. No indicator is used

1762. In redox titration, which one serve as both titrant and indicator function :
A. KMnO4 B. Iodine
C. AgNo3
D. Potassium dihromate

1763. Redox reaction are important in :
A. Purfying metals
B. Producing gases
C. Protecting metals from corrossion
D. All of the above

1764. In idometric titration , iodine is usually titrated with standard :
A. Thiosulfate solution
B. Potassium permagnate
C. Agno3
D. Disodium salt of EDTA

1765. How many moles of oxalate is needed to completely neutralize 0.1 normal 200 ml potassium permagnate solution :
A. 2 B. 3
C. 4 D. 5

1766. How many moles of KMnO4 is needed for complete oxidation of 1mol of KI in basic medium :
A. 2 B. 4
C. 6 D. 10

1767. Which one is redox reaction :
A. NaCl + KMnO3 - > NaNO3 + KCL
B. Ca2CO4 + HCL -> CaCl2 +C2H2O4
C. Both a&b
D. Zn+Ag2CN -> 2Ag +Zn (CN)2

1768. What is the colour of KMnO4 :
A. Red B. Blue
C. Green D. Purple

1769. By which titration concentration of Vitamin C is determined :
A. Redox titration
B. Precipitation titration
C. Acid - base titration
D. Complexometric titration

1770. In the reaction of KMnO4 and oxalic acid . Which one is reducing agent :
A. Oxalic acid is reducing agent
B. KMnO4 is reducing agent
C. Both are reducing agent
D. Both are oxidizing agent

1771. As the soultion's potenial changes with addition of titrant , the indicator chages its:

A. Oxidation state B. Colour
C. Both a&b D. pH of the solution

1772. Potassium permagnate is not considered as a primary standard solution because :

A. Low molar mass
B. Only react in acidic solution
C. It is not highly soluble in water
D. Its solution are unstable

1773. The titration in which E0 is consider :

A. Precipitation titration
B. Acid -base titration
C. Complexometric titration
D. Oxidation-reduction titration

1774. For the complete oxidation of 1.25 mol Cu2S, the moles of KMnO4 required is :

A. 2 B. 10
C. 6 D. 3

1775. How many moles of potassium permagnate us required to react with one mole of sulphide acidic medium :

A. 1/3 B. 3/5
C. 1/5 D. 1/1

1776. What is the standard reduction potential of indicator phenosafrannin :

A. 0.28 B. 0.36
C. 0.53 D. 0.75

1777. In the oxidized form indicator Diphenylamin colur is voilet but when is reduced it become :

A. Red B. Blue
C. Green D. Colourless

1778. What is the standard reduction potenial Eo of indicator. methylene blue :

A. 0.28 B. 0.36
C. 0.53 D. 0.75

1779. What is the colour of indigotetra sulfonate in oxidzed form :

A. Red B. Blue
C. Green D. Voilet

1780. When starch react with iodine form :

A. Blue colour complex
B. Dark red colour complex
C. Purple colour complex
D. Does not react

1781. Iodometry involve :

A. Direct titration of iodine
B. Indirect titration of iodine
C. Back titration of iodine
D. Substitution titration of iodine

1782. Iodimetry involves :

A. Direct titration of iodine
B. Indirect titration of iodine
C. Back titration of iodine
D. None

1783. In the strongly acidic solution , potassium permahnate reduce to :

A. Mn2+ B. Mn3+
C. Mn4+ D. Mn4+

1784. Which one is self indicator :

A. KMnO4 B. Cerium (IV)
C. Both a&b D. None of the above

1785. Find strongest oxidizing agent :

A. Potassium permagnate
B. Potassium dichromate
C. Bromine
D. Chlorine

1786. In the titration of mohr's salt with potassium dichromate which indicator is used :

A. Diphenylamine
B. methylene blue
C. Phenolphthalein
D. No indicator is needed

1787. For the determmination of halogen containing compound which titration is used :

A. Acid - base titration
B. Precipitation titration
C. Redox titration
D. None

1788.The reaction between N2O4 (Nitrogen tetraoxide) and hydrazine (N2H4) is redox reaction.This reaction is very useful:

A. Rocket propulsion system
B. Engine making
C. vaccum system
D. None

1789. When a reagent act as both an oxidizing agent as well as reducing agent , it is said to undergoing :
A. auto - oxidation
B. Disproportionation
C. Both a&b
D. Redox - reagent

1790. In the determination of calcium in a sample of calcium carbonate which indicator is used :
A. Methyl red
B. Nitroferroin
C. Phenolphthalein
D. All of the above

1791. In the standard hydrogen electrode zinc rod is dipped in a solution of :
A. Zn2+ ion B. Ag+ ion
C. Cd2+ ion D. All

1792. In Galvanic cell the electrode at which the reduction occur is called :
A. Anode B. Cathode
C. Both a&b D. None

1793. The potentiometer is a device for measuring :
A. Voltage B. pH
C. Temprature D. All

1794. Potassium iodate is a powerful :
A. Oxidising agent B. Reducing agent
C. Both a&b D. None

1795. KMnO4 is a :
A. Self indicator B. Specific indicator
C. External indicator D. Internal indicator

1796. NH4CN is a :
A. Internal indicator B. External indicator
C. Self indicator D. Specific indicator

1797. When starch react with iodine produce :
A. Deep blue complex
B. Dark red colour
C. Voilet colour
D. Gryish - yellow colour complex

1798. Nitroferroin indicator colour in reducing agent :
A. Red B. Blue
C. Green D. Purple

1799. Assay of hydrogen peroxide performed by wich titration :
A. Acid - base titration
B. Precipitation titration
C. Redox titration
D. All of the above

1800. Electrode Potential Have Potency:-
A. Lose Electrons B. Gain Electrons
C. Both D. None

1801. The Potential Of Substance Is Known As :-
A. Oxidation Potential
B. Redox Potential
C. Reduction Potential
D. A And C

1802. Cu2+ Have A Tendency To :-
A. Accept Electrons B. Donate Electrons
C. Both D. None

1803. Potential Of A Single Electrode Cannot Be Measured, With Another Electrode Whose Potential Is Known:-
A. Reference Electrode
B. Hydrogen Electrode
C. Calomel Electrode
D. None

1804. In A Potentiometric Dvm ________
A. Voltage Is Compared
B. Current Is Compared
C. Resistance Is Compared
D. Power Is Compared

1805. Potensiometry Is The Method Used For:-
A. Electroanlytical Chemistry
B. Analytical Chemistry
C. Pharmaceutical Chemistry
D. None

1806. Salt Bridge Making By Which Substance:-
A. Kcl B. Cacl2
C. Mgso4 D. H2o

1807. Which Of The Following Has Not Part Of Potentimetric :-
A. Electrode
B. Salt Bridge
C. Analytical Solution
D. Electric

1808. Zn Zn2+ + 2E-

A. Oxidation B. Reducation
C. Redox D. None

1809. Cu2+ + 2E- Cu

A. Oxidation B. Reduction
C. Redox D. Precipitation

1810. Potentiometry Is An......... Method Of Analysis.

A. Spectroscopic B. Analytical
C. Electroanalytical D. None

1811. There Is A Linear Relationship Exit Between The Ph And ...... Of Solution.

A. Colour B. Turbidity
C. Potential D. None

1812. Hydrogen Electrode Can Be Used As:-

A. Reference B. Indicator
C. Both D. None

1813. Antimony Electrode Is An :-

A. Indicator Electrode
B. Secondary Reference Electrode
C. Reference Electrode
D. None

1814. Which Of The Following Metal Is Used In Redox Electrode :-

A. Platinum B. Bismuth
C. Hydrogen D. None

1815. Electrode Are Used In Potentiometry

A. Reference Electrode
B. Indicator Electrode
C. Hydrogen Electrode
D. A And B

1816. Advantage Of Ag/Agcl Electrode

A. Thermal Stability B. Less Toxicity
C. Both D. None

1817. Disadvange Of Ag/Agcl Electrode

A. Electrode Is Large Soluble In Kcl
B. Easy To Prepare Than Sce
C. Disposal Difficulties
D. All Of The Above

1818. Redox Titration Use To Determine

A. Concentration Of Substrance
B. Mass Of Substance
C. Analyte
D. All Of These

1819. In This Equation E=E0 –Rt/Nf Ln A Mn+ , E= ?

A. Electrode Potential
B. Energy
C. Standard Potential Of The Electrode
D. None

1820. Universal Gas Constant Is -

A. 8.314 J/K.Mol B. 0.08421 Mol
C. 83.14 J/K.Mol D. All Of These

1821. Which Of The Folloing Is Faraday Constant Is

A. 96485.33 C / Mole
B. 9834 C/ Mole
C. 96485.33 C/ Mole
D. 76485.8 C / Mol

1822. Potentiometry Measured System Consist Of ;

A. Reference Electrode
B. Indicator Electrode
C. Both
D. None

1823. Determination Of Ph Of Unknown By Which Equation

A. E1=Irl1 B. E1=Iel1
C. E1=Irml1 D. All Of These

1824. Which Of The Following Is Used To Determine End Point;

A. A Normal Titration
B. First Derivative
C. Second Derivative
D. All Of These

1825. Applications Of Potentiometric Titration

A. Acid-Base Titration
B. Redox Titration
C. Precipitation Titration
D. All Of Above

1826. Which Of The Following Cathodic Reaction

A. Gain Of Positive Charge
B. Lose Of Positive Charge
C. No Change Of Charge
D. None Of The Above

1827. In Poteniomeric Titration , The Change In The Electrode Potential Upon

A. Addition Of The Titrant
B. Addition Of The Titrate
C. Both
D. No Effect

1828. Which Of The Following Instruments Used To Measurement Of Potentials:-

A. Electronic Instrument
B. Non- Electronic Instrument
C. Automatic Instrument
D. All Of These

1829. Which Is Independent Of The Composion Of The Solution:-

A. Reference Electrode
B. Hydroden Electrode
C. Sample Electrode
D. Cell Electrode

1830. Which Of The Following Instrument Advantage Has High Resistance Of The Glass:-

A. Electronic Instrument
B. Non Electronic Instrument
C. Automatic Instrument
D. All Of These

1831. The Final Category Of Automatic Titrators Are Known:-

A. Differential Titrator
B. Simple Titrator
C. Compound Titrator
D. All Of These

1832. What Is The Reference Electrode Used In Titration

A. Reference Electrode
B. N – Calomel Electrode
C. Hydrogen Electrode
D. All Of The These

1833. E.M.F Of The Cell Is Proportional To The The :-

A. Change In Solvent
B. Change In Titrant
C. Change In Electrode Potential
D. No Effect

1834. Potentiometric End Point Detection :-

A. Edta Titration
B. Hcl Titration
C. Complex Formation
D. None Of These

1835. Calculate The Standard Potential Of The Reaction Fe 2+ = Fe 3+ + E

A. E0 = -0.76V B. E0 = 0.76V
C. E0 = -0.70V D. E0 = -0.23V

1836. Calculate The Standard Potential Of This Reaction Ce4+ + E- = Ce3+

A. E0 = -0.60V B. E0 = -1.76V
C. E0 = 1.16V D. E0 = 0.76V

1837. Calculate The Standard Potential Of This Reaction Ce4+ + Fe2+ = Ce3+ + Fe

A. E0 = -1.76V B. E0 = -1.76V
C. E0 = -1.76V D. E0 = 0.85V

1838. Which Of The Following Equilibrium Constant For Ce4+ + E- = Ce3+

A. E = Ce4+ /Ce3+ - 0.0591/1LOG (Ce3+/Ce4+)
B. Both
C. E = Ce4+ /Ce3+ + 0.0591/1LOG (Ce3+/Ce4+)
D. None Of These

1839. Which Of The Following Equilibrium Constant For Fe 2+ = Fe 3+ + E

A. E = Fe 2+/Fe 3+- 0.0591/1 Log(Fe 2+/Fe 3+)
B. E = Fe 2+/Fe 3+
C. E = Fe 3+/Fe 2+- 0.0591/1LOG(Fe 2+/Fe 3+)
D. All Of These

1840. E.M.F. Of A Cell As Given Ecell =

A. Ecell = Ereference + Eindicator
B. Ecell = Eindicator + Ejuction
C. Ecell = Ereference + Ejuction
D. Ecell = Ereference + Ejuction + Eindicator

1841. What Is The Standard Electrode Potential Of Hydrogen

A. Zero B. Infinity
C. One D. None

1842. Which Of The Following Indicator Use In Neutralization Redox Titration

A. Glass Electrode B. Mercury-|| Electrode
C. Silver Electrode D. Pt Electrode

1843. In Which Of Following Electro-Analytical Method Is Potential Vs Volume Of Titrant
A. Conductometry B. Potentiometry
C. Amperometry D. Polarghaphy

1844. In Potential Vs Volume Of Titrant Is ?
A. No Current Flow I.E. I = 0
B. Potential = Constant
C. V = Constant
D. Temperature = Constant

1845. Which Of The Following Analytical Methods Use To Measured Electrical Potential ;
A. Coulometer
B. Spectroscopy
C. Potentiometey
D. Spectrophotometry

1846. What Is Included In The Karl Fischer Reagents?
A. Odine , So2
B. Iodine , Pyridine , So2 , Methanol
C. Odine, Pyridine , So2
D. Methanol, So2

1847. In Diazotizatin Titration , Reference Electrode Is
A. Glass Electrode
B. Hydrogen Electrode
C. Ag - Ag Electrode
D. Saturated Calomel Electrode

1848. Faraday Is Unit Of
A. Charge Standard Hydrogen Electrode
B. Current
C. Potential
D. Voltage

1849. The Primary Reference Electrode Is
A. Standard Hydrogen Electrode
B. Pt Electrode
C. Hydrogen Electrode
D. All Of The Above

1850. What Is The Molar Concentration Of Normal Hydrogen Electrode
A. 0.0 B. 0.4
C. 0.1 D. 0.6

1851. The Accurate Method Of Detection Of End Point In Potentiometric Titration
A. Method Of Detection
B. Method Of Reflection
C. Derivatisation Method
D. Method Of Precipitation

1852. Measurement Of Ph Is An Examples For The Direct Reading
A. Potentiometric B. Precipitation
C. Conductometry D. None Of These

1853. The Potential Of Standard Hydrogen Electrode Was
A. Arbitrarily Defined
B. Practical Defined
C. Experimentally Defined
D. Turbidometry Defined

1854. The Potential Of Saturated Ag-Agcl At 25 Degre C Relative To The Normal Hydrogen Electrode
A. 0.10 Volt B. 0.09 Volt
C. 0.199 Volt D. 0.5 Volt

1855. In Potentiometric Titration The Graph Drawn By Against Volumes Is Maximum
A. Initial Point
B. Mid Point
C. Equivalent Point
D. End Point

1856. The Potential Of Standard Silver Electrode Is
A. 0.224 Volt B. -0.224 Volt
C. 0.0 Volt D. 0.50 Volt

1857. Example Of Solid State Electrode Is
A. Fluoride Electrode
B. Pt Electrode
C. Hydrogen Electrode
D. Glass Electrode

1858. In Potentiometric Titration At The End Point
A. Rate Of Change Of Potential Is Maximum
B. Potential Is Maximum
C. Rate Of Change Of Potential Is Maximum
D. Potential Is Minimum

1859. Sodium Ion Error Is Associated With
A. Pt Electrode
B. Fluoride Electrode
C. Hydrogen Electrode
D. Glass Electrode

1860. Potential Of Saturated Calomel Electrode Is

A. 0.0 Volt B. 0.1 Volt
C. 0.2458 Volt D. 2.34 Volt

1861. In Potentiometry Curve Is Obtained By Plotting

A. Emf Vs Ml Of Titrant
B. Emf Vs Current
C. Current Vs Ml Of Titrant
D. None Of These

1862. Karl Fischer Reagent Is Used In Determination Of

A. Hcl B. Naoh
C. H2o D. Nacl

1863.Which Of The Following Is Nernst Equation

A. E = E0 + (Rt / Nf)In Am
B. E = E0 + (Rnt / Nf)In Am
C. E = E0 - (Rt / Nf)In Am
D. E = E0 + (Rt / Nrf)In Am

1864. In Nernst Equation E = E0 + (Rt / Nf)In Am , Eo = ?

A. Electrode Potential
B. Electricity
C. Standard Electrode Potential
D. Voltage

1865. In Nernst Equation E = E0 + (Rt / Nf)In Am, E – ?

A. Electrode Potential
B. Electricity
C. Standard Electrode Potential
D. Voltage

1866. The Potential Of Electrode Depend Upon

A. Concentration Of The Ion
B. Don't Depend On Concentration
C. Depend On Current
D. None Of These

1867. Which Of The Glass Electrode Used In Responsive Electrode

A. Hydrogen Electrode
B. Pt Electrode
C. Mercury Electrode
D. All Of The These

1868. The E.M.F Of The Cell May Expressed By The Equation

A. E = Kr + (Rt / F)In Am
B. E = K / (Rt / F)In Am
C. E = K + (Rt / F)In Am
D. E = K - (Rt / F)In Am

1869. In This Equation E = K + (Rt / F)In Am , K = ?

A. Constant
B. Depend On Concentration
C. Depend On Charge Particle
D. Independent Of Charge

1870. Potentiometric Titration Is A Laboratory Method Used To

A. Determine The Concentration
B. Determination Of Voltage
C. Determination Of Current
D. None Of These

1871.Potentiometric Titration Used In Characterization Of

A. Acid B. Base
C. Amphoteric D. All Of The Above

1872. Which Of The Following Electrode Is Used As A Reference Electrode?

A. Hydrogen Electrode
B. Calomel Electrode
C. Pt Electrode
D. None Of These

1873. How To Determine The Endpoint Of Potentiometric Titration?

A. Combination Electrode
B. Pair Of Electrode
C. By Two Electrode
D. All Of The Above

1874. Which Of The Following Chemical Indication In Potentiometric Titration

A. Colour Change
B. PPT Formation
C. No Any Of Chemical Indication
D. Complex Formation

1875. In Potentionmetric Titration , Reference Electrode Is Independent Of

A. Concentration Of Analyte
B. Concentration Of Solvent
C. Concentrations Of Solute
D. Concentration Of Dilution

1876. The Potential That Develops At Each End Of Salt Bridge Is

A. Junction Potential
B. Equivalent Potential
C. Electrode Potential
D. None Of The Above

1877. Which Of Following Reaction Occurred In Standard Hydrogen Electrode

A. H2 = 2H 2e B. H2 = 2H-
C. 2H+ + 2e = H2 D. 2H = H2

1878. Which Of The Following Membrane Used In Glass Membrane Electrode

A. Na20 B. Al203
C. Sio2 D. All Of The Above

1879. Which Of The Following Inside Glass Bulb Used In Glass Membrane Electrode

A. Solution Of HCL B. Solution Of KCL
C. Both D. None F These

1880. The Potential Of The Calomel Electrode Depends Upon The Concentration Of

A. Kcl B. Nacl
C. Kbr D. All Of The Above

1881. A Single Measurement Of Electrode Potential Is Used To Determine?

A. Concentration B. Voltage
C. Potential D. All Of The Above

1882. The Silver - Silver Chloride Electrode Used To Measured ?

A. Concentration Of Chloride In Solution
B. Potential Of Solution
C. Concentration Of Bromide In Solution
D. None Of These

1883. The Total Area Of Platinum Foil Is About

A. 1 Cm2 B. 5 Cm2
C. 10 Cm2 D. 8 Cm2

1884. Which Of Following Mixture Used To Cleaned The Platium Electrode

A. Hot Water B. Cold Water
C. Hot Chrome D. Cold Chrome

1885. The Electrode Can't Be Used In The Presence Of

A. Oxidising Agents B. Redusing Agent
C. Both D. Amphotheric

1886. A Calomel Half-Cell Is One In Which Mercury And Other

A. Calomel B. Platinum
C. Hydrogen D. None

1887. The Potential Relative To The Standard Hydrogen Electrode

A. 25oc B. 35oc
C. 20oc D. 15oc

1888. The Electrode Reaction Is -

Hg2cl2 + 2e- = 2 Hg + ?

A. Cl- B. 3 Cl-
C. 2cl- D. 2 E-

1889. The Silver- Silver Chloride Electrodes Is Consists Of

A. Silver Wire B. Aluminium Wire
C. Soda Ash D. Pt Wire

1890. A Hydrogen Electrode Can Obviously Be Used As

A. Indicator Electrode
B. Modify Electrode
C. Reference Electrode
D. Equivalent Electrode

1891. Which Of Following Glass Electrodels Most Widely Used

A. Silver Ion B. Hydrogen Ion
C. Sodium Ion D. Platinum Ion

1892. The Hydrogen Electrode Can Be Used In The Ph Range

A. Ph 3-8 B.
C. Ph 5 – 6 D.

1893. The Indicator Electrode Is Also Known As

A. A Thick Glass Bulb
B. Glass Electrode
C. A Thin Glass Bulb
D. None

1894. Which Of Following Is Important For Construction Of The Glass Electrode

A. Nature Of Solution
B. Nature Of The Glass
C. Nature Of Ion
D. Nature Of Solvent

1895. How Much Per Cent Of Sio2 Was University Used For The Manufacturing Of Glass Electrode

A. 60 % B. 50 %
C. 72 % D. 80 %

1896. Na2o How Much Per Cent Of Na2o Was University Used For The Manufacturing Of Glass Electrode

A. 22% B. 1%
C. 45% D. 10%

1897. How Much Per Cent Of Cao Was University Used For The Manufacturing Of Glass Electrode

A. 5% B. 4%
C. 6 % D. 2%

1898. In E.M.F Equation E = K + (Rt / F)In Am At A Temperature Of 250C By The Expression

A. E = Kr + 0.0591 Ph
B. E = K + 0.0591 Ph
C. E = K - 0.0591 Ph
D. E = Kf + 0.0591 Ph

1899. The Glass Electrode Are Now Available As

A. Combination Electrode
B. Mixed Electrode
C. Compound Electrode
D. All Of The Above

1900. The Glass Electrode Can Be Used In The Presence Of

A. Strong Oxidants B. Strong Redutants
C. A And B D. Weak Base

1901. Which Of The Following Agents Useto Washed Glass Electrode After Each Measurement

A. Distilled Water B. Ethanol
C. Purified Water D. Methanol

1902. The Glass Electrode Should Not Allowed To

A. Cold B. Moistured
C. Dry D. All Of The Above

1903. A Hydrogen Electrode Can Obviously Be Used As

A. Reference Electrode
B. Indicator Electrode
C. Pt Electrode
D. Calmol Electrode

1904. Which Titration A Silver Electrode Will Be Used

A. Redox Titration
B. Ppt
C. Complexometric Titration
D. Acid Base Titration

1905. Which Type Of Membrane Electrode Of The Pressed Disc (Or Pellet)

A. Complexometric B. Radiation
C. Crystalline D. Filter

1906. Crystalline Membrane Electrode Is Illustrated By

A. Silver Shulphide
B. Hydrogen Floride
C. Nitrogen Sulphide
D. Sodium Chloride

1907. Which Kind Of Electrode Is Referred To As A Liquid-Membrane Electrode

A. Calomel Electrode
B. Pt Electrode
C. Hydrogen Electrode
D. None Of These

1908. Which Of The Enzyme Used In Hydrolysis Of Usea In Urea Electrode

A. Urease B. Urokinses
C. Urea D. All Of The Above

1909. Which Of Following Enzyme Penicillin Can Likewise Used To Determined Enzyme Based Electrode

A. Urease B. Urokinses
C. Penicillinase D. None

1910. Which Of Following Solution Of Gases Used To Analyse Gas Sensing Electrode

A. Carbon Dioxide B. Nitrogen Dioxide
C. Ammonia D. All Of The Above

1911. The Response Time Of An Electrode Is Defined As The Time Taken For The Cell E.M.F To A Reach A Value Which Is

A. 1 Millivolt B. 10 Millivolt
C. 0.1 Millivolt D. None

1912. What Is TISAB?

A. Total Ionic Strength Adjuster Buffer
B. Total Ion Solid Acid Base
C. Total Cationic Strength Adjuster Buffer
D. Total Ions Solvent Basic

1913. Which Of Following The Most Satisfactory Method Used To Measured E.M.F. Of A Cell

A. Poggendoff's Competition Method
B. Electrodecompletemethod
C. Hydrogen Competition Method
D. Ions Exchange Method

1914. In Nernst Equation , Glass Electrode Potential For A Given Ph Value Will Be Dependent Upon

A. Pressure B. Voltage
C. Temperature D. None Of These

1915. In Direct Potentiometry , What Is Measured In The Use Of A Ph Meter

A. Concentration Of Potassium
B. Concentration Of OH -
C. Concentration Of Phosphorus D. Concentration Of H+

1916. What Is The Region Of Ph In Resulting Solution Willexert A Buffering Action

A. Ph 5 – 6 B. Ph 7-8
C. Ph 3-4 D. Ph 1-2

1917. What Is Evaluate By Gran's Plot Procedure?

A. Initial Concentration Of The Test Solution
B. Potential
C. Initial Concentration Of The Standard
D. Voltage

1918. What Is Measured When The Electrode System Must Be Connected To A Potentiometric Voltmeter.

A. Potential Of Cell B. Voltage
C. E.M.F. D. Equivalent Points

1919. What Is The Potential Difference Developed At The End Point.

A. 100-200 Millivolt
B. 200-250 Volt
C. 200-300 Millivolt
D. 100-150 Volt

1920. Which Of Following Is Example Of Redox Couple .

A. Cr 3+ B. Cr2O7 2-
C. Mn 2+ D. All Of The Above

1921. Which Of The Following System Consists Of Two Identical Pura Platium Wires ?

A. Metallic B. Trimettalic
C. Bimetallic D. None Of These

1922. The Procedure InvolvedMeasurement Of The E.M.F Between Two Electrode Is

A. Potentiometry
B. Direct Potentiomtry
C. Condustometry
D. Indirect Potentiometry

1923. Which Of Electrode Does Not Respond Readily To Changes In Potential During Oxidation-Reduction:-

A. Pt B. Calomel
C. Tungsten D. Hydrogen

1924. Which Of Following Type Of Curve Obtained In The Neutralization Curve For An Acid?

A. S-Shape B. C-Shape
C. D-Shape D. L-Shape

1925. Which Electrode Is Used To Quantity Is The Change In E.M.F. At Constant Current.

A. Unpolarized Electrodes
B. Hydrogen Electrode
C. Polarized Electrode
D. Pt Electrode

1926. Which Of The Following Graphs Is Ploted, When E.M.F. Reading Obtained With The Normal References Electrode- Indicator Electrode Pair Against VolumeOf Titrant

A. Neutralization Curve
B. Condustometric Curve
C. Potentiometric Curve
D. None Of These

1927. The Following Can Be Used As Indicator Electrode By

A. Hydrogen
B. Saturated Calomel
C. Glass
D. Silver-Silver Chloride

1928. The Glass Membrane Of Glass Electrode Has

A. High Resistance
B. Low Resistance
C. Low Melting Point
D. High Conductance

1929. The Inner Side Of Glass Electrode Is Filled With

A. 0.1N Hcl B. 1N Hcl
C. 0.1N Kcl D. 10N Hcl

1930. In A Glass Membrane Electrode

A. H+ Is More Sensitive Then Divalent Ion
B. H+ Is Least Sensitive
C. Di Valent Is More Sensitive Then H+ Ions
D. None Of These

1931. The Relation Between Concentration , Temperature And Potential Of Solution Is Given By

A. Iikovic Equation
B. Nernst Equation
C. Henderson Equation
D.Hassalbach Equation

1932. How To Determine End Point In Potentiometric Titration

A. Rate Of Change Of Potential Is Minimum
B. The Potential Is Maximum
C. Rate Of Change Of Potential Is Maximum
D. The Potential Is Minimum

1933. Standard Hydrogen Electrode Can Be Used As

A. Primary Reference Electrode
B. A And C Both
C. Secondary References Electrode
D. Indicator Electrode Only

1934. At The End Point Of Potentiometry Titration

A. D Emf/Dv Is Maximum
B. D Ph/Dv Is Maximum
C. D Emf/Dv Is Minimum
D. D Ph/Emf Is Maximum

1935. The Gran's Plot Procedure Is Relatively Simple Method For

A. Fixing An End Point
B. Relative Potential
C. Fixing An Equivalent Point
D. None Of These

1936. Which Of The Following Is Advanced Form Of Titration Because Titration In Form Of Accuracy.

A. Potentiometric B. Neutralization
C. ConductometrucD. All Of The Above

1937. Which Method Used To Find Out Actual End Point Of Samples :-

A. Conductometry B. Voltameter
C. Potentiometry D. Gravimeter

1938. Which Of Following Potentiometric Titration Is Not Involve In Chemical Reaction

A. Neutralization Reaction
B. Potentiometric Reaction
C. Oxidation-Reduction Reaction
D. Free Radicalreaction

1939. How Much Amount Of The Equivalent Point Volume Required For Greatest Accuracy

A. 30 Percent B. 20 Percent
C. 15 Percent D. 13 Percent

1940. Which Of Following Is Not Used As A Indicator Electrode ?

A. Hydrogen Electrode
B. Antimony Electrode
C. Glass Electrode
D. Calomel Electrode

1941. The Potential Of The Immersed Electrode Is Thus Controlled By

A. The Ratio Of Concentration
B. The Ratio Of Voltage
C. The Ratio Of Potential
D. Can't Control

1942. The Chromium In The Substance Is Convertinto

A. Chromate B. Dichromate
C. Both D. Dichromate

1943. What Is Colour Of The Manganese (111) Pyrophosphate Complex

A. Reddish-Voilet B. Blue
C. Green D. Red

1944. Which Of Following Ph Range Of The Change In The Equivalent Point.

A. Ph Between 6 And 7
B. Ph Between 9 And 10
C. Ph Between 7 And 8
D. Ph Between 1 And 2

1945. The Pyrophosphate Complex Is Unstable At Which Ph

A. Ph Between 6 And 8
B. Ph Between 3 And 4
C. Ph Above 8
D. Ph Between 6 And 8

1946. Which Equation Is Related To Potentiometry

A. E = E0 - Log(H+) B. A =€Bc
C. E =E0 + Log (H+) D. All Of The Above

1947. Which Of Following Curve In Potentiometric Method Of Analysis

A. Current-Potential Curve
B. Potential-Volume Curve
C. Conductance-Volume Curve
D. None Of These

1948. The Potential Of The Mercury Indicator Depend Upon

A. Total Mercuryconcentration
B. Potential Of Ions
C. Total Hydrogen Concentration
D. Voltage Of Electrode

1949. In Titration Assembly, The Electrode System Consists Of

A. Mercury Electrode
B. Reference Electrode
C. Saturated Calomel
D. All Of The Above

1950. Potentiometric Method Can Be Used To Determined The End Point Of

A. Non-Aqueous Titration
B. Potentiometric Titration
C. Aqueous Titration
D. Geometric Titration

1951. An Electronic Millivoltmeter Or A Ph Meter Can Be Used To Measured

A. The E.M.F. Of The Titration Cell
B. Potential
C. The E.M.F. Of The Potential
D. Volumetric Potential

1952. Which Equation Is Related To Potential .

A. Nernst Equation
B. Beer's Law
C. Llkovic Equation
D. All Of The Above

1953. In Which Potentiometric Titration Mercury-Mercury (11) Electrode Use

A. Acid-Base
B. Potentiometric
C. Complexometry
D. Voltage

1954. How To Obtained Balance In Potentiometric Titration ?

A. By Detector
B. By Supply Voltage
C. By Changing The Pot Setting
D. By Transformation

1955. What Is The Accuracy Of A Potentiometric DVM Is

A. Zero
B. Medium
C. Low
D. High

1956. Which Electrode Used In End Point Detection With Dual Polarized Electrodes:-

A. Platinum Electrode
B. Twin Platinum Electrode
C. Reference Electrode
D. All Of The Above

1957. Which Indicating System Use In Potentiometric Determinations Of Halide ?

A. Silver Wire
B. Mercurous Sulfate Electrode
C. Both A And B
D. Hydrogen Ions

1958. Which Is One Of The Most Widely Used Chelating Agent

A. EDTA
B. EDTA-
C. EGTA
D. All Of The Above

1959. What Is EDTA ?

A. Ethylenediamine tetraacetic Acid
B. Ethylene diamine
C. Ethydiamine tetraacetic Acid
D. All Of The Above

1960. Which Of Following Titration method Use Gold Redox Electrode?

A. Gravimetric
B. Conductometric
C. Potentiometric
D. Neutralization

1961. What Is Current Density Of Platinum Redox Electrode ?

A. 0 Ma/Cm2
B. 0.5 Ma/Cm2
C. 0.2 Ma/Cm2
D. 1.0 Ma/Cm2

1962. What Is Recommended To Use As An Auxiliary Electrode ?

A. Platinum wire
B. Hydrogen Ions
C. Hydrogen Electrode
D. Salt Bridge

1963. What Is Potential Of Reference Electrode (Silver- Silver Electrode)

A. -19 Mv
B. 5 Mv
C. 19 Mv
D. 15 Mv

1964. What Is Disadvantage Of Mercury-Coated Indicating Electrodes?
A. Consumed Time By Amalgam Formation
B. Complicated Processes
C. Expensive
D. Time Consumed

1965. What Is The Purpose Of Indicator Electrode ?
A. To Absorbed Electrons
B. To Regulate Electrons
C. To Transmit Electrons
D. To Stimulate Electrons

1966. Whis Is E = I ×R
A. Ph Electrode B. Ohm's Law
C. Potentiometry D. None Of These

1967. Junction Potential Are Caused By The Unequal Mobilies Of Ions In Solution
A. Indicator Electrode
B. Hydrogen Electrode
C. Junction Potential
D. Pt Electrode

1968. Which Of The Following References Electrode In Half Reaction

Hg2Cl2 (L) + 2e- = 2 Hg (L) + 2Cl- (G)
A. Saturated Calomel Electrode (S.C.E.)
B. Pt Electrode
C. Hydrogen Electrode
D. All Of The Above

1969. Potentiometry Is One Type Of
A. Electrochemical Analysis Method
B. Electric Analysis Method
C. Chemical Analysis Method
D. None Of These

1970. What Is Advantage Of Using Small Cells ?
A. Light Weight B. Constant Voltage
C. High Voltage D. All Of The Above

1971. Nitric Acid Is A Good
A. Oxidizing Agent B. Reducing Agent
C. Both A And B D. Rectant

1972. Which Titration Is Based On Formation Of Complex Ion In Processes:-
A. Acid Base Titration
B. Complaxometric Titration
C. Potentiometry Titration
D. All Of These

1973. Which Statement Is True For Ligand :-
A. Form Coordinated Bond With Metal Ion
B. Electron Donar Pair
C. Both
D. None

1974. What Are The Types Of Ligand Found In Complexometric Analysis :-
A. Monodenate B. Pentadenate
C. Multidinate D. All Of The Above

1975. Hardness Of Water Is Determined By :-
A. Sedimentation
B. Complaxometric Titration
C. Acid Base Titration
D. Gravimetry Analysis

1976. Complexometric Titration Is Based On Which Of The Following :-
A. Trimetric Assay B. Bimetry Assay
C. Potential D. Current

1977. EDTA Is Example Of :-
A. Hetradenate Ligand
B. Bidenate Ligand
C. Pentadenate Ligand
D. Multidinate Ligand

1978. Calcium Cyclamate Is Assayed By:-
A. Acid Base Titration
B. Non Aqueous Titration
C. Precipitation Titration
D. Complexometry Titration

1979. The Bond Formed By Complex Containing One Ligand :-
A. Covalent Bond B. Co-Ordinate Bond
C. Ionic Bond D. None

1980. Ligand Having More Than One Electron Donating Group Are Called :-
A. Chelating Agent
B. Complex
C. Sesquesting Agent
D. All

1981. The Solubility Of Metal Complex With Bi Or Polyvalent Metal Ions Is Called :-
A. Hydrophilic Group
B. Hydrophobic Group
C. Both
D. None

1982. In Complexometic Titration End Point Determine By :-
A. Spectrophotometry
B. Amperemetric Titration
C. Potentiometry Titration
D. All

1983. Ammonium Fluoride Will Mask............By Complex Formation:-
A. Aluminium
B. Iron
C. Titanium
D. All

1984. EDTA Forms Complex With Most Of Cation In Chelating Agent :-
A. 1:1
B. 1:2
C. 2:1
D. 2:3

1985. Which Of The Following Is Sequestering Agent :-
A. Ethylenediamine Tetra Acetic
B. Aluminium
C. Dimethyl Glyoxime
D. Salicyldoxime

1986. Which Of The Following Is A Chelating Agent :-
A. EDTA
B. Dimethyl Glyoxime
C. Salicyladehye
D. A&B

1987. For Determination Of End Point In Complexometric Titration Which Types Of Indicator Is Used :-
A. Pka
B. Pkb
C. Pm
D. None

1988. Sodium Lactate Injection Is Assayed By:-
A. Tetrabututyl Ammonium Hydroxide
B. Perchloric Acid
C. Sodium Methoxide
D. Calcium Gluconate

1989. Which Of The Following Are Assayed By Complexometric Titration :-
A. Magnesium Trisilicate
B. Calcium Lactate
C. Sodium Calcium Edentate
D. Progesterone Injection

1990. Zinc Undeocenoate Is Estimated By:-
A. Complexometry
B. Diazotization
C. Precipitation
D. Acid Base Titration

1991. What Are The Types Of Comlexometry Titration:-
A. Direct & Indirect Titration
B. Replacement Titration
C. Back Titration
D. All Of These

1992. Examples Of Complxometric Indicator In Following:-
A. Morderant Black ||
B. Phenopthalin
C. Erichrome Black T
D. Both A&C

1993. What Is The Ph Range For Sodium Alizarin Sulphonate:-
A. 4.6
B. 4.69
C. 4
D. 5

1994. Which Of The Following Indicator Are Not Gives Red To Blue Colour At 6-7 Ph Range:-
A. Solochrome Black T
B. Morderant Black ||
C. Erichrome Black T
D. Methyl Orange

1995. Xylenol Range Indicator Gives Which Colour :-
A. Blue To Black
B. Red To Orange
C. Lemon To Yellow
D. Blue To Red

1996. Which Metal Are Detected By Catachol Violet Indicator Ph Range 8-10:-
A. Mn
B. Mg
C. Fe
D. All Of These

1997. When Ph Range Are 12 And Change Colour Violet To Blue So What Will Be The Indicator
A. Crystal Violet
B. Ammonium Purpurate
C. Alizarin
D. Phenol Red

1998. What Are The Application Of Comlexometry Titration:-
A. Determination Of Calcium
B. Detriminston Of Magnesium
C. Determination Of Hard Water
D. All

1999. What Is Pm Indicator:-
A. Dye To Form Complex
B. Chelate Metal Complex
C. Both
D. None

2000. What Are The Property Of EDTA:-
A. Water Soluble
B. Non Hygroscopic
C. Sequestering Agent
D. All Of The Above

2001. Which Factors Influencing The EDTA Reaction:-
A. Nature & Activity Of Ion
B. Ph
C. Presence Of Ion
D. All

2002. Definition Of Chelating Agent:-
A. Ligand Have 1 Electron Accepting Group
B. Ligand Have Electron
C. Ligand Have More Than 1 Electron Donating Group
D. Ligand Have Proton

2003. What Are The Examples Of Unidenate Ligand:-
A. Ammonia (NH3) B. Halide Ion (Cl,F,I)
C. Cyanide Ions D. All Of These

2004. Which Masking Agent Is Not Use In Comlexometry:-
A. Pottasium Iodide
B. Triethanolamine
C. Pottasium Cynide
D. Tetrahydrocannabinol

2005. Pottasium Iodide Is Use In Complaxometry For Masking Which Agent:-
A. Mercury B. Aluminium
C. Titanium D. Cyanide

2006. The End Point Of Complaxometry Is Shown By Which Of The Following:-
A. Acid Base Titration
B. Colorimeter
C. Pm Indicator D. Ph Meter

2007. Ammonium Purpurate (Murexide) Is Used For Determination Of :-
A. Sodium B. Silver
C. Calcium D. Iron

2008. Which Indicator Shows Blue Colour At End Point
A. Mordant Black ||
B. Erichrome Black T
C. Solochrome Black T
D. All

2009. What Are The Objective For Complexometric Titrations:-
A. Stability Of Metal Ligand Complex
B. PM Indicator
C. Theory Of Metallochrometic Indicators
D. Both B &C

2010. Number Of Bond Formed By Ligand Are Known As Which Of Following:-
A. Complex Bond B. Denticity
C. Corrdinate Bond D. Ionic Bond

2011. The Higher The Complex Stability Constant .... In The Carcinogenic Activity Of
A. Ligand:-A. Greater
B. Lesser
C. Moderant
D. No Effect

2012. The Epemirazation Of Tetra Cycline Is .... Reaction:-
A. Unidenate B. Multidenate
C. Both A & B D. Hexadenate

2013. Which Of These Chelate:-
A. Hemoglobin B. Chlorophyll
C. Cisplatin D. Povidone- Iodine

2014. Sequestering Agent Are :-
A. Ligand Which Form Soluble Chelate
B. Ligands Which Form Complex
C. Insoluble In Water
D. Soluble In Organic Solvent

2015. Replacement Titration Are Used When:-
A. Back Titration End Point Not Sharp
B. Direct Titration Is Not Possible
C. Both
D. None

2016. Mordant Black Is Used In Which Titration:-
A. Replacement Titration
B. Back Titration
C. Direct Titration
D. Acid Base Titration

2017. Xylenol Orange Is Prepared From Which Reagent :-
A. O-Cresol Sulphonapthalein
B. HCHO
C. Iminodiacetic Acid
D. All Of These

2018. IUPAC Name Of Eriochrome Black T :-

A. Sodium 1- (1 Hydroxy -2napthylazo)-6 Nitro-2-Napthol-4-Sulphonate
B. Sodium 1- (1 Hydroxy -2napthylazo)-6 Nitro-2-Napthol-6-Gluconate
C. Sodium 1- (1 Hydroxy -2napthylazo)
D. Sodium 1--6 2-Napthol-6-Gluconate

2019. Which Of The Following IUPAC Are Name Of Fast Sulphon Black F:-

A. 1-Hydroxy-8--Naphthalene-6-Disulfonic Acid
B. 1-Hydroxy--6-Disulfonic Acid
C. 1-Hydroxy-8--Naphthalene-Disulfonic Acid
D. None

2020. What Are The Synonym Of Solochrome Dark Blue :-

A. Erichrome Blue Black RC
B. Erichrome Blue RC
C. Solochrome Blue Black RC
D. None Of These

2021. What Are The Pka Value Of Murexide Indicator At Colour (Red –Violet):-

A. 9.9 B. 9.2
C. 10.3 D. 3.3

2022. Metal Indicator Is Also Know As

A. Metal-Ion Indicator
B. Pm Indicator C. Metalic Indicator
D. None Of These

2023. The Complexometric Titration Curve Ploted Between

A. Ph Vs Concentration
B. Pm Vs 0.1 M EDTA
C. Log(Ph)
D. All Of The Above

2024. How To Detect End Point In Acid-Base Complexometric Titration

A. By Ph Sensitive
B. By Indicator
C. By Metal Sensitive
D. By Metalic Ion

2025. In The EDTA Titration , Pm = ?

A. -Log (M N+) B. Log(Mn-)
C. Log (M N +) D. Log(M+N)

2026. What Is A Point Of Inflexation Occurs ?

A. End Point B. Initial Point
C. Equivalent Point D. Finnal Point

2027. Equivalent Point Determined In Magnitude Of Change Of The Concentration Of The Metal Ion By

A. Amperometric
B. Potentiometric
C. Spectrophotometric
D. All Of The Above

2028. End Point Determined In Magnitude Of Change Of The Concentration Of The Metalion By

A. Amperometric
B. Potentiometric
C. Spectrophometric
D. All Of The Above

2029. Potentiometric Titration Method Used To Determined

A. End Point
B. Equivalent Point
C. A And B
D. Concentration Of Charge

2030. The Precipitation Of Hydroxide Of The Metal Is

A. Acid Salt B. Amphotheric Salt
C. Basic Salt D. Ppt

2031. Substitution Titration May Be Used For

A. Metal Ions B. Ppt Titration
C. Pt Ions D. Complexation

2032. Which Form Of EDTA Complexs That Are More Stable

A. Magnesium B. Calcium
C. A And B D. Potassium

2033. A Standard Solution Of Sodium Hydroxide Used In

A. Acid Base Titration
B. Potentiometric End Point
C. Cation Anions Titration
D. All Of The Above

2034. Fluoride May Be Determined By Precipitation As

A. Lead Chorofluride
B. Lead
C. Chorofluride
D. Fluoride

2035. The Lead Is Titrated With EDTA By Using
A. Xylenol Orange Indicator
B. Methyl Blue Indicator
C. Blue Orange Indicator
D. Methyl Orange Indicator

2036. Which Of Following Can't Be Titrated Complexometrically ?
A. Silver And Gold B. Iron And Gold
C. Silver Andiron D. Gold And Calcium

2037. The Sulphate May Be Determined By Precipitation As
A. Barium Sulphate B. Lead Sulphate
C. Both D. None

2038. Which Precipitate May Be Determined Phosphate ?
A. Mgpo4 6H20 B. Mg(NH4)PO4 6H20
C. Capo4 6H20 D. All Of The Above

2039. What Is The Radio Of Stability Constant Of EDTA Complexes Of Metals M And N Must Be Such That
A. Km / Kn More Then 10power6
B. Km/Kn Is Equal To 10
C. Km/Kn Less Than10
D. Km / Km Is Zero

2040. The Back Titration With Standard Magnesium Ion Solution In The Presence Of
A. Chrome Black
B. With Blank
C. Solochrome Black
D. Pt Electrode

2041. What Is Use Of Masking Agents In A Mixture Can Often Be 'Masked'
A. No Longer React With EDTA
B. Order Masked
C. React With EDTA
D. Colour Masked

2042. Which Of Following Is Not Form Stable Cyanide Complexes With The Cations
A. Cd B. Na
C. Zn D. Ag

2043. An EDTA Titration Depend Upon ...... Determination Of The End Point.
A. The Concentration
B. The Temperature
C. The Precise
D. The Voltage

2044. Which Metal Ion Indicator Affect The Coloured Change Of Indicator
A. Hydrogen Ion B. Potassium Ion
C. Pt Ions D. Calcium Ion

2045. Which Metel Ions Can't React With Murexide To Form Complex ?
A. Cu B. Co
C. Ni D. Cl

2046. The Direct EDTA Titration Of Calcium At Ph=?
A. Ph= 10 B. Ph= 15
C. Ph= 11 D. Ph = 20

2047. The Colour Change In The Direct Titration Of Nickel At Ph 10-11 Is
A. Yellow To Blue – Violet
B. Blue To Violet
C. Violet To Blue
D. Yellow To Blue

2048. Solochrome Black Is Also Known As
A. Erichrome Black T
B. Erichrome T
C. Black T
D. Chrome Black

2049. When Calcium Ions Are Titrated With EDTA At Ph ?
A. Ph Between 4 And 6
B. Ph Between 10 And 12
C. Ph Between 12 And 14
D. Ph Between 8 And 10

2050. A Sharp Colour Change Wine Red To Pure Blue Obtained When EDTA IsTitrated With?
A. Potassium Ions B. Calcium Ions
C. Sodium Ions D. Chloride Ions

2051. What Is The Combining Ratio Between Calcium And The Indicator Is
A. 1:1 B. 1:3
C. 2:3 D. 1:4

2052. Which Compound Is More Stable Between Sodium Or Magnesium And The Indicator Is ?
A. Calcium Compound
B. Both Are Equally Stable
C. Magnesium Compound
D. None Of These

2053. The Metal Ions Indicator "Thymolphthalein Complexone"Is Also Know As
A. Thymolphthalexone
B. Phthalexone
C. Thymolphthalexol
D. Thymol Blue

2054. The Colour Change From Blue To Colourless, When Thymolphalexone Titrated With
A. Sodium
B. Calcium
C. Magnesium
D. Chloride

2055. Which Of Following Colour Change, When Calcium Is Titrate With Thymolphalein Complexone ?
A. Blue To Colour Less
B. Blue To Slight Pink
C. A And B(Both)
D. No Change Of Colour

2056. Which Of The Following Electrode Use Detection Of End Point In Potentiometric Titration ?
A. Mercury Electrode
B. Hydrogen Electrode
C. Calomel Electrode
D. Pt Electrode

2057. The Determination Of Cyanide By Titration With.......Which Involves Formation OfComplex.
A. Standard Potassium Nitrate Solution
B. Potassium Ions
C. Standard Silver Nitrate Solution
D. Sodium Ions

2058. Which Of Following Metal Interfere In The Determination Of Calcium And Magnesium:-
A. Co , Ni
B. Hg, Mn
C. Cu , Zn
D. All Of The Above

2059. How Much Mole Of Copper Solution Titrate With Standard EDTA Solution To Change Colour ?
A. 1 Mole Cu2+
B. 3 Mole Cu3+
C. 2 Mole Cu2+
D. 1 Mole Of Co2

2060. Which Of The Following Colour Change ,If Copper Titrate With Standard EDTA Solution
A. From Purple To Dark Green
B. From Green To Blue
C. From Purple To Blue
D. From Yellow To Blue

2061. The Cyanide Complexes Of Zine And Cadmium May Be Demasked With
A. Formaldehyde Solution
B. Formic Acid
C. Formaldehyde-Acetic Acid Solution
D. Acetic Acid

2062. Which Of Following Reaction Is Correct M 2+ + 4CN- =
A. [M(CN)4] 2-
B. [M(CN)2]
C. [M(CO)2]-
D. [M(CN)6]

2063. Which Reagent Used In Formation Of Complex
A. Ligand + Metal Ion
B. Metal Ions + Acid
C. Metal Ions + Indicator
D. Acid Or Base + Ligand

2064. Complexometric Titration May Be Electrically
A. Positive
B. Neutral
C. Negative
D. All Of The Above

2065. What Is Ligand ?
A. Electron Pair Donor
B. H+ Donor
C. Electron Pair Acceptor
D. Accept 0H-

2066. The Formation Of A Coordination Is Known As
A. Gravimetric Titration
B. Polarography
C. Complexometric Titration
D. Precipitation Formation

2067. Which Of Following Options Related To EDTA ?
A. Tetraprotic Acid
B. Monoprotic Acid
C. Diprotic Acid
D. Triprotic Acid

2068. EDTA Is Used As A Titrant To Determine
A. Water Hardness
B. Hardness Of Metal
C. Moisture
D. End Point

2069. The Metal Ion Is Known As
A. Central Metalatom
B. End Metal Of Complex
C. Initial Metal Atom
D. All Of The Above

2070. The Anion Or Neutral Molecule Is Known As
A. Anion Ligand
B. Ligand
C. Metal Ions
D. Complexation

2071. Central Metal Atom Act As a
A. Lewis Acid
B. Neutral
C. Lewis Base
D. Electron Donor

2072. Techniques use for the separation of mixture.
A. Magnetic attraction
B. Paper chromatography
C. Filtration
D. All of these

2073. Separating funnel use for the separation of
A. Mixture of oil and water
B. Mixture of kerosen oil and water
C. both A and B
D. None of these

2074. Chromatography technique was introduced by
A. Michael tsweet
B. Alice Huang
C. Hedy Lamarr
D. None of these

2075. Chromatographic techniques are
A. TLC
B. Column Chromatography
C. Paper Chromatography
D. All of these

2076. Chromatography use for the
A. Blood test
B. Urine tast
C. Seprate the butter from cream
D. Separate the colour in dye

2077. Congratulations is the process of separation of........... Matrial from a liquid.
A. Insoluble Matrial
B. where filteration dont work well
C. Both A and B
D. None of these

2078. Separation of butter from cream technique use for
A. Centrifugation
B. Filteration
C. Evaporation
D. Crystallization

2079. Distillation use to seprate of
A. Separation of acetone and water
B. Distillation of alcohol
C. To separate colours in dye
D. Both A and B

2080. If a solid particals is dissolved in water. Which methods is used for separating it?
A. Distillation
B. Filteration
C. Evaporation
D. Decantation

2081. settling down of the insoluble solid partical in a liquid is called.
A. decantation
B. Sieving
C. sedimentation
D. filteration

2082. Which one is homogeneous mixture?
A. nitrogen-oxygen mixture
B. mist
C. sand-water mixture
D. Tiny pieces of stones are

2083. It is the process vapor is convented in the water form called...
A. condensation
B. Evaporation
C. Filteration
D. None of these

2084. If the Iron mix with the substance it's separated from the mixture by:
A. magnetic separation
B. Filteration
C. sedimentation
D. Sieving

2085. What is air?
A. pure substance
B. the compound of oxygen and nitrogen
C. heterogeneous mixture
D. homogeneous mixture

2086. Mixture of two liquid like water and oil is seprated by
A. Filteration
B. Separating funnel
C. Evaporation
D. Distillation

2087. Cream formation phenomenon is
A. Permanent
B. Reversible
C. Irreversible
D. Steady state

2088. Extraction reagent Acetylacetone boiling point is

A. 120°c B. 139°c
C. 100°c D. 149°c

2089. Sepration of salt form sea water isprocessing of

A. Distillation B. Magnetic sepration
C. Evaporation D. None of these

2090. Which one method used to separate substances differing in colour, size and shape from a solid mixture ......

A. Handpicking
B. decantation
C. sieving
D. magnetic separation

2091. method use for separate the seeds from the fruit juice is ....

A. filtration B. crystallization
C. sieving D. winnowing

2092. Which one mixtures are not uniform in appearance and composition.

A. Heterogeneous
B. Homogeneous mixture
C. Both A and B
D. None of these

2093. The process liquid convented into vapour is called

A. Evaporation B. Sieving
C. Both A and B D. None of these

2094. Which one process is a separating the component of substances from a liquid mixture by selecting evaporation and condensation.

A. Evaporation B. filtration
C. Distillation D. None of these

2095. State whether 'True'

A. Rock salt is an impure substance.
B. Filtration is used to make fruit juice
C. Filtration is used to make fruit juice
D. All of these

2096. Name of process by water is separated from rice and pulses after washing them.

A. Sedimentation B. Handpicking
C. Both A and B D. None of these

2097. Which method is mainly used to separate small pieces of stones from pulses at home?

A. Filteration B. Distillation
C. Handpicking D. None of these

2098. Which kind of substance is use to loading the clay particles suspended in muddy water?

A. Sedimentation B. Filteration
C. Distillation D. None of these

2099. Which is separation techniques is dependent on difference in volatility

A. Distillation
B. Magnetic separation
C. Crystallization
D. Fractional crystallization

2100. Crystallization exploits difference in which factors?

A. Specific heat B. Melting point
C. Boiling point D. Bubble point

2101. separation by polymer membrane is called

A. Exploits the difference in volatility
B. Exploits the difference in flowability
C. Exploits the difference in diffusivity
D. Exploits the difference in permeability

2102. Which one the separation techniques exploits differences in electric charge and diffusivity?

A. Chromatography B. Distillation
C. Electrophoresis D. Filteration

2103. What is the size of equipment determined by?

A. Rate of mass transfer from one phase to another
B. The number of reactions taking place
C. Rate of heat transfer from one phase to another
D. The amount of byproduct formed

2104. Which of the following is not an important property that governs the extent of separation?

A. Polarizability B. Temperature
C. Vapor pressure D. Radius of gyration

2105. Which of the following methods are to be applied to separate Oxygen rich components and Nitrogen rich components?

A. Zone melting

B. Distillation

C. Crystallization

D. Magnetic separation

2106. How to you will separate o-Xylene and m-Xylene products of same compounds

A. Crystallization

B. Distillation

C. Polymer membrane

D. Electrophoresis

2107. How is Oil and Hexane separated?

A. Distillation

B. Crystallization

C. Separating funnel

D. None of these

2108. How to mixture of isopropyl alcohol and water can be separat?

A. One step distillation

B. Two step distillation

C. Two step crystallization

D. Separating funnel

2109. How to mixture of iron and copper filling can be separated?

A. Magnetic separation

B. Crystallization

C. Evaporation

D. Distillation

2110. How can the DNA fragments be separated from DNA?

A. Crystallization B. Distillation

C. Electrophoresis D. Zone melting

2111. Which manners are chemical or biochemical plant is not operated in?

A. Continuous

B. Semi-continuous

C. Batch-wise

D. Discontinuous

2112. separation process is not required in a manufacturing process.

A. When there is a decomposition reaction

B. When the byproducts are in form of gases

C. When there is a complete conversion

D. When the reaction is reversible

2113. only 5% of Ethylene is converted to Ethylene glycol, why is there a need of 7separation process?

A. feed more reactant to the reacting mixture

B. recover the unreacted Ethylene Glycol

C. To remove the ethylene glycol formed

D. start an intermediate reaction

2114. How is the Diethyl Ether removed in the manufacturing of ethanol from ethylene?

A. Directly removed

B. Low pressure flash drum

C. Crude distillation column

D. Light-ends tower

2115. Chemical reactions require feed mixtures from non-renewable resources like coal, petroleum. What is used in place of non-renewable sources?

A. Sunlight B. Biodiesel

C. Biomass D. Microorganisms

2116. What is a condition of operation for biochemical plant?

A. Metallic catalyst

B. Elevated temperature

C. Chemical catalyst

D. Non-pathologic state of the organism

2117. Which is the separation techniques is not use to the process of manufacturing of citric acid ?

A. Ultrafiltration B. Crystallization

C. Ion-exchange D. Distillation

2118. What is the separation technique is used when a separation operation is accompanied by chemical reaction that facilitates separation?

A. Distillation

B. Reactive distillation

C. Fractional distillation

D. Fractional crystallization

2119. Which is the machines do not require a chemical separation technique?

A. The washing machine
B. Water cooler
C. Refrigerator
D. Coffee machine

2120. Which of the following is NOT an importance of separation process?

A. Reduces the operating cost
B. Reduces the probability of side reactions
C. Reduces the risk of explosion
D. Increases the speed of the reaction

2121. Which of the following is NOT used to represent a chemical process?

A. Block flow diagram
B. Flow chart
C. Process-flow diagram
D. None of these

2122. How to geted salt out of a solution (separating salt from water) we should try...

A. Melting it
B. Using a magnet
C. Evaporate of the water so the salt is left behind
D. Using the solute to redissolve it

2123. If wants to get the iron filings out of some sand, what could she use to separate these two solids

A. A magnet B. Evaporation
C. Decanting D. None of these

2124. Evaporation means going from a liquid convented into ....

A. Solid B. Gas
C. Liquid D. None of these

2125. Condensing means going from a gas to a ....

A. Solid B. Gas
C. Liquid D. None of these

2126. If I will pour the water off after I will boil the potatoes, what is this an example of? [I Shall separating the solid potatoes from the liquid hot water]

A. Decoutage B. Double glazing
C. Decanting D. Decarting

2127. If i will making lip balm. I have pour my cooked mixture by some muslin (fabric). What should I doing to the mixture? [I am going separate the solid particals from the liquid bits: the liquid can fit through the tiny holes in the muslin fabric]

A. Decanting it B. Filtering it
C. Mixing it D. Serrating it

2128. I will put dirty or tap water into afunnel with a paper lining. Clean water comes out of the funnel into beaker and solid dirt gets left behind on the paper. It is an example of ___________

A. Filteration B. Distillation
C. Evaporation D. None of these

2129. If the rain falls, this is because the water vapor in form of the clouds is condensing into liquid

A. Hydrogen B. Water
C. Oxygen D. None pf these

2130. Which of the following is NOT a mixture

A. Water
B. A boiled sweet
C. Hot chocolate made with milk
D. Coffee made up with hot water

2131. Which of the following mixtures can not be separated into its components by DECANTING?

A. Beans in hot water
B. Coffee in hot water
C. Sand in water
D. None of these

2132. If something has been dissolved in water, how to separate it from the water again?

A. By decanting it
B. By dissolving it in milk
C. By evaporating the water
D .None of these

2133. Which methods of separating a solid from a liquid?

A. Decanting, filtering and dissolving
B. Decanting, filtering and evaporating
C. Decanting and dissolving
D. All Of these

2134. Crystallization is the process that sepration of the
A. Dissolved solids into a solution
B. Impossible liquid
C. Liquid in solution
D. None of these

2135. Separating funnel use to seprate
A. Two immiscible liquid
B. Miscible liquid
C. Both A and b
D. None of these

2136. What is the Bunsen burner...
A. Cooling device
B. Heating device
C. Use for filtration
D. Separating device

2137. Bunsen burner was discovered by
A. Robert Bunsen
B. Thomas Alva Edison
C. Michael Faraday
D. Galileo Galilei

2138. Bunsen burner base is made up of
A. Aluminium B. Silver
C. cast Iron D. Stainless Steel

2139. Bunsen burner Nipple made of
A. Brass rod B. Iron
C. Stainless steal D. None of these

2140. Blue flame also known as
A. coolest" flame B. medium flame
C. hottest flame D. None of these

2141. The temperature of medium flame is
A. 200°C B. 300°c
C. 400°c D. 500°C

2142. The hottest flame known as
A. Riaring blue B. Blue flame
C. Yellow Flame D. Orange flame

2143. wash-bottle container use for the
A. Keep distilled water
B. Keep Tablet
C. Keep Capsul
D. Keep Eye drops

2144. stirring rod also known as
A. Glass rod B. stir rod
C. Both A and B D. None of these

2145. Buner tube made up of
A. Metal B. Plastic
C. Rubber D. None of these

2146. Which one glassware use to major the urin sample
A. Volumetric flask
B. Beaker
C. graduated cylinder
D. None of these

2147. Glassware use for make 100 ml of 10% sol. is
A. Volumetric flask B. Beaker
C. Both a and b D. None of these

2148. suction device used to draw up liquids is a:
A. Volumetric flask B. Safety bulb
C. Beaker D. None of these

2149. If the pipette with a bulged-out portion in the middle is
A. Mohr pipette B. Serological pipette
C. Volumetric pipette D. None of these

2150. The destruction of all kind of micro-organisms Called
A. Sanitation B. Sterilization
C. Antisepsis D. All of these

2151. Ug is a unit use to describe for
A. Time B. Weight
C. Volume D. Length

2152. pH 2 is 1000 time more acidic than of ph
A. pH3 B. pH5
C. pH4 D. None of these

2153. For preparing of blood RBC must be use
A. EDTA blood B. oxalated blood
C. citrated blood D. clotted blood

2154. Which one reagent is not routinely use to preserve tissue in a life-like manner:
A. Formic acid
B. Zenker's fluid
C. 40% formaldehyde dissolved in water
D. None of these

2155. What is formula of calculating dilution
A. c1v1=c2v2 B. c1=c2-v
C. Both A and B D. None of these

2156. Formula of dilution (c1v1=c2v2) in c1 stand for
A. initial solution's concentration
B. volume
C. diluted solutions' concentration
D. All of these

2157. In the formula c1v1=c2v2 in c2 is
A. initial solution's concentration
B. Volume
C. Diluted solution's concentrated
D. All of these

2158. Who is invented mass spectrometers
A. J.J Thompson B. Aston
C. Nikola Tesla D. None of these

2159. the sample that has to be analysed is bombarded in the mass spectroscopy With which one
A. Protone B. Neutrons
C. Electrons D. All of these

2160. Mass spectrometer Is separates ions by the
A. Mass
B. Mass to charge ratio
C. Charge
D. None of these

2161. Full form of CARE
A. cromic acid Cleaning mixture
B. Calcium acetate cleaning mixtures
C. Both A and B
D. None of these

2162. Graduated flask size 5 have a tolerance
A. 0.04ml B. 0.05ml
C. 0.06ml D. 0.15ml

2163. Gradated flask size 100 have tolerance
A. 0.06ml B. 0.15ml
C. 0.30ml D. 0.80ml

2164. Which is not correct capacity of the Graduated flask
A. 1ml B. 2ml
C. 300ml D. 500ml

2165. Which one is not correct pipette capacity
A. 1ml B. 5 ml
C. 15 ml D. 25 ml

2166. Pipette capacity 10 ml have a tolerance
A. 0.01ml B. 0.04ml
C. 0.06ml D. None of these

2167. Pipette capacity 100ml have a tolerance
A. 0.01ml B. 0.04ml
C. 0.06ml D. 0.12ml

2168. Which one Reference masses use as the working reference standards or as high - precision analytical weights.
A. Class M B. Class S
C. Class S-I D. Class J

2169. Which one reference masses use as microweight standards for microbalances.
A. ClassM B. ClassS
C. ClassJ D. None of these

2170. Measuring of large volumes of liquids Convenient unit employ
A. Cubic decimeter B. Cubic centimeter
C. Both A and B D. Nine of these

2171. For measuring of smaller volumes of liquid
A. (cm3) B. (dm3)
C. Both A and B D. None of these

2172. According to British standards institution a subsidiary standards tempture is
A. 20°C B. 25°C
C. 27°C D. 30°C

2173. What is the coefficient of cubical expansion of soda glasses as about
A. 0.000030 Per 1°c B. 0.000010 Per1°C
C. 0.00020 Per1°c D. 0.000040 Per1°C

2174. Cofficient of cubical expansion of borosilicate glass about
A. 0.000010 Per 1°C
B. 0.000020 Per 1°C
C. 0.000030 Per 1°C
D. 0.000040 Per 1°C

2175. Which one Apparatus used to measure volume of liquids
A. Measuring cylinder
B. Measuring tapes
C. Jar
D. Cylinder

2176. 1 liter is equal to
A. 100ml B. 1000ml
C. 10mm D. 10 kg

2177. It's Volume measured by help of a curve made in measuring cylinder called
A. Meniscus curve B. Round curve
C. Slanting curve D. None of these

2178. Volume of liquids can be measured by using different instruments which one will be
A. Cylinders B. Volumetric flasks
C. Both A and B D. None of these

2179. Highest tempture Of polythene(L.D.) that tempture it Can't be melted of brack..
A. 80-90°c B. 100-110°c
C. 120-130°c D. None of these

2180. What is the melting point of platinum electrodes
A. 1000°C B. 1200•c
C. 1559°C D. 1773°C

2181. Total weight loss of pure pt at temperature 900°c
A. 0.00 B. 0.08
C. 0.81 D. None of these

2182. Weight loss of platinum 99% and iron 1% By manufacturer of Equipment At 1200°c
A. 0.01 B. 0.04
C. 0.08 D. 0.81

2183. Hot plate is heat the material by
A. Electrically heated
B. Gaseous fuels
C. Vapor
D. All of these

2184. Burners is heated the substance by the
A. Electrically B. Gaseous fuels
C. Vapor D. None of these

2185. Burners fuels are available in the form of
A. Natural gas
B. Liquidfied petroleum
C. Bottled gas
D. All of these

2186. Electric ovens have maximum tempture
A. 110 -140°c B. 250-300°c
C. 300-500°c D. None of these

2187. Microwave oven use for the
A. Drying B. Heating
C. Both Aand B D. None of these

2188. Which one Process is not related to microwave oven
A. Determination of moisture contact
B. Heating of substance
C. Drying of substance
D. Remove the impurities

2189. Maximum tempture of the Muffle furnances..
A. 500°c B. 800°c
C. 1200°c D. 1500°c

2190. Muffle furnaces Heated the substance by
A. Electrically B. Gaseous
C. Liquid substances D. None of these

2191. Air baths have a maximum tempture limited up to
A. 120•c B. 180°c
C. 250°c D. 400°c

2192. Air baths use for the
A. Drying solids B. Vaporization of acid
C. Evaporation D. All of these

2193. Air baths can be made up of
A. Nickel B. Copper
C. Both A and B D. None of these

2194. Beaker tongs are made up of
A. Solid nickel
B. Nickel steel
C. rustless ferro-alloy
D. All of these

2195. Handling capacity of beaker tongs are
A. 10 -20ml B. 100 -500 ml
C. 100 - 2000 ml D. 1-1000 ml

2196. A desiccator use for the
A. Strange of the object in dry atmosphere
B. Ensure the absorption
C. Major the drying rate of substance
D. None of these

2197. Desiccator is covered by the
A. Glass container
B. Iron container
C. Stainless steal container
D. Both A and B

2198. Stirring apparatus use for the
A. Heating B. Cooling
C. Mixing D. None of these

2199. StIrring rod is made From
A. Glass rod 3-5 mm in diameter
B. Iron rod 2-5mm in diameter
C. Stainless steal 6-10mm in diameter
D. None of these

2200. Funnel can be use like
A. Simplest apparatus for filteration
B. Transfer of liquid ane apparatus to another
C. Mixing
D. Both A and B

2201. Example of reagents are
A. Colline reagent
B. Fenton's reagents
C. Million's reagents
D. All of these

2202. Reagents use for the detection of
A. Parsent of another substances in molecule
B. Absence of another substance in molecule
C. Measurement of the concentration of substance
D. All of these

2203. Purification is the process that is use for
A. Recrystallisation From water
B. Filteration
C. Both A and B
D. None of these

2204. The Process is faster than filtration but not so effective
A. Decanting B. Centrifuging
C. Crystallization D. None of these

2205. Crystallization process is used For the
A. Purify sugar
B. Purify fertilizers
C. Separate salt from solution
D. Both A and B

2206. Anhydrous agent is used for remove water from ethanol distillate can be
A. Iodine B. Hydrocarbon
C. Calcium chloride D. None of these

2207. Only one kind of atom is found in
A. organic compounds
B. inorganic compounds
C. pure substances
D. All of these

2208. Water May be separated from sea water By the
A. Centrifugation
B. Separating funnel
C. Fractional distillation
D. Simple distillation,

2209. separatation of insoluble particles from liquids is called
A. Drying B. Filteration
C. Sieving D. All of these

2210. When the tip of funnel touches side of beaker it avoids
A. Splashing B. Bubbling
C. Bumping D. All of these

2211. cover one fourth Part of the filter paper with precipitate filter paper should be
A. Large B. Medium
C. Small D. Very small

2212. Filter paper Should be folded
A. One time B. Two time
C. Three time D. Five time

2213. Concentration polarization may be reduced by
A. By the pre filtration of solution
B. Back washing periodically
C. Reducing the flow rate per surface area
D. All of these

2214. What is the angle of the filter paper ,when it's keep into the funnel
A. 30° B. 40°
C. 60° D. 80°

2215. Direct dryers are known as
A. Batch driers
B. Semi-batch driers
C. Continuous driers
D. None of these

2216. Cabinet/ Tray driers are
A. Direct dryers B. Indirect dryers
C. Both A and B D. None of these

2217. It's necessary to know about the dryer size and
A. Time of drying B. Heat of drying
C. Speed of drying D. All of these

2218. Constant drying conditions include
A. Temperature constant
B. Humidity constant
C. Velocity constant
D. All of these

2219. What is drum dryer called f it will open to the atmosphere?
A. Open dryer B. Box dryer
C Trough dryer D. Trench dryer

2220. Which material is not used in drying in a freeze dryer?
A. Seafood
B. Dyes
C. Pharmaceuticals
D. None pf these

2221. Which dryer used radiation for drying?
A. Drum dryer B. Microwave dryer
C. Heat exchanger D. Nucleator

2222. In the drying process the final product found in the form of
A. Slurry B. Solution
C. Solid D. All of these

2223. Condition that is the highly critical for drying operation
A. Moisture B. Tempture
C. Ph D. Volume

2224. Drying is as essential offer
A. Crystallization B. Evaporation
C. Mixing D. Size reduction

2225. The sepration principal of GLC is
A. Absorption B. Partataion
C. Ion exchange D. Interaction

2226. The sepration ofprincipal in GLC Is gas liquids Chromatography
A. Absorption B. Partataion
C. Ion exchange D. Gel permeation

2227. Measurements of pH is an example of
A. Conductometry B. Amperimetry
C. Biamperometry D. Potentiometry

2228. Best example of the solid state electrode
A. Cakomek electrode
B. Hydrogen electrodes
C. Fluoride electrodes
D. All of these

2229. Compression is done by process
A. Cutter mill B. Roller mill
C. Hammer mill D. Colloidal mill

2230. Impact is done by process
A. Cutter mill B. Roller mill
C. Hammer mill D. None of these

2231. Attrition process is the done by
A. Hammer mill B. Colloidal mill
C. Roller mill D. All of these

2232. Impact and attrition process done by
A. Ball mill B. Fluid energy mill
C. Both A and B D. None of these

2233. What Is the final products size of cutter mill
A. 0.5-0.01cm B. 1-30 micron
C. 30-50 micron D. None of these

2234. What is the final product size of roller mill
A. 0.5- 0.01cm B. 1 - 30 micron
C. 30-50 micron D. None of these

2235. Roller mill use for
A. Soft material B. Abrasive Matrial
C. Friable matrial D. Both B and C

2236. Fluid energy mill is not use for
A. Vitamin B. Antibiotics
C. Enzymes D. Soft material

2237. What is the actions of ball mill
A. Crushing
B. Impact and attrition
C. Compression
D. All of these

2238. What is the action of End and Edge runner mill
A. Crushing B. Shearing
C. Both A and B D. None of these

2239. Ball mill not use for the
A. Hard product B. Abrasive products
C. Both A and B D. None of these

2240. What is the final product size of ball mill
A. 0.01cm B. 0.10cm
C. 0.05cm D. None of these

2241. End and Edge Runner mill use for
A. Fibrous B. Tough
C. Sticky Matrial D. All of these

2242. What is the partical size of compression
A. 100-80000 micron
B. 50-8000 micron
C. 50-10000 micron
D. 1-50 micron

2243. Coarse powder must be pass through by sieve no
A. 10 B. 22
C. 44 D. 85

2244. Fine powder can be pass through the sieve no
A. 10 B. 22
C. 44 D. 85

2245. What is the SI unit of tempture
A. Degree Celsius B. Degree Fahrenheit
C. Kelvin D. None of these

2246. Zero kelvin(K) equals to
A. 37°c B. -273°c
C. +273°c D. Both A and B

2247. The wet bulb tempture is the always.
A. Lower than the dry bulb tempture
B. Higher Then the dry bulb tempture
C. Equally to the dew point tempture
D. None of these

2248. Humidity can be major by
A. Gravimetric method
B. Hygrometer
C. Tempture based
D. All of the these

2249. Which one method most accurate for humidity measurement
A. Gravimetric Method
B. Tempture Based
C. Hygrometer
D. Both A and B

2250. Tray dryer use for the
A. Drying of chemicals
B. Power
C. Continuous
D. Both A and B

2251. Tray dryer not suitable for
A. Continuous process
B. Batch process C. Both A and B
D. None of these

2252. Fluidized bed dryer use for the
A. Drying of tables
B. Plastic Matrial
C. Coal
D. All of these

2253. Tunnel dryer use for the drying of
A. Gelatine B. Plastic
C. Inorganic salt D. Coal

2254. Rotary dryer not use for the
A. Continuous process
B. Batch process
C. For short drying(30 min)
D. None of these

2255. Drying of the biological products, blood products, enzymes and antibiotics wgich one dryer use
A. Freeze dryer B. Spray dryer
C. Tray dryer D. Tunnel dryer

2256. Sublimation pressure of the freeze dryer is
A. 0.1 -0.3mm-Hg B. 0.5-0.7 mm-Hg
C. 0.2-0.7mm-Hg D. None of these

2257. Spray dryer generally use for the
A. Milk product
B. Drying of the paraffin wax gelatin
C. Both A ab B
D. None of these

2258. Drum dryer have
A. Single drum B. Double drum
C. Twin drum D. All of these

2259. What is the frequency range of of microwave vacum dryer
A. 300-3000 MHZ B. 10-100 MHZ
C. 200-2000 MHZ D. 500-5000 MHZ

2260. Pan dryer widely use for, the
A. Slurries B. Solution
C. Filter cake D. All of these

2261. Drying for the paste or Sludges dryer use for
A. Vacuum dryer B. Rotary dryer
C. Turbo dryer D. FBD

2262. The crystallization process is consist of major events know as
A. Nucleation B. Crystal growth
C. Both A and B D. None of these

2263. What is the nucleation

A. Solute molecule dispersed in solvent
B. Solvent dispersed in solute
C. Mass transfer of solute from the liquid solution
D. Both A and C

2264. According to super saturation method In Tank crystallizer use for

A. Cooling B. Evaporation
C. pH D. None of these

2265. Which one crystallization equipment not belong to Cooling process

A. Tank crystallizer B. Magma crystallizer
C. Swenson walker crystallizer
D. Krystal crystallizer

2266. Magma crystallizer working on the method of

A. Evaporation B. Cooling
C. Both A and B D. None of these

2267. Tank crystallizer's uses for

A. Globar salt B. Synthatic sponge
C. Both A and B D. None of these

2268. Which is not Processing of size reduction

A. Impact B. Attrition
C. Cutting D. Elutriation

2269. Dry mill Should be Contain maximum moisture

A. <2% B. <3%
C. <4% D. <5%

2270. Mill use for the low melting drug

A. Hammer mill B. Fluid energy mill
C. Cutter mill D. Ball mill

2271. Light is generally use in radiant heat dryer

A. Uv rays B. Infrared light
C. Sun light D. None of these

2272. Chromatography is used to separate

A Solution B Atom
C Mixture D Molecule

2273. Partltion cofficient (Kp = S1/S2) In s1 is

A Solubility of substance A in solvent 'a'
B Solubility of substance A in solvent` b`
C Both A and B
D None of these

2274. Two phase aqueous extraction requires

A Low water content and low surface tension
B High water content and low surface tension
C Low water content and high surface tension
D High water content and high surface tension

2275. In Two phase aqueous extraction ....are usedto create two (or more) aqueous phases.

A Natural hydrophilic polymers
B Synthetichydrophilic polymers
C Hydrophobic polymers
D Both A and B

2276. Determination of lead(II)by method

A Thiocynate method
B Dithizone method
C Both A and B
D None of these

2277. The extraction of cpbalt from hydrochloric acid using.................... In meta -xylene

A Alamine336 B Nickel
C Cobalt D Hydroxyoximes

2278. Nickel can be extracted using............. and tributyl phosphate in hudro corbon diluent

A Alkyl amines
B Phasphoric acid
C Tributyl phosphate
D Non of these

2279. Palladium and platinum can be extract by using

A Dialkyl sulfides
B Alkyl amine
C Tributyl phosphate
D All of above

2280. The process of settling down of particals of a solid in liquid known as

A Sublimation B Decantation
C Sedimentation D Precipitation

2281. Which are the following is essential to perform winnowing activity?

A Soil B Wind
C Water D None of these

2282. Hand picking method is effective in
A Gaseous mixture
B Liquid mixture
C Solid mixture
D None of these

2283. Salt is obtained from sea water by using which the following process.
A Sedimentation B Evaporation
C Condensation D Congratulations

2284. Which of the following method use to seprate two miscible liquid?
A Separating funnel
B Filtration
C Sieving
D Winnowing

2285. washing machine dries clothes work on the principal of
A Filteration B Evaporation
C Centrifugation D None of these

2286. Which one belong to Duhring's rule
A. Crystallization B. Evaporation
C. Filteration D. Distillation

2287. Filter fraction done by the following mechanism
A. Sieving or screening
B. Electrostatic attraction
C. Entrapment
D. All of these

2288. Clarification is the process use when the solid contant of the product
A. Doesn't exceeded 1%
B. Doesn't exceeded 7%
C. Doesn't exceeded 15%
D. All of these

2289. Fixed oil should be extracted by using
A. Vacuum still B. Molecule still
C. Water still D. All of these

2290. Total 100 squares in a 1 inch^2 area is termed
A. 100 mesh sieve B. 15 mesh sieve
C. 20 mesh sieve D. 10 mesh sieve

2291. What are the factors affecting the evaporation
A. Surface area of liquid
B. Tempture
C. pH
D. Both A and B

2292. Vacuum pan use for the
A. Thermo labile products
B. Viscous matrial
C. Use for suger
D. All of these

2293. Evaporating still use for the
A. Thermo labile Matrial
B. Use for liquor
C. None viscous
D. All of these

2294. Vartical tube evaporator use for
A. Suger B. Havy chemicals
C. Salt D. All of these

2295. Climbing film (kestner tube) evaporator use for
A. Insuline B. Vitamin
C. Blood plasma D. All of these

2296. Falling film evaporator use for
A. Viscous liquids B. Insuline
C. Blood plama D. Bone of these

2297. Rotary film evaporator use for
A. Low viscous liquids
B. High viscous liquid
C. Vitamin
D. All of these

2298. Mixtures are divided into the
A. Positive mixture
B. Negative mixtures
C. Natural mixtures
D. All of these

2299. Positive mixture are
A. Irreversible Mixing
B. Reversible Mixing
C. Both A and B
D. None of these

2300. Example of positive mixture
A. Sugar in water
B. Two immiscible liquid
C. Emulsion
D. Cream

2301. Propeller mixtures rotated at

A. <8000 rpm B. <2000 rpm
C. <4000 rpm D. <1000 rpm

2302. Propeller mixture use for the

A. Glycerin B. Liquid paraffin
C. Castor oil D. Low viscous liquids

2303. Rotation of paddle mixture is

A. 100 rpm B. 50 rpm
C. 10 rpm D. 200 rpm

2304. Which one is not a liquid mixture

A. Propeller mixture
B. Turbine mixture
C. Paddle mixture
D. Tumbling mixture

2305. Which one is not semi solid mixture

A. Sigma blade
B. Planetary motion mixtures
C. Colloidal mixture
D. Turbine mixture

2306. If the solid move with streamline flow and strike of filtermedium.. Mechanism of filteration known as

A. Straining B. Impingement
C. Entanglement D. Attractive Force

2307. Mechanism of filteration in partical become entangled in mass of fiber due to small Size of Partical than pore size process known as

A. Straining B. Entanglement
C. Impingement D. Attractive fource

2308. Surface filteration also know as

A. Screen filteration B. Cake filteration
C. Depth filteration D. None of these

2309. What is the principal of super centrifuge

A. Sedimentation B. Sieving
C. Filteration D. All of these

2310. Plate and frame filtration work on the principal of

A. Surface filtration
B. Sedimentation
C. Sieving
D. None of these

2311. Ultra centrifuge use for the

A. Sepration of solid from liquids
B. Blood plasma sepration
C. Use for anhydrous product
D. All of these

2312. What is the speed of high speed centrifuge

A. 1000 rpm B. 3000 rpm
C. 10000rpm D. 5000 rpm

2313. Cartidge filters work on the principal of

A. Sieving B. Filteration
C. Centrifuge D. None of these

2314. Cartidge filter use for the

A. Plasma Sepration
B. Manufacturing of ophthalmic products
C. Manufacturing of enzymes
D. Emulsion

2315. Filteration centrifuge use for the

A. Blood plasma sepration
B. Collidal research
C. Obtained anhydrous product
D. Emulsion

2316. Which one equipment use for the sepration of cream from the milk

A. De laval clarifire
B. Super centrifuge
C. Perforated basket type
D. All of these

2317. What is the wave -Length of IR lamp

A. 1μm B. 5 μm
C. 10 μm D. 20 μm

2318. What is the wave -length Of ceramic rods and panels

A. 5 to 20 μm B. 20 to 50 μm
C. 2 to 4 μm D. 5 to 15 μm

2319. Simple distillation use for

A. Preparation of distilled water
B. Water for injection
C. Both A and B
D. None of these

2320. Flash distillation use for the

A. Preparation of distilled water
B. Water for injection
C. Petroleum eather sepration
D. All of these

2321. Absolute alcohol is the prepared by the the method
A. Simple distillation
B. Azeotropic Distillation
C. Flash distillation
D. Steam distillation

2322. Sepration of immiscible liquids to the method
A. Simple distillation
B. Steam distillation
C. Flash distillation
D. All of these

2323. Sepration of vitamin from the distillation method by the process
A. Azeotropic Distillation
B. Extractive distillation
C. Steam distillation
D. Molecular distillation

2324. Dry -distillation is known as
A. Destructive distillation
B. Steam distillation
C. Simple distillation
D. Flash distillation

2325. Obtaining fresh water from the sea -water for making pyrogen free process knows as
A. Destructive distillation
B. Steam distillation
C. Flash distillation
D. Compression distillation

2326. Which one process use to the refining of fixed oil
A. Molecular distillation
B. Simple distillation
C. Steam distillation
D. None of these

2327. Sepration of of miscible liquid like acetone and water process use
A. Simple distillation
B. Compression distillation
C. Flash distillation
D. Fractional distillation

2328. Gelsication term is use for
A. Vacuum drying B. Freeze drying
C. Turbo drying D. None of these

2329. Working principal of the freeze drying is
A. Evaporation of water
B. Sublimation of water from ice phase to gas phases
C. Liquefaction of ice to water
D. None of these

2330. Which one light is Most widely used in radiant heat dryer
A. Radio waves B. Sunlight
C. Uv rays D. Infrared light

2331. Size reduction of plant like rouwolfia can be size rduced the best way
A. Cutter mill B. Ball mill
C. Hammer mill D. None of these

2332. Which one is not a filter aid
A. Gelatin B. Carbon
C. Diatomite D. Asbestos

2333. Modified type of sweet land Filter is
A. Leaf filter B. Edge filter
C. Cartridge filter D. None of these

2334. Mixer belong to the agitator mixer
A. Planetary mixer B. Sigma bladder
C. Both A and B D. Ribbon blender

2335. Indicator Cresol red produce colour in acid
A. Red B. Yellow
C. Green D. Blue

2336. Indicator cresol red give produce colour with alkaline solution
A. Red B. Green
C. Yellow D. None of these

2337. What should be the pH range of acid solution that indicator Brilliant cresyl blue produce red colour
A. 0.0-1.0 B. 0.2-1.8
C. 0.5-2.5 D. 0.8-1.9

2338. Indicator methyl red produce colour with acid solution
A. Red B. Yellow
C. Green D. Orange

2339. Methyl red produce colour with alkali solution
A. Green B. Blue
C. Red D. Yellow

2340. What is the chemical name of indicator cresol red (base)
A. 1-cresolsulphonphthalien
B. 1-Cresol
C. Phenolphthalein
D. None of these

2341. What is the pk'in vallue of thymol blue indicator
A. 1.5 B. 1.7
C. 2.1 D. 7.3

2342. Phenol red produce the cilour with the alkaline solution
A. Blue B. Green
C. Orange D. Red

2343. Indicator bromocresol green produce colour with alkaline solution
A. Yellow B. Blue
C. Green D. None of these

2344. Nitramine produce orange -brown colour in solution of
A. Acid solution B. Alkaline solution
C. Both A and B D. None of these

2345. What is the chemical name of phenolphthalein
A. Thymol phthalein B. Phenolphthalien
C. Both A and B D. None of these

2346. Indicator use in the complexometric titration
A. Rose bengal B. Eosin
C. Crystal violet D. Murexide

2347. Indicators use for the aqueous titration method
A. Methyl orange B. Methyl red
C. Methyl yellow D. All of these

2348. Indicator 1-napthol use for titration
A. Complexometric B. Nonaqueous
C. Aqueous D. All of these

2349. Methyl red indicator use for titration
A. Aqueous B. Nonaqueous
C. Complexometric D. Both A and B

2350. Xylenol orange indicator use in titration
A. Complexometric B. Nonaqueous
C. Precipitation D. Aqueous

2351. Which one indicator not use in the precipitation titration
A. Eosin B. Alizarin red
C. Rose bengal D. Zincon

2352. Indicator nitramine give the colour in acid solution
A. Red B. Orange
C. Blue D. Colourless

2353. What is chemical name of natural red indicator
A. Aminodimethylaminotoluphenazonium chloride
B. Phenolphthalien
C. Both A and B
D. None of these

2354. Ethyl red indicator produce colour with alkaline solution
A. Red B. Orange
C. Blue D. Yellow

2355. What should be it's pH range of solution that indicator
A. 6.8 -8.0 B. 1.2-5.5
C. 8.5-9.5 D. 5.5-6

2356. For the drug benzocaine which one titrant use
A. 0.1M NaNO2
B. 0.1cerric ammonium sulphate
C. Both A and B
D. None of these

2357. For drug paracitamol, which one titrant use
A. 0.1M Carric ammonium sulphate
B. 0.05M disod. edetate
C. 0.1M NaNO2
D. None of these

2358. Titration of paracitamol comes under the reaction
A. Complexometric titration
B. Redox titration
C. Idometry titration D. None of these

2359. Drug ascorbic acid comes under the reaction
A. Complexometric titration
B. Redox titration
C. Nitrite titration
D. Iodometry titration

2360. The organic solvent most commonly used in conventional liquid liquid extraction?
A. Ethyl acetate
B. Methyl tert-butyl eather
C. Hexane
D. All of these

2361. Liquid -Liquid extraction Known as
A. Solvent extraction
B. Solutes extraction
C. Both
D. None of these

2362. Which is not a extraction reagent
A. Acetylacetone
B. 2-naphthol
C. 8 -hydroxyquinoline
D. Dimethylglyoxime

2363. In liquid-liquid extraction, if the feed flow rate is F, what is the maximum flow rate of solvent in the following ternary system: (Feed point e, solvent point a)
A. F*(eb/ba) B. F*(ed/da)
C. F*(ec/ca) D. F

2364. Gibbs phase rules is
A. P+V=C+2 B. [A]1/[A]2=contact
C. PV=C+2 D. None of these

2365. In the Gibbs phase rules V stand for
A. No. of phase B. No. Of components
C. Solvent D. Degree of freedom

2366. Formula of distribution coefficient
A. [A]1 / [A]2 = Contact
B. K=0.6993w/V
C. PV=C+2
D. None of these

2367. 1. A measure of the degree of molar polarization of a compound is
A. Electrostatic capacity C
B. Partition coefficient K
C. The dielectric constant D
D. None of these

2368. Which plays a deciding role in the choice of solvents in liquid-liquid extraction process
A. The dielectric constant D
B. Partition coefficient K
C. Both of above
D. None of above

2369. . From given list which is least polar solvent
A. Hexane
B. Carbon tetrachloride
C. Cyclohexane
D. Water

2370. The simplicity of extraction process is decided by
A. The dielectric constant
B. Partition coefficient
C. Electrostatic capacity
D. None of these

2371. Out of given list, in which condition the extraction should be easy?
A. Whenever a value of K is 0.1
B. Whenever a value of K is 0.5
C. Whenever a value of K is 10
D. Whenever a value of K is 50

2372. In which process the feed and extracting solvent pass through the cascade in opposite directions?
A. Single-stage extraction system
B. Co-current extraction system
C. Counter-current extraction system
D. None of these

2373. The half-life of penicillin G atPH2.0, 20°C is,
A. 10 minutes B. 30 minutes
C. 15 minutes D. 60 minutes

2374. The solution of known concentration called as
A. Analyte B. Titrant
C. Standard solution D.None of these

2375. The solutions of unknown concentration but known volume called as
A. Analyte B. Titrant
C. Standard solution D. Both B and C

2376. Pure water molecule contains
A. Only water molecules
B. hydronium ions only
C. Water molecules, hydronium ions, and hydroxide ions
D. Both A and B

2377. Carminic acid produce purple color with

A. Alkalis B. Acid
C. Weak Acid D. None of these

2378. What is the substance in that Phenolphthalein changes colors

A. Acid B. Water
C. Alkalis D. None of these

2379. M is stand for

A. Molarity B. Normality
C. Molality D. None of these

2380. What is the range of pH scale

A. 0-1 B. 0-5
C. 0-12 D. 0-14

2381. Acid base titration known as

A. Composition reaction
B. Neutralization reaction
C. Decomposition reaction
D. All of these

2382. It is the number of moles of solute, parsent in per kilogramOf solvent known as

A. Normality B. Molarity
C. Molality D. None of these

2383. Titrimetric calculations is

A. NaVa=NsVs B. MaVa=MsVs
C. NaVs=VaNs D. Both A and B

2384. In the equation(NaVa=NsVs) Na stand for

A. Normality of analyte
B. Normality of standard solution
C. Both A and B
D. None of these

2385. In the equation (MaVa=MsVs) Ms stand for

A. Molarity of standard solution
B. Normality of standard solutions
C. Molarity of analyte
D. None of these

2386. What will be results when the reaction between the HCl +NaOH

A. Water + salt B. Salt
C. Onlt Acid D. None of these

2387. It's involves the formation of colored precipirate at the end point known as

A. Mohr's method B. Volhard's method
C. Fajan's method D. None of these

2388. An acid is a substance which when dissolved in water gives H+ ions and a base is a substance which on dissolution in water give OH- ions. This theory is given by:

A. Arrhenius
B. Bronsted-lowry
C. Both a and b
D. Lewis

2389. An acid is a substance that can donate a proton and a base is a substance that can accept a proton. This theory is given by:

A. Arrhenius B. Bronsted-lowry
C. Lewis D. All of the above

2390. Acids act as electron pair acceptors and bases act as electron pair donors. This theory is given by:

A. Arrhenius B. Bronsted-lowry
C. Lewis D. None

2391. The parts by weight of that substance which is chemically equivalent to 1.008 parts by weight of hydrogen (or 8 parts by weight of oxygen or 35.45 parts by weight of chlorine) is known as:

A. Molecular weight
B. Equivalent weight
C. Molecular mass
D. None

2392. For an monobasic acid equivalent weight is equal to its:

A. Molecular mass
B. Molecular weight
C. Equivalent weight
D. None

2393. Hcl,hbr,HI,hclo4 are:

A. Dibasic acids
B. Tri basic acids
C. Monobasic acids
D. Tetrabasic acids

2394. The number of ionisable hydrogen atoms present in a molecule of an acid is known as:

A. Acidity B. Molecular weight
C. Basicity D. Equivalent weight

2395. Amount of solute per 100 parts of solution is known as:

A. Percentage
B. Parts per billion
C. Parts per million
D. Parts per thousand

2396. Number of parts of solute per million parts of solution is known as:

A. Percentage
B. Parts per billion
C. Parts per million
D. Parts per thousand

2397. Amount of solute in grams present in one litre of the solution is called:

A. Concentration B. Strength
C. Molarity D. Molality

2398. Number of gram equivalents of a solute present in per litre of solution is called:

A. Molarity B. Formality
C. Molality D. Normality

2399. Number of moles of a solute present in per litre of solution is called:

A. Molarity B. Formality
C. Molality D. Normality

2400. Which of the following glycoside linkage foud in maltose ?

A. Glucose (â - 2 b) fructose
B. Glucose (a1 - 4) glucose
C. Galactose (b1 - 4) glucose
D. Glucose (b1 - 4) glucose

2401. which of the following is an aldotriose ?

A. Dihydroxyacetate B. Glyceraldehyde
C. Ribulose D. Erythrose

2402. The glycoside linkage in cellobiose is

A. a 1 - 4 B. b 1 - 4
C. a1 - 6 D. b 1 - 6

2403. Which of the following sugar a positive result with seliwonoff test .

A. Sucrose B. Glucose
C. Galactose D. Mannose

2404. A pentose sugar reported to be present in heart cells is ?

A. Xylose B. Arabinose
C. Lyxose D. Xylulose

2405. Majority of monosachharides found in human body are of ?

A. L - type B. D - type
C. DL type D. None

2406. How many number of asymmetric carbon atoms is present in moleculor formula of Hexoser?

A. 4 B. 5
C. 2 D. 3

2407. Aqueqous solution of fructose is also called as ?

A. Fructopyranose B. Laevulose
C. Fructofurnose D. None of them

2408. When D fructose undergoes a condensation reaction with phenylhydrazine it gives

A. D - fructose phenylhydrazone
B. D- fructose semicarbazone
C. D - fructose Oxime
D. Both (a) and (b)

2409. When sucrose is heated to 210° c it it forms a brown mass calked as

A. Sucrosates B. Sucrose octacetate
C. caramel D. All of the above

2410. A molecule of Amylopectin which contain 1500 glucose residues and is branched after every 30 residues . How many residues ends are there !

A. 0 B. 1
C. 2 D. 5

2411. Which of the following compound is responsible for coordinatrd regulation of glucose and glycogen metabolism?

A. NAD+
B. Fructose 2,6 bisphosphate
C. Acrtylel CoA
D. Fructose 1,6 bisphosphate

2412. Cellulose fibers resembles with protien structure in the form of

A. B sheets B. a helices
C. B turns D. None of the above

2413. Glucagon and epinephrine

A. Inhibits gluconeogenesis and stimulates glycolysis

B. Stimulates gluconeogenesis and glycolysis
C. Stimulates glconeogenesis and inhibit glycolysis
D. Inhibits glucneogenesis and glyoclysis

2414. The NA6 substrate is hydrolysed by human lycozyme to form
A. 6 glucosamnie + 6 Acetic acid
B. NAG4 + NAG2
C. NAG3 + NAG2
D. NAG3

2415. Which of the following Mucopolysacharides is non sulfated and most abundant in tissue ?
A. Hyaluronic acid B. Heparin
C. keraten suplhate D. Dermatan suphate

2416. Which of the followin gives a Negative reaction with Barfoed's test
A. Glucose B. Maltose
C. Erthromycin D. Fructose

2417. N - Acetyl Neuromini acid is
A. Sugar B. Amino sugar acid
C. Amino sugar D. Sugar alcohol

2418. Which of the following does not form Osazone crystals?
A. Galactose B. Maltose
C. Lactose D. Sucrose

2419. Which of the following tests is not bsed on reactor of carbohydrates with strong acid?
A. Molisch B. Bendict's
C. Bial's D. Saliwonoff's

2420. Mucioc acid and Gluconic acid are
A. Glycosides
B. Sugar acids
C. Amino sugar acids
D. Sugar alcohols

2421.All tests are positive for Lactose expect
A. Benedict's B. Barfoed
C. Molisch D. Osazone

2422. Which of the follwing is a keto tertrose?
A. Xylose B. Erythrose
C. Fructose D. Sedoheptulose

2423. Choose an Aldo pentose
A. Glyceraldehyde B. Dihydroxyacetate
C. Erthryose D. Arabinose

2424. Choose asugar abundantely present in Honey
A. Maltose B. Fructose
C. Ribulose D. Lactose

2425. Which out of the following is a fructosan?
A. Glycogen B. Agar
C. Inulin D. Celluloae

2426. What is the moleculor formula of cellobiose
A. $C12H22O12$ B. $C12H24O12$
C. $C14H22O12$ D. $C12H26O18$

2427. A polysachharide formed by B1-4 glycoside linkage between glucose residuals
A. Inulin B. Amylase
C. Agar D. Cellulose

2428. a-D glucose and b-D glucose are
A. stereo isomers
B. Anamers
C. Ketoaldose isomers
D. Optical isomers

2429. Uses of starch includes :
A. To treat textile fibres
B. Manufacturing of dextrins
C. In coating and sizing paper
D. All of the above

2430. Inulin is found in the roots of
A. Chichory B. Dahlia
C. Dandelion D. All of the above

2431. Gun cotton is obtained when
A. All OH groups are replaced with ONO2
B. All O groups are replaced with ONO2.
C. Both (a) and (b)
D. None

2432. Cotton is traeted with strong NaoH solution anf wash from alkali then product formed is .
A. Ethyl cellulose B. Mercised cotton
C. Inulin D. None of the above

2433. What are the test that are carried out for carbohydrates .

A. Molisch 's test B. Anthrone test
C. Fehling 's test D. All of the above

2434. Amylopectin is composed of chains of units.

A. 20 to 24 D glucose
B. 24 to 30 D glucose
C. 22 to 30 D glucose
D. 20 to 22 D glucose

2435. Relative sweetness of which artifical sugar is highest ?

A. Cyclamate B. Nectrain
C. Sachharin D. Invertase

2436. Lactose ia also hydrolysed by an enzyme that hydrolyses B glycodides .

A. Lactonic acid B. D Galactose
C. Emulsion D. Both (a) and (b)

2437. Lactose reacts with phenylhydrazine in presence of acetic acid to produce

A. Emulsion B. Lactosazone
C. Inulin D. All of the above

2438. In extraction of sugar solution washed beets are cut by specially shaped knives called.

A. V shape knife B. Cutters
C. Difuses D. Coseltes

2439. Lactose reacts with Dmethyl sulphate in alkaline soltion to form.

A. Pentamethyl lactose
B. Octamethyl lactose
C. Caramel
D. Tetramethyl lactoe

2440. On oxidation of lactose with Bromine water it yields ?

A. Monocarboxyli acid
B. Lactobionic acid
C. Lactonic acid
D. All of the above

2441. Sucrose in aqueqous solution reacts with hydroxides of calicum, rarium, strantium to produce.

A. Fructose B. Invertase
C. Sucrosates D. None of the above

2442. The percentage of amylopectin in natural starch is ?

A. 70 to 80 B. 80 to 90
C. 60 to 90 D. 60 to 80

2443. When starch reacts with iodine it forms deep blue colour due to

A. Hydrolysis of starch
B. Decomposition of dextrins
C. Presence of amylopectin
D. Inclusion complex

2444. Cellulose dissolves in very special reagents like

A. Schweitzer's reagent
B. Cross and Bermi reagent
C. Mixtur of NaoH and carbon disulphide
D. All of the above

2445. One projection commonly used for repsentation of D and L Glyceraldehyde is known as:

A. Enantiomers
B. Robert projection
C. Fischer projection
D. Both (a) and (b)

2446. The simpler way of drawing fischer projection is to use

A. Horizontal lines B. Vertical lines
C. Diagonal lines D. All of the above

2447. In aldotroses how many optical isomers are posible

A. 2 to 6 B. 2 to 4
C. 2 to 8 D. only 2

2448. The D and L- erthryose are mirror images so also be called

A. Mesoisomers B. Enantiomers
C. Superimposible D. None of the above

2449. Aldohexoses contain how many numbers of asymmetric carbon atom

A. 2 B. 4
C. 3 D. 1

2450. How many optical isomers are possible in Epimers

A. 6 to 16 B. 4 to 16
C. 2 to 16 D. 8 to 16

2451. What is a Deoxy sugar
A. Hydroxyl group is replaced by hydrogen atom
B. Hydroxyl atom is replaced by hydroxyl group
C. Both (a) and (b)
D. None of the above

2452. In process of conversion of aldose with higher aldose it is first reacted with
A. HCN B. HCL
C. H2SO4 D. None of the above

2453. The process of epimerisation is related to
A. Conversion of aldose into lower aldose
B. conversion of aldose into epimeric aldose
C. Conversion of ketose into aldose
D. Conversion of aldose into higher ketose

2454. Glucose can be occured from
A. sucrose B. starch
C. cellulose D. All of the above

2455. Glucose reacts with acetic anhydride in presence of pyridine to form
A. Hexaacetate B. Tetracetate
C. pentacetate D. Triaacetate

2456. Oxidation of gluconic acid with nitric acid gives
A. a - gluconic acid B. Gluconic acid
C. b - gluconic acid D. Both (b) and (d)

2457. The structure of glucose is
A. Pentahydroxy Heptanal
B. pentahydroxyhexanal
C. Pentahydroxyoctanal
D. pentahydroxypental

2458. D glucose reacts with thiols to form
A. Dimethyl mercaptane
B. Ditioacetates
C. Mercaptals
D. Both (b) and (c)

2459. Action of strong alkali on D glucose leads to
A. Reddish brown produtcts
B. Brown resinous products
C. Crystal green products
D. Orange brown products

2460. D - glucose enolate anion after stabilized with resonance to form a
A. Enetriol B. Enediol
C. Enepentol D. Both (b) and (c)

2461. Uses of glucose include
A. Production of food , candy
B. As prserviours
C. Silvering of mirror
D. All of the above

2462. Calcium fructostate is removed by filtartion and converted to Fructose by passing
A. a- D glucose B. CO2
C. H2SO4 D. None of the above

2463. D - fructose undergoes a condenstion reaction with senicarbazide
A. Cyanomannitol B. Semicarbazone
C. D fructose D. None of the above

2464. D fructose undergoes a condenstion reaction with hydroxylamine to form an oxime called
A. a- glucose oxime
B. D- glucose oxime
C. D - fructose oxime
D. L - fructose oxime

2465. D glucose and D fructose form identical osazones an treatment with
A. H2SO4
B. Alcohol
C. Phenyl hydrazine
D. Hydrazine

2466. D fructose reacts with acetic anhydride in pyridine solution to form
A. Anomeric pentacetates
B. cationic pentacetaes
C. Anomeric octaacetates
D. All of the above

2467. In manufacturing process of sucrose juice is traeted with high pressure steam and 2-3 % lime and this process is known as ?
A. Juice purification B. Defecation
C. Carbonation D. Decolorisation

2468. Sucrose is decolorised by treating with
A. Nitric acid B. Sulphur dioxide
C. Alcohol D. carbon dioxide

2469. Which of the following sugars is a tetrose?

A. Galactose B. Idose
C. Fructose D. Erthryose

2470. Which of the following sugar is pentose

A. Ribose B. Threose
C. Gulose D. Mannose

2471. Which of the follwing sugars is found in RNA ?

A. Glucose B. Xylose
C. Ribose D. Therose

2472. Which of the following sugars is found in DNA ?

A. d - ribose B. d - xyllulose
C. d - ribulose D. 2-deoxy-d-ribose

2473. Which of the follwing is sugar alcohol?

A. Gluconic acid
B. Maltose
C. Mannitol
D. Chondrotion suphate

2474. What is the blood concentration of glucose in healthy human

A. 6.0 - 6.5 mm B. 3.4 - 5.0 mm
C. 5.0 - 6.5 mm D. 4.5 - 5.0 mm

2475. Drug compressiblity about 27% by addition of

A. Glidant B. starch
C. Binderc D. Talc

2476. Which are the examples of heptoses in monosachharides

A. T glucoheptose B. Glucoheptase
C. None of the aboveD. Both of the above

2477. Which of the following products is not derived from cellulose?

A. rayon B. Insulin
C. Gun cotton D. paper

2478. The monosachharides obtained by hydrolysis of starch is

A. D glucose B. Maltose
C. D - galactose D. D - ribose

2479. Starch is a

A. trsaccharide
B. also called amylose
C. mixture of amylose + amylopectin
D. also called amylopectin

2480. The reagent that can be used to differentiate an aldose and a ketose is

A. Bromine water B. Fehling's solution
C. Tollen's reagent D. None of these

2481. Which of the following compounds reduces tollen's reagent ?

A. Glucose B. Sucrose
C. Methanol D. Acetic acid

2482. Which of the following carbohydrates will not give a red percipitate of cu2o when heated with benedict's soution

A. Maltose B. Glucose
C. Sucrose D. Fructose

2483. A reducing sugar will

A. React with fehling's test
B. not react with fehling's test
C. Have fewer calories
D. always be a ketone

2484. By approximately what factor is the sweetness of sachharin greater than that of sugar

A. 5 B. 50
C. 500 D. 1000

2485. Mutarotation is term related to

A. Interconversion of anomers
B. Reltionship of D and L families
C. Hydrolysis of sucrose
D. Numbervof monosachharides in a carbohydrates

2486. All of the following monosachharides give the same osazone except

A. Galactosec B. Glucosec
C. Fructose D. Mannose

2487. Which of the following statements is false about an aldohexose ?

A. It is a monosachharide
B. It contain a potential aldehyde group
C. a-D-Glucopyranose is an aldohexose
D. Fructose is an aldohexose

2488. a-D-Glucopyranose is a(n) :

A. Hemiacetal B. Hemiketal
C. Acetal D. Ketal

2489. Glucose reacts with acetic anhydride in the presence of pyridine to form
A. Tetracetate B. Pentaacetate
C. Monoacetate D. Triacetate

2490. Oxidation of gluconic acid with nitric acid gives
A. Gluconic acid B. a - gluconic acid
C. Both (a) and (b) D. b - gluconic acid

2491. Action of strong alkali on D glucose leads to
A. Crystal green product
B. Brown resinous product
C. Reddish brown product
D. Orange blue product

2492. D glucose reacts with thiols to form
A. Dimethyl meracarptal
B. Mercaptals
C. Dithioacetates
D. Both (a) and (b)

2493. The pancretic secretion also contains maltose which convert into
A. Maltose to glucose
B. Maltose to galactose
C. Fructose to glucose
D. None of the above .

2494. PH of stomach is
A. 0.5 to 1.5 B. 3.5 to 6
C. 1.5 to 3.5 D. 9.0 to 7.5

2495. Saliva contains a carbohydrate which is known as
A. Lipase B. Salivary amylase
C. Salivary Maltose D. Bilirubin

2496. Saliva a mixed secretion of several glands contains a pH of
A. 6.4 to 6.9 B. 6.4 to 6.5
C. 6.1 to 6.9 D. 6.0 to 7.0

2497. Dentram is used as
A. Plasma substitute B. Haemoglobin
C. sugar subsitute D. None of the above

2498. Maltose on hydrolysis yields
A. Glucose + Glucose
B. Fructose
C. Glucose + Fructose
D. fructose + fructose

2499. what are the sources of impurities in pharmaceutical chemicals ?
A. Raw materials employed manufacture
B. Reagents used in manufacturing.
C. Method of the process used in manufacture
D. All of the above

2500. What are the methods used to purify inorganic substances ?
A. cleaning
B. Change in manufacturing process
C. Washing and drying
D. All of the above

2501. Limit test of chloride is based on reaction between silver nitrate and soluble b chlorides to obtain.
A. Chloride Nitrate B. Nitrate
C. Silver chloride D. All of the above .

2502. If the turbidity from chloride sample is less than standard turbidity the sample will.
A. fail the limit test
B. Pass the limit test
C. Again limit test will occur
D. None of the above

2503. In standard solution of limit test for chloride, what is the concentartion of sodium chloride
A. 1ml of 0.05845 w/v
B. 1 ml of 0.05845 v/w
C. 1ml of 0.005848 w/v
D. 1 ml of 0.005845 v/w

2504. Limit test for sulphate is carried out in presence of
A. Dilute Nitric acid
B. Dilute Sulphuric aci
C. Dilute Hydrochloric acid
D. None of the above

2505. Potassium sulphate is added to limit test for suplhate .
A. Increasing heat of test
B. Increasing sensitivity of test
C. Increasing speed of test
D. Increasing turbidity of test

2506. Why alcohol is used in limit test for sulphate ?

A. To prevent saturation

B. To prevent super saturation

C. To produce more uniform opalscence

D. All of the above.

2507. Standard solution taken for limit test for suphate contains

A. 1 ml of 0.01089% wlv

B. 1 ml of 0.1029% w/w

C. 1ml of 0.01089% v/v

D. 1 ml of 0.1029% v/w

2508. In limit test of Iron the ferrous compounds are formed from

A. Pink to greenish

B. Pale pink to deep reddish purple

C. Orange to deep red

D. Deep reddish purple to pale pink .

2509. Limit test for iron is based on reaction of iron in ammonical solution in presencec of

A. Hydrochloric acid B. Ascorbic acid

C. citric acid D. Sulphuric acid

2510. The colour formed in limit test for iron gets destroyed by

A. Oxidising agents and alkalies

B. Reducing agents and alkali

C. Both (a) and (b)

D. None of the above .

2511. Standard solution of iron is prepared by adding

A. Adding 0.173 g of ferric ammonium sulphate

B. Adding 0.173 g of Fe2NHSO4

C. Adding 0.173 g of NH2FESO4

D. All of the above

2512. Limit test for Heavy metals is done with reaction of Hydrogen sulphide to form

A. Metal sulphide B. Ferric sulphides

C. copper sulphides D. All of the above

2513. In limit test of heavy metals which colour is produced

A. Blackish colour B. Whitesh colour

C. Brownish colour D. Yellowish colour

2514. What is the usual limit of impurities in limit test of heavy metals as per IP

A. 22 PPM B. 20 PPM

C. 24 PPM D. 18 PPM

2515. According to IP limit test of heavy metals is done by 3 methods in which 1st method is used For :

A. Turbidity and opalscence solution

B. Do not give clear colourless solution

C. Clear colourless solution

D. None of the above

2516. The 3rd method for limit test of heavy metals according to IP gives

A. Not a clear solution

B. Translucent and turbid solution

C. Clear colourless solution in NaoH

D. Both (b) and (c)

2517. In limit test of heavy metals Method 1 standard solution contains pH .

A. 3 to 4 B. 2 to 3

C. 4 to 5 D. 2 to 4

2518. In limit test for heavy metals in volatile oils test is passed when

A. Darkening in colour occurs

B. Clear , transparent colour occurs

C. crystal clear colour occurs

D. No darkening in colour occurs

2519. Before carrying out limit test for Iron they should be oxidised with

A. Nitric acid and ferric chloride

B. Nitrous acid and ferrous acid

C. Nitrogen oxide and ferric chloridev

D. Nitric acid and ferrous acid

2520. In limit test of lead as per B.P how many standard solutions are taken

A. 2 B. 1

C. 3 D. None

2521. Acetic acid is a good solvent for lead and help in limit test as

A. Insolubiling lead

B. Making lead soluble

C. Increasing the rate of limit test

D. All of the above

2522. In limit test of Arsenic a gas is passed over mercuric bromide then which colour gas is produced ?

A. Brown to yellow
B. yellow to brown
C. Orange to brown
D. Red to brown

2523. Reduction of arsenic to arsine can be achieved by .

A. stannous chloride and zinc
B. Combined action of zinc ,acid and potassium iodide
C. Potassium iodide
D. All of the above

2524. Foreign particle that affect the purity of pharmacuetical substances are called as

A. Impurities B. pollutant
C. scum D. contamination

2525. Chemical substances inside a confined amount of liquid gas or solid which differ from chemical composition of material is known as

A. Impurities B. poisoning
C. Diliement D. Uncleanliness

2526. Impurities which obstruct working nature of material is called

A. Constructive impurities
B. Bracking
C. Destructive impurities
D. All of the above

2527. Impurities is complete removed means we reduce the entropy of system to

A. Infinite B. 1
C. 0 D. None of the above

2528. Pericipated CaCo3 may be prepared by interaction of calcium chloride with

A. Sodium carbonate
B. Sodium nitrate
C. Calcium nitrate
D. All of the above

2529. Which are not the sources of impurities in pharmaceutical chemical are ?

A. Raw materails used in manfucaturing
B. Chemical process is used in manufacturing
C. Reagents used in manufacturing
D. Addition of pure compound

2530. Suspended solid that are completely soluble in water and are present as particle are known as

A. chemical impurity
B. Suspended impurities
C. Dispersed impurities
D. All of the above

2531. Impurities resulting from living matter like bacteria and thereby produced including pyrogens is known as

A. Chemical B. physical
C. Biological D. Both (a) and (b)

2532. Impurities that are completely dissolved in water are called as

A. Misicible B. soluble
C. saturated D. All of the above

2533. Impurities which are generally present in raw material

A. Arsenic B. Lead
C. Heavy metal D. All of the above

2534. If reagent are used in manufacturing process are not completely removed by washing there may lead entry into final product then those impurities are known as

A. Raw materials containing impurities
B. chemical impurities
C. Reagent impurities
D. None of the above .

2535. 2 or more element that are not bounded together chemical then this is called

A. Impure B. Admix
C. Dirty D. None of the above

2536. The presence of wanted particulate matter can arise in a number of ways like

A. Glass B. porcelin
C. Inclusion of dirt D. All of the above

2537. The description characteristion, quantitaion of identified and unidentified impurities present in drug compound is known as

A. Impurity data B. Impurity monitoring
C. Impurity profiling
D. Identity of impurity

2538. What are the main types of impurity
- A. Bi product impurity
- B. Degardation product impurity
- C. Transformed product impurity
- D. All of the above .

2539. We can isolate impurities from which process
- A. Column chromtography
- B. HPLC
- C. TLC
- D. All of the above

2540. Which are not methods are used to purify inoragnic substances ?
- A. Washing
- B. Drying
- C. Recryastalltion
- D. Extraction

2541. Phase transformation during manufacturing and storage result in solid state impurities represente by various unwanted polymorphic forms after drug product is known as
- A. Amorphous impurity
- B. Polymorph impurity
- C. polymer impurity
- D. None of the above

2542. Unidentified impurities occurs from the manufacturing process such as starting material, intermedaite by product is known as
- A. Drug impurities
- B. Process impurity
- C. Both (a) and (b)
- D. Organic impurities

2543. Impurities can arise in API or drug product formulation during manufacturing or storage of drug is known as
- A. Organic impurities
- B. Inorganic impurities
- C. Biological impurities
- D. Microbiolgical impurities

2544. Purity and impurities both are different because of
- A. Contamination
- B. Pollution
- C. Adulteration
- D. All of the above

2545. Quntitative or semi quntaitative test designed to identify and control small quantities of impurity is known as
- A. Control test
- B. Limit test
- C. Purity test
- D. All of the above

2546. Name the apparatus used for carrying and limit test
- A. Conical flask
- B. Volumetric flask
- C. Nessler's cylinder
- D. Measuring cylinder

2547. Pharmaceutical buffer system could be categorized in
- A. 1
- B. 2
- C. 3
- D. None of the above

2548. Fluorides inhibits carries formulation via
- A. Increased acid solubility of enamel
- B. Bacterial inhibition
- C. Decreased acid solubility of enamel
- D. Both (a) and (b)

2549. Which of the following substrates derived from adipose tissues contributes to net Gluconeogenesis in mammalian liver?
- A. Alanine
- B. Glutamate
- C. Glycerol
- D. Pyruvate

2550. Which of the following substrates derived from adipose tissues contributes to net Gluconeogenesis in mammalian liver?
- A. Alanine
- B. Glutamate
- C. Glycerol
- D. Pyruvate

2551. Which of the following statements is incorrect ?
- A. Aerobically, oxidative decarboxylation of pyruvate forms acetate that enters the citric acid cycle.
- B. In anaerobic muscle, pyruvate is converted to lactate.
- C. Reduction of pyruvate to lactate generates a coenzyme essential for Glycolysis.
- D. Under anaerobic conditions pyruvate does not form because Glycolysis does not occur.

2552. The steps of Glycolysis between glyceraldehyde 3-phosphate and 3-phosphoglycerate involve all of the following except
- A. ATP synthesis
- B. Catalysis by phosphoglycerate kinase
- C. Oxidation of NADH to NAD+
- D. Formation of 1,3 biphosphoglycerate

2553. The oxidation of 3 mol of glucose by the pentose phosphate pathway may result in the production of

A. 2 mol of pentose, 4 mol of NADPH, and 8mol of CO

B. 3 mol of pentose, 4 mol of NADPH, and 3mol of CO2.

C. 3 mol of pentose, 6 mol of NADPH, and 3mol of CO2.

D. 4 mol of pentose, 3 mol of NADPH, and 3mol of CO2.

2554. How many ATP molecules can be derived from each molecule of acetyl CoA that enters the Krebs' Cycle?

A. 6 B. 12

C. 18 D. 3

2555. – All of the following vitamins except one participate in the TCA cycle

A. Pantothenic acid B. Lipoic acid

C. Folic acid D. Riboflavin

2556. Which of the following enzymes is Thiamine dependent and essential for glucose oxidation in the brain?

A. Pyruvate dehydrogenase complex

B. Acetyl Co A carbooxylase

C. Transaldolase

D. Succinyl CoA thiokinase

2557. The reaction catalyzed by phosphofructo kinase is

A. Inhibited by Fructose 2,6 bisphosphate

B. Activated by high concentration of ATP

C. A regulatory step of glycolysis

D. All of the above

2558. Pyruvate carboxylase requires ———— as a coenzyme.

A. FMN B. Biotin

C. NAD+ D. TPP

2559. In erythrocytes the most abundantly found Phospho ester is

A. Glucose 6 phosphate

B. fructose 1,6 bisphosphate

C. Fructose 6 phosphate

D. 2,3 bisphosphoglycerate

2560. Formation of Galactose-1-P from Galactose is catalyzed by

A. Hexokinase

B. Aldolase

C. Galactokinase

D. Galactose-1-P Uridyl transferase

2561. All the following enzymes except one require NADP+ as a coenzyme

A. Glucose- 6-phosphate dehydrogenase

B. Cytosolic Isocitrate dehydrogenase

C. Malic enzyme

D. Glucose-6-phophatase

2562. Which of the following product of Triglyceride breakdown and subsequent beta oxidation would undergo gluconeogenesis

A. Propinoyl CoA

B. Acetyl CoA

C. Aceto acetate

D. Beta hydroxy butarate

2563. which of the following reactions generate ATP ?

A. Glucose to Glucose 6 phosphate

B. Pyruvate to lactate

C. Phosphophenol pyruvate to pyruvate

D. Glucose 6 phosphate to fructose 6 phosphate

2564. Glucose enters muscle cell generally by ?

A. Simple diffusion

B. Facilitated diffusion using a specific glucose transporter

C. Co transport with sodium

D. Co transport with Amino acids

2565. - Which one of the following compounds is common to both the oxidative phase and the non- oxidative phase of the pentose phosphate pathway?

A. Xylulose 5 phosphate

B. Gluose 6 phosphate

C. Ribulose 5 phosphate

D. Glyceraldehyde 3 phosphate

2566. Mc Ardle's syndrome causes muscle cramps and muscle fatigue with increased muscle glycogen. Which of the following enzyme is deficient?

A. Hepatic hoxokinase

B. Muscle phosphorylase

C. Muscle debranching enzyme

D. Muscle Hexokinase

2567. During starvation, the major source of blood glucose is

A. Hepatic gluycogenolysis
B. Gluconeogenesis
C. Muscle Glycogenolysis
D. Dietry glucose from intestine

2568. Hexokinase has a considerably lower km for

A. Glucose B. Fructose
C. Galactose D. Mannose

2569. In the fasting state there is considerable release of———from the muscles.

A. Glycine B. Alanine
C. Valine D. Glutamic acid

2570. A galactosemic child will manifest all except

A. Hepatomegaly B. splenomegaly
C. Catarqct D. Mental retardation

2571. Which one of the following reactions is unique to gluconeogenesis-?

A. Lactate<———>Pyruvate
B. Oxaloacetate—>Phosphoenol pyruvate
C. Glucose-6-phosphate— >Glucose
D. Phosphoenol pyruvate–>Pyruvate

2572. The main stores of glycogen are found in

A. Adipose tissue B. Skeletal muscle
C. Brain D. Erthrocytes

2573. Succinyl co A is cleaved by

A. Succinate dehydrogenase
B. Succinate Thiokinase
C. Succinate lyase
D. Succinate Thioesterase

2574. Arsenate binds to

A. Free amino end of enzyme
B. SH linkages
C. Free carboxyl end
D. Any of the above

2575. All are intermediates of glycolysis except

A. Glucose-6 phosphate
B. Fructose 1, 6 bisphosphate
C. Fructose-6- phosphate
D. Glycerol – 3- phosphate

2576. The key regulatory enzyme of HMP pathway is

A. Glucose- 6-phosphate dehydrogenase
B. Transaldolase
C. Transketolase
D. Glucose-6-phophatase

2577. The net production of ATP in glycolysis during anaerobic condition is:

A. 2 from glucose and 3 from glycogen
B. 2 from glucose and 4 from glycogen
C. 3 from glucose and 4 from glycogen
D. 3 from glucose and 2 from glycogen

2578. Which of the followings does not generate free glucose during the enzymatic breakdown of glycogen in skeletal muscles?

A. Phosphorylase
B. α-1-6-amyloglucosidase
C. Debranching enzyme
D. glucose-6-phosphatase

2579. Which of the followings promotes glucose and amino acid uptake by muscle?

A. Adrenaline B. Insulin
C. Glucagon D. Cortisol

2580. In a tissue that metabolizes glucose via the pentose phosphate pathway, C-1 of glucose would be expected to end up principally in

A. Carbon dioxide
B. Glycogen
C. Phosphoglycerate
D. Pyruvate

2581. Which one of the following enzymes catalyzes the phosphorylation of the substrate with the use of inorganic phosphate-?

A. Hexokinase
B. phospho fructokinase
C. Gkyceraldehyde 3-phosphate dehydrogenase
D. Phospho glycerate kinase

2582. The major glycolytic product produced under normal circumstances by erythrocytes required for unloading of oxygen to the peripheral tissues is

A. 2,3bisphosphoglycerate
B. 2,3bisphosphoglycerate
C. Lactate
D. pyruvate

2583. Which of the following explains why individuals with hyperlipidemia should minimize their intake of sucrose and high fructose syrup?

A. Fructose metabolism is faster than glucose

B. After initial modification fructose is cleaved by a specific Enolase

C. Fructose is ultimately converted to galactose

D. Fructose can be phosphorylated by hexokinase in adipose cells

2584. A medical student developed hemolytic anemia after taking the oxidizing Antimalarial drug primaquine. This severe reaction is most likely due to

A. Glucose-6- phosphate dehydrogenase deficiency

B. Concomitant Scurvy

C. Diabetes

D. Glycogen phosphorylase deficiency

2585. Which of the following enzymes is associated with Glycogen synthesis?

A. Amylo- (1, 4->1,6) – transglycosylase

B. Phosphorylase

C. Amylo-1,6-glucosidase

D. Glucose-6- phosphatase

2586. The citric acid cycle is inhibited by which of the following?

A. Fluroacetate B. Aerobic conditions

C. Malic acid D. Flurouracil

2587. It is very important to feed the baby very soon after birth, because during the first few hours after birth the enzyme Phosphoenolpyruvate carboxykinase is present in very low amounts, and this fact compromises:

A. Gluconeogenesis

B. Glucose phosphorylation

C. Glycogenesis

D. Glucogenolysis

2588. Which statement BEST describes the fate of Propionyl-CoA in mammalian systems?

A. Propionyl-CoA is metabolized via are action sequence that involves vitamin B12 and biotin.

B. Propionyl-CoA is converted to acetyl CoA

C. Propionyl-CoA and acetyl CoA condense to form a 5 carbon precursor of a TCA cycle intermediate.

D. Propionyl-CoA is oxidized to Malonate and CoAq

2589. Anaplerotic reactions are those that result in replenishing intermediates in the TCA cycle. Which of the following enzymes catalyzes an Anaplerotic reaction?

A. Malate dehydrogenase

B. pyruvate carboxylase

C. Pyruvate kinase

D. citrate syntthase

2590. Which of the following enzymes catalyzes a reaction that involves a decarboxylation reaction?

A. Pyruvate dehydrogenase

B. Isocitrate dehydrogenase

C. α-keto glutarate dehydrogenase

D. All of the above

2591. Which of the following statements about the pentose phosphate pathway is incorrect?

A. It generates 36 mol of ATP per mole of glucose consumed.

B. It generates 6 moles of CO2for each mole of glucose consumed

C. It is a reductive pathway; it consumes NADH.

D. It provides precursors for the synthesis of nucleotides

2592. An enzyme used in both glycolysis and gluconeogenesis is:

A. 3-phosphoglycerate kinase.

B. Glucose 6-phosphatase.

C. Hexokinase.

D. Phosphofructokinase-1.

2593. Which of the following is a coenzyme in the reaction catalyzed by glyceraldehyde 3-phosphate dehydrogenase?

A. ATP B. Cu2+

C. Heme D. NAD+

2594. In an anaerobic system that is metabolizing glucose as a substrate, which of the following compounds would you expect to increase in concentration following the addition of fluoride?

A. 2-phosphoglycerate

B. Glucose
C. Phosphoenolpyruvate
D. Pyruvate

2595. Which of the following is not an intermediate of the citric acid cycle?
A. Acetoacetate B. Citrate
C. Oxalosuccinate D. Succinyl CoA

2596. -Cellular isozymes of pyruvate kinase are allosterically inhibited by:
A. High concentrations of AMP.
B. High concentrations of ATP.
C. High concentrations ofFr1,6 bisphosphate
D. Low concentrations of acetyl-CoA.

2597. All are correct about pyruvate dehydrogenase complex except one-
A. The formation of acetyl CoA from pyruvate is an irreversible step
B. Pyruvate dehydrogenase is switched off when Acetyl co A is in excess
C.)Phosphorylation switches off the activity of the complex.
D. Pyruvate as well as ADP (a signal of low energy charge) inhibits the complex.

2598. Why Phosphofructokinase rather than hexokinase is the pacemaker of Glycolysis?
A. Glucose 6-phosphate is not solely a glycolytic intermediate
B. Hexokinase has low km for glucose
C. Hexokinase is inhibited by feed back inhibition
D. None of the above

2599. Temporary hardness of water removed by
A. bioling B. lime process
C. deionized water D. All of the above

2600. Permanent hard water is softend by
A. addition of soluble carbonate
B. polyphosphate chelation
C. Zeolitev
D. All of the above

2601. Sterile water for injection is stored in
A. Type 1 B. Type 2
C. Both (a) and (b) D. None of these

2602. Water attack test can be applied for
A. borosilicate glass
B. treated sodalime glass
C. general purpose soda lime glass
D. soda lime glass

2603. Aldohexoses contain how many numbers of asymmetric carbon atom.
A. 2 B. 3
C. 4 D. 5

2604. what is a Deoxy sugar
A. Hydrogen atom is replaced by hydroxyl group
B. Hydroxyl group is replaced by hydrogen atom
C. Both a and b
D. None of the above

2605. Glycogen are example of
A. hetropolysachharides
B. Trisachharides
C. Homopolysachharides
D. Monosachharides

2606. which are the examples of disachharides
A. Maltose B. Trehlose
C. Rotinose D. Rassinose

2607. Carbohydrates (Glucagon) is first discoverd by
A. Robert brown B. Alexander flemming
C. Claude Bernard D. Loius pasteur

2608. Which sachharide yield 2 to 10 monosachharides units on hydrolysis
A. Disachharides
B. Oligosachharides
C. Monosachharides
D. Polysachharides

2609. Which is hexoses monosachharides are also known as
A. Glucose and fructose
B.Glucose and ribose
C. Ribose and fructose
D. None of the above

2610. How many optical isomers are possible in epimers
A. 2 to 16 B. 4 to 16
C. 8 to 16 D. 6 to 16

2611. The D and L erthrose are mirror images so also be called
A. Mesoisomers B. Enantiomers
C. Superimposible D. None of the above

2612. In aldotroses how many optical isomers are possible

A. 2 to 6 B. 2 to 8

C. 2 to 4 D. only 4

2613. The simpler way of drawing fischer projection is to use

A. Horizontal lines B. Diagonal lines

C. Vertical lines D. All of the above

2614. One projection commonly used for representation of D and L glyceraldehyde is known as

A. Robert projection

B. Fischer projection

C. Enantiomers

D. Both (a) and (b)

2615. Which is pentose are also known as monosachharides

A. Ribose B. Fructose

C. Glucose D. Lactose

2616. Which formula is monosachharides tetroses

A. C6H11O6 B. C6H10O6

C. Both D. None of the above

2617. Insulin contains how many amino acids

A. 51 B. 68.

C. 5 D. 58.

2618. Glucose is reaboserbed in the

A. Proximal Tubule B. Distal tubule

C. Collecting duct D. Loop of Henle

2619. Lactose reacts with Dimethylsulphate in alkaline solution to form

A. Octamethyl lactose

B. Hexamethyl lactose

C. Caramel

D. Tetramethyl lactose

2620. The percentage of amylopectin in natural starch is

A. 70 to 80% B. 60 to 90 %

C. 80 to 90 % D. 60 to 80 %

2621. Lactose reacts with phenylhydrazine in prsence of acetic acid to produce

A. Octamethyl lactose

B. Tetramethyl lactose

C. Pentamethyl lactose

D. Caramel

2622. Lactose reacts with phenylhydrazine in presence of acetic acid to produce

A. Emulsion B. Lactosazone

C. Insulin D. All of the above

2623. Lactose is also hydrolysed by an enzyme that hydrolyses B glycosides

A. Emulsion B. Lactonic acid

C. D galactose D. Both (a) and (b)

2624. D glucose and D fructose form identical osazones on treatment with

A. H2SO4 B. Alcohol

C. Hydrazine D. Phenyl hydrazine

2625. What is the bond that links monosachharides in polysachharides ?

A. Nuclear bond B. Metallic bond

C. Glycosidic bond D. Ionic bond

2626. What is the plant cell walls mainly composed of

A. Polysqchharides B. Enzymes

C. monosachharides D. Viatmins

2627. What is colour of starch -I2 complex

A. Grey colour B. Blue colour

C. Red colour D. Pink colour

2628. D fructose undergoes a condensation reaction with Hydrosylamine to form an Oxime called

A. a - glucose oxime B. D fructose oxime

C. D glucose oxime D. L glucose oxime

2629. Calcium fructosate is removed by flitration and converted to fructose by passing

A. a-d glucose B. H2so4

C. CO2 D. NH3

2630. D glucose enolate amion after stabilized with resonance to form an

A. Enetriol B. Enediol

C. Enepentol D. Eneoctal

2631. D fructose undergoes a condensation reaction with semicarbazide

A. D - Fructose B. Cyanomannitol

C. Semicarbazone D. None of the above

2632. Polymer of fructose is

A. Inulin B. Mannitol

C. Dextrose D. Starh

2633. What is cellulose polymer as a

A. Heteropolymers
B. Homopolymers
C. Nucleotide
D. Nucleoside

2634. Which of the following sugars is a monosachharides ?

A. Starch B. Maltose
C. Sucrose D. Mannose

2635. Which of the following is a sugar alcohol ?

A. Mannitol B. Gluconic acid
C. Maltose D. Dextrose

2636. Which of the following sugars is found in DNA

A. D ribulose B. 2 deoxy d ribose
C. d Xylulose D. D ribose

2637. How many molecules of ATP are produced when one molecule of glucose gets completely oxidised ?

A. 32 B. 36
C. 24 D. 38.

2638. Range of renal threshold value for glucose is from

A. 120 to 160 mg % B. 160 to 180 mg %
C. 100 to 120 mg % D. 180 to 200 mg%

2639. Main site of glycolysis is

A. Muscles B. Kidney
C. Spleen D. Brain

2640. Main site for gluconeogenesis are

A. Brain B. liver
C. Lungs D. Pancreas

2641. Main site for glucogenesis are

A. Pancreas B. Liver and muscles
C. Liver and Brain D. Thymus

2642. In erythrocytes , the most abundantly found phosphate ester is

A. Glucose -1- P
B. Glucose -6-p
C. Fructose -6-p
D. 2,3 diphosphoglyceratev

2643. Fructose -6-p is converted into F1, 6 Diphosphate with help of enzyme

A. Phosphofructokinase
B. phosphoglucokinase
C. phospholactokinase
D. Xylulose 5P

2644. Which catalyses the reaction of gkucose - 1-phosphate to glucose -6- phosphate

A. Phosphogkucomutase
B. Phoaphogmycerate
C. phospomutase
D. Phosphoglucose

2645. Liver gkucagon is very _____ in glucogenosis

A. High B. Very high
C. Low D. Reduce

2646. Liver glucagon is very _______ in Von Gierkets disease

A. Low B. Medium
C. High D. None of the above

2647. Ptyalin acts on starch and glycogen producing limited quntities of

A. Lactose B. Maltose
C. Fructose D. Galactose

2648. Carbohydrates are not digested in the

A. Stomach B. Mouth
C. small intestine D. Duedoneum

2649. Fructose is metabolized by

A. fructose 1-phosphate pathway
B. fructose 6-phosphate pathway
C. glyceraldehyde 3-phosphate pathway
D. both (a) and (b)

2650. A common way that cells capture the energy released during the breakdown of large molecules is to add electrons to smaller, specialized molecules that can accept them. This process of electron acceptance is otherwise known as

A. biosynthesis B. metabolism
C. reduction D. catalysis

2651. Humans are unable to digest

A. starch
B. complex carbohydrates
C. denatured protien
D. cellulose

2652. Gluconeogenesis requires a higher amount of ATP equivalents as compared to that produced by glycolysis because

A. gluconeogenesis releases energy as heat
B. glycolysis releases energy as heat
C. glycolysis occurs in the mitochondria while gluconeogenesis occurs in the cytosol
D. all of the above

2653. Which of the following is carried out when cAMP functions as a second messenger?

A. Acts second in importance to AMP
B. .Activates all cytosolic protein kinases
C. Activates the cAMP-dependent protein kinase
D. Acts outside the cell to influence cellular processes

2654. The production or break down of __________ is often coupled with the metabolic reactions of biosynthesis and catabolism.

A. aspirin B. DNA
C. ATP D. CO2

2655. Which of the following statements about the energy needs of cells is false?

A. Without a continuous input of energy, cell disorder will increase
B. The laws of thermodynamics force cells to acquire energy
C. Many cellular reactions have an associated activation energy
D. The most usable energy for cells comes from the rapid combustion of glucose

2656. In lysozyme catalysis, which of the following does not contribute?

A. The abnormally high pKa of Glu35
B. The strained conformation of the D sugar
C. Formation of a covalent intermediate at Asp52
D. Formation of a covalent intermediate at Ser195

2657. Cellulose fibers resemble with the protein structure in the form of

A. β-sheets B. α-helices
C. β-turns D. None of these

2658. During vigorous exercise, pyruvate produced by glycolysis is converted to

A. acetate
B. lactate
C. monosodium phosphate
D. pyruvic acid

2659. Glucagon and epinephrine

A. inhibits gluconeogenesis and stimulates glycolysis
B. stimulates gluconeogenesis and glycolysis
C. stimulates gluconeogenesis and inhibits glycolysis
D. inhibits gluconeogenesis and glycolysis

2660. The NAG6 substrate is hydrolyzed by human lysozyme to form

A. 6 glucosamines + 6 acetic acids
B. NAG4 + NAG2
C. NAG3 + NAG3
D. NAG3

2661. Gluconeogenesis uses

A. 3 ATPs and 2 GTPs per glucose
B 2 ATPs and 1 GTPs per glucose
C. 3 ATPs and 3 GTPs per glucose
D. 4 ATPs and 2 GTPs per glucose

2662. The conversion of pyruvate to oxaloacetate

A. requires biotin
B. involves the fixation of carbon dioxide
C. occurs in the mitochondria
D. all of the above

2663. Hydrolysis of lactose yields

A. galactose and fructose
B. galactose and glucose
C. glucose and fructose
D. fructose and galactose

2664. Two major products of pentose phosphate pathway are

A. nicotinamide adenine dinucleotide and ribose 5-phosphate
B. flavine adenine dinuclueotide and glucose 5-phosphate
C. FAD and CoA
D. NADPH and NAD

2665. A catabolic intermediate which stimulates phosphofructokinase would stimulate

A. gluconeogenesis
B. glycolysis
C. glycogen synthesis
D. none of these

2666. Pyruvate is initially converted to which of the following in the gluconeogenesis?

A. Glycerol
B. Phosphoenol pyruvate
C. Oxaloacetate
D. Acetyl CoA

2667. Boat and chair conformations are found

A. in pyranose sugars
B. in any sugar without axial -OH groups
C. in any sugar without equatorial -OH groups
D. only in D-glucopyranose

2668. Which of the following can act as precursors for gluconeogenesis?

A. Lactate B. Glycerol
C. Alanine D. All of these

2669. a-amylose is similar to

A. β-sheets B. β-turned coils
C. α-helicesD. the hydrophobic core

2670. Storage polysaccharide made by animals is

A. amylopectin B. glycogen
C. cellulose D. collagen

2671. The glycosidic bond

A. in maltose is not hydrolyzed in lactose intolerant humans
B. in sucrose is hydrolyzed by bees
C. joins glucose and fructose to form sucrose
D. both (b) and (c)

2672. The ultimate source of energy that sustains living systems is

A. glucose B. oxygen
C. sunlight D. carbon dioxide

2673. Citric acid accumulation would

A. stimulate phosphofructokinase activity
B. stimulate fructose 1,6 diphosphatase activity
C. inhibit phosphofructokinase activity
D. both (b) and (c)

2674. Which of the following is not involved in the biosynthesis of DNA?

A. Energy from ATP
B. Mononucleotides
C. Carbonic anhydrase
D. Enzymes

2675. Which of the following would be considered a part of metabolism?

A. Biosynthetic pathways that build DNA
B. Catabolic pathways that break down complex carbohydrates
C. The capture of light energy for use in making glucose
D. All of the above

2676. Insulin

A. stimulates gluconeogenesis and glycolysis
B. stimulates gluconeogenesis and inhibits glycolysis
C. inhibits gluconeogenesis and glycolysis
D. inhibits gluconeogenesis and stimulates glycolysis

2677. Patients suffering from Von Gierke's disease are unable to perform gluconeogeneis because they have a defective

A. lactate dehydrogenase
B. glucose 6 phosphatase
C. pyruvate carboxylase
D. none of these

2678. The multistep pathways of metabolism are efficient because they

A. locate all of the enzymes for a pathway in the same place within the cell
B. use the same substrate for all of the enzymes in the pathway
C. use the same enzyme for all of the substrates in the pathway
D. spread the enzymes for a pathway into several different organelles

2679. Metabolic reactions that break down complex molecules into smaller compounds, thereby releasing usable energy for the cell, are best described as

A. biosynthetic B. catabolic
C. catalytic D. photosynthetic

2680. Fructose diphosphate accumulation would

A. inhibit glycolysis and gluconeogenesis
B. stimulate glycolysis and gluconeogenesis
C. stimulate glycolysis and inhibit gluconeogenesis
D. inhibit glycolysis and stimulate gluconeogenesis

2681. Aldolases splits fructose 1,6 biphosphate into

A. glyceraldehyde 3- phosphate
B. glyceraldehyde 3- phosphate and dihydroxyacetone phosphate
C. dihydroxyacetone phosphate
D. none of the above

2682. What would be the molecular formula for a polymer made by linking ten glucose molecules together by dehydration synthesis, if molecular formula for glucose is C6H,206?

A. C60H100O50 B. C60H120O60
C. C60H102O51 D. (C6H12O6)10

2683. Glycolysis reactions take place in

A. cytoplasm B. cell membrane
C. cell wall D. plasmids

2684. Which of the following enzymes plays an important role in the Cori " cycle?

A. Glucokinase
B. Glucose-6-phosphate dehydrogenase
C. Lactate dehydrogenase
D. Glucose isomerase

2685. Regulated metabolic pathways are

A. compartmentalized in eukaryotes
B. usually regulated at the first step
C. committed after the first step
D. all of these

2686. Glycogen degradation requires the enzyme name

A. glycogen phosphorylase and phosphoglucomutase
B. glycogen phosphorylase and glycogen-debranching enzyme
C. glycogen synthase and phosphorylase
D. none of the above

2687. The hormones, glucagon and epinephrine, stimulate glycogen breakdown to G-6-P

A. only in the liver
B. using ATP as the phosphoryl donor
C. directly, by binding to glycogen phosphorylase
D. indirectly, by first stimulating adenylate cyclase to make cAMP

2688. What is the cause of the genetic disease known as Galactosemia?

A. Deficiency in lactase
B. Absence of galactose 1-P uridyl transferase
C. Absence of lactose synthetase
D. Non functioning of semnase

2689. Which of the following does not occur during gluconeogenesis?

A. The carboxylation of pyruvate to oxaloacetate
B. The conversion of pyruvate to phosphoenolpyruvate (PEP)
C. The decarboxylation of oxaloacetate to phosphoenolpyruvate
D. The conversion of PEP to fructose bisphosphate

2690. Which of the following characteristic enzymes of gluconeogensis is not found in the cytosol?

A. Pyruvate carboxlyase
B. Fructose-l,6-bisphosphatase
C. Both (a) and (b)
D. Glucose-6-phosphatase

2691. What is the consensus N-glycosylation site in a protein sequence?

A. Asn-Xaa-(Ser or Thr)
B. (Ser or Thr)-Asn-Ala
C. Thr-(Asn or Gln)-Ala
D. None of these

2692. The process not involved in the formation of glucose by gluconeo-genesis is

A. the conversion of oxaloacetate to glucose
B. the conversion of lactate to pyruvate
C. the dephosphorylation of glucose-6-phosphate
D. all of the above

2693. Each reaction in a metabolic pathway is

A. reversible
B. irreversible
C. catalyzed by a specific enzyme
D. controlled by the end product

2694. Minimum number of carbon required for a monosaccharide

A. 1 B. 3
C. 2 D. 4

2695. Which Biomolecules simply refers as "Staff of life" in the given....

A. Protein B. Lipids
C. Carbohydrate D. Vitamins

2696. The reagent used for distinguishing a reducing monosaccharide from a reducing disaccharide is ...

A. Benedict's reagent
B. Barfoed's reagent
C. Fehling's reagent
D. Selwinoff's reagent

2697. Example for "Fructosan" is ....

A. Inulin B. cellulose
C. chitin D. Starch

2698.The following Sugar exhibits inversion of optical rotation on heating with dilute acid ....

A. Glucose B. sucrose
C. Lactose D. Fructose

2699. Reducing agents used in Brich reduction is

A. $LiAlH_4$ B Na/ROH
C. $AlCl_3$ D PCl_5

2700. Pyridine is ....basic than alkylamine

A. More B Less
C. Equal D None

2701. Clemmensen reduction of a ketone is carried out in the presence of which of the following

A. Zn-Hg and HCl
B $NaBH_4$
C. $LiAlH_4$
D H_2 and Pt as catalyst

2702. One of which does not example of organic addition reaction

A. Halogenation B Hydration
C. Dehydration D Hydrohalogenation

2703. Formation of a single product from two reactant molecules is known as

A. Elimination reaction
B Substitution reaction
C. Addition reaction
D Rearrangement reaction

2704. Alcohol are treated with Cr_2O_7 by refluxing gives

A. Carboxylic Acid B Ketone
C. Alkane D Aldehyde

2705. Which will react faster in the SN2 nucleophilic substitution reaction

A. CH= CH_2 – CH_2 – Br
B CH_2 = CH- CH_2 = Br
C. CH_2 = CH- CH_2 – Br
D CH_2-CH=CH_2=Br

2706.Whichofthefollowingorganicreactionusedto convertaprimaryamidetoaprimaryamineusi nga halogen

A. Reimer-Tiemann reaction
B Clemmensen reduction
C. Hofmann rearrangement reaction
D Kolbe-Schmitt reaction

2707. Formation of free radicals are occur in free radical reaction which of the following step

A. Initiation Step B Propagation Step
C. Termination Step D Both A and B

2708.Whichoneofthefollowingstepfreeradicalsar eformedandwhichattackreactantsmolecule stogeneratemore and more free radicals.

A. Initiation Step B Propagation Step
C. Termination Step D Both A and B

2709. Choose the following statements regarding the SN2 mechanism is not true

A. Its usually second order
B SN2 reactions are bimolecular
C. Its occurs in one step
D Its occur in two steps

2710. Choose the following most reactive compound by the SN1 mechanism

A. CH_2= $CHCH_2Br$ B
C. $CH_3CH_2CH_2Br$ D Both A and C

2711. Choose the following statements regarding the E2 mechanism is not true

A. E2 mechanism are always bimolecular
B E2 mechanism usually occur in one step
C. E2 mechanism are generally second order
D E2 mechanism usually occur in two step

2712. Which of the following does not have alpha hydrogen
A. Formaldehyde
B Acetone
C. acetaldehyde
D Phenyl acetaldehyde

2713. The number of structure isomers of C6H14 is:
A. 4 B 5
C. 6 D 7

2714. An isomer of ethanol is:
A. methanol B diethyl ether
C. acetone D dimethyl ether

2715. Formation of a single product from two reactant molecules is known as
A. Addition reaction
B Elimination reaction
C. Substitution reaction
D Oxidation

2716. Commercial sources of alkanes include
A. Coal B Natural gas
C. Petroleum D all of above

2717.Theionicbondisformedduetoelectrostaticatt ractionbetweenstableionsformedbycomple tetransfer of electron from one atom to another
A. Electrovalent bond
B Covalent bond
C. Metallic bond
D None of the above

2718. When two electronegative atoms react together is known as
A. Covalent bond B Metallic bond
C. Both D None of the above

2719. Which type of bond is frequently encountered in inorganic compounds
A. Electrovalent bond
B Covalent compound
C. Both
D None of the above

2720. Which of the following are type of covalent bond
A. Sigma bond B Pi bond
C. Both D None of the above

2721. Which type of bond is formed by the linear or end to end overlap of orbital
A. Sigma bond
B Pi Bond
C. Electrovalent bond
D None of the above

2722. Which type of bond is formed by parallel or side to side overlap of P Orbital
A. Pi Bond B Sigma bond
C. Both D None of the above

2723. The hybrid formed by combining one S and three P orbital
A. Sp Hybridization
B Sp2 Hybridization
C. Sp3 Hybridization
D None

2724. Which compounds showing the characteristics of smell and inflammation
A. Ionic bond B Electrovalent
C. Covalent bond D None of the above

2725. Which theory responsible for the formation of covalent bond
A. The valency bondtheory
B The molecule bond theory
C. Both
D None of the above

2726. Which electron are loosely held in the pair of electron in a sigma bond
A. Pi electron
B Non bonding electron
C. Sigma bond
D Both A and B

2727. Which bond are more reactive and easily broken
A. Pi bond B Sigma bond
C. Both D All of theabove

2728.Theprocessofmixingofpureorbitaltogivease tofnewequivalentorbitalisknownas
A. Hybridization B Molecule orbital
C. Bonding orbital D None of the above

2729. Which compound are soluble in water but insoluble in organic compound
A. Electrovalent bond
B Ionic bond
C. Metallic compound
D None of the above

2730. Thevsharingofanelectronpairoccursbetwee n twoelectronsonefromeachoftwoatom

A. Coordinate covalent bond
B Pi bond
C. Ionic bond
D Sigma bond

2731. The angle between the two orbital is

A. 109°28 B 110°28
C. 111° D 105°

2732. Which type of orbital whenever carbon is bonded to four other atom or group

A. Sp Hybridization
B Sp2 Hybridization
C. Sp3 Hybridization
D Both A and B

2733. Which type of bond present in Methane

A. Pi Bond
B Covalent bond
C. Electrovalent bond
D Sigma Bond

2734. The energy Required to break any of four bond is the

A. 100 kcal B 102kcal
C. 104 kcal D 102 kcal

2735. In ethylene how much C-H single covalent bond are present

A. Two B Four
C. Three D One

2736. Whenever carbon is bonded to three other atoms or group it always use

A. Sp Hybridization
B Both A and C
C. Sp2 Hybridization
D Sp3 Hybridization

2737. Which of these atoms measure of its power to attract elecctron that is sharing in covalent bond

A. Electronegativity
B Electron postivity
C. Electron affinity
D None of the above

2738. Distance of the valence electron from the nucleus

A. Atomic Radius B Bond length
C. Atomic Diameters D Both A and B

2739. The magnitude of the positive energy charge on the nucleus is called

A. Atomic mass B Atomic number
C. Atomic Radius D None of the above

2740. The bond which appear to have a positiv end and a negative end is said to be

A. Electrovalent bond
B Non Polar Bond
C. Polar Bond
D None of the above

2741. There is no positive and negative end such bond are known as

A. Semi-polar Bond
B Non Polar Bond
C. Polar Bond
D Both A and B

2742. Which bond is formed between the C-Cl bond

A. Polar bond
B Non Polar bond
C. Semi Polar bond
D None of the above

2743. The angle between H-o-H is

A. 103° B 102°
C. 104° D 108°

2744. The formula of Dipole moments

A. Charge×time B Charge×Distance
C. Charge×Radius D None of the above

2745. Non Polar molecules do notpossess

A. Polarization B Covalent bonds
C. Vanderwalls force D Dipole moments

2746. All carbon carbon bond in benzene have same bond length

A. 1.54 A° B 1.44°
C. 1.65° D 1.76°

2747. The difference in energy between the hybrid and the most stable resonance structure is known as

A. Resonance energy
B Electric Energy
C. Both
D None of the above

2748. At which energy Benzene is said to be stabilize

A. 42 kcal/mol B 40 kcal/mol
C. 44 kcal/mol D 38 kcal/mol

2749. Which of the statement is true about Resonance

A. Resonance is actual structure
B Resonance hybrid are less stable
C. It involves the delocalization of electron
D Resonance are more reactive

2750. The force of attraction is known as

A. Hydrogen Bond B Covalent bonds
C. Both D None of the above

2751. At which condition the breakup of the Hydrogen bond between the water molecules

A. If non Polar molecules dissolve in alcohol
B If polar molecules dissolve in water
C. If non Polar molecules were to dissolve in water
D All of the above

2752. In stable organic compounds carbon always formed

A. 1 bond B 3 bond
C. 2 bond D 4 bond

2753. Acetylene consists of

A. Three sigma and two Pi bond
B One sigma and one Pi bond
C. Four sigma and three Pi Bond
D Two Sigma and two Pi bond

2754. Fromaldehyde is a

A. Co-Planar molecule
B Non-Planar Molecule
C. Planar molecules
D Both A and B

2755. The maximum bond length between carbon carbon present in

A. $CH2=CH2$ B $CH3-CH3$
C. Both D None of the above

2756. In which molecule greatest dipole moments present

A. CH3Cl B CH3Br
C. CH3F D CH3I

2757. Displacement mechanism includes the effects

A. Inductive effects
B Mesomeric effect
C. Electromeric effect
D All of the above

2758. The permanent effect whereby polarity is induced on the carbon atom is known as

A. Mesomeric effect
B Hyperconjugative
C. Inductive effects
D Electromeric effect

2759. The molecule which shows inductive effects contains

A. Single bond B Double bond
C. Triple bond D All of the above

2760. Which effect takes place when the molecule is exposed to an attack by electrophilic reagent

A. Electromeric effect
B Inductive effects
C. Mesomeric effect
D None of the above

2761 In which effect polarity is caused by complete transfer of an electron pair to one of two atom joined by multiple bond

A. Inductive effects
B Electromeric effect
C. Mesomeric effect
D None of the above

2762. In inductive effects permanent effect depends on the

A. Attacking Reagent
B Structure of substrates molecules
C. Both
D None of the above

2763. In which effect temporary polarization causes

A. Inductive effects
B Mesomeric effect
C. Electromeric effect
D Hyperconjugative

2764. In inductive effects the order of alkyl group are

A. Primary>secondary>tertiary
B Secondary>primary>tertiary
C. Tertiary>secondary>primary
D Both A and B

2765. The Carbonium ion containing

A. 1°carbon atom
B 2°carbon atom
C. 3° carbon atom
D All of the above

2766.TheformulamassofGlucoseishowmuchtime largerthantheformulamassofitsempiricalfo rmula

A. Two times
B Three times
C. Four times
D Six times

2767.If a compound has an empirical formula of CH2 and a molar mass of 70.13g/molit's molecular formula is

A. C5H10
B CH2
C. C10H5
D C6H12

2768. For the compound C11H24 theempirical formula is

A. C2H6
B C5H10
C. C11H24
D C3H6

2769. Which of the following group belong to +I group

A. OH
B COOH
C. OCH3
D CH3

2770. Which of the following is strongest -I group

A. N(CH3)2
B F
C. NH3
D O

2771. What does the symbol *P* represent in a QSAR equation?

A. pH
B. plasma concentration
C. partition coefficient
D. prodrug

2772. Arrange these species in their decreasing order of Nucleophilicity

A. C>D>B>A
B B>A>C>D
C. A>B>C>D
D C>A>B>D

2772. Which of the following molecule can act as a Nucleophilic and an Electrophilic

A. CH3NH2
B CH3OH
C. CH3CN
D None of the above

2773. Select the correct order of Basicity

A. CH3CH2>CH2=CH>HC=C>OH
B CH3CH2>OH>HC=C>CH2=CH
C. CH3CH2>HC=C>CH2=CH>OH
D All of the above

2774. Point on incorrect statements

A. Resonance structure should have equal energy
B In Resonance there should be the same number of electron pair
C. InResonancetheconstituentatom shouldbeinsame position
D All statement are correct

2775. Resonance structure of molecules have

A. Identical bonding
B Identical arrangement of atom and near by same energy
C. Different bonding
D the different number of paired and unpaired electron

2776. Shifting of electron of a multiple bond under the influence of a reagent is called

A. I effect
B P effect
C. M effect
D T effect

2777. Which of the following is not a planar molecule

A. H2C=C=CH2
B H2C=C=C=CH2
C. H2C=C=O
D NC-HC=CH-XN

2778. Choose the correct statement

A. I effect operate in Both sigma and Pi bond
B I effect create net charge in molecule
C. I effect transfer electron from one carbon to Another
D I effect create partial charge and it is distance dependent

2779. Which of the following are electrophile

A. BF3
B NH4
C. I-
D None of the above

2780. Which of the following statements are true

A. RO- is a stronger nucleophile than OH
B RO is weaker Nucleophile than OH
C. RCOO is a stronger nucleophile than OH
D None of the above

2781. Which among following statements are correct

A. Homolytic bond fission takes place in non polar solvent
B Cation and anion is produced Homolytic bond Fission
C. Energy needed for hemolytic bond fission is less than that required for the hetrolytic bond fission.
D None of the above

2782. Which of the following are Electrophile

A. CH B R-O-R
C. BF3 D None of the above

2783. Which of the following are Nucleophile

A. BF3 B CN
C. AlCl3 D None of the above

2784. Find out the correct statement regarding Resonance energy

A. It is eqal to the energy of least stable structure
B It is eqal to the difference in energies of the most stable canonical structure and resonance hybrid
C. It is eqal to energy of Resonance Hybrid
D None of the above

2785. Which statement true about Carbene

A. It is obtained by photolysis of diazomethane or ketone
B It can exist as single or triplet
C. Both are true
D None of the above

2786. Which of the following compound react with Lewis base Cl in Lewis acid base reaction.

A. OH B AlCl3
C. CH3 D All of the above

2787. Choose the strongest Base

A. HCOO- B NO2CH2COO-
C. FCH2COO- D MeCOO-

2788. Which of the following molecule have highest dipole moments

A. CH3Cl B CCl4
C. CH2Cl2 D None of the above

2789. Select the most acidic compound

A. P-nitrophenol
B O-hydroxybenzoic acid
C. P-hydroxybenzoic acid
D Both A and C

2790. Hyperconjugation involves overlap of which orbital

A. P-P B S-P
C. Both D None

2791. Which of the following molecule contains acidic hydrogen

A. 2,4 hexanedione B Butane
C. Pentane D 4,2 butanedione

2792. Select the molecule which conatain lowest dipole moments

A. 2-Butyne B Cis butyne
C. 1-butyne D All of the above

2793. Select the molecule which contains zero dipole moments

A. C6H6 B C4H8
C. C5H10 D C3H6

2794. Which molecule have both sigma and Pi bond

A. NaCN B NO2
C. SO2 D None of the above

2795. Choose the correct Hybridization about aromatic nitrogen

A. Sp Hybridization
B Not Hybridization
C. Sp2 Hybridization
D Sp3 Hybridization

2796. Choose the correct option of paramagnetic

A. Co B N2
C. No D O2

2797. Maximum covalent shown by which compound

A. AlCl3 B Sncl2
C. FeCl2 D MgCl2

2798. IF7 Structure shown by

A. Pentagonal Bipyramid
B Octahedral
C. Square Bipyramid
D Tetrahedral

2799. Peroxide ion is

A. Dimagnetic B Has bond order
C. Both D None of the above

2800. During the formation of chemical bond result in Energy

A. Increses B Decrease
C. Not effect D Any other effect

2801. Ductility and Malleability metal ion due to

A. The capacity of layer of metal ion to slide over the Other
B The presence of electrostatic force.
C. The crystalline structure in Metal
D None of the above

2802. In the cleavage of homolytic bond the formation of which chemical species

A. Anion B Cation
C. Atom D Free radical

2803. In chemical bond the energy stored in which form

A. Potential Energy
B Thermal energy
C. Chemical Energy
D All of the above

2804.Triplet excitation energy is required for which type of cleavage

A. Hetrolytic B Homolytic cleavage
C. Both A and B D None of these

2805. Hetrolytic cleavage required the type of energy

A. Singlet B Doublet
C. Triplet D All of the above

2806. Rateconstant of reaction depends on

A. Temperature
B Enzyme
C. Activation energy
D All of the above

2807. In which Carbon-Halogen bond consists highest bond energy

A. C-Br B C-F
C. C-Cl D C-I

2808. Prepration of Alkyl halide from alchol thereactants generally used

A. Pyridine B SoCl2
C. Both A and B D None of the above

2809. Ethane is formed when Nascent hydrogen react with

A. Butyl chloride B Methyl chloride
C. Ehtyl chloride D None of the above

2810. The intermolecular forces attraction are strong in

A. P-dichlorobenzene
B O-dichlrobenzene
C. M-dichlorobenzene
D. All of the above

2811. Uses of Hexachlroetane is

A. Repellent B Plasticizer
C. Fungicider D All of the above

2812. Which of the following method of preparation of Chlorobenzene

A. Grignard reagent
B Aldol condensation
C. Raschig Process
D None of these

2813. How many chlorine atom consists in the formula of DDT?

A. 3 B 7
C. 5 D 6

2814. Trichloromethane is IUPAC name of

A. Chloroform B Tartaric acid
C. Formic acid D None of the above

2815. Chloroform have the maineffect on

A. Peripheral systems
B Central Nervous system
C. Both A and B
D. None of the above

2816. A formula with the lowest whole ratio of element in a compound is called

A. Empirical formula
B. Molecular formula
C. Chemical formula
D Ionic formula

2817. A chemical formula which shows the atom present in a molecule of compound is known as

A. Empirical formula
B Ionic formula
C. Molecular formula
D Covalent formula

2818. All are empirical formula except

A. N2O B C3H8
C. N2O4 D Na2SO4

2819. Main source of organic compounds is

A. Animal B Fossils
C. Coal D Plants

2820. Carbon which burn with smoky flame are called

A. Aliphatic B Aromatic
C. Allicyclic D Aldehyde

2821. Isomerism shown by propene is

A. Cis-trans isomerism
B Geometricisomerism

C. Both a and b
D None of the above

2822. In laboratory the first organic compounds synthesis by

A. Kolbe B Grignard
C. Wohler D None of the above

2823. Organic compounds do not synthesis from inorganic compounds is related to which theory

A. Bayer theory B Vital force theory
C. Both a and b D None of the above

2824. First organic compounds which synthesis in laboratory are

A. Alcohol B Hexane
C. Urea D Acid

2825. Polymer are organic compound which contains

A. Low molecular weight
B Moderate molecule weight
C. High molecule weight
D All of the above

2826. Organic compounds generally soluble in

A. Polar solvent
B Water
C. Non Polar solvent
D Any other solvent

2827. The Process in which larger molecule with high molecular weight breaks down into smaller molecules with lower molecules weight is known as

A. Sterio isomerism B Pyrolysis
C. Both a and b D None of the above

2828. Tetrahedral geometry occurs in whichHybridization

A. Sp3 B Sp
C. Sp2 D All of the above

2829. EhoxyEthane consists

A. Only sigma bond B Covalent bonds
C. Only Pi bond D All of the above

2830. In Cyno group which type of Hybridization can be seen

A. Sp2
B Not show Hybridization
C. Sp
D Sp3 Hybridization

2831. Which is not heterocyclic compound

A. Pyridine B Thiophene
C. Furan D Anilline

2832. C5H12 has total no of isomer is

A. Five B Four
C. Six D Three

2833. General formula of cycloalkene is

A. CnH2n-2 B CnH2n+3
C. CnH2n-3 D None of the above

2834. Group of atom or single atom which give the properties of compound is called

A. Isomerism
B Name reaction
C. Functional group
D None of the above

2835. In industry methane is used as power generation isusually

A. Expensive B Cheper
C. Rare D None of the above

2836. In organic compound generally low melting point shown by

A. Strong intermolecular forces
B Consist of pi and sigma bond
C. Weak intermolecular forces
D. All of the above

2837. Acetic acid is also known as

A. Butanoic acid B Hexonoic acid
C. Pentanoic acid D Ehanoic acid

2838. Boiling point of ethanol is

A. 86°C B 72° C
C. 78°C D 90°C

2839. Choose the strongest acid

A. CH3COOH B ClCH2COOH
C. Br2CH2COOH D FCH2COOH

2840. CaC2O4 is a salt of

A. Fumic acid B Tartaric acid
C. Acetic acid D None of the above

2841. When we do the sulphonation of benzoic acid which compound mainly produces

A. M-sulphobenzoic acid
B P-Sulphobenzoic acid
C. O-Sulphobenzoic acid
D. All of the above

2842. Oxidation of bezyl chloride gives

A. Benzene B Benzoic acid
C. Anilline D Toluene

2843. When we treated acetic anhydride with sodium acetate the product formed

A. Benzaldehyde B Acetyl chloride
C. Alcohol D Acetamide

2844. When acid anhydride is Hydrolyzed theproduct formed is

A. Alcohol B Carboxyllic acid
C. Ketone D All of the above

2845. Acetylation of ethyl amine gives

A. N-ethyl acetamide
B. Acetamide
C. Acetylene
D. Propyl acetamide

2846. What will be the product CH3OH+CO

A. Ethyl formate
B Acetic acid
C. Methyl formate
D Formic acid

2847. Fruity like smell shown by

A. Acid B Ether
C. Alcohol D Ester

2848. In biodiesel the chemical reaction occurs are

A. Transesterification B Fermentation
C. Sublimation D All of the above

2849. When we do Reduction of nitroalkanes the yield are

A. Acid B Amines
C. Alcohol D Diazocompound

2850. Which reason is not responsible for the host of optical activity of quartz?

A. Fusion B Vaporisation
C. Dissolution D Condensation

2851. Which of the following state exhibits optical activity?

A. Liquid B Gaseous
C. Crystalline D All of the above

2852. Which of the following is the reason for differences in Enantiomer?

A. Physical properties
B Action on plane polarised light
C. Chemical properties
D. All of the above

2853. Which of the following is first substance to exhibit the phenomenon of optical activity

A. Glass B Quartz
C. Nicol D All of the above

2854. Which of the following is the reason for vanishing the crystalline form of structure

A. Fusion B Solution formation
C. Vaporisation D All of the above

2855. Crystal form of Quartz which are non superimpossible to each other known as

A. Enantioceps B Enantiospecies
C. Enantiomorps D All of the above

2856. Which of the following structure is not able torotate the plane polarised light

A. Asymmetric structure
B Symmtric Structure
C. Both A and B
D None of the above

2857. The two form are non superimpossible mirror image of each other such pair are known as

A. Meso compound B Diastromorp
C. Enantiomorps D None of the above

2858. Which of the following statements about enantiomer are incorrect

A. All enantiomer are levorotatary
B All enantiomer are rotate plane polarised light in a counter clock wise directions
C. Both A and B
D None of the above

2859. A carbon having four different monovalent atom or group is known as

A. Chiral carbon
B Chiral centre
C. Both A and B
D Chiral molecule

2860. Achiral or non chiral molecule are those

A. Which possess a plane of symmetry
B Superimpossible image
C. Both A and B
D None of the above

2861. If a molecule can be divided into equal halves in any plane then it is called

A. Racemix mixture B Plane of symmetry
C. Chiral molecule D None of the above

2862. From which Rotation optical isomer in a molecule containing Nnumber of different chiral carbon

A. 2n B 2n-1
C. 2n-2 D None of these

2863. A compound is optically inactive whose molecule is superimpossible on its mirror image even though it contain chiral central

A. Mesocompound B Chiral centre
C. Both A and B D None of the above

2864. Which of the following molecule is optically inactive

A. Planar molecules
B Coplanar molecule
C. Symmetry
D None of the above

2865. Which of the following compound possess alternative axis of symmetry

A. 1,3 disec butyl cyclobutane
B Truxillic acid
C. Both A and B
D None of the above

2866. Which of the molecule possesses neither a plane nor central of symmetry

A. 3,4,3,4 tetramethyl spiro dipyrolidium p-sulphur
B Truxillic acid
C. 1,3 di sec butyl cyclobutane
D None of the above

2867. There are few molecule which do not contain any chiral carbon atom but are still chiral such are called

A. Disymmtric B Racemix mixture
C. Symmtric D None of the above

2868. Which of the following form of tartaric acid is consider optical inactive

A. Dextrotartaric acid
B Levotartaric acid
C. Mesotartaric acid
D None of the above

2869. Which of the formula is used demonstrated plane of symmetry

A. Tetrahedral formula
B Plane formula
C. Both A and B
D Trigonal formula

2870. Transform of compound having a central of symmetry

A. Dimethylketopyridine
B Dimethylketopiperaziene
C. Diethyloxopiperaziene
D Both A and B

2871. Which of the following reasons is responsible for differences in the enantiomer having identical chemical properties

A. Action towards optical active compound
B Activity of Enantiomer
C. Action of plane polarised light
D None of the above

2872. When enantiomer react with opticalactive with reagent with ____ rate?

A. Similar B No reaction
C. Different D None of the above

2873. The Geometrical structure of the molecule should not superimpossible on its mirror image it must exist

A. Enatiomorps form B Diastromorp
C. Both A and B D None of the above

2874. Which type of compound cannot exhibit geometrical isomerism

A. Single bonded B Double bonded
C. Triple bonded D Cyclic Compounds

2875. The sterioisomerism which is due to restricted rotation about single bond is known as

A. Atropisomerism B Isomerism
C. Biphenyl D None of the above

2876. Which molecule always possesses a plane or centre of symmetry andhence optical inactive

A. Planar B Coplanar
C. Both A and B D None of the above

2877. What manufacturing industry regularly uses or produces products are Racemix mixture

A. Automotive B Pharmaceutical

C. Plastic D Textile

2878. Select the correct pair of compound which are tautomer

A. Vinyl alcohol and ethanol

B Propane and 3 propanol

C. Butane and 4 Butanol

D None of the above

2879. In Ethane the total no of conformations are

A. Infinite B 7

C. 3 D 4

2880. Which compound is isomeric with trimethyl amine are

A. 2-Propamime B 2-propamine

C. 3-propamine D Both A and B

2881. Least stable conformation in n-butane

A. Fully eclipsed B Eclipsed

C. Straight D None of the above

2882. Which of the following is not the method of Racemix Modification

A. By mixing of enantiomer

B ByRacemisation

C. By synthesis

D None of the above

2883. Which of the following molecule do not has any chiral central

A. 2,3 Heaxadiene B 2,4 Pentadiene

C. 2,3 Pentadiene D All of the above

2884. Which of the following is not considered criteria of Chirality

A. Centre of symmetry

B Chiral centre

C. Optical activity

D None of the above

2885. Chiral molecule consists which of the following properties

A. Plane of symmetry

B Centre of symmetry

C. Superimpossible mirror image

D All of the above

2886. Which type of project we get staggered and Eclipsed Eclipsed conformations

A. Newsman projection

B Sawhorse Projection

C. Both A and B

D None of the above

2887. Which of the following is an alkane which can exhibit optical activity

A. Pentane B Neopentane

C. 3-methyl pentane D None of the above

2888. Compound having Chirality formed mirror image are

A. Superimpossible

B Non superimpossible

C. Racemix mixture

D None of the above

2889. Which of the following is an example of optical active compound without Chirality

A. Tartaric acid B Sulphonium salt

C. Diphenic acid D Glycerdehyde

2890. No of atom present in chiral carbon

A. 4-Monovalent atom

B 4-Divalent atom

C. 4-trivalent atom

D None of the above

2891. In R and S configuration priority is given to the group depend on;

A. Atomic weight

B Atomic number

C. Valence electrons

D None

2892. In R and S configuration which of these group will given the highest priority?

A. I(iodine) B Br(bromine)

C. Cl(chlorine) D H(hydrogen)

2893. Which order of arrangement according to the priority os correct for R and S configuration?

A. Br>I>H>Cl B Cl>H>I>Br

C. I>Br>Cl>H D H>I>Br>Cl

2894. In R and S configuration R stands for;
A. Right B Rectus
C. Ramus D None

2895. In R and S configuration S stands for;
A. Sinister B Semister
C. Smister D None

2896. In R and S configuration R represent which direction?
A. Anti clockwise B Counter clockwise
C. Clockwise D None

2897. Which of the following can be specified by prefix RS?
A. Racemic modification
B Meso structure
C. Distereomers
D None

2898. In newmann projection molecule bind to how many C-atom?
A. Four B Three
C. Two D None

2899. From C-atom in newmann projection formulae form an angle of;
A. 109.5° B 108°
C. 120° D 60°

2900. In newmann projection formulae front atom forms how many sogma bonds?
A. Three B Two
C. Four D Zero

2901. Which of these is confirmation of n-butane?
A. Staggered B Gauche
C. Eclipsed D All of the above

2902. Isomer of 1,2-cyclopentadiol are;
A. Enantiomers B Meso structure
C. Distereomers D None

2903. Which of the following is not a chiral molecule;
A. Cis 1,2-cyclopentadiol
B Trans 1,2-cyclopentadiol
C. Both (a) & (b)
D None

2904. Which of these configuration is sepprable into enantiomers?
A. Cis-diols B Trans-diols
C. R-diols D S-diols

2905. Which of the following is a meso compound?
A. Trans-1,2 dimethyl cyclopropane
B Cis-1,2 cyclopentadiol
C. Trans-1,2 cyclopentadiol
D None

2906. Which of the following is not the confirmation of cyclohexane?
A. Half chair B Chair
C. Twist boat D Both (a) & (b)

2907. Confirmation of cyclohexane arise due to;
A. Rotation around C-C bond
B Breaking of C-C bond
C. Different Orientation of atom
D None

2908. Energy required for the interconversion of half chair form of cyclohexane;
A. 5.5kcal/mole B 7kcal/mole
C. 11kcal/mole D 6.8kcal/mole

2909. Energy required for the interconversion of the twist boat form of cyclohexane;
A. 8.2kcal/mole B 6.5kcal/mole
C. 5.9kcal/mole D 7.1kcal/mole

2910. Which of these confirmation has lowest energy?
A. Chair B Twist boat
C. Half chair D Boat

2911. Which of the following confirmation is leas stable?tl
A. Twist boat B Chair
C. Half chair D Boat

2912. 99.9% of cyclohexane molecule exist in which confirmation at any one time?
A. Twist boat B Boat
C. Chair D Chair

2913. In which form of cyclohexane hydrogen lies in the rough plane off ring us known as;
A. Axial hydrogen B Equatorial hydrogen
C. Planer hydrogen
D Hemispherical hydrogen

2914. Each of six C-atom of cyclohexane has;

A. One equatorial & one planer H-atom

B Oen equatorial & one axial H-atom

C. One planar & one axial H-atom

D None

2915. Cyclohexane molecule is estimated to be in the boat form at any given time in what percentage?

A. Over 99%

B Approximately 50%

C. Between 90% & 99%

D Less than 1%

2916. In which position methyl group in cyclohexane should exist for minimum repulsion?

A. Axial B Equatorial

C. Planar D Both (a) & (b)

2917. In which position methyl groupof cyclohexane should exist for maximum repulsion?

A. Axial B Planar

C. Equatorial D Both (b) & (c)

2918. Energy of the confirmation is lower if the methyl group is in;

A. Axial position

B Planar position

C. Equatorial position

D None

2919. Which order of the groups is correct for equatorial position in the cyclohexane?

A. Propyl>butyl>methyl>ethyl

B Butyl>propyl>ethyl>methyl

C. Methyl>ethyl>propyl>butyl

D Ethyl<butyl<propyl<methyl

2920. The bond angle between carbon atom in cyclohexane?

A. 60° B 90°

C. 109.5° D 120°

2921. Total no of isomer in C3H6O that are either cyclic or chiral

A. 6 B 4

C. 3 D 5

2922. Drug contain chiral carbon except

A. Omeprazole B Esomeprazole

C. Ketoprophen D Predinisolone

2923. Choose the wrong statement about 5 Memberb ring

A. It is more stable than 4 members ring

B It is more stable than 7 members ring

C. It is more stable than 6 members ring

D All above statement are False

2924. Which of the following is not a five member ring?

A. Pyridine B Furan

C. Pyrrole D Thiophene

2925. Choose the most Resonance stblized ring?

A. Furan B Thiophene

C. Pyrrole D Pyridine

2926. Which elementpresent in the furan ring

A. Sulphur B Oxygen

C. Nitrogen D All of the above

2927. Smallest angle in the pyridine ring is

A. 116° B 120°

C. 114° D 122°

2928. Which Hetro atom present in Pyridinering?

A. Nitrogen and sulphur

B Nitrogen and oxygen

C. Nitrogen

D Oxygen

2929. Mammals synthesize nicotinic acid through

A. Reduction

B Oxidation and Reduction

C. Oxidation

D None of these

2930. The extent or angle of rotation of palne polarised light or the optical activity of a substance is measured in an instrument known as

A. Analyser B. Voltmeter

C. Polarimeter D. None of the above

2931. The polarised light is passed through 1 decimeter of solution have concentration of 1 gram per millilitre is called

A. Specific Rotation

B. Enantiomer

C. Optical inactive

D. Levorotatary

2932. The wavelength of light use for theoptical activity of Sodium D is

A. 540 mu B. 589mu

C. 640mu D. 248mu

2933. In 1811 which substance firstly exhibit the phenomenon of optical activity

A. Glass B. Quartz

C. Plastic D. Steel

2934. Example of optical activity due to molecular structure are

A. Sodium chloride B. Barium

C. Glucose D. Zinc Sulphate

2935. Enantiomer having identical properties except

A. Boiling point

B. Melting Point

C. Refractive indices

D. Optical towards optical compound active

2936. When two enantiomer are mixed in eqimolecular quantities it results in formation of optical inactive compounds called

A. Racemix mixture B. Plane of symmetry

C. Meso form D. None of the above

2937. A plane of symmetry may be demonstrated successfully with the help of

A. Two dimensional B. Three dimensional

C. Both A and B D. One dimensional

2938. Chiral molecule contains chiral central except

A. Tartaric acid B. 2,3 pentadiene

C. Lactic acid D. Propionic acid

2939. The term Chirality is proposed by

A. Kelvin B. Jack and jones

C. Einstein D. None of the above

2940. Compounds which have different arrangements of atoms in space while having same atoms bonded to each other are said to have

A. Position isomerism

B. Functional group isomerism

C. Chain isomerism

D. Sterioisomerism

2941. Reducing agents used in Brich reduction is

A. LiAlH4 B Na/ROH

C. AlCl3 D PCl5

2942. Pyridine is ....basic than alkylamine

A. More B Less

C. Equal D None

2943. Clemmensen reduction of a ketone is carried out in the presence of which of the following

A. Zn-Hg and HCl

B NaBH4

C. LiAlH4

D H2 and Pt as catalyst

2944. One of which does not example of organic addition reaction

A. Halogenation B Hydration

C. Dehydration D Hydrohalogenation

2945. Formation of a single product from two reactant molecules is known as

A. Elimination reaction

B Substitution reaction

C. Addition reaction

D Rearrangement reaction

2946. Alcohol are treated with Cr2O7 by refluxing gives

A. Carboxylic Acid B Ketone

C. Alkane D Aldehyde

2947. Which will react faster in the SN2 nucleophilic substitution reaction

A. CH= CH2 – CH2 – Br

B CH2 = CH- CH2 = Br

C. CH2 = CH- CH2 – Br

D CH2-CH=CH2=Br

2948. Which of the following organic reaction used to convert a primary amide to a primary amine using a halogen

A. Reimer-Tiemann reaction

B Clemmensen reduction

C. Hofmann rearrangement reaction

D Kolbe-Schmitt reaction

2949. Formation of free radicals are occur in free radical reaction which of the following step

A. Initiation Step

B Propagation Step
C. Termination Step
D Both A and B

2950. Which one of the following step free radicals are formed and which attack reactants molecules to generate more and more free radicals.

A. Initiation Step B Propagation Step
C. Termination Step D Both A and B

2951. Choose the following statements regarding the SN2 mechanism is not true

A. Its usually second order
B SN2 reactions are bimolecular
C. Its occurs in one step
D Its occur in two steps

2952. Choose the following most reactive compound by the SN1 mechanism

A. CH2= CHCH2Br B
C. CH3CH2CH2Br D Both A and C

2953. Choose the following statements regarding the E2 mechanism is not true

A. E2 mechanism are always bimolecular
B E2 mechanism usually occur in one step
C. E2 mechanism are generally second order
D E2 mechanism usually occur in two step

2954. Which of the following does not have alpha hydrogen

A. Formaldehyde
B Acetone
C. Acetaldehyde
D Phenyl acetaldehyde

2955. The number of structure isomers of C6H14 is:

A. 4 B 5
C. 6 D 7

2956. An isomer of ethanol is:

A. Methanol B diethyl ether
C. Acetone D dimethyl ether

2957. Formation of a single product from two reactant molecules is known as

A. Addition reaction
B Elimination reaction
C. Substitution reaction
D Oxidation

2958. Commercial sources of alkanes include

A. Coal B Natural gas
C. Petroleum D all of above

2959. The ionic bond is formed due to electrostatic attraction between stable ions formed by complete transfer of electron from one atom to another

A. Electrovalent bond
B Covalent bond
C. Metallic bond
D None of the above

2960. When two electronegative atoms react together is known as

A. Covalent bond B Metallic bond
C. Both D None of the above

2961. Which type of bond is frequently encountered in inorganic compounds

A. Electrovalent bond B Covalent compound
C. Both D None of the above

2962. Which of the following are type of covalent bond

A. Sigma bond B Pi bond
C. Both D None of the above

2963. Which type of bond is formed by the linear or end to end overlap of orbital

A. Sigma bond
B Pi Bond
C. Electrovalent bond
D None of the above

2964. Which type of bond is formed by parallel or side to side overlap of P Orbital

A. Pi Bond B Sigma bond
C. Both D None of the above

2965. The hybrid formed by combining one S and three P orbital

A. Sp Hybridization B Sp2 Hybridization
C. Sp3 Hybridization
D None

2966. Which compounds showing the characteristics of smell and inflammation

A. Ionic bond B Electrovalent
C. Covalent bond D None of the above

2967. Which theory responsible for the formation of covalent bond

A. The valency bondtheory

B The molecule bond theory

C. Both

D None of the above

2968. Which electron are loosely held in the pair of elrctron in a sigma bond

A. Pi electron

B Non bonding electron

C. Sigma bond

D Both A and B

2969. Which bond are more reactive and easily broken

A. Pi bond B Sigma bond

C. Both D All of theabove

2970. The process of mixing of pureorbital to give a set of new equivalent orbital is known as

A. Hybridization B Molecule orbital

C. Bonding orbital D None of the above

2971. Which compound are soluble in water but insolble in organic compound

A. Electrovalent bond

B Ionic bond

C. Metallic compound

D None of the above

2972. Thevsharing of an electron pair occurs between two electrons one from each of two atom

A. Coordinate covalent bond

B Pi bond

C. Ionic bond

D Sigma bond

2973. The angle between the two orbital is

A. 109°28 B 110°28

C. 111° D 105°

2974. Which type of orbital whenever carbon is bonded to four other atom or group

A. Sp Hybridization

B Sp2 Hybridization

C. Sp3 Hybridization

D Both A and B

2975. Which type of bond present in Methane

A. Pi Bond

B Covalent bond

C. Electrovalent bond

D Sigma Bond

2976. The energy Required to break any of four bond is the

A. 100 kcal B 102kcal

C. 104 kcal D 102 kcal

2977. In ethylene how much C-H single covalent bond are present

A. Two B Four

C. Three D One

2978. Whenever carbon is bonded to three other atoms or group it always use

A. Sp Hybridization

B Both A and C

C. Sp2 Hybridization

D Sp3 Hybridization

2979. Which of these atoms measure of its power to attract elecctron that is sharing in covalent bond

A. Electronegativity

B Electron positivity

C. Electron affinity

D None of the above

2980. Distance of the valence electron from the nucleus

A. Atomic Radius B Bond length

C. Atomic Diameters D Both A and B

2981. The magnitude of the positive energy charge on the nucleus is called

A. Atomic mass B Atomic number

C. Atomic Radius D None of the above

2982. The bond which appear to have a positiv end and a negative end is said to be

A. Electrovalent bond

B Non Polar Bond

C. Polar Bond

D None of the above

2983. There is no positive and negative end such bond are known as

A. Semi-polar Bond

B Non Polar Bond C. Polar Bond

D Both A and B

2984. Which bond is formed between the C-Cl bond

A. Polar bond
B Non Polar bond
C. Semi Polar bond
D None of the above

2985. The angle between H-o-H is

A. 103° B 102°
C. 104° D 108°

2986. The formula of Dipole moments

A. Charge×time B Charge×Distance
C. Charge×Radius D None of the above

2987. Non Polar molecules do not possess

A. Polarization
B Covalent bonds
C. Vanderwalls force
D Dipole moments

2988. All carbon carbon bond in benzene have same bond length

A. 1.54 A° B 1.44°
C. 1.65° D 1.76°

2989. The difference in energy between the hybrid and the most stable resonance structure is known as

A. Resonance energy
B Electric Energy
C. Both
D None of the above

2990. At which energy Benzene is said to be stabilize

A. 42 kcal/mol B 40 kcal/mol
C. 44 kcal/mol D 38 kcal/mol

2991. Which of the statement is true about Resonance

A. Resonance is actual structure
B Resonance hybrid are less stable
C. It involves the delocalization of electron
D Resonance are more reactive

2992. The force of attraction is known as

A. Hydrogen Bond B Covalent bonds
C. Both D None of the above

2993. At which condition the breakup of the Hydrogen bond between the water molecules

A. If non Polar molecules dissolve in alcohol
B If polar molecules dissolve in water
C. If non Polarmolecules were to dissolve in water
D All of the above

2994. In stable organic compounds carbon always formed

A. 1 bond B 3 bond
C. 2 bond D 4 bond

2995. Acetylene consists of

A. Three sigma and two Pi bond
B One sigma and one Pi bond
C. Four sigma and three Pi Bond
D Two Sigma and two Pi bond

2996. Fromaldehyde is a

A. Co-Planar molecule
B Non-Planar Molecule
C. Planar molecules
D Both A and B

2997. The maximum bond length between carbon carbon present in

A. CH2=CH2 B CH3-CH3
C. Both D None of the above

2998. In which molecule greatest dipole moments present

A. CH3Cl B CH3Br
C. CH3F D CH3I

2999. Displacement mechanism includes the effects

A. Inductive effects
B Mesomeric effect
C. Electromeric effect
D All of the above

3000. The permanent effect whereby polarity is induced on the carbon atom is known as

A. Mesomeric effect
B Hyperconjugative
C. Inductive effects
D Electromeric effect

3001. The molecule which shows inductive effects contains

A. Single bond B Double bond
C. Triple bond D All of the above

3002. Which effect takes place when the molecule is exposed to an attack by electrophilic reagent

A. Electromeric effect
B Inductive effects
C. Mesomeric effect
D None of the above

3003. In which effect polarity is caused by complete transfer of an electron pair to one of two atomjoined by multiple bond

A. Inductive effects
B Electromeric effect
C. Mesomeric effect
D None of the above

3004. In inductive effects permanent effect depends on the

A. Attacking Reagent
B Structure of substrates molecules
C. Both
D None of the above

3005. In which effect temporary polarization causes

A. Inductive effects
B Mesomeric effect
C. Electromeric effect
D Hyperconjugative

3006. In inductive effects the order of alkyl group are

A. Primary>secondary>tertiary
B Secondary>primary>tertiary
C. Tertiary>secondary>primary
D Both A and B

3007. The Carbonium ion containing

A. 1°carbon atom
B 2°carbon atom
C. 3° carbon atom
D All of the above

3008. The formula mass of Glucose is how much time larger than the formula mass of its empirical formula

A. Two times B Three times
C. Four times D Six times

3009. If acompound has an empirical formula of CH2 and a molar mass of 70.13g/mol it's molecular formula is

A. C5H10 B CH2
C. C10H5 D C6H12

3010. For the compound C11H24 the empirical formula is

A. C2H6 B C5H10
C. C11H24 D C3H6

3011. Which of the following group belong to +I group

A. OH B COOH
C. OCH3 D CH3

3012. Which of the following is strongest -I group

A. N(CH3)2 B F
C. NH3 D O

3013. What is the geometry of central oxygen atom in the ozone molecule

A. Trigonal planar B tetrahedral
C. Linear D None of the above

3014. Which of the following molecule can act as a Nucleophilic and an Electrophilic

A. CH3NH2 B CH3OH
C. CH3CN D None of the above

3015. Select the correct order of Basicity

A. CH3CH2>CH2=CH>HC=C>OH
B CH3CH2>OH>HC=C>CH2=CH
C. CH3CH2>HC=C>CH2=CH>OH
D All of the above

3016. Point on incorrect statements

A. Resonance structure should have equal energy
B In Resonance there should be the same number of electron pair
C. In Resonance the constituent atom should be in same position
D All statement are correct

3017. Resonance structure of molecules have

A. Identical bonding
B Identical arrangement of atom and nearby same energy
C. Different bonding
D The different number of paired and unpaired electron

3018. Which of the following is not a planar molecule

A. H2C=C=CH2
B. H2C=C=C=CH2
C. H2C=C=O
D NC-HC=CH-XN

3019. Choose the correct statement

A. I effect operate in Both sigma and Pi bond

B I effect create net charge in molecule

C. I effect transfer electron from one carbon to Another

D I effect create partial charge and it is distance dependent

3020. Which of the following are electrophile

A. BF3 B NH4

C. I- D None of the above

3021. Which of the following statements are true

A. RO- is a stronger nucleophile than OH

B RO is weaker Nucleophile than OH

C. RCOO is a stronger nucleophile than OH

D None of the above

3022. Which among following statements are correct

A. Homolytic bond fission takes place in non polar solvent

B Cation and anion is produced Homolytic bond fission

C. Energy needed for homolytic bond fission is less than that required for the hetrolytic bond fission.

D None of the above

3023. Which of the following are Electrophile

A. CH B R-O-R

C. BF3 D None of the above

3024. Which of the following are Nucleophile

A. BF3 B CN

C. AlCl3 D None of the above

3025. Find out the correct statement regarding Resonance energy

A. It is equal to the energy of least stable structure

B It is equal to the difference in energies of the most stable canonical structure and resonance hybrid

C. It is equal to energy of Resonance Hybrid

D None of the above

3026. Which statement true about Carbene

A. It is obtained by photolysis of diazomethane or ketone

B It can exist as single or triplet

C. Both are true

D None of the above

3027. Which of the following compound react with Lewis base Cl in Lewis acid base reaction.

A. OH B AlCl3

C. CH3 D All of the above

3028. Choose the strongest Base

A. HCOO- B NO2CH2COO-

C. FCH2COO- D MeCOO-

3029. Which of the following molecule have highest dipole moments

A. CH3Cl B CCl4

C. CH2Cl2 D None of the above

3030. Select the most acidic compound

A. P-nitrophenol

B O-hydroxybenzoic acid

C. P-hydroxybenzoic acid

D Both A and C

3031. Hyperconjugation involves overlap of which orbital

A. P-P B S-P

C. Both D None

3032. Which of the following molecule contains acidic hydrogen

A. 2,4 hexanedione B Butane

C. Pentane D 4,2 butanedione

3033. Select the molecule which conatain lowest dipole moments

A. 2-Butyne B Cis butyne

C. 1-butyne D All of the above

3034. Select the molecule which contains zero dipole moments

A. C6H6 B C4H8

C. C5H10 D C3H6

3035. Which molecule have both sigma and Pi bond

A. NaCN B NO2

C. SO2 D None of the above

3036. Choose the correct Hybridization about aromatic nitrogen

A. Sp Hybridization

B Not Hybridization

C. Sp2 Hybridization

D Sp3 Hybridization

3037. Choose the correct option of paramagnetic

A. Co B N2

C. No D O2

3038. Maximum covalent shown by which compound

A. AlCl3 B Sncl2

C. FeCl2 D MgCl2

3039. IF7 Structure shown by

A. Pentagonal Bipyramid

B Octahedral

C. Square Bipyramid

D Tetrahedral

3040. Peroxide ion is

A. Dimagnetic B Has bond order

C. Both D None of the above

3041. During the formation of chemical bond result in Energy

A. Increses B Decrease

C. Not effect D Any other effect

3042. Ductility and Malleability metal ion due to

A. The capacity of layer of metal ion to slide over the Other

B The presence of electrostatic force.

C. The crystalline structure in Metal

D None of the above

3043. In the cleavage of homolytic bond the formation of which chemical species

A. Anion B Cation

C. Atom D Free radical

3044. In chemical bond the energy stored in which form

A. Potential Energy

B Thermal energy

C. Chemical Energy

D All of the above

3045. Triplet excitation energy is required for which type of cleavage

A. Hetrolytic B Homolytic cleavage

C. Both A and B D None of these

3046. Hetrolytic cleavage required the type of energy

A. Singlet B Doublet

C. Triplet D All of the above

3047. Rate constant of reaction depends on

A. Temperature B Enzyme

C. Activation energy D All of the above

3048. In which Carbon-Halogen bond consists highest bond energy

A. C-Br B C-F

C. C-Cl D C-I

3049. Prepration of Alkyl halide from alchol the reactants generally used

A. Pyridine B SoCl2

C. Both A and B D None of the above

3050. Ethane is formed when Nascent hydrogen react with

A. Butyl chloride B Methyl chloride

C. Ehtyl chloride D None of the above

3051. The intermolecular forces attraction are strong in

A. P-dichlorobenzene

B O-dichlrobenzene

C. M-dichlorobenzene

D All of the above

3052. Uses of Hexachlroetane is

A. Repellent B Plasticizer

C. Fungicider D All of the above

3053. Which of the following method of preparation of Chlorobenzene

A. Grignard reagent

B Aldol condensation

C. Raschig Process

D None of these

3054. How many chlorine atom consists in the formula of DDT?

A. 3 B 7

C. 5 D 6

3055. Trichloromethane is IUPAC name of

A. Chloroform B Tartaric acid

C. Formic acid D None of the above

3056. Chloroform have the main effect on

A. Peripheral systems

B Central Nervous system

C. Both A and B

D None of the above

3057. A formula with the lowest whole ratio of element in a compound is called

A. Empirical formula
B Molecular formula
C. Chemical formula
D Ionic formula

3058. A chemical formula which shows the atom present in a molecule of compound is known as

A. Empirical formula
B Ionic formula
C. Molecular formula
D Covalent formula

3059. All are empirical formula except

A. N2O   B C3H8
C. N2O4   D Na2SO4

3060. Main source of organic compounds is

A. Animal   B Fossils
C. Coal   D Plants

3061. Carbon which burn with smoky flame are called

A. Aliphatic   B Aromatic
C. Allicyclic   D Aldehyde

3062. Isomerism shown by propene is

A. Cis-trans isomerism
B Geometric isomerism
C. Both a and b
D None of the above

3063. In laboratory the first organic compounds synthesis by

A. Kolbe   B Grignard
C. Wohler   D None of the above

3064. Organic compounds do not synthesis from inorganic compounds is related to which theory

A. Bayer theory   B Vital force theory
C. Both a and b   D None of the above

3065. First organic compounds which synthesis in laboratory are

A. Alcohol   B Hexane
C. Urea   D Acid

3066. Polymer are organic compound which contains

A. Low molecular weight
B Moderate molecule weight
C. High molecule weight
D All of the above

3067. Organic compounds generally soluble in

A. Polar solvent
B Water
C. Non Polar solvent
D Any other solvent

3068. The Process in which larger molecule with high molecular weight breaks down into smaller molecules with lower molecules weight is known as

A. Sterio isomerism   B Pyrolysis
C. Both a and b   D None of the above

3069. Tetrahedral geometry occurs in which Hybridization

A. Sp3   B Sp
C. Sp2   D All of the above

3070. Ehoxy Ethane consists

A. Only sigma bond   B Covalent bonds
C. Only Pi bond   D All of the above

3071. In Cyno group which type of Hybridization can be seen

A. Sp2
B Not show Hybridization
C. Sp
D Sp3 Hybridization

3072. Which is not heterocyclic compound

A. Pyridine   B Thiophene
C. Furan   D Anilline

3073. C5H12 has total no of isomer is

A. Five   B Four
C. Six   D Three

3074. General formula of cycloalkene is

A. CnH2n-2   B CnH2n+3
C. CnH2n-3   D None of the above

3075. Group of atom or single atom which give the properties of compound is called

A. Isomerism   B Name reaction
C. Functional group D   None of the above

3076. In industry methane is used as power generation is usually

A. Expensive   B Cheper
C. Rare   D None of the above

3077. In organic compound generally low melting point shown by

A. Strong intermolecular forces
B Consist of pi and sigma bond
C. Weak intermolecular forces
D All of the above

3078. Acetic acid is also known as

A. Butanoic acid B Hexonoic acid
C. Pentanoic acid D Ehanoic acid

3079. Boiling point of ethanol is

A. 86°C B 72° C
C. 78°C D 90°C

3080. Choose the strongest acid

A. CH3COOH B ClCH2COOH
C. Br2CH2COOH D FCH2COOH

3081. CaC2O4 is a salt of

A. Fumic acid B Tartaric acid
C. Acetic acid D None of the above

3082. When we do the sulphonation of benzoic acid which compound mainly produces

A. M-sulphobenzoic acid
B P-Sulphobenzoic acid
C. O-Sulphobenzoic acid
D All of the above

3083. Oxidation of bozyl ohloride gives

A. Benzene B Benzoic acid
C. Anilline D Toluene

3084. When we treated acetic anhydride with sodium acetate the product formed

A. Benzaldehyde B Acetyl chloride
C. Alcohol D Acetamide

3085. 145 When acid anhydride is Hydrolyzed the product formed is

A. Alcohol B Carboxyllic acid
C. Ketone D All of the above

3086. Acetylation of ethyl amine gives

A. N-ethyl acetamide B Acetamide
C. Acetylene D Propyl acetamide

3087. What will be the product CH3OH+CO

A. Ethyl formate B Acetic acid
C. Methyl formate D Formic acid

3088. Fruity like smell shown by

A. Acid B Ether
C. Alcohol D Ester

3089. In biodiesel the chemical reaction occurs are

A. Transesterification
B Fermentation
C. Sublimation
D All of the above

3090. When we do Reduction of nitroalkanes the yield are

A. Acid B Amines
C. Alcohol D Diazocompound

3091. Which reason is not responsible for the host of optical activity of quartz?

A. Fusion B Vaporisation
C. Dissolution D Condensation

3092. Which of the following state exhibits optical activity?

A. Liquid B Gaseous
C. Crystalline D All of the above

3093. Which of the following is the reason for differences in Enantiomer?

A. Physical properties
B Action on plane polarised light
C. Chemical properties
D All of the above

3094. Which of the following is first substance to exhibit the phenomenon of optical activity

A. Glass B Quartz
C. Nicol D All of the above

3095. Which of the following is the reason for vanishing the crystalline form of structure

A. Fusion B Solution formation
C. Vaporisation D All of the above

3096. Crystal form of Quartz which are non superimpossible to each other known as

A. Enantioceps B Enantiospecies
C. Enantiomorps D All of the above

3097. Which of the following structure is not able torotate the plane polarised light

A. Asymmetric structure
B Symmtric Structure
C. Both A and B
D None of the above

3098. The two form are non superimpossible mirror image of each other such pair are known as

A. Meso compound
B Diastromorp
C. Enantiomorps
D None of the above

3099. Which of the following statements about enantiomer are incorrect

A. All enantiomer are levorotatary
B All enantiomer are rotate plane polarised light in a counter clock wise directions
C. Both A and B
D None of the above

3100. A carbon having four different monovalent atom or group is known as

A. Chiral carbon B Chiral centre
C. Both A and B D Chiral molecule

3101. Achiral or non chiral molecule are those

A. Which possess a plane of symmetry
B Superimpossible image
C. Both A and B
D None of the above

3102. If a molecule can be divided into equal halves in any plane then it is called

A. Racemix mixture
B Plane of symmetry
C. Chiral molecule
D None of the above

3103. From which Rotation optical isomer in a molecule containing Nnumber of different chiral carbon

A. 2n B 2n-1
C. 2n-2 D None of these

3104. A compound is optically inactive whose molecule is superimpossible on its mirror image even though it contain chiral central

A. Mesocompound
B Chiral centre
C. Both A and B
D None of the above

3105. Which of the following molecule is optically inactive

A. Planar molecules B Coplanar molecule
C. Symmetry D None of the above

3106. Which of the prism is used in plane polarised light

A. Nicol prism B Glass prism
C. Quartz D All of the above

3107. The substance which rotates the plane polarised light to the left is called

A. Dextrorotatry B Levorotatary
C. Both A and B D None of these

3108. In which condition the light is totally cutt off and nothing is visible

A. When two prism are perpendicular to each other
B When two prism are similar directions
C. When two prism are in opposite directions
D None of the above

3109. Which compound do not rotate the plane polarised light in any direction

A. Optical inactive
B Optical active
C. Racemix mixture
D None of the above

3110. Which of the following is reasons of optical inactivity of molecules

A. Plane of symmetry
B Alternative symmetry axis of symmetry
C. Chirality
D All of the above

3111. How many optical isomer are possible in a compound with one chiral compound

A. 5 B 4
C. 2 D 3

3112. The number of Racemix form of molecules having different chiral carbon

A. 2n B 2n-1
C. 2n+1 D None of the above

3113. To possess an N-fold alternating action of symmetry molecule is rotated to which angle

A. 90° B 180°
C. 360° D 120°

3114. Which of the following compound possess alternative axis of symmetry

A. 1,3 disec butyl cyclobutane
B Truxillic acid
C. Both A and B
D None of the above

3115. Which of the molecule possesses neither a plane nor central of symmetry
A. 3,4,3,4 tetramethyl spiro dipyrolidium p-sulphur
B Truxillic acid
C. 1,3 di sec butyl cyclobutane
D None of the above

3116. There are few molecule which do not contain any chiral carbon atom but are still chiral such are called
A. Disymmtric B Racemix mixture
C. Symmtric D None of the above

3117. Which of the following form of tartaric acid is consider optical inactive
A. Dextrotartaric acid
B Levotartaric acid
C. Mesotartaric acid
D None of the above

3118. Which of the formula is used demonstrated plane of symmetry
A. Tetrahedral formula
B Plane formula
C. Both A and B
D Trigonal formula

3119. Transform of compound having a central of symmetry
A. Dimethylketopyridine
B Dimethylketopiperaziene
C. Diethyloxopiperaziene
D Both A and B

3120. Which of the following reasons is responsible for differences in the enantiomer having identical chemical properties
A. Action towards optical active compound
B Activity of Enantiomer
C. Action of plane polarised light
D None of the above

3121. When enantiomer react with optical active with reagent with ____ rate?
A. Similar B No reaction
C. Different D None of the above

3122. The Geometrical structure of the molecule should not superimpossible on its mirror image it must exist
A. Enatiomorps form
B Diastromorp
C. Both A and B
D None of the above

3123. Which type of compound cannot exhibit geometrical isomerism
A. Single bonded B Double bonded
C. Triple bonded D Cyclic Compounds

3124. The sterioisomerism which is due to restricted rotation about single bond is known as
A. Atropisomerism B Isomerism
C. Biphenyl D None of the above

3125. Which molecule always possesses a plane or centre of symmetry andhence optical inactive
A. Planar B Coplanar
C. Both A and B D None of the above

3126. What manufacturing industry regularly uses or produces products are Racemix mixture
A. Automotive B Pharmaceutical
C. Plastic D Textile

3127. Select the correct pair of compound which are tautomer
A. Vinyl alcohol and ethanol
B Propane and 3 propanol
C. Butano and 4 Butanol
D None of the above

3128. In Ethane the total no of conformations are
A. Infinite B 7
C. 3 D 4

3129. Which compound is isomeric with trimethyl amine are
A. 2-Propamime B 2-propamine
C. 3-propamine D Both A and B

3130. Least stable conformation in n-butane
A. Fully eclipsed B Eclipsed
C. Straight D None of the above

3131. Which of the following is not the method of Racemix Modification
A. By mixing of enantiomer
B By Racemisation
C. By synthesis
D None of the above

3132. Which of the following molecule do not has any chiral central

A. 2,3 Heaxadiene B 2,4 Pentadiene
C. 2,3 Pentadiene D All of the above

3133. Which of the following is not considered criteria of Chirality

A. Centre of symmetry
B Chiral centre
C. Optical activity
D None of the above

3134. Chiral molecule consists which of the following properties

A. Plane of symmetry
B Centre of symmetry
C. Superimpossible mirror image
D All of the above

3135. Which type of project we get staggered and Eclipsed Eclipsed conformations

A. Newsman projection
B Sawhorse Projection
C. Both A and B
D None of the above

3136. Which of the following is an alkane which can exhibit optical activity

A. Pentane
B Neopentane
C. 3-methyl pentane
D None of the above

3137. Compound having Chirality formed mirror image are

A. Superimpossible
B Non superimpossible
C. Racemix mixture
D None of the above

3138. Which of the following is an example of optical active compound without Chirality

A. Tartaric acid B Sulphonium salt
C. Diphenic acid D Glycerdehyde

3139. No of atom present in chiral carbon

A. 4-Monovalent atom
B 4-Divalent atom
C. 4-trivalent atom
D None of the above

3140. In R and S configuration priority is given to the group depend on;

A. Atomic weight
B Atomic number
C. Valence electrons
D None

3141. In R and S configuration which of these group will given the highest priority?

A. I(iodine) B Br(bromine)
C. Cl(chlorine) D H(hydrogen)

3142. Which order of arrangement according to the priority os correct for R and S configuration?

A. Br>I>H>Cl B Cl>H>I>Br
C. I>Br>Cl>H D H>I>Br>Cl

3143. In R and S configuration R stands for;

A. Right B Rectus
C. Ramus D None

3144. In R and S configuration S stands for;

A. Sinister B Semister
C. Smister D None

3145. In R and S configuration R represent which direction?

A. Anti clockwise B Counter clockwise
C. Clockwise D None

3146. Which of the following can be specified by prefix RS?

A. Racemic modification
B Meso structure
C. Distereomers
D None

3147. In newmann projection molecule bind to how many C-atom?

A. Four B Three
C. Two D None

3148. From C-atom in newmann projection formulae form an angle of;

A. 109.5° B 108°
C. 120° D 60°

3149. In newmann projection formulae front atom forms how many sogma bonds?

A. Three B Two
C. Four D Zero

3150. Which of these is confirmation of n-butane?

A. Staggered B Gauche
C. Eclipsed D All of the above

3151. Isomer of 1,2-cyclopentadiol are;

A. Enantiomers B Meso structure
C. Distereomers D None

3152. Which of the following is not a chiral molecule;

A. Cis 1,2-cyclopentadiol
B Trans 1,2-cyclopentadiol
C. Both (a) & (b)
D None

3153. Which of these configuration is sepprable into enantiomers?

A. Cis-diols B Trans-diols
C. R-diols D S-diols

3154. Which of the following is a meso compound?

A. Trans-1,2 dimethyl cyclopropane
B Cis-1,2 cyclopentadiol
C. Trans-1,2 cyclopentadiol
D None

3155. Which of the following is not the confirmation of cyclohexane?

A. Half chair B Chair
C. Twist boat D Both (a) & (b)

3156. Confirmation of cyclohexane arise due to;

A. Rotation around C-C bond
B Breaking of C-C bond
C. Different Orientation of atom
D None

3157. Energy required for the interconversion of half chair form of cyclohexane;

A. 5.5kcal/mole B 7kcal/mole
C. 11kcal/mole D 6.8kcal/mole

3158. Energy required for the interconversion of the twist boat form of cyclohexane;

A. 8.2kcal/mole B 6.5kcal/mole
C. 5.9kcal/mole D 7.1kcal/mole

3159. Which of these confirmation has lowest energy?

A. Chair B Twist boat
C. Half chair D Boat

3160. Which of the following confirmation is leas stable?tl

A. Twist boat B Chair
C. Half chair D Boat

3161. 99.9% of cyclohexane molecule exist in which confirmation at any one time?

A. Twist boat B Boat
C. Chair D Chair

3162. In which form of cyclohexane hydrogen lies in the rough plane off ring us known as;

A. Axial hydrogen
B Equatorial hydrogen
C. Planer hydrogen
D Hemispherical hydrogen

3163. Each of six C-atom of cyclohexane has;

A. One equatorial & one planer H-atom
B Oen equatorial & one axial H-atom
C. One planar & one axial H-atom
D None

3164. Cyclohexane molecule is estimated to be in the boat form at any given time in what percentage?

A. Over 99%
B Approximately 50%
C. Between 90% & 99%
D Less than 1%

3165. In which position methyl group in cyclohexane should exist for minimum repulsion?

A. Axial B Equatorial
C. Planar D Both (a) & (b)

3166. In which position methyl groupof cyclohexane should exist for maximum repulsion?

A. Axial B Planar
C. Equatorial D Both (b) & (c)

3167. Energy of the confirmation is lower if the methyl group is in;

A. Axial position
B Planar position
C. Equatorial position
D None

3168. Which order of the groups is correct for equatorial position in the cyclohexane?

A. Propyl>butyl>methyl>ethyl
B Butyl>propyl>ethyl>methyl

C. Methyl>ethyl>propyl>butyl
D Ethyl<butyl<propyl<methyl

3169. The bond angle between carbon atom in cyclohexane?

A. 60° B 90°
C. 109.5° D 120°

3170. Total no of isomer in C3H6O that are either cyclic or chiral

A. 6 B 4
C. 3 D 5

3171. 232 Drug contain chiral carbon except

A. Omeprazole B Esomeprazole
C. Ketoprophen D Predinisolone

3172. Arranged the following heterocyclic compound in increasing order of their basicity?

A. Thiirane>oxirane>aziridine
B. Thiirane >aziridine>oxirane
C. Oxirane>thiirane>aziridine
D. Oxirane>aziridine>thiirane

3173. What kinetics follow Gabriel ring closure method .

A. Seond order B. Zero order
C. Mixed order D. First order

3174. Which of the following heteroyclic compound act as a anti-caner agent.

A. Oxirane and thiirane
B. Oxirane and azirine
C. Oxirane and azirine
D. None of this

3175.Which of the following statement is correct.

A. Three membered heterocyclic compound are more reactive than cyclopropane derivative
B. Three membered heteroclic compound are less reactive than cyclopropande derivative
C. The chemical property of heterocyclic compound are similar to that of cyclopropane derivative
D. All the above statement are correct

3176. Which type of spectroscopy is used to determine the bond distance and bond length of heterocyclic compound.

A. IR spectroscopy
B. UV spectroscopy
C. Microwave spectroscopy
D. Mass spectroscopy

3177. Aziridine is prepared by.

A. Hoch-campbell method
B. Ring closure method
C. From diazoalkane
D. From II-mercaptoethanol

3178. Which heterocyclic compound is used for the manufacture of plastic

A. Oxaziridine B. Oxirane
C. Thirane D. Diazirine

3179. What ever the condition like photochemical and thermal,the major reaction is the formation of two radical fragmentation CH3 and CHO. Who revealed the statement.

A. Kwaski and coworkes
B. Woodward and Hoffmann
C. Hassner and coworkes
D. Nishiwaki et al

3180. Alpha,beta –epoxyethane has been designated as.

A. Thirane B. Aziridine
C. Oxirane D. Thirane and oxirane

3181. furan is less aromatic then pyrrole that can be proved by which of the following reaction .

A. Resinification B. Metalation
C. Acylation . D. Diels reaction -alder

3182. How many different ether isomer are possible for C3H6O .

A. 4 B. 10
C. 6 D. 8

3183. Name the heterocyclic compound that have been as light and heat stabilizer for polyvinyl chloride.

A. Aryloxypropane sulphide
B. Dithioglycidyl thiophosphate
C. Acrylonitrile
D Ethylene sulphide

3184. Dithioglyidyl thiophosphate are used as.

A. Tuberculosis

B. Strong insecticidal effect

C. Fire extinguishers

D. Polymers

3185. Which of the following reagent undergo mercuration of furan by heating with mercuric chloride.

A. Aqueous sodium hydroxide

B. concentrated sodium acetate

C. Aqueous sodium acetate

D. None of this

3186. Which of the following compound gives more than one oxirane upon epoxidation with Ag2O\heat

A. CH3-C(CH3)=CH2

B. CH(CH3)=CH(CH)3 cis type

C. CH(CH3)=CH(CH3) trans type

D. C(CH3)(C2H5)=C(CH3)(C2H5)

3187. Write the IUPAC name of the following heterocyclic compound.

A. 4-phenyl-1H-123-triazole

B. 4 –benzyl-123-triazole

C. 4-benyl-123-nitroentane

D. None of this

3188. Identify the structure of ferulic acid

A. 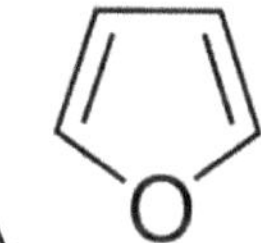

B. (C5H8O4)n

C. O OH O

D. O O H

3189. Name the heterocyclic compound that inhibit "Tuberculosis"

A. Aziridine

B. Dithioglycidol

C. Epoxides

D. Ethylene

3190. What is the dipole movement of Azirines

A. 3.15 D and 3.18 D

B. 2.10 D and 2.43 D

C. 2.51 D and 2.56 D

D. 2.80 D and 2.89 D

3191. Which of the fllowing five membered ring is most resonance .

A. Pyrrole >thiophene>furan.

B. Thiophene >pyrrole >furan

C. Pyrrole >furan >thoiphene

D. Furan >pyrrole>thiophene

3192. Which of the following statement is correct.

A. Thiophene is less aromatic than furan

B. Pyrrole is more reactive than furan

C. Thiophene undergo dies alder reaction.

D. Thiophene does not undergo dieldo alder

3193. What "prefix" is used for "tin" in the nomenclature of heterocyclic compound.

A. Stiba

B. Stanna

C. Bora

D. Plumba

3194. What is the reactivity order in the following five membered heterocyclic compound.

A. Pyrrole

B. Thiophene

C. Furan

D. Pyridine

3195. What is the name of rection .

A. Gattermann reaction

B. Reimer tiemann reaction

C. Blanc's chloromethylation

D. Friedal craft reaction

3196. Electrophiic substitution in furan usually occure at.

A. C (2) atom

B. C (3) atom

C. 0 atom

D. Both A and C

3197. Which is the correct order of reactivity toword electrophiles

A. Furan > pyrrole >thiophene

B. Thiophene >pyrrole >furan

C. Furan >thiophene >pyrrole

D. Pyrrole > furan > thiophene

3198. C5H10O4 acid? complete the following reaction.

-3H2O

A.

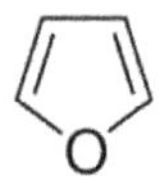

B. (C5H8O4)n

C.

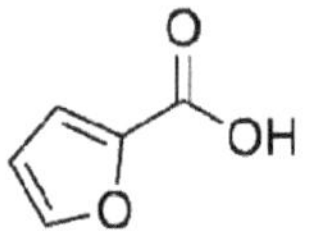

D.

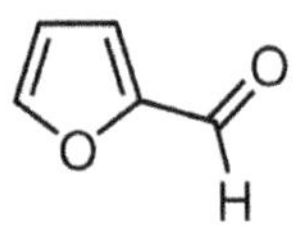

3199. Which is the correct structure of "rose oil"

A.

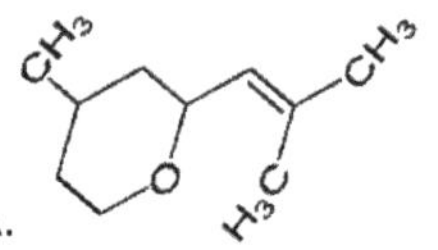

B.

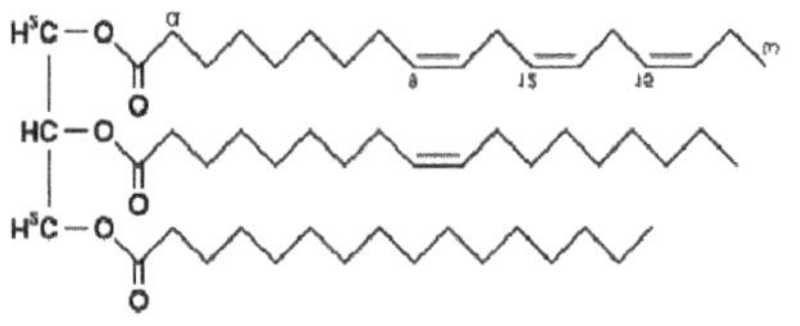

C.

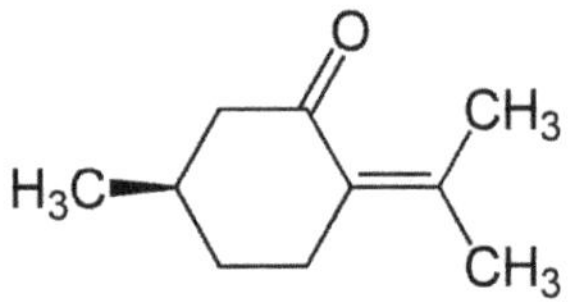

D.

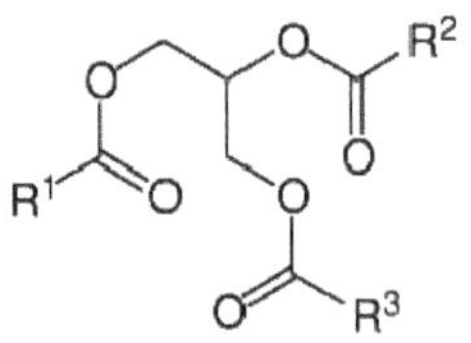

3200. The derivative of furan are prepared from .

A. Acetylation reation

B. Ethylacetoacetate

C. By ά-acylaminocarbonayl compound

D. By thiourea

3201. Pyrrole is less basic than pyridine the orbital having the long pair of electron on nitrogen in pyrrole is.

A. S B. P

C. Sp2 D. Sp3

3202. Which heterocyclic compound forms the trimer when they contact with dilute acid for a brief period.

A. Indole B. Furan

C. Pyrrole D. Pyrrodine

3203. Reaction of spongy nickel or palladium oxide on phenol gives which of the following product

A. 2-acetyl furan B. 2-arylfuran

C. Tetrahydrofuran D. All the above

3204. Two elimination product can be formed during elimination reaction one of the product in major amount can be identified according to.

A. Hoffmann's rule

B. Saytzeff's rule

C. Markonokowff's rules

D. Anti –markonikowff's rule

3205. Anisole can be prepared by the action of methyl iodide on sodium phente the reaction is called

A. Wiliamson's reaction

B. Wurtz's reaction

C. FiHig's reaction

D. Eturd's reaction

3206. Indole undergo mannich reaction with formaldehyde and dimethyl amino , it give which type of product

A. 3-formyl indole B. Gramine

C. 3-acetyl indole D. None of this

3207. Furan is available from furfural by the oxidic hydrolysis of polysaccharide .At what temperature the furfural give furan.

A. At 2000C by the steam distillation with metal oxide.

B. At 4000C by the steam distillation with metal oxide.

C. At 500C by the evaporator or steam distillation with metal oxide .

D. At 1000C by the evaporator method with metal oxide.

3208. The most appropriate reagent that can bring about the following transformation.

A. Sncl4 or Pd-Pdo

B. Air in presence of (o)

C. Aqueous KOH

D. Raney Ni or Pd – Pdo

3209. Which of the following five membred heterocyclic compound are highly volatile and unstable when they come in contact with the air.

A. Thiophene B. Isoxazole
C. Furan D. Imidazole

3210. Name one heterocyclic compound which act as antidepressant ,Antibiotic and pesticides

A. Pyridine B. Thiazole
C. Acridine D. Isoxazole

3211. Pyrrole is obtained by passing a mixture of acetylene through red hot tube by the use of which of the following reagent

A. Freon B. Carbon dioxide
C. Ammonia D. Hydrogen

3212. Which element is present as hetero atom in pteridine

A. Oxygen
B. Sulphar
C. Nitrogen
D. Sulphar and nitrogen

3213. What is the boiling point of the pyrrole .

A. 1390C B. 1310C
C. 1800C D. 1200C

3214. Which of the following plant is the natural source of pyrrole.

A. Bile pigment
B. Ficus religiose
C. Ocimum tenuiflorum
D. Azadirachta indica

3215. Mycobacterium tubercurosis and Escherichia coil produce nicotinic acid by condensation of which of the following compounds

A. Acetylene
B. Glyceraldehyde -3 phosphate
C. Pyrrole
D. Amino acid

3216. What is the name of the following reaction

A. Chichibabin synthesis
B. Houben – hoesh synthesis
C. Dealkylation of alkylpyrrole
D. Bonneman cyclization

3217. At which position of pyrrole electrophilic substitution reaction is most preferred .

A. Third B. First
C. Second and first D. Second

3218. Pyrrole react with chloroform in presence of aqueous potassium hydroxide to give 2-formyl pyrrole and 3-chloropyridine .Name the reaction.

A. Friedal craft acylation
B. Nitration
C. Reamer –Tiemann reaction
D. Gattermann synthesis

3219. Name the notable drug which containing pyrazole ring.

A. Celecoxib and stanozole
B. Trimethoprin
C. Sulfamethoxypyridazine
D. Pipofezine

3220. was isolated from seed of watermelons Name the natural pyrazole which.

A. Sodium persulfate
B. Sodium alanine
C. 1-pyrazolyl alanine
D. Diazomethane

3221. Name the natural indole was which occurs in plant growth hormone .

A. Tryptophan
B. Indole -3-acetic acid
C. Bracine
D. Indole -1- acetic acid

3222. Name the reaction which is based on condensation reaction between ά -halo with arylamine in presence of acid .

A. Madeling indole synthesis
B. Reissert synthesis
C. Trans indigo
D. Bischler indole synthesis

3223. How many steps involved in the mechanism of bischler indole synthesis .

A. 8-steps B. 4-steps
C. 2- steps D. 6-steps

3224. At which temperature "lipp synthesis" is carrid out.

A. 1200C – 1700C B. 1900C – 2000C
C. 1600C – 2000C D. 1600C – 1700C

3225. Name the synthesis which on reacting with O – amino – chlorostyrene and sodium ehoride at 1600C- 1700C give indole

A. By lipp synthesis
B. Fischer indole synthesis
C. Bischler indole synthesis
D. By reissert synthesis

3226. Which of the following is correct structure of isatin .

A.

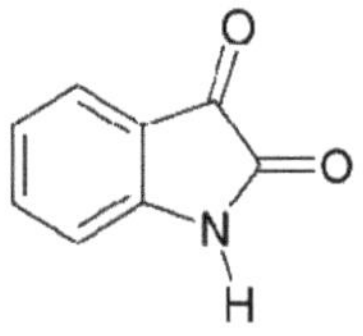

B.

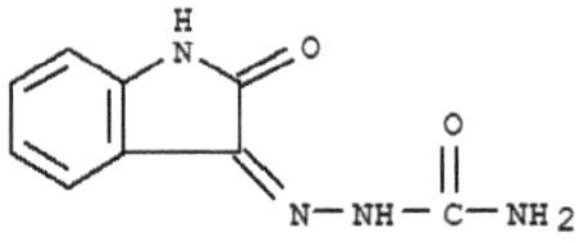

C.

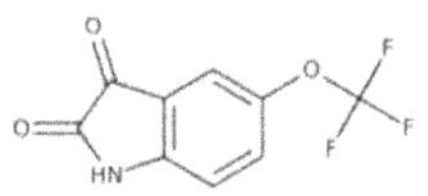

D.

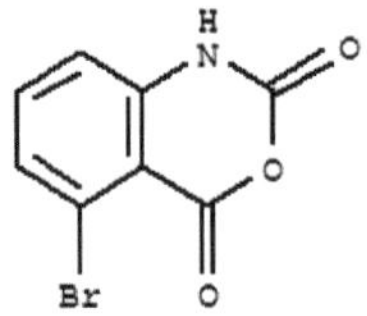

3227. Which is the best method of preparation of indole

A. Fischer indole synthesis
B. Reissert synthesis
C. Madeling indole synthesis
D. Lipp synthesis

3228. Which of the following is correct

A. Indole is a parent substance of dye indigotin
B. Indole is strong basic in nature
C. Indole is crystalline solid withmelting 1000 C
D. Indole has six resonance hybrid structure

3229. Dimerisation of indole is carried out using

A. Zinc sulphate B. Formaldehyde
C. Hydrochloric acid D. Chloro quinoline

3230. O-acylaminotoluene react with strong potassium t-butoxide to give

A. Two ketoester B. Oxindole
C. Phenyl indole D. Indole

3231. Indole is biosynthesized by which pathway.

A. Amino acid pathway
B. Shikimate pathway
C. Acetate pathway
D. None of this

3232. Name the scientist who give the original structure of indole in 1869.

A. Adoll von Baeyer
B. Leo baekelend
C. Stephan moulton babcock.
D. Joseph achille lebel

3233. Which of the following IUPAC name of the gramine .

A. 3- dimethylamino methyl indole.
B Dimethylamino -2-methyl indole
C. 3- methylamino dimethyl indole.
D. 3-di methylamino -4- dimethyl indole

3234. Which of the following is the structure of gra mine.

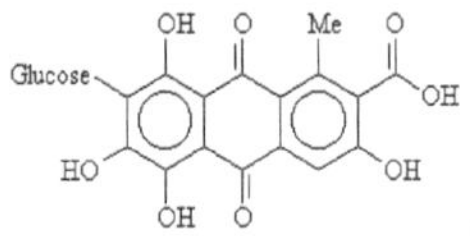

A.

B.

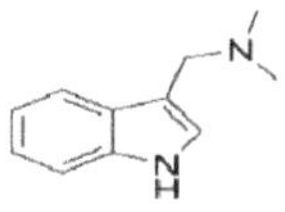

C. 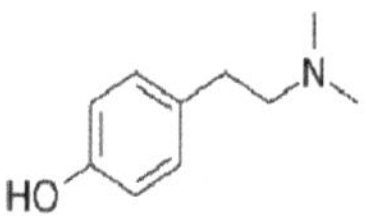 HO

D.

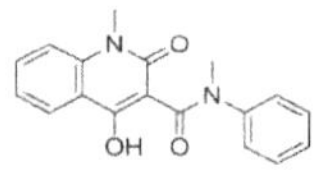

3235. Which of the following reaction is usefull for the synthesis of 3-substitution indole.

A. Diazocoupling
B. Reimmer –tieman reaction
C. Gatterman reaction
D. Mannich reaction

3236. Name the heterocyclic compound which are found in "Riboside"

A. Thiazole B. Pyrazole
C. Imidazole D. Pteridine

3237. Imidazole is the natural product of

A. Pyrimidine B. ά-amino acid
C. Vitamin B12 D. Growth hormone

3238. Name of the compound which can act both as a base and as an acid .

A. Imidazole B. Oxazole
C. Pyrazole D. Indole

3239. Polybenzimidazole (PBI) contain imidazole fused to a benzene ring act as .

A. Insecticidal and herbicidal
B. Bactericidal
C. Fire retardant
D. All of the above

3240. Name of the compound which do not undergo "friedal –craft's acylation

A. Indole B. Pyrrole
C. Pyridine D. Imidazole

3241. Oxamide is formed by imidazole by which of the following reagent.

A. Oxalic acid B. Hydrogen peroxide
C. Formic acid D. All of the above

3242. 1,3 –diazacyclopenta -2,4 – diene is the IUPAC name of which compound .

A. Imidazole B. Thiophene
C. Furan D. Pyrazole

3243. Name the synthesis method for oxazole which involve dehydration of ά- acylamino ketone.

A. Knorr pyrrole synthesis
B. Hantzsch synthesis
C. Robinson –gabriel synthesis
D. Bischler synthesis

3244. Which is the smallest angle in pyridine ring.

A. 116.70 B. 124.00
C. 118.10 D. 115.00

3245. Synthesis of acrolien is done by which method.

A. Knoevenagel condensation
B. Claisen condensation
C. Aldol condensation
D. Dieckmann condensation.

3246. Which of the following catalyst can be used in the synthesis of pyridine by bonneman cyclization .

A. Niekel based catalyst
B. Cobalt catalyst
C. Silver or platinum based catalyst
D. Vanadium oxide

3247. What is the name reaction of following reaction.

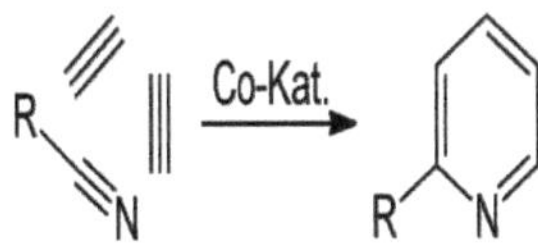

A. Chichibabin synthesis
B. Dealkylation
C. Hantzsch pyridine
D. Bonnemann of alkylation

3248. Pyridine react with hot solution of HNO3 in presence of sulphuric acid which product is formed.

A. 3-nitropyridine
B. 2,4,6 –trinitropyridine
C. 2,3-dinitropyridine
D. None of this

3249. Name the comound which is obtained from light oil by treating with dilute sulphuric acid.

A. Pyrimidine B. Oxazole
C. Thiophene D. Pyridine

3250. Which of the following is the derivative of pyridine.

A. Isatin B. 2,4-picoline
C. Phenyl hydrazone D. Furoic acid

3251. Dreaw the structure of ά-picoline.

A.

B.

C. 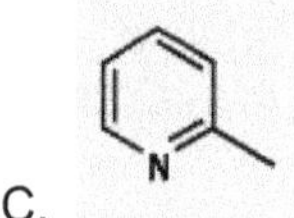

D. 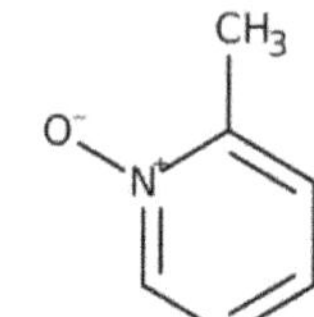

3252. Chichibabin reaction is the nucleophilic substitution reaction of which hetercyclic compound.

A. Quinoline B. Indole
C. Pyridine D. Thiazole

3253. Name the reaction which on react with pyridine with sodamide in presence of toluene, it gives 2-aminopyridine

A. Reaction with NaOH and KOH
B. Chichibabin
C. Both A andB
D. Metalation

3254. Pyridine undergoes nucleophilic substitution with excess of NaNH2 at 1000C to give which of the following.

A. 2,6-diaminopyridine
B. 3,5-diaminopyridine
C. 3-aminopyridine
D. 2,5-diaminopyridine

3255. Pyridine is heating with which of the following reagent to form 2-pyridone.

A. NaOH B. NaCl
C. Both A and d D. KOH

3256. What is the name of the following reaction.

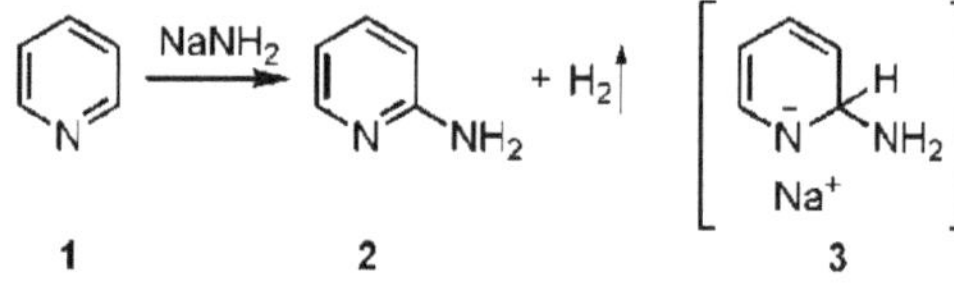

A. Chichibabin reaction
B. Hantzsch pyridine synthesis
C. Dealkylation reation
D. Bonnemann reaction

3257. Dihydropyridine is obtained by the condensation of two molecule of beta – carbonyl compound with one molecule of aldehyde and one molecule of ammonia. give the name of the reaction.

A. From acetylene
B. From 1,5 –diketone
C. From pentamethylene diamine hydrochloride.
D. Hantzsch synthesis

3258. Name of the heterocyclic compound which is a colorless hygroscopic liquid having odour and develop yellowish color on exposureto air.

A. Isoquinoline B. Pyridine
C. Acridine D. Quinoline

3259. Which of the following is correct .

A. Quinoline is soluble in organic solvent like acetone and chloroform
B. Quinoline is highly aromatic heterocyclic compound having strong odour
C. It is the most stable and occur in nature as quinoline.
D. All of the above

f. HNO_3
c. H_2SO_4, 0 °C
80%
NO_2 ... N + 9:1 ... NO_2

3260. Name the below reaction.

A. Pfitizinger synthesis
B. Friedlander synthesis
C. Skraup synthesis
D. Knorr quinoline synthesis

3261. How many mechanism of steps involved in the synthesis of skraup synthesis

A. 4 B. 2
C. 3 D. 8

3262. In the "skraup synthesis"glycerol gives acrolein by the addition of which reagent .

A. Conc.HCL B. Δ,NH3
C. Conc.H2SO4 D. KOH

3263. Name the reagent which upon addition it produce the reaction less violent in the "skraup synthesis".

A. Conc.H2SO4 B. Ferrous sulphate
C. Arsenic acid D. Nitrobenzene

3264. In the skraup synthesis, Michael addition of aniline to acroline .what product it gives

A. Quinoline B. Propionaldehyde
C. Glycerol D. None of this

3265. Friedlandar reaction is the synthesis method of which heterocyclic compound .

A. Acridine B. Pyridine
C. Indole D. Quinoline

3266. What is the name of the following reaction.

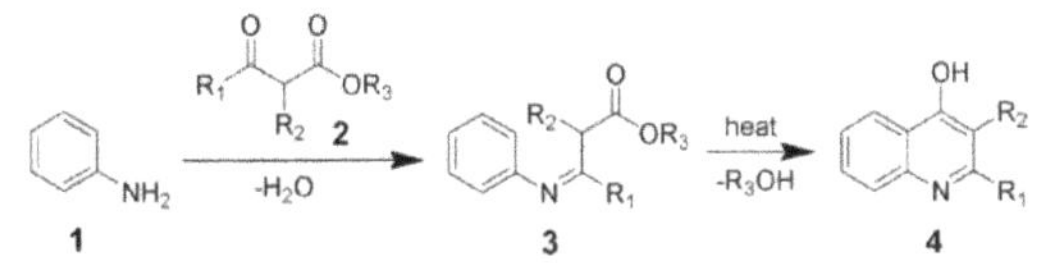

A. Conrad – limpach synthesis
B. Doebner – miller synthesis
C. Knorr quinoline synthesis
D. Pfitziner synthesis

3267. Which is the correct structure of "cinnamon aldoxine"

A. 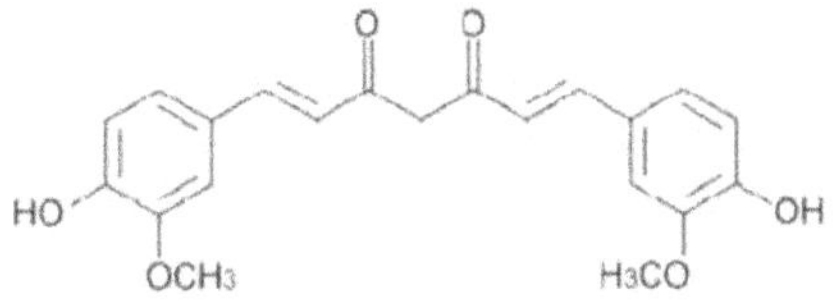
B. 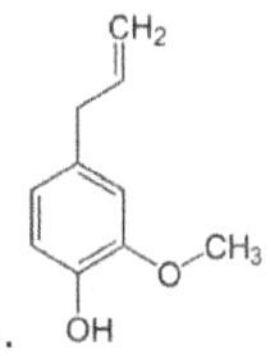
C. 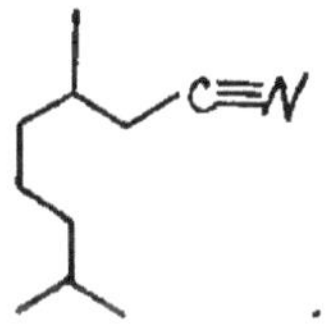
D.

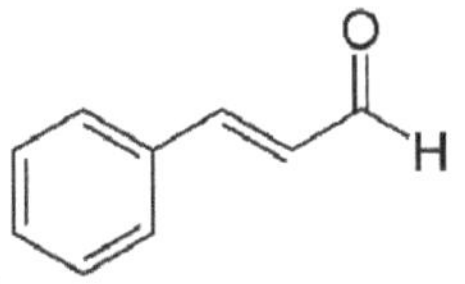

3268. Name the synthesis of isoquinoline which undergoes beckmann's rearregement.

A. From cinnamaldehyde
B. Bischler napieralski
C. Piotet –spengler reaction
D. Pomeranz –fritsch reaction

3269. Name the below reaction

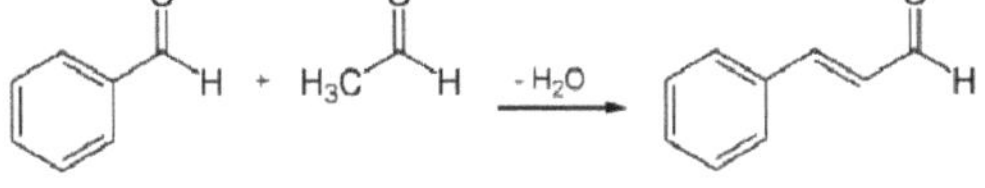

A. Bischler naieralski
B. Piotet –spengler reaction
C. From cinnamaldehyde
D. Pomeranz –fritsch reaction.

3270. Which of the following compound derived naturally from the aromatic amino acid tyrosine .

A. Acridine B. Quinoline
C. Pyridine D. Isoquinoline

3271. Which of the following heterocyclic compound are also known as "white oil"

A. Quinoline B. Oxazole
C. Pyrazole D. Isoquinoline

3272. Name the scientist who was first extracte the "quinoline " from coal tar .

A. Charless gerharat
B. Friedlieb Ferdinand
C. August Hoffmann
D. leo Baekeland

3273. Name the reagent which on addition with quinine ,strychnine and cinchonine form a quinoline compound .

A. Potassium hypochloride
B. Potassium bromide
C. Potassium hydroxide
D. All of the above

3274. Name the scientist who obtained a compound called as "Quinoline" by dry distilling quinine ,strychinine or cichonine with potassium hydroxide

A. Charless Gerhardt
B. August Hoffmann
C. Leo Baekeland
D. None of this

3275. Hoogewerf and van dorp isolated isoquinoline comound from coal tar by which method.

A. Evaporation
B. Fractional distillation
C. Condensation
D. Fractional crystallization

3276. Name the scientist who exploiting the fact that isoquinoline is more basic than quinoline.

A. Friedliet Ferdinand
B. Weissgerber
C. Hoogewerf and van dorp
D. Charles Gerhardt

3277. Name the scientist who was first isolated and identified the compound known as "benzene"

A. Michael faraday
B. Hoogewerf and van dorp
C. Lew Baekeland
D. Weissgerber

3278. The word benzene is derived by which naturally accuring compound .

A. Gum acacia B. Gum Benjamin
C. Gum rosin D. All of the above

3279. Which of the following is the best method of identification test for benzene ,toluene and xylene

A. Coloumn chromatography
B. Reaction with KMno4
C. Gas chromatography
D. All of the above

3280. Name the below reaction .

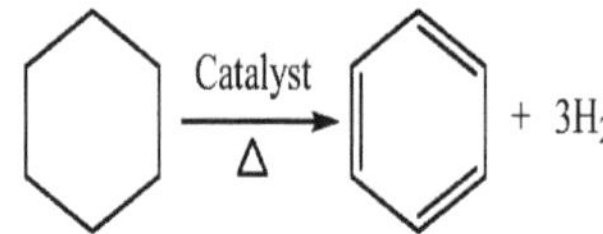

A. Dehydrogenation of cyclohexane
B. Hydrogenation of cyclohexane
C. From cyclohexane
D. None of this

3281. Name the catalyst which are used in the dehydration of cyclohexane to form a benzene.

A. Silicon dioxide (SiO2)
B. Aluminium oxide (Al3O3
C. Organo –nikle
D. Platinum or palladium

3282. According to the kekule structure for benzene which is the C-C bond length.

A. 1.08Å B. 1.48 Å
C. 1.40Å D. 1.09Å

3283. Which of the following is the IUPAC name of cumene.

A. Isopentylbenzene
B. Isobutylbenzene
C. Isopropylbenzene
D. Cyclopropylbenzene

3284. What is the IUPAC name of styrene.

A. Mesitylene B. Isodurene
C. Hexylbenzene D. Vinylbenzene

3285. Which of the following compound are the clan of "non-benzoid aromatic compound"

A. Ferrocene B. Anthraene
C. Naphthacene D. Phenol

3286. Write the example of Anti - Aromatic compound.

A. Annulenne
B. Anthracene
C. Cyclopentadienone
D. Azulene

3287. Arrange the following aromatic compound in the increasing order of their "boiing point"

A. M-xylene>Durene>Phennanthrene>toluene
B. Phennanthrene>Durene>M-xylene>toluene
C. Toluene>M-xylene>Durene>Phennanthrene
D. Durene>toluene>M-xylene>Phennanthrene

3288. Hydrocarbon is formed by strongly heating the sodium salt of an aromatic carboxylic acid by which of the following rection .

A. KOH B. HCL
C. Soda lime D. Aq.KOH

3289. ἀ-tetralone is obtained by cyclization reaction with hydrofluoric acid by which of the following reaction.

A. Gama –phenylpetanoic acid
B. Phenylpropanole
C. Gama-phenylbutanoic acid
D. None of this

3290. Write the name of the following aromatic compound.

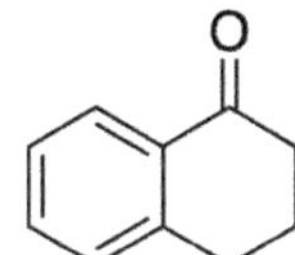

A. α̇-Benzolone B. α̇-Pentaetone
C. α̇-Ketone D. α̇-tetralone

3291. Name the below reaction

Zn(Hg), HCl

A. Clemmensen reduction reaction
B. Wurtz –fitting reaction
C. Friedalcrafft alkylation
D. Decarboxylation reaction

3292. Among the following test in which the benzene are not responsible .

A. Bromine test B. Ignition test
C. Baeyer's test D. Permanganate test

3293. Benzene react with bromine in presence of ferric bromide (FeBr3) to form bromobenzene and hydrogen bromide (HBr) in the halogenation, FeBr3 act as a

A. Reducing agent B. Acid catalyst
C. Basic catalyst D. All of the above

3294. Name the catalyst which act as a mild deliquescent in the iodination of benzene .

A. Aluminium chloride
B. Potassium sulphate
C. Sodium nitrate
D. AgClO4

3295. Which chemical reaction of benzene does not required the presence of any catalyst

A. Sulfonation B. Halogenation
C. Nitration D. Iodination

3296. Oxidation of benzene in air in the presence of vanadium pentoxide ,it give which of the following product.

A. Phthalic anhydride
B. Potassium permanganate
C. Maleic anhydride
D. All f the above

3297. How many number of pie (^) electron is present in benzene.

A. 9 B. 7
C. 8 D. 6

3298. Which intermidate is formed in wolff's raction .

A. Carbocation B. Ketone
C. Carbanion D. Carbine

3299. What type of oxidizing agent convert the CH3 group of toluene to an a aldehyde in "etard reaction".

A. Nitric acid
B. Hydrogen peroxide
C. Potassium nitrate
D. Chromyl choride

3300. The product of friedal craft's acylation reaction are.

A. Halobenzene
B. Arylketone
C. Alkybenzene
D. Alkylamine

3301. Name which reagent is used to partially reduced the benzene ring in the aromatic compound.

A. Ammonia alcohol mixture
B. Lithium and alcohol mixture
C. Liquid ammonia and propanol mixture
D. All of the above

3302. Name the aromatic compound which act as a agriculture insecticide and cause neurotoxine in human.

A. Heptachlor
B. Fennthion
C. Gammaxene
D. Omethoate

3303. Benzaldehyde can be prepared from benzene with carbon monoxide and hydrochloric acid in presence of.

A. Zinc chloride
B. Kmno4
C. Carbon tetrachloride
D. Aluminium chloride

3304. Predict the name of the below reaction.

$+ CO + HCl \xrightarrow[CuCl]{AlCl_3}$

A. Wolff-kishner reduction
B. Gatterman-koch reaction
C. Chlromethlation
D. Claisen condensation

3305. Benzene is obtained which method other than fractional distillation method.

A. From petroleum
B. From catalytic dehydrogenation
C. From oppenouer oxidation
D. From gem-dihalide

3306. Name the process which are used for the larger scale production of benzene and it's homologues

A. Anti platforming B. Non-platforming
C. Platforming D. All of the above

3307. Which type of source is used to obtained benzene or toluene by hydrodealkylation.

A. Mercury source B. Palladium source
C. Rhodium source D. Platinum source

3308. Tolu balsan is known as .

A. Benzene B. Cumene
C. Toluene D. Chloroform

3309. Toluene is prepared from which method .

A. From fat's and oil
B. Petroleum and coal
C. Chlorine and benzene
D. None of this

3310. Which of the following is the commercial method for the preparation of phenol.

A. Hock method
B. From diazonium salt
C. Dows process
D. By decarboxylation

3311. Among the dihydroxybenzene ,the B.P.decrase in the following order .

A. Resorcinol>phenol>quinol>catechol
B. Quinol >phenol>resorcinol>catechol
C. Phenol>quinol>resorcinol>catechol.
D. Catechol>phenol>quinol>resorcinol.

3312. Identify this structure

OH
HO OH

A. Pyrogallol B. Phloroglucinol
C. Hydroquinone D. Catechol

3313. Aryl halides react with hot sodium hydroxide and then on acidic hydrolysis it gives which of the following compound

A. Aniline B. Benzene
C. Toluene D. Phenol

3314. Name the method of preparation which react with hot sodium hydroxide solution and then on acidification the phenol is formed.

A. Dow process
B. Baeyer-villiger oxidation
C. Cumne hydroperoxide
D. Benzene sulfonic acids

3315. What is the reagent which will react with sodium phenoxide to give phenol in "dow process"

A. NaCl B. NaOH
C. KOH D. HCl

3316. Phenol of the following by product is formed in the cumene hydroperoxide preparation

A. Acetaldehyde B. Acetone
C. Ketone D. Ethanol

3317. Name the reagent which react with cumene to give phenol.

A. Chlorine B. Hydrogen
C. Oxygen D. Sulphar

3318. Sodium salicylate can be prepared from which of the following reaction .

A. Phenol,chloroform and AlCl3
B. Phenol,sodium nitrate
C. Phenol,carbon and tetrachloride
D. Phenol ,soda lime and NaOH.

3319. Phenol is stronger aidic than water and weaker acidic than_

A. Ethanol B. Carboxylic acid
C. Both A and B D. Methanol

3320. Which of the following is more acidic

A.

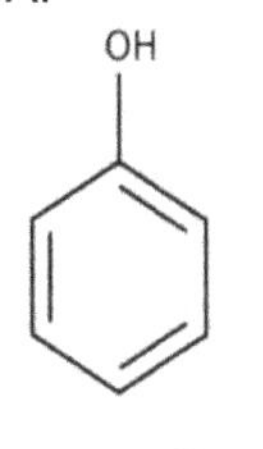

OH

O_2N

B.

OH

O_2N NO_2

NO_2

C.

CH_3

OH

D.

3321. Among the ortho,meta and para group of phenol ,which one is the more acidic in nature .

A. Meta group

B. Ortho group

C. Para group

D. Ortho and para group

3322. Name the reagent which does not react with phenol.

A. PBr B. Aq.NaOH

C. K2S2O8 D. CrO3

3323. Reaction of phenol with dimethyl sulphate in presence of aqueous sodium hydroxide give which of the following product.

A. Phenoxic acetic acid

B. Anisole

C. Phenoxyethyl

D. Phenoxy sulphate

3324. Name the agent that can be used in the formation of ether by phenol in presence of dimethyl sulphate

A. Aq.NaCl B. Cocen.NaOH

C. Cocen.KOH D. Aq,NaOH

3325. When phenol react with sodium hydroxide it gives which of the following product.

A. Sodium phenoxide

B. Sodium salicylate

C. Sodium benzoate

D. None of this

3326. In which of the following reaction phenol do not give the product.

A. Elb oxidation

B. Kolbe reaction

C. Fischer esterification

D. Reimer – tiemann reaction

3327. Reaction of potassium persulfate on phenol gives which of the following product .

A. Mixture of catechol and quinol

B. Mixture of catechol and quinol

C. p-quinol

D. None of this

3328. Which of the following is the product of "Elb oxidation"

A. Sodium salicylate

B. 2,4-dihydrobenzaldehyde

C. Hydroxybenzaldehyde

D. Catechol

3329. Name the reagent that converts phenol into P-quinone

A. Aq.KHCO3 B. OH-

C. Na2Cr2O7 D. H2O

3330. p-quinone is the product of which of the following reaction .

A. Elb oxidation

B. Condensation with phthalic anhydride

C. Fischer reaction

D. Kolbe reaction

3331. What will be the product if sodium phenoxide is heated with CO2 under pressure of 1250C

A. p-nitrosophenol

B. Sodium salicylate

C. Vaniline

D. Protocatechol

3332. Name the reaction that give sodium salicylate and salicylic acid as a product when sodium phenoxide or phenol heating with CO2under pressure .

A. Kolbe reaction

B. Reduction of the aromatic ring

C. Nitrosation

D. None of this

3333. Resorcinol on heating with CO2in pressure of aqueous KHCO3 what product is formed.

A. 2,4 –dihydroxybenzoic acid

B. p-hydroxybenzaldehyde

C. o-hydroxybenzaldehyde

D. All of the above

3334. Which of the following is the major product of reamer – tiemann reaction of phenol

A. p-quinone

B. 2,4 –dihydroxybenzoic acid

C. o-hydroxybenzaldehyde

D. Protocatechol

3335. Identify the structure of protocatechol .

A.

B.

C.

D.

3336. by heating phenol with conc.H2SO4 which of the Phenolphthalein is obtained following reagent .

A. Phthalic acid B. Benzyl alcohol

C. Benzoic acid D. Chromate ion

3337. Name the product that are obtained through condensation with phthalic anhydride

A. 2-methyl -4-nitrosophenol

B. Salicylic acid

C. Phenolphthaine

D. None of this

3338. Moleculelar formula of phenolphthalein is

A. C24H14O4 B. C20H14O4

C. C20H14O5 D. None of this

3339. At which PH the phenolphthalation does not show the presence of any color .

A. 7.4 B. Above 8.5

C. 7.9 D. Below 8.5

3340. Which of the following is the structure of phenolphthalein .

A.

B.

C.

D.

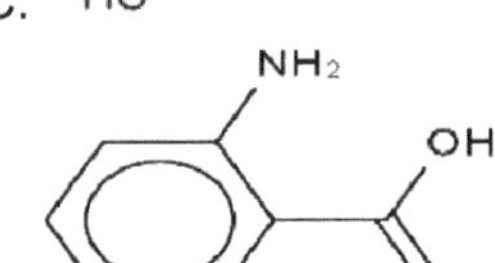

3341. Which of the following is the correct product formed from diazo coupling reaction of phenol .

A. Ortho para –dihydroxyazobenzene
B. Both A and B
C. Para- hydroxyazobenzene
D. None of this

3342. Phenol is reduced with H2 in presence of Ni, it give which of the following product?

A. 2,4-Dibromophenol
B. Cyclohexanol
C. 2-methyl-4-nitrosophenol
D. All of the above

3343. Which of the following statement is true about the nitration reaction

A. ortho-nitrophenol is less reactive than P-nitropheno
B. O-nitrophenol has a lower solubility in water but a high volatility
C. P-nitrophenol is formed greater as compair to ortho-nitrophenol
D. All of the above

3344. Phenol intract with concentrated nitric acid ,it give which of the following product

A. Picric acid
B. Salicylic acid
C. Ortho –nitrophenol
D. All the above

3345. Picric acid is formed by which reaction

A. Sulfonation
B. Nitration
C. Schotten –baumann reaction
D. Friedel –craft's reaction

3346. In which reaction of phenol ,the product formed is temperature dependent .

A. Kolbe reaction
B. Oxidation
C. Reamer-tiemann reaction
D. Sulfonation

3347. In the sulfonation of phenol which product is thermodiamically more stable

A. Ortho-isomer B. Meta-isomer
C. Para-isomer D. Both A and C

3348. At which temperature the ortho-sulfonate product are obtained in the higher energy level .

A. 1000C B. 250C
C. 2000C D. 2000C

3349. Phenol react with excess of water it give which of the following product

A. 2,4,6-Tribromophenol
B. m-bromophenol
C. 2,4-dibromophenol
D. All the above

3350. Name the solvent that may undergo monobromination of phenol at lower temperature

A. Carbon tetrachloride
B. Bromine water
C. Hydrogen bromide
D. None of this

3351. Carbon disulhate react with phenol at lower temperature, it give which of the following product

A. 2,4-Dibromo-6-methylphenol
B. M-bromophenol
C. 2,4,6-tribromophenol
D. p-bromophenol

3352. Name the below reaction

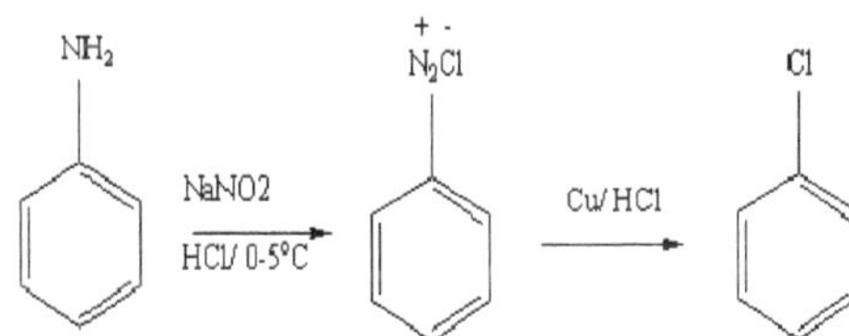

A. Schotten – baumann reaction
B. Gattermann reaction
C. Nitration
D. Formation of resins

3353. An intermediate product is formed when phenol reacts with hydrogen cyanide and HCl in presence of cyanide and HCl in presence of AlCl3,which on hydrolysis it gives which type of product

A. m-and p-hydroxybenzaldehyde
B. o-and m-hydroxybenzaldehyde
C. p-hydroxybenzaldehyde
D. All of the above

3354. Condensation reaction between phenol and formaldehyde which can be catalyzed either by acid and base then what type compound is formed.

A. Bakelite B. Cyclohexanol
C. Cyclohexane D. None of this

3355. Name the synthetic resin which is formed from condensation reaction of phenol with formaldehyde.

A. Polyurethane B. Polyester resins
C. Duroplate D. Bakelite

3356. Bakelite was developed by

A. E.D jammis B. Leo Baekeland
C. Milan randie D. Albert Ladenburg

3357.Polyoxybenzylmethylmethylenglycolanhydride is also known as.

A. Thiolyte B. Polyketone
C. Bakelite D. Benzoxazine

3358. Bakelite is formed when phenol react with which of the following reactant .

A. Hydrogen B. Sulphuric acid
C. Nitric acid D. Formaldehyde

3359. Bakelite is the type of .

A. Thermosetting plastic
B. Oleum
C. Thermoplastic polymer
D. All the above

3360. Phenol in a dilute aqueous solution used as a raw material for the manufacture of.

A. Cyclohexanol B. Benzoxazines
C. Bakelite D. Cyclohexane

3361. Name the constituent of phenol which is used for the treatment of inhibitor skin marked by itching..

A. Chlor –trimeton
B. Cuticura ointment
C. Benadryl
D. Atarax

3362. Name the below reaction

NaOH, H_2O , reflux 3 hrs. 82%

A. Williamson synthesis
B. Wurtz 's synthesis
C. Grignad synthesis
D. Kolbe's synthesis

3363. Williamson synthesis produce ether by reacting which of the following .

A. Alkooxide with alkyl halide
B. Alcohol with metal
C. Both A and B
D. Alkoxide with aldehyde

3364. In which base the Williamson synthesis reaction fail.

A. Sodium ethoxide + iodomethane
B. Sodium ethoxide + iodoethane
C. Sodium ethoxide +2-iodo-methylpropane
D. Sodium ethoxide + 2- iodoproprane

3365. Arrange the following primary alkyl halides according to their order of reactivity.

A. RBr>Rd>RI B. RBr > RI >RCl
C. RCl>RBr>RI D. RI>RBr>RCl

3366. Mercuric acetate on treatment with alkane in alcoholic solution the A product is formed then this A product is converted into ether by using reducing agent .name the B of the following reaction.

A. A is mercuration adduct and B is +NaBH4
B. A is mercuration adduct and B is Na2SO4
C. A is oxymercuric and B is Na2SO4
D. All of the above

3367. Oxymmercuration adduct is converted into ether by which of the following reducing agent.

A. Na2SO4 B. NaCl
C. NaOH D. NaBH4

3368. The diapole moment of diethyl ether is .

A. 1.10 D B. 1.25D
C. 1.18D D. 1.20D

3369. What will be the product ,if secondary and tertiary alkyl ether is heated with concentrated H2SO4

A. Alkene B. Alkane
C. Alkyne D. All of the above

3370. Which of the following "Lewis acid " form stable complex with ether

A. AlF3+ B. Fe 2+ and Fe3+
C. Cu2 D. BF3

3371. Ether used as a solvent because they react only with which of the following reactant .

A. Oxidising agent B. Acid
C. Reducing agent D. Bases

3372. Which of the following is the name of the reaction .

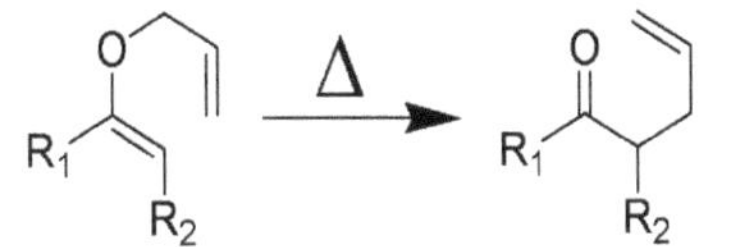

A. Pinacol rearrangement
B. Faworskit rearrangement
C. Claisen rearrangement
D. Wolf's rearrangement

3373. What will be the smell of diethyl ether.

A. Sweet smell B. Vinger
C. Roften egg. D. Fish like smell

3374. When ether is expose to air ,which of the following product is formed .

A. Alkynes
B. Alkene
C. Oxide
D. Peroxide of diethyl ether

3375. A chiral molecule is/ ion is .

A. Suerinposable on it's mirror image
B. Non - Suerinposable on it's mirror image
C. Both A and B
D. None of this

3376. The mirror image of a chiral molecule is.

A. Configurational isomer
B. Diasteroisomer
C. Enantiomers
D. All of the above

3377. Which of the following show the asymmetrical behaviour .

A. Glyceraldehydes B. Styrene
C. Benzanillides D. Triproylborane

3378. Atoms which of the following are superimposable abd show no optical activity.

A. Glyceraldehydes
B. 1,1-dichloroethane
C. Lactic acid
D. Alanine

3379. Which of the following morecule are chiral.

A. H–C(=O)–C(H)(OH)–CH_2OH
B. Cl(H)C=C(H)Cl
C. CH_3–CH(OH)–CH(CH_3)–CH_3
D. Br–CH_2–CH_2–Br

3380. Which of the following statement about enantiomer are not true.

A. All (+) enantiomer are levorotatory
B. Enantiomer rotate plane polarized light in opposite direction
C. Enantiomers rotate plane polarized right in opposite direction
D. All R enantiomer are dextrorotatory .

3381. Name the molecule that exist as a pair of enantiomer .

A. 2-cyclohex-1-ol
B. 2-bromopropane
C. Cis -1,2-dichlorocyclobutane
D. 1-bromo -3-methylbutane

3382. Which of the following is capable of existing as a pair of enatiomers .

A. 2-methylhexane
B. 3-methylpentane
C. 3-methylhexane
D. 2- methylpentane

3383. Name the device that block all the components except those wave that are polarized in one particular direction .

A. PCE-151 B. Tachometer
C. Polarizer D. All of the above

3384. A polarimeter is a device used to measure are.

A. Angle of rotation
B. Polarization direction
C. Optical activity
D. All of the above

3385. Plane polarized light are analyzed by optical device of which is made up.

A. Graphite B. Calcite
C. Both A and B D. Cermet

3386. Which of the following wavelength is mostly used in the polarimeter.
A. Sodium D line
B. Potassium lamp
C. Tungsten carbide
D. Tungsten lamp

3387. A Calcite material is used for the construction of which device .
A. Polarized B. Spectrometry
C. Both A and B D. None of this

3388. The wave forming ordinary image are.
A. Partially polarized B. Unpolarized
C. Plane polarized D. Any of above

3389. Name the device that convert unpolarized light into polarized.
A. Calcite prism B. Toumaline crystal
C. Both A and B D. Nicol prism

3390. Nicol prism based on the action of .
A. Double refraction B. Refraction
C. Reflection D. Scattring

3391. A optically active material are
A. Change the direction of refracted light
B. Change the direction of propogation of light
C. Change the direction of the plane of polarization
D. All of the above

3392. The property to rotate the plane of polarized light is known as .
A. Dichroism
B. Double refreaction
C. Opticaly activity
D. Polarization

3393. Plane of vibration is defined only for are.
A. Unpolarized B. Plane polarized
C. Both A and B D. None of this

3394. Name the phoomena tha suggest light may be a transverse wave .
A. Diffraction
B. Reflection
C. Photo electric effect
D. Polarization

3395. Whih of the following cannot be polarized .
A. Ultrasonic wave B. Radio wave
C. Infrared ray D. Ultraviolet rays

3396. Identify which type of polarisation depend on temperature.
A. Interfacial B. Ionic
C. Electronic D. Orientational

3397. The difference in pharmacologic activity between the two enantiomer of a drug is represented by
A. Eudysmic ratio B. Eudismic ratio
C. Both A and B D. None of this

3398. Name the chiral compound tha has no desired activity or may even be toxic ,
A. Distomer B. Enantiomer
C. Eutomer D. Diastereomer

3399. Which of the following chiral compound antagonize the effect of eutomer
A. Enantiomer B. Distomer
C. Diastereomer D. All of the above

3400. Amino acid an example of
A. Distomer B. Enantiomer
C. Eudysmic ratio D. Eutomer

3401. Which of the following amino acid can not be incorporated into protein in the human body
A. D –aspartate B. D –serine
C. Both A and B D. None of this

3402. A achiral species which can converted to a chiral in two steps is known as.
A. Optical activity B. Proprochiral
C. Plane polarized D. Unpolarization

3403. The amount of enantiomer in a mixture on be excepted by which method .
A. Eutomer excess B. Optical purity
C. Both C and D D. Enantimeric excess

3404. The formula of enantiomeric excess is
A. [(d+L)(d- L)}X100
B. [(d)/(d-L)] X 100
C. [(d-L)/(d+L)] X100
D. [(d+L)/(d)]X 100

3405. Optical purity is defined as the .

A. Sum of rotation of mixture and rotation of pure enantiomer

B. Product of rotation of mixture and rotation of pure enantiomer

C. Ratio of rotation of pure enantiomer to rotation of mixture

D. Ratio of rotation of mixture to rotation of pure enantoimer

3406. Which of the following can exist as a diastereomers

A. 2-Butane B. Lactic acid

C. Ethane D. 1-butane

3407. What is meant by 94% enantiomeric excess

A. The product contain an enantiomer which is 94% pure

B The product contain 97% of one enantiomer and 3% of the other enatiomer

C. The product contain 94% of enantiomer and 6% of other product

D. The product contain 94%of enantiomer and 6% of other product

3408. If a chemical rection produce the two enantiomer of a chiral product in unequal amount than it is said to be.

A. Enantiomeric excess

B. Enantioselective

C. Prochiral

D. All of the above

3409. If the molecule is chiral the faces are said to be.

A. Diastereotopic B. Enantiotopic

C. Both A and B D. None of this

3410. If the molecule is achiral the faces are said to be.

A. Diastereotopic B. Enantiotopic

C. Iodolactonisation D. Prochiral

3411. Asymmetric synthesis also known as

A. Diastereoselective synthesis

B. Enantiospecificity synthesis

C. Enantioselective synthesis

D. None of this

3412. Diasteroselectivity ca be explained by

A. Fisher projection

B. Felkin –ahn model

C. Optical purity

D. Newman projection

3413. Name the compound that contain stereogenic carbon and can exist in both R and S form.

A. Epinephrine B. Pseudoepinephrine

C. Thalidomide D. All of the above

3414. Which of the following chiral compound cause external and internal abnormalities in fetus if it is given to pregnant woman.

A. Atoruastatin B. Thalidomide

C. Both A and B D. None of this

3415. The asymmetrical catalytic oxidation propranolol is done by which reagent.

A. Platinum propoxide

B. Titanium propoxide

C. Titanium propoxide

D. None of this

3416. Shi epoxidation of alkenes is done by which catalyst .

A. Glucose derived chiral catalyst

B. Sucrose derived chira catalyst

C. Fructose derived chiral catalyst

D. A of the above

3417. T – butyl hydroperoxide and titanium isopropoxide oxidizing agent is used for the synthesis of which chiral comound .

A. Propranolol B. Naproxen

C. Penicillamin D. None of this

3418. The asymmetrical synthesis of captopril is done by which reagent

A. NaOH and NH3 B. NaCl and NH3

C. NaCl and NH4 D. NaOH and NH4

3419. Captopril is formed by 3-acetylthio-2-methylpropanoyl chloride followed by aminolysis under besic condition using which reagent .

A. D –proine
B. L –proline
C. L –propaline
D. All of the above

3420. Captopril belongs to which category of drug

A. Angiotensin 2 blocker
B. Renin inhibitor
C. Angiotensin converting enzyme inhibitor
D. Alpha plus beta blocker

3421. W]]]]hich of the following is the most important role of protecting group in the functional group .

A. Split the functional group into different groups of other molecule
B. Block the reactivity of a functional group by converting it into a different group
C. Block the action of single functional group
D. All of the above

3422. A protecting groups in the organic synthesis are .

A. Higher energy level and most stable
B. Lower energy level with highly reactive
C. Cheap ,stable and easy to remove in high yield
D. None of this

3423. Name the protecting group for alcohol .

A. Acetyl r or ketals
B. Ethers
C. Ester
D. All of the above

3424. Which of following the is the commonly used ketal

A. Hexyl derivative
B. Methylbutane pyranyl
C. Tetrahydropyranyl
D. Methoxy propyl

3425. Methoxymethyl is a used as a protecting group for which of the following functional group .

A. For ketone
B. For alcohol
C. For ether
D. For carboxylic acid

3426. Acetals and ketal are simply removed by treatment of which agent

A. Alkaline NaOH
B. Aqueous acid .
C. Both A and B
D. None of this

3427. Alcohol may be simply converted to ethers by which of the following group of chemical compound

A. Hydrogen
B. Carbon
C. Hydrogen halide
D. Alkyl halide

3428. In which condition the ether are more stable

A. Strong base
B. Mildly acidic
C. Mildly acidic
D. Mildly and strong base

3429. Ether do not react with which of the following agent .

A. Oxidizing agent
B. Reducing agent
C. Both A and B
D. None of this

3430. Name the agent which converted to alcohols under neutral condition by catalytic hydrogenolysis

A. Benzyl hexnal
B. Benzyl ether
C. Butyl ether
D. Benzyl propyl ether

3431. Name the protecting group for alcohol that may hydrolyzed with dilute acid .

A. Butyl ether
B. Benzyl ether
C. Both A and B
D. t-butyl ether

3432. Name the protecting group for primary alcoholic group

A. Tri-phenylmethyl
B. Propyl methane
C. Tetrahexyl methyl
D. Butanol

3433. Which of the following is most stable protecting of primary alcoholic groups.

A. t-butylether
B. Tri-phenylmethyl
C. Propylmethyl ether
D. Benzyl ether

3434. Which of the following reagent is the inert for ether .

A. Sulfa metallic reagent
B. Sulfahydroxy metallic reagent
C. Organo –metllic reagent
D. All of the above

3435. Trichloroacetate and pivoloate is used as a protecting group for which of the following compound .

A. Esters for alcohol
B. Ketones for alcohol
C. Ketones for alcohol
D. None of this

3436. Name the protecting group for 1,2 and 1,3 diols

A. Aceroxiances
B. Dioxlanes and dioxanes
C. Both A and B
D. Acetoxane

3437. 1,2 acetanoid formation is usually favoured over 1,3 –acetonides which is done by

A. Alcoholic ether
B. Cyclic acids
C. Mild aqueous acid
D. Acetylnitrils

3438. Which of the following is the example of cyclic acetals and ketals

A. Isopropylidene
B. Benzylidene acetals
C. Cycloalkylidene acetals
D. All of the above

3439. Name the cycloalkylidene acetals which is easier to cleave than acetonides

A. Cyclomethylidences
B. Cycopentylidenes
C. Both A and B
D. Cyclohexylidenes

3440. Name the cycloalkylidene acetals which is slightly harder to cleave than acetonides

A. Cyclohexylidenes
B. Cycopentylidenes
C. Cyclomethylidences
D. None of this

3441. Benzylidene acetals are hydrogenolysed slower than which compound

A. Benzyl alcohol
B. Isopropylidene
C. Acetonides
D. Olefins and benzyl ether

3442. Name the method which have been used to protect alcoholic group

A. Aryl ether
B. Acetals and silyl ether
C. Both A and B
D. Acetaldehyde

3443. Which of the following reagent is capable of reducing ester to alcohol and that is highly reactive in nature

A. Sodiumbroohydride
B. Sodium tetrahydroborate
C. Lithium aluminium hydride
D. Sodium tetrahydridoborate

3444. Methoxymethlene acetals are the example of.

A. Cyclic carboxylic acid
B. Cyclic acetals and ketals
C. Cyclic carbonate
D. Cyclic ortho ester

3445. Which of the following proteting group is quite stable toward hydrolysis

A. Thioacetals and thioketals
B. Acyclic acetals
C. Acylic ketones
D. None of this

3446. Which of the following shows above good ideal property of protecting group

A. Protected compound must be highly hydrophobic and provide suitable purification

B. Should be created a new chiral centre at the molecule
C. Should be protected compound in good yield
D. All of this above

3447. Arrange the following protecting group for alcohol –ether in the increasing order of their reactivity towards .
A. Tri-butyldiphenyl silyl ether >tri-isopropylsilyl ether>tri-butyldimethylsilyl ether >tri-ethylsilyl ether
B. tri-butyldimethylsilyl ether> tri-ethylsilyl ether> tri-isopropylsilyl ether> Tri-butyldiphenyl silyl ether
C. Tri-butyldiphenyl silyl ether> tri-ethylsilyl ether> tri-isopropylsilyl> tri-butyldimethylsilyl ether
D. None of this

3448. Name the protecting group for amines .
A. Acetaphenyl amine
B. Dihydroxyl amine
C. Dimethylphenyl amine
D. p-methoxphenyl amine

3449. Which of the following is the example of amide protection .
A. Vinyloxyamide
B. Allylexyamide
C. Trifluoroacetamide
D. All of the above

3450. Amines carbonate protection is done by
A. Allyloxycarbonyl (Alloc)
B. Vinyloxycarbonyl (voc)
C. Both A and B
D. Trichlorocarbonyl

3451. Name the carbonyl protecting group.
A. Acetal protection B. Dithiane protection
C. Both A and B D. None of this

3452. Which protecting group are selectively enough to protect primary as well as secondary and tertiary alcohol
A. Silyl ethers protection
B. Ester protection
C. Ether protection
D. None of this

3453. In which of the following example of silyl ether are acid and water labile.
A. Tri-iseprопylsilyl ether
B. Tertiary butyldiphenyl silyl ether
C. Acetenoid
D. Trimethylsilylether

3454. Carbonates cleavage are removed by.
A. Acid B. Base
C. Strong acid D. Neutral

3455. Hydroxyl carbonates are converted into 1,2-diols by the action of which reagent.
A. Triphosgene B. Imidazole DMF
C. DMF D. None of this

3456. Ethyl glycol and propyl glycol is used as a
A. Protection of alcohol
B. Protection of ester compound
C. Protection of diol
D. Protection of carbonyl

3457. The most common group for the protection of acid is.
A. Ketone B. Ester
C. Ether D. Aldehyde

3458. Which is the example of the carboxylic acid protection
A. Benzyl ether
B. Acyclic acetals
C. Trichlorocarbonyl
D. Tetrahydropyranyl ester

3459. What would happens if tetrahydropyranyl ester is used as a carboxylic acid protection
A. Formation of RCOOH
B. Formation of 2RCooH
C. Formation of RCOO-
D. None of this

3460. Trimethylsilyl ester is formed by the reaction of carboxylic acid with trimethylsilyl chloride by the action of which reagent
A. Ethanol B. Pyridine
C. Pyrimidine D. All of the above

3461. Name the protecting group which is used for both alcohol and amine

A. t-butyl carbamate
B. Carbamates
C. 9-fluorenylmethyl carbonate
D. Benzyl carbamate

3462. Pyridine and NaHCO3 is used for the formation of which of the following carbamate reaction.

A. Benzyloxycarbonyl
B. 9-fluorenylmethyl carbonate
C. Both A and B
D. None of this

3463. For the protection of alcohol which of the following acetals may be mostly preferred

A. Tetrahydroxypyranyl derivatve
B. Methoxyethoxymethyl derivative
C. Both A and B
D. None of this

3464. A protecting agent are mostly attack at which position of chemical compound

A. Nucleophilic position
B. Electrophilic position
C. Both A and B
D. None of this

3465. Sodium hydride, diazomethane and tetrahydrofuran are formed by which of the following compound

A. Trimethyl butylether
B. Butylether
C. Trihydroxy ether
D. Methyl ether

3466. Methoxy methyl chloride is used as a ether protecting group which is considered a

A. Toxic compound
B. Carcinogenic compound
C. Both A and B
D. All of the above

3467. Primary amine get converted into benzyloxyxarbonyl compound by reacting with which of the following agent .

A. Sodium crystals
B. Aqueous sodium nitrate
C. Sodium hydroxide
D. Alkoholic potassium oxide

3468. Benzyloxycarbonyl compound is mostly preferred protecting group for which functional atom

A. Amides B. Diols
C. Amines D. Ethers

3469. Formamide ,acetamide and benzamide is the protecting group for amineswhich amide is generally cleaved under in which solution .

A. Strong acidic and basic condition
B. Strong basic condition
C. Strong acidic condition
D. None of this

3470. Name the protecting group for primary amines

A. Benzyl ether B. Sodium hydride
C. Triphogene D. Phthalimide

3471. Anaesthetic agents contraindicated in hypertension is

A. Propofol
B. Ketamine
C. Thiopentane sodium
D. Diazepam

3472. Which of the following is correct regarding color coding of anaesthetic gases

A. Oxygen- Black with gray shoulders
B. Nitric oxide-blue
C. Cyclopropane-Red
D. Helium- orange

3473. Contraindications to vasoconstrictors in local anaesthetic is

A. Regional anesthesia
B. Spinal anesthesia
C. Epidural anesthesia
D. Digital nerve block

3474. Preferred muscle relaxant in a patient with liver dysfunctio/ Renal failure is

A. Rocuronium B. Pancuronium
C. Atracuronium D. Vecuronium

3475. LSCS can be carried out under all the following techniques of anaesthesia except

A. Spinal anesthesia
B. Caudal anesthesia
C. Combined spinal Epidural anesthesia
D. General anesthesia

3476. The laryngeal mask airways used for securing the airway of a patient in all of the following condition except

A. During CPR
B. In a difficult attribution
C. large tumor patient in a oral cavity
D. Child undergoing on elective eye surgery

3477. All of the following are the disadvantages of anesthetic ether except

A. Induction is slow
B. Affects blood pressure & is liable to produce arrhythmias
C. Induction is slow
D. Irritant nature of ether increase salivary and bronchial secretion

3478. Which one of the following anesthetic agents cause a rise in intra cranial pressure

A. Propofol
B. Lignocaine
C. Sevoflurane
D. Thiopentone sodium

3479. One of the fastest acting inhalation agents is

A. Sevoflurane B. Ether
C. Halothane D. Isoflurane

3480. Which of the following agents is not used to provide induced hypotension during surgery

A. Esmol
B. Hydralazine
C. Mephentermine
D. Sodium nitropruside

3481. Which of the following agents is used for treatment of postoperative shivering

A. Suxamethonium
B. Pethidine
C. Atropine
D. Thiopentone sodium

3482. Which of the following intravenous agents is the most suitable for day care surgery

A. Diazepam B. Propofol
C. Morphine D. Ketamine

3483. Which one of the following local anesthetic belongs to the ester group-

A. Bupivacaine B. Procaine
C. Lignocaine D. Mepivacaine

3484. Which of the following statement is not true about etomidate

A. An intravenous anesthetic
B. Precipitate coronary insufficiency
C. Inhibits cortisol synthesis
D. Causes pain at site of injection

3485. Which one of the following antibacterials should not be used with d- tuberculosis

A. Lefotaxime B. Doxycycline
C. Streptomycin D. Norfloxacin

3486. Which one of the following muscle relaxanthas the maximum duration of action

A. Atracurium B. Vecuronium
C. Rouronium D. Doxacurium

3487. Which of the following is not an indication for endotracheal intubation

A. Pneumothorax
B. Maintenance of a patent airway
C. To provide positive pressure ventilation
D. Pulmonary toileting

3488. Which of the following anesthetic agents does not trigger malignant hyperthermia

A. Thiopentone B. Suxamethonium
C. Isoflurane D. Halothane

3489. Which of the following side effect is commonly seen with fentanyl

A. Pain in abdomen B. Hypertension
C. Trachycardia D. Chest wall rigidity

3490. Which of the following is not true about xenon anesthesia

A. Non explosive
B. Slow-induction & slow recovery
C. Low blood gas solubility
D. Minimal cardiovascular side effects

3491. Which of the following in anesthesia will produce decreased EEG activities

A. Nitric oxide B. Early hypoxia
C. Ketamine D. Hypothermia

3492. Last muscle to be rendered akinetic with a retrobulbar anesthetic block is

A. Superior Rectus
B. Superior oblique
C. Inferior oblique
D. Levator palpebral superioris

3493. Which of the following neuromuscular blocking agent has the shortest onset of action

A. Vecuronium B. Mivacurium
C. Succinylcholine D. Rapacuronium

3494. Which of the following inhalation agents has the minimum blood gas solubility coefficient

A. Desflurane B. Sevoflurane
C. Nitrous oxide D. Isoflurane

3495. Methemoglobinemia caused by

A. Procaine B. Bupivacaine
C. Prilocaine D. Lignocaine

3496. Merits of nasotracheal intubation

A. Good oral hygiene
B. Less infection
C. Less mucosal damage & bleeding
D. More movement or displacement of endotracheal tube

3497. The cardinal features of general anesthesia are-

A. Loss of all sensation, especially pain
B. Sleep, unconsciousness & amnesia
C. Immobility and muscle relaxant
D. All of the above

3498. Most common nerve used for monitoring during anesthesia is

A. Ulnar B. Radial
C. Facial D. Median

3499. Side effects of oxygen therapy are all except

A. Absorption atelactasis
B. Increased pulmonary compliance
C. Endothelial damage
D. Decreased vital capacity

3500. The following modes of ventilation may be used for wearing of patients fron mechanical ventilation except

A. Assist- control ventilation (ACV)
B. Pressure support Ventilation (PSV)
C. Synchronized intermittent mandatory ventilation (SIMV)
D. Controlled Mechanical Ventilation (CMV)

3501. Tissue plasm in activator

A. Helps in wound healing
B. Allergy response
C. Immunity
D. Dissolves clot in blood vessels

3502. Which of the following will not coagulate when placed separately on four slides

A. Blood serum
B. Blood plasma
C. Blood from pulmonary vein
D. Blood from lymphatic tissue

3503. The vitamin essential for blood clotting is -

A. Vitamin A B. Vitamin B
C. Vitamin C D. Vitamin K

3504. What prevwnts clotting of blood inblood vessel

A. Serotonin B. Fibrinogen
C. Heparin D. Fibrin

3505. Clumping of Cells in known as

A. Clotting B. Mutathione
C. Agglutination D. Glutathione

3506. Which of the following is correct -

A. Lymph=plasma+WBC'S+RBC'S
B. Plasma=Blood-Lymphocytes
C. Neuron=Cyton+Dendron+Oxon+Syropse
D. Blood=Plasma+RBC'S+WBC'S+Platelets

3507. Antibiotics are useful against -

A. Virus
B. Bacteria
C. Autoimmune disease
D. Fungi

3508. Antigen presenting cell are-

A. T cells B. B Cells
C. Macrophages D. Mast cell

3509. Which of the following plasma protein is involved in coagulation of blood

A Albumin B. Globulin
C. Fibrinogen D. Amylase

3510. In the Clotting mechanism pathway Thrombin activates

A. XI, VIII V B. XI, IX, X
C. VIII, X, V D. IX, VIII, V

3511. Which of the following drug have strong electronegative charges

A. Heparin B. Glucuronic Acid
C. Danaparoid D. Ancrod

3512. Which of the following are oral anticoagulants -

A. Warfarin Sodium B. Phenindione
C. Acenocoumaral D. All of the above

3513. Heparin is powerful & instantaneously acting Coagulant effective in

A. In vivo B In vitro
C. Both A & B D None of the above

3514. In higher dose Heparin inhibits platelets

A. Aggregation B. Agglutition
C. Sedimentation D. Turbidity

3515. Danaparoid are conventionally given by-

A. I. V. Route B. Oral
C. Topical D. I. M. Route

3516. A hemorrhagic disease was described in the year-

A. 1930 B. 1924
C. 1926 D. 1920

3517. First Clinical use of bishydroxycoumarin was made in-

A. 1941 B. 1943
C. 1940 D. 1946

3518. Warfarin & its congeners act as anticoagulants in

A. Vivo B. Vitro
C. Both A& B D. None of the above

3519. Carboxylation is essential for the ability of the clotting factors to bind

A. Ca2+ B. K+
C. Na++ D. Mg++

3520. The inhalation anesthetic agents used today generally are-

A. Hydrocarbons & ethers
B. Cyclopropane
C. Carbon & esters
D. None of these

3521. Which was the first anesthetic agent used-

A. Nitric oxide B. Methyl Xanthines
C. Nitrous oxide D. Ethyl Oxide

3522. The first use of the nitrous oxide as a surgical anesthetic was in-

A. 1820 B. 1844
C. 1829 D. 1835

3523. Whom demonstrated the first use of nitrous oxide as a surgical anesthesia in 1844

A. Horace Wells B. Harry Boston
C. William Bortan D. None of the above

3524. In which hospital Horace wells attempted to demonstrate the anesthetic action

A. Massachusetts Hospital
B. Wolk billian Hospital
C. Hartford hospital
D. None of the above

3525. Physical properties of diethyl ether is-

A. Inflammable B. Flammable
C. Explosive D. Both B&C

3526. In which year the use of nitrous oxide was minimal

A. 1860 B. 1850
C. 1840 D. 1870

3527. In specific areas of the Central nervous system is believed to be responsible for anesthetic state

A. Blocking of Neurons
B. Neuronal Depression
C. Neuronal Ganglia
D. None of the above

3528. Excitation of the pyramidal cells helps to maintain
A. Unconsciousness
B. Consciousness
C. Excitatory
D. Inhibitory

3529. The anesthetic agent which is an inhibitor of NMDA glutamate receptors is
A. Thiopental B. Halothane
C. Ketamine D. Sevoflurane

3530. An ideal anesthetic drug would -
A. Induces anesthesia smoothly & rapid recovery
B. Possess a wide margin of safety
C. Has a minimal adverse effect
D. All of the above

3531. First Benzodiazepine to be discovered is-
A. Diazepam B. Lorazepam
C. Clonazepam D. Librium

3532. The organ most resistant to geneeal anesthesia is -
A. Spinal cord B. Medulla Oblongata
C. Medullary cortex D. Cerebellum

3533. Which produces Dissociative anesthesia -
A. Propanidid
B. Thiopentone sodium
C. Fentanyl Droperidol
D. Ketamine

3534. Which of the intravenous anesthetics has antiemetic action-
A. Thiopental B. Propofol
C. Ketamine D. Fentanyl

3535. Which of the following agents is used to accelerate recovery from the Sedative actions of IV Benzodiazepine
A. Naloxone B. Flumazenil
C. Katamine D. Fomepizole

3536. The intravenous anesthetic which causes minimal cardiovascular & respiratory depressant effect is-
A. Propofol B. Thipental
C. Etomidate D. Midazolam

3537. Which of the following general anesthetic belongs to inhalants
A. Thiopental B. Ketamine
C. Desflurane D. Propofol

3538. Sevoflurane has largely replaced halothane& isoflurane as an inhalation anesthetic of choice because
A. Inductin is achieved more rapidly & smoothly
B. Recovery is more rapid
C. Low post-anesthetic organ toxicity
D. All of the above

3539. The limitation of Sevoflurane is-
A. High incidence of coughing & laryngospasm
B. Chemically I stable
C. Centrally mediated sympathetic activation
D. Hepatotoxicity

3540. Who is the father of modern anesthesia
A. W. T. G. Morton B. Clark
C. Sigmund Freud D. Pasteur

3541. Which of the following anesthetics Decreases Methionine synthase activity & Cause Megaloblastic anaemia
A. Desflurane B. Halothane
C. Nitrous oxide D. Sevoflurane

3542. Which of the following inhaled anesthesia can produce hepatic necrosis
A. Sevoflurane B. Desflurane
C. Halothane D. Nitrous oxide

3543. Which of the following drug is metabolised by plasma cholisterase
A. Bupivacaine B. Lidocaine
C. Ropivacaine D. Tetracaine

3544. Wgich of the following factors is the most important determined of the spread of epidural block-
A. Age of the patient
B. Height of patient
C. Site of injection
D. Volume of injection

3545. Which of the following is not true about xenon anesthesia -
A. Non- explosive
B. Minimal cardiovascular side effects
C. Slow induction & slow recovery
D. Low blood gas solubility

3546. A 20 year old patient with early pregnancy was admitted for medical termination of pregnancy in day care facility what will be the anesthetic induction agent of choice -

A. Thiopentone B. Ketamine
C. Propofol D. Diazepam

3547. In General, the last muscle to be rendered akinetic with a retrobulbar anesthetic block is-

A. Superior rectus B. Superior Oblique
C. Inferior oblique D. None of the above

3548. Which of the following drugs is contraindicated in a patient with raised intracranial pressure -

A. Thiopentane B. Propofol
C. Midazolam D. Ketamine

3549. Which of the following fluorinated anesthetic corrodes metal in vaporizers& breathing system-

A. Sevoflurane B. Isoflurane
C. Influrane D. Halothane

3550. LSCS can be carried out under all the following techniques of anesthetic except-

A. Spinal Anesthesia
B. Spinal Epidural Anesthesia
C. Caudal Anesthesia
D. General anesthesia

3551. Which anesthetic agent boils at a room temperature -

A. Desflurane B. Ketamine
C. Propofol D. Diazepam

3552. Which of the following symptoms is seen in a patient administered with 20-40% of nitrous oxide

A. Sweating B. Paresthesia
C. Floating sensation D. None of the above

3553. Local anesthetic act by inhibiting

A. Motor fibers only
B. Motor& Sensory fibers
C. Only Sensory Fibers
D. None of the above

3554. To correlate changes in depth of anesthesia is

A. Electroencephalograph
B. Electrophoresis
C. Electrocardiograph
D. Electrolyte balance

3555. Which of the given drugs used as preanesthetic agents to alter the ECG-

A. Concomitant Drugs
B. Contraindicated Drugs
C. Highly Degradabke drugs
D. None of the above

3556. During the period of anesthetic administration a patient has-

A. Regular Respiratory Rate
B. Irregular Respiratory rate
C. Regular Heart Beat
D. None of the above

3557. A level of adequate surgical anesthesia generally has begun due to

A. Exhibits Elevation in blood pressure
B. Increase Respiration rate
C. Increase jaw tension
D. All of the above

3558. Depth of anesthesia progresses response can not be decrease by-

A. Monitoring reflexes, blood pressure
B. Respiration Rate
C. Contraction of lungs
D. None of these

3559. The production & maintenance of the anesthetic state is believed by-

A. Dependant on concentration
B. Partial pressure
C. BothA & B
D. None of the above

3560. Anthral acts as purgative due to

A. Irritant action
B. Bulk formation in intestinal lumen
C. Osmotic action
D. Emollient action

3561. True about lactulose is

A. Blood ammonia
B. 10% absorbed
C. Osmotic laxative
D. Diasaccharide of lactose & sucrose

3562. Which purgative cause hypokalemia

A. Liquid paraffin B. Bisacodyl
C. Castor oil D. Osmotic purgatives

3563. Osmolality ORS recommended by WHO is
A. 245mOSM/L B. 300mOSM/L
C. 270mOSM/L D. 260mOSM/L

3564. Which of the following laxatives lowers blood ammonia level in hepatic encephalopathy
A. Bisacodyl B. Liquid paraffin
C. Lactulose D. Magnesium Sulfate

3565. Stimulant purgatives are contraindicated in the following
A. Bed Ridden patients
B. Before abdominal radiography
C. Subacute intestinal Obstruction
D. All of the following

3566. The success of oral rehydration therapy of diarrhoea depends upon which of the following process in the intestinal mucosa
A. Sodium pump mediated Na+ absorption
B. Glucose coupled Na+ absorption
C. Bicarbonate coupled Na+ absorption
D. Passive Na+ diffusion

3567. The concentration of sodium ion in the standard WHO oral rehydration solution is-
A. 40mMoles/L B. 60mMoles/L
C. 90mMoles/L D. 110mMoles/L

3568. The new formula WHO-ORS Differs from the older standard formula
A. Lower Na+& Glucose concentration
B. Higher K+ Concentration
C. No basic salt
D. Both B&C

3569. Which of the following statement is true about new formula WHO-ORS
A. Na+ion concentration of 75mm/L
B. Glucose concentration is 75mm/L
C. Total Osmolarity is 245mOSM/L
D. All of the above

3570. Apart from Diarrhoea oral rehydration solution has been employed in -
A. Severe Vomiting B. Heat strokes
C. Burn Cases D. Both B&C

3571. Bisacodyl is-
A. Bulk forming
B. Stool Softener
C. Stimulant Purgatives
D. osmotic Purgatives

3572. Diarrhoea is side effect of
A. Osemeprazole B. Sucralfate
C. Metoclopramide D. Misoprostol

3573. Antacid drug that typically causes diarrhoea
A. Sodium Bicarbonate
B. Magnesium Hydroxide
C. Calcium Bicarbonate
D. Aluminium Hydroxide

3574. Not true about the composition of ORS
A. Nacl-3.59 B. Kcl-1.5gm
C. Bicarbonate - 2gm D. Glucose-20gm

3575. Which of the following oil is not a laxative
A. Corn oil B. Liquid paeaffin
C. Olive oil D. Glycerin

3576. Which one of the following methods is not a route of administration for laxative
A. Chocolate B. Pessary
C. Chewing Gum D. Suppositories

3577. Which one of the following foods does not help in constipation
A. Bran Flakes B. White Rice
C. Plums D. Brown Rice

3578. According to the NHS which of the following is the most effective laxative -
A. Irritant
B. Lubricant
C. Bulking
D. They are all the same

3579. Which of the following herbs doesn't have laxatie properties
A. Henna B. Senna
C. Cascara D. Aloe

3580. Serotonin stimulants are used to treat anxiety & depression but also serve function in constipation due to their-
A. Laxative effect B. Purgatives effect
C. Cathartics effect D. None of these

3581. The volatile anesthetic isoflurane, desflurane, enflurane & halothane each contain

A. Symmetric carbon

B. Both A& B

C. Asymmetric carbon

D. None of th above

3582. The process of making an object free from living organism including bacterial & fungal spores & viruses is known as

A. Sterilization B. Disinfectant

C. Tyndallization D. None of the above

3583. Which of the following induces action of thymine

A. Infra- Red rays B. UV rays

C. Gamma rays γ D. None of the above

3584. A chemical agents that kills the microorganisms & is commonly applied to substances used on inanimate objects are-

A. Antiseptics B. Sanitizer

C. Disinfectants D. Antibiotics

3585. An agents that prevents the bacteria are known as-

A. Bactericidal B. Antibiotics

C. Antimicrobial D. Bacteriostatics

3586. Which of the following is the characteristic of sanitizers-

A. Destroys all microbial forms

B. Prevents growth of microorganisms

C. Reduces the microbial population of safe levels

D. Kills the bacteria

3587. Which of the following is not a chemical agent for microbial control

A. Radiations B. Antibiotics

C. Antiseptics D. Germicide

3588. Which of the following method of sterilization has no effect on spores-

A. Drying B. Autoclaving

C. Pasteurisation D. Disinfectant

3589. Bacterial concentration of phenol is

A. 2% B. 4%

C. 1% D. 8%

3590. Lysol is a-

A. Antiseptic B. Sterlizers

C. Antibiotics D. Disinfectant

3591. Steam exposure of a material at 100°C for 20 minutes for three consecutive days is known as

A. Tyndallization B. Crystallization

C. Pasteurisation D. Sterilization

3592. Which of the following was the first widely used antiseptic & disinfectant

A. Lysol B. Phenol

C. Formaldehyde D. Ethylene oxide

3593. Which is the most important surface active disinfectant -

A. Cationic Compounds

B. Anionic Compounds

C. Both A& B

D. None of the above

3594. Aldehydes, which are most powerful disinfectant following -

A. Formaldehyde B. Glutaraldehyde

C. Both A & B D. None of the above

3595. Disinfectant is less effective than

A. Sterilisers B. Antimicrobials

C. Antibacterials D. Antiseptics

3596. Disinfectant work by destroying the cell qall of microbes or interfering with-

A. Excretion B. Defecation

C. Metabolism D. Absorption

3597. Disinfectant kill more germs than-

A. Pesticides B. Sanitizers

C. Sterilisers D. None of the above

3598. The most cost effective home disinfectant is-

A. Sodium hypochloride

B. Choline bleach

C. Sodium Chromoglycate

D. Sodium Chromate

3599. Chlorine Bleach is effective against most common pathogens

A. Tuberculosis B. Entarococcus

C. Staphylococcus D. All of the above

3600. Laxative, purgative or or aperients are substances that loosen stools & increases
A. Bowl movement
B. Constipation
C. Diarrhoeal movement
D. None of the above

3601. Laxative may be administered by........ Route
A. Oral B. Rectal
C. Both A & B D. Parientral

3602. Dietary Fibres metamucil are the example of-
A. Bulk- Forming agents
B. Emolient agents
C. Saline Laxative agents
D. All of the above

3603. Which of the following used in chronic idiopathic constipation & bowl syndrome
A. Lubiprostone B. Tegaserod
C. Prucalopride D. None of the above

3604. Osmotic laxativs are effective in-
A. Below the counter
B. Over the counter
C. Between the counter
D. None of the above

3605. Wheat Bran consist of dietary fibers about-
A. 20% B. 30%
C. 40% D. 70%

3606. Which of the following is not action of bulk forming laxatives
A. Stimulate local peristalsis
B. Decreases water content of faces
C. Absorb water in intestines
D. Swells

3607. Lactulose is broken down by-
A. Colonic Bacteria
B. Osmotically active products
C. Disaccharide of fructose
D. None of the above

3608. Lubricant laxatives can be given in-
A. Bulk Form
B. Emulsified Form
C. Suspended Form
D. None of the above

3609. Dioctyl sodium sulfosuccinate is an-
A. Cationic Detergent B. Emulsifying agent
C. Anionic Agents D. Wetting agent

3610. Surfactant laxatives act as-
A. Sweeting agent B. Binding agent
C. Wetting agent D. Spreading agent

3611. Purgatives are used for-
A. Colonic Cleansing
B. Food/drug poisoning
C. Abdominal X-ray
D. All of the above

3612. Prostaglandins are naturally occuring fatty acid derivatives of-
A. 20- carbon, cyclopentano
B. 40-carbon Cyclopentano
C. 10-carbon cyclopentano
D. 20- Carbon hexapentano

3613. 20-carbon cyclopentano fatty acids are
A. Polyunsaturated B. Monounsaturated
C. Saturated D. Polysaturated

3614. Who reported the human seminal fluid possessed relaxant effect on smooth muscles-
A. Kurzrok&Lieb B. Von Euler
C. Goldblatt D. None of the above

3615. The human Seminal Fluid possessed relaxant effect on smooth muscles in the year
A. 1935 B. 1940
C. 1965 D. 1931

3616. Who identified the activeconstituent as a lipophillic acidic substance
A. Von Euler B. Kurzrok& Lieb
C. Goldblatt D. None of the above

3617. Who realized that van Eulers Prostaglandin was actually mixture of fatty acids
A. Kurzrak & Lieb
B. Bergstrom&Samulsson
C. Goldblatt
D. None of the above

3618. The first report of the structure of the Prostaglandin was actually stimulated relating to chemical & biological properties in-
A. 1965 B. 1972
C. 1962 D. 1961

3619. Which of the following substitution pattern Prostaglandin possess -
A. 15α-Hydroxy group
B. 18α- hydroxy group
C. 16α- hydroxy group
D. 13α-hydroxy group

3620. On the nature & stereo chemistry of oxygen substituents of prostaglandin
A. 9th position B. 11th position
C. BothA&B D. 13th position

3621. Diagnostic agents includes chemical compounds of-
A. Organic nature B. Inorganic Nature
C. Structural Moiety D. All of the above

3622. Diagnostic agents depend upon their-
A. Constitution & Functional group
B. Chemical Nature
C. Inorganic Nature
D. None of the above

3623. Important class of diagnostic agents for quantitative determination -
A. Dyes&stain B. Gum & Acacia
C. BothA&B D. None of the above

3624. Important examples of diagnostic agents for quantitative determination are-
A. Functioning of thyroid gland
B. Metabolism & Excretion
C. Digestion
D. All of the above

3625. Different part of body organ systems involved in diagnostic agents are-
A. Liver B. Brain
C. Kidney D. All of the above

3626. The major classes of diagnostic agents are-
A. Inorganic & Organic Compounds
B. Dyes & Stains
C. Radioactive Tracers
D. All of the Following

3627. Diagnostic agents are special compounds having reaction -
A. Quantitative
B. Qualitative
C. BothA&B
D. Potentiometric reaction

3628. In eadiological contrast media, Barium sulphate not having-
A. Low systemic toxicity
B. Low water solubility
C. Lack of osmotic activity
D. High Water Solubility

3629. In the biosynthesis of prostaglandin members of PGG&PGH series are-
A. Cycloendoperoxide
B. Cyclopentane
C. Cyclohexaoxide
D. None of the above

3630. Which of the following precursor derived in the cyclopentane ring of prostaglandin -
A. Fatty Acid B. Fructose
C. Glycerol D. Mannitol

3631. Naturally occuring prostaglandins contain number of
A. Single bond B. Triple bond
C. Double bond D. None of the above

3632. In prostaglandin the most common fatty acids in humans is-
A. Eicosatrienoic acid
B. Arachidonic acid
C. Apetonic acid
D. Linolenic acid

3633. Arachidonic Acid is derived from -
A. Dietary Linoleic Acid
B. Ingested from the diet
C. Esterified to phospholipids
D. All of the above

3634. Various initiating factors of prostaglandin interact with-
A. G-protein couple receptor
B. Membrane binding receptor
C. Phospholipase receptor
D. None of the above

3635. A polypeptide produced by leukocytes in prostaglandin biosynthesis is-
A. Interleukin-2 B. Interleukin - 1
C. Interleukin-3 D. Leukotrine-2

3636. Arachidonic acid with cyclooxygenase interaction occur in the presence of-
A. Hydrogen B. Barium
C. Oxygen D. Zinc

3637. PGD2 is formed by the action of-
A. Glutathione-S-Transferase
B. Glutathione - P-Transferase
C. Glutathione-N-Transferase
D. None of these

3638. NSAIDS inhibits prostaglandin biosynthesis which prevent -
A. Swelling B. Inflammation
C. Headache D. Bacterial Infection

3639. The isoform of COX was first purified in-
A. 1986 B. 1977
C. 1970 D. 1976

3640. The isoform of the COX was first Cloned in-
A. 1988 B. 1989
C. 1987 D. 1990

3641. Which out of the following alcohols is used for waxes-
A. Cholesterol B. Glycerol
C. Cetyl Alcohol D. Sphingol

3642. Choose the Dienoic fatty acid of the following
A. Oleic acid B. Linolenic acid
C. Stearic acid D. Acetic acid

3643. Which of the following is not a glycerophospholipid-
A. Cardiolipim B. Plasmalogen
C. Lecithin D. Sphingomylein

3644. Which out of the following enzyme is defective in Gaucher's disease -
A. β- Glucocerebrosidase
B. Sphingomyleinase
C. HexosaminidaseA
D. β- Galactocerebrosidase

3645. Choose the following Glycerophospholipid that acts as a precursor for second messenger -
A. Phosphatidyl Choline
B. Phosphatidyl anositol
C. Phosphatidyl Serine
D. Phosphatidyl ethanolamine

3646. Which out of the following is not a derived lipid-
A. Ketone Body
B. PGE2
C. Diacylglycerol
D. Galactosyl Ceramide

3647. Cholesterol is transported from extra hepatic tissues to liver by which of the following lipoproteins-
A. Cyclomicrons B. VLDL
C. LDL D. HDL

3648. All are non-essential fatty acids except -
A. Palmitic acid B. Linolenic acid
C. Oleic acid D. Stearic acid

3649. Which of the following is an animal sterol-
A. Ergo Sterol B. Stigmasterol
C. Sitosterol D. Cholesterol

3650. Which of the following is an ω'6 fatty acids
A. α Linolenic acid B. Elaidic acid
C. Oleic acid D. Arachidonic acid

3651. A polar derivative of cholesterol is-
A. Bile salt B. Oestrogen
C. Vitamin D D. Progesterone

3652. Acetyl number is a-
A. Measure of unsaturation of a fat
B. Degree of rancidity
C. Measure of a volatile fatty acids
D. Measure of - OH groups

3653. All are conditions of hypercholesterolemia except -
A. Anaemia
B. Diabetes Mellitus
C. Hypothyroidism
D. Nephrotic syndrome

3654. Which of the following is an intermediate for both the synthesis of phospholipids & Triacylglycerols
A. Diacyl Glycerol B. Cholesterol
C. Cholines D. Inositol

3655. Which fatty acid would have the least melting point out of the following -
A. Stearic acid B. Anachidonic acid
C. Timnodonic acid D. Palmitic acid

3656. Which are not a source of glycerol -
A. Diet B. Adipolysis
C. Glycolysis D. Glycogenolysis

3657. Which out of the following is a glycerophospholipids

A. Cardiolipin
B. Galactosyl ceramide
C. GM2
D. Sphingomyclin

3658. Which out of the following enzyme is defective in Niemann pick's disease -

A. β-Glucocerebosidase
B. HexosaminidaseA
C. Sphingomyelinase
D. β- Galactocerebosidase

3659. Choose a lipid that acts as a precursor for Glycerophospholipids-

A. Cholesterol
B. Sphingosine
C. N-acetyl Neuraminic acid
D. Phosphatidic acid

3660. All except one are fatty acids with 18 carbon atoms-

A. Oleic acid B. Linolenic acid
C. Palmitic acid D. Stearic acid

3661. For which out of the following compounds cholesterol serves as a precursor-

A. Bile pigments B. Bile salts
C. Vitamink D. Triacyl Glycerol

3662. Which out of the following is a hydroxy fatty acid-

A. α Linolenic acid B. Linolenic Acid
C. Palmitic acid D. Cerebronic acid

3663. The iodine number of Linolenic acid is-

A. 1 B. 6
C. 4 D. 3

3664. Which of the following is not a derived lipid-

A. Arachidonic acid B. Diacyl Glycerol
C. HDL D. Vitamin D

3665. Which of the following is not an essential fatty acid-

A. Arachidonic acid B. Linolenic acid
C. Acetic acid D. Palmitic acid

3666. COX2 rapidly inducible & expressedby-

A. Hormonal factor B. Growth Factor
C. Thyroidal factor D. None of these

3667. COX-3 is selectively inhibited by-

A. Antipyretic drugs
B. Analgetic drugs
C. Both A & B
D. Anti asthamatic drugs

3668. Sometimes COX-3 Potentially inhibited by-

A. NSAIDS B. Anti inflammatory
C. Anti allergic D. None of the above

3669. Cyclooxygenase-1 contains-

A. 430to433amino acids
B. 599to602 amino acid
C. 470to472 amino acids
D. 535to537 amino acid

3670. In cyclooxygenase-2 structure -

A. 603 to 604 amino acids
B. 604 to 605 amino acids
C. 612 to 613 amino acids
D. 622 to 623 amino acids

3671. Both COX-1&COX-2 Isoform contain-

A. 60%homology within the species
B. 60% homology without the species
C. 70%homology within the species
D. 70% homology without the species

3672. Crystal structure of COX-2 is-

A. Dimensional B. Radiographic
C. Both A&B D. Two Dimensional

3673. With both Isoforms displaying similar ability to convert arachidonic acid to-

A. PGH2 B. PGF2
C. PGG2 D. PGD2

3674. Which one of the following accepts wider range of fatty acids-

A. COX-2 B. COX-1
C. COX-3 D. None of the above

3675. COX-2 Metabolites -

A. C-18 fatty acids B. C-22 fatty acids
C. C-20 fatty acids D. Both A& C

3676. Which one of the following selective inhibitors do not bind with Arg-120-

A. COX-1 B. COX-3
C. COX-2 D. PGH2

3677. Function of COX-1 to produce prostaglandin that are involved in normal

A. Cellular activity B. Kinetic activity
C. Potential activity D. None of these

3678. Function of COX-2to produce prostaglandin at-
A. Radial Cells B. Inflammatory cells
C. Unit Cells D. Lypolysed cell

3679. Selective COX-2 Inhibitions may eliminate side effects associated with NSAIDS are-
A. Gastric effect B. Nausea
C. Renal effect D. Both A&C

3680. Prostaglandin are rapidly inactivated by-
A. Oxidative&Reductive
B. Oxidative & Hydrolysis
C. Reductive & Hydrogenesis
D. All of the following

3681. Enzymes normally involved in prostaglandin are-
A. β&ω amino acids B. α&ω fatty acids
C. B&ω fatty acids D. λ&ω fatty acids

3682. Dicarboxyllic acid derivatives only containing
A. 20 carbon atoms B. 16 carbon atoms
C. 17 carbon atoms D. 14 carbon atoms

3683. PGE2&PGE1 are the major excreted metabolites of
A. Amino acids B. Dicarboxyllic acid
C. Linolenic acid D. None of these

3684. Which route PGE2 will stimulate the endometrium of gravid uterus -
A. Intravenously B. Rectally
C. Intravaginally D. Parentrally

3685. PGE2 is available as-
A. Dinoprostone B. Monoprostone
C. Cycloprostone D. BothA&C

3686. Which drug is well established in antithrombolytic activity -
A. Triflusal B. Indobufen
C. Aspirin D. Dipyridamole

3687. Aspirin irreversibly deactivate
A. WBC COX-1 B. Platelet COX-1
C. RBC COX-1 D. Leukocyte COX-1

3688. Half life of aspirin in stomach is-
A. 15-20 min B. 10-15 min
C. 20-25 min D. 25-30 min

3689. Which of the following differ from their pharmacological effect -
A. Aspirin B. Triflusal
C. Clostazol D. Dipyridamole

3690. Which are usually termed as local hormones -
A. Eicosanoids B. Prostaglandin
C. Corticotropin D. Calcitonin

3691. Which drug helps to maintain the potency of the ductus arterious-
A. Epoprostinol Sodium
B. Misoprostol
C. Alprostadil
D. Probucol

3692. Which of the following drug help in potency pending Surgical manipulation-
A. Misoprostol B. Epoprostinol Sodium
C. Probucol D. Alprostadil

3693. Alprostadil is given by which form for erectile disfunction -
A. Tablet B. Capsule
C. Injection D. Opthalmic

3694. Direct insertion of Alprostadil into the urethra in the form of-
A. Suppositories B. Capsule
C. Tablet D. All of the above

3695. Which of the following deug cause vasodilation & prevent platelet aggregation
A. Misoprostil
B. Epoprostinol sodium
C. Alprostadil
D. Probucol

3696. The endogenous substance of arachidonic acid metabolism is known as-
A. Tetracycline B. Prostaglandin
C. Prostacyclin D. None of the above

3697. Prostacyclin is much less active than-
A. 6-keto prostaglandin F1α
B. 7-keto Prostaglandin F1α
C. 6-keto prostaglandin F2α
D. 7-keto prostaglandin F2α

3698. The drug which inhibit gastric acid secretion but also entraces mucosal resistance known as-
A. Alprostadil B. Gemfibrozil
C. Theofibrate D. Misoprostol

3699. The drug which rapidly & largely absorbed is-
A. Misoprostol B. Alprostadil
C. Epoprostinol Sodium
D. Probucol

3700. The half life of Misoprostol is-
A. 30-40mins B. 20-40mins
C. 10-20mins D. 40-50mins

3701. Misoprostol almost excreted in urine about -
A. 80% B. 85%
C. 90% D. 75%

3702. The following offer a bright prospect for the treatment of immune system & hypertension is-
A. Prostaglandin B. Eicosanoids
C. Cardiac Steroids D. Inotropic Drugs

3703. The patient with elevated blood cholesterol are bound with
A. α- Lipoproteins B. β- Lipoproteins
C. Phospholipids D. Fatty acids

3704. Fibric acid is a structural analogue of-
A. Theofibrate B. Probucol
C. Alprostadil D. Gemfibrozil

3705. Theofibrate Causes-
A. Plasma Concentration
B. Secretion Of Bile
C. Regression of Xanthines
D. None of the above

3706. Sulphur containing Bis-Phenol is a structural moiety of-
A. Probucol B. Theofibrate
C. Gemfibrozil D. Etofyline

3707. Probucol minimises LDL-Cholesterol up to-
A. 40% B. 20%
C. 30% D. 10%

3708. Activated platelets released
A. Eicosanoids B. Cyclooxygenase
C. Prostaglandin D. Thromboxane

3709. Anti Thrombotic effects are mediated through irreversible inhibition of-
A. Cyclooxygenase
B. Thromboxane
C. Prostacyclin
D. Eicosanoids

3710. The enzyme which is necessary for thromboxane Synthesis -
A. TXA1 B. TXA2
C. TXAA D. TXA3

3711. TXA2 have ability to bind & activate -
A. β-receptor B. γ- receptor
C. G-protein coupled receptor
D. α- receptor

3712. What is the symbol π in a QSAR equation?
A. The hydrophobicity of the molecule
B. The electronic effect of a substituent
C. The substituent hydrophobicity constant
D. A measure of the steric properties for a substituent

3713. Thromboxane production is increased in-
A. Asthma B. Tuberculosis
C. Cancer D. Hypertension

3714. Omega-3 fatty acids are the group of-
A. Eicosanoids B. Prostanoids
C. Thrombocytes D. None of the above

3715. The first local anesthetic cocaine was used by-
A. Carl Koller B. Willstatter
C. Muller D. None of these

3716. The first local anesthetic was used in-
A. 1885 B. 1874
C. 1884 D. 1890

3717. Amylocaine esters of basic alcohols with benzoic acid were prepared in-
A. 1906 B. 1909
C. 1904 D. 1905

3718. Anesthetics essentially afford anesthesia by blocking nerve conductance in
A. Motor Neurons B. Sensory Neurons
C. Sensory Organ D. Nerve Fibre

3719. Local Anesthetics exert their action at selective site of-
A. K(+) channel B. Ca(+) Channel
C. Na(+) channel D. Li(+) Channel

3720. Which of the following local Anesthetics is a surface anesthetic-
A. Procaine B. Butamben
C. Orthocaine D. Cocaine

3721. One of the following local Anesthetics having twice duration of action than that procaine-
A. Tetracaine Hydrochloride
B. Procaine
C. Cocaine
D. Orthocaine

3722. Which of the following used in opthalmology & induces no initial irritation-
A. Proxymetacaine HCl
B. Procaine
C. Orthocaine
D. Butamben

3723. Relative contraindications for the administration of ketamine hydrochloride include all of the following
A. Age<5 years
B. History of epilepsy
C. Raised intracranial tension
D. Recent anterior myocardial infraction

3724. Concentration of Dissociative Sedation & analgesia described by Robert & Roserbaum in 1971 is-
A. 5 to 20% N2O B. 20 to 30% N2O
C. 30 to 50% N2O D. 50 to 70% V

3725. Nitrous oxide is carried in the blood stream by-
A. Haemoglobin B. White blood cells
C. Red blood cells D. Serum

3726. Chloroxylenol has-
A. Local Anesthetic property
B. Local Anesthetic & antiseptic Action
C. Antiseptic Action
D. Antibiotic Action

3727. Rapid Onset of inhalation on general anesthesia are-
A. Blood solubility B. Cerebral Blood flow
C. Antiseptic Action D. All of the above

3728. Which factor of the following contributes to short duration of Anesthetic action of single dose thiopenral
A. Rapid Biotranformation
B. Rapid accumulation on body fat
C. High lipid solubility
D. Ability to enter & leave brain tissue

3729. Lidocaine produces its antiarrythmic effect by-
A. Increasing A-V Conduction
B. Decreasing Cardiac Excitability
C. Increasing Cardiac Conduction
D. Increasing spontaneous pacemaker activity

3730. The organ most resistant to GA is
A. Spinal cord B. Medullary Cortex
C. Medulla oblongata D. Cerebrum

3731. Cardiac arrythmias are most commonly seen during administration of-
A. Thiopental B. Halothane
C. Ethyl Ether D. Nitrous Oxide

3732. Which produces Dissociative anesthesia -
A. Propanidid
B. Fentanyl Droperidol
C. Thiopentone Sodium
D. Ketamine

3733. Problems associated with Nitrous Oxide anesthesia is-
A. Behavioural problem
B. Sensitises the heart to adrenaline
C. Prolonged difficult Induction
D. Tachycardia & arrythmias

3734. Methemoglobinemia is a complicated on following the administration of-
A. Lignocaine B. Benzocaine
C. Prilocaine D. Procaine

3735. Krtamine is a-
A. Short general Anesthetic agent
B. Local Anesthetic agent
C. Antidepressive agent
D. Hypnotic agent

3736. A dentist who first used ether as ageneral Anesthetic was-
A. Martin B. Morton
C. Morrison D. Murroy

3737. Which of the following Anesthetic drugs produces powerful stimulation of the cerebral cortex-
A. Cocaine B. Procaine
C. Lidocaine D. Tetracaine

3738. The dentist who first used nitrous oxidefor the abolition pain due to dental extraction was-

A. Harpes David B. Harvey Willian
C. Horace wells D. Hunter john

3739. The drug combination which produces neuroleptanalgesia is-

A. Daroperidol+fentadyl
B. Daroperidol+Ketamine
C. Daroperidol+Ether
D. Daroperidol+Thiopental Sodium+Nitrous oxide

3740. The drug not belonging to amide group

A. Procaine B. Xylocaine
C. Lignocaine D. Bupivacaine

3741. Local Anesthetic are-

A. Cocaine B. Procaine
C. Lignocaine D. Bupivacaine

3742. In the second stage of anesthesia the pupil is

A. Constricted B. Partially dilated
C. Normal in size D. Totally dilatd

3743. Hallucination are seen after anesthesia -

A. Ketamine B. Thiopentone
C. Tentanyl D. Nitrous oxide

3744. Which of tge following agents sensitises the myocardium to catecholamines

A. Isoflurane B. Ether
C. Halothane D. Propofol

3745. In which of the following stage general anesthesia surgery is done-

A. Stage-1 B. Stage-2
C. Stage-3 plane2 D. Stage-3Plane3

3746. After I. V. administration of which of the following Anesthetic agent there is rapid recovery & less headache -

A. Propofol B. Diazepam
C. Droperidol D. Miclazolam

3747. Which among the following is not used for surface anesthesia

A. Lignocaine B. Procaine
C. Tetracaine D. Benzocaine

3748. Nitrous oxide is-

A. A good analgesic but poor Anesthetic
B. A good Anesthetic & a good analgesic
C. A good analgesic & a good Anesthetic
D. A poor analgesic & poor Anesthetic

3749. General Anesthetic most likely to cause bronchodilation is-

A. Thiopentone B. Krtamine
C. Propofol D. Fentanyl

3750. About anticaine all are true except -

A. Plasma half life- is 90 min
B. Is amide which is metabolized in liver
C. More breaks down causes more toxicity
D. Mandibullar infuration is more effective than nerve block

3751. Attachment of erythrocyte to surface of virally infected cell is termed as

A. Interference
B. Hemadsorption
C. Neutralisation
D. Complement Fixation

3752. A duration of time, a specific antibody develops, becoming detachable in blood know as-

A. Serology B. Blood culture
C. Seroconversion D. Antibody production

3753. The device used to study the activity of brain is-

A. EEG B. ECG
C. Autocatalyser D. Dialyser

3754. Cross Sectional image of internal body structure can be obtained by using this medical technique

A. ECG B. CAT
C. NMR D. EEG

3755. Blood dialysis is also called -

A. Artificial Lung B. Artificial kidney
C. Artificial Heart D. Artificial Brain

3756. During amniocentesis chromosomal abnormalities to the fetus can be detected by taking the sample of

A. Foetal blood
B. Mother's blood
C. Body fluid from the mother
D. Fluid surrounding the fetus

3757. Who is considered as the father of electrocardiography-

A. Jenner B. Purcell
C. Housefield D. Einthovan

3758. Which one of the following is an imaging technique

A. MRI Scan B. ELISA
C. Widal test D. ECG

3759. The technique used to detect foetal movement is-

A. PET B. CT Scan
C. ECG D. Ultrasound scan

3760. First human EEG recorded by-

A. Purcell B.
C. Hans Berger D.

3761. ELISA is used to detect viruses where the key reagent is

A. Catalase B. DNA Probe
C. RNAase D. Alkaline phosphate

3762. Cornea transplantation is successful because

A. Cornea is easy to preserve
B. Cornea is easy available
C. Cornea is not linked up with blood vascular r & immune system
D. The technique involved is very simple

3763. The matrix of formed elements in the blood is

A. 45% B. 50%
C. 55% D. 65%

3764. The matrix of blood is known as-

A. Plasma B. Serum
C. RBC&WBC D. WBC&Platelets

3765. The ratio of WBC & RBC is

A. 1:60 B. 1:600
C. 1:6000 D. 1:60000

3766. During blood coagulation thromboplastin is released by-

A. RBC
B. Blood plasma
C. Leukocyte
D. Clumped platelets & damaged tissues

3767. The normal level of Hb per 100ml of blood in women is

A. 14g B. 18g
C. 20g D. 10g

3768. Blood circulation was first explained by

A. Jenner B. William Harvey
C. Mendel D. Pasteur

3769. What is the name of the iron containing protein that gives red blood vessels their colour

A. Hemocyanin B. Pyrite
C. Haemoglobin D. Myoglobin

3770. Which of the following are not components of blood-

A. Aorta B. Capillaries
C. Pulmonary vein D. Heart

3771. Which of the following cations is required for the conversion of prothrombin into active thrombin by thromboplastin -

A. Ca2+ B. Fe2+
C. Mg2+ D. Mn2+

3772. Classic opioid receptors are all except

A. Alpha B. Mu
C. Kappa D. Delta

3773. Mu receptors are responsible for

A. Mediate spinal analgesia
B. Supra-spinal analgesia
C. Respiratory depression
D. Hallucination

3774. Activation of delta receptors produces all except

A. Respiratory depression
B. Affective behavior
C. Increase GI motility
D. Spinal analgesia

3775. Sigma receptors are least considered because

A. Doesn't activated by morphine
B. Doesn't blocked by naloxone
C. Both A and B
D. Activated by morphine and block by naloxone

3776. Precursor comp. For the synthesis of buprenorphine

A. Di-hydrothebainone
B. 3,4-dimethoxy-phenylacetic acid
C. Bengal chloride
D. Thebaine

3777. In morphine, at which position saturation of double bond give more potent compund

A. C-6 B. C-7
C. C-3 D. C-1

3778. Which one of the following when reacts with dienophile gives 6,14-endoetheno-tetrahydro derivatives

A. fentanyl citrate B. Thebaine
C. Alphaprodine D. Lofentanil

3779. Which one of the following is extremely potent mu agonist

A. Etorphine B. Morphine
C. Dihydro codeine D. Dihydro morphine

3780. Precursor compound in the synthesis of the fentanyl citrate is

A. 2-phenylacetonitrile
B. Propionyl chloride
C. Benzyl chloride
D. Phenyl acetonitrile

3781. 1,3-dimethyl-4-phenyl-4-(piperidine) propanoate is

A. Ketobemidone B. Loperamide
C. Alphaprodine D. Lofentanil

3782. The 14.beta-hydroxyl group on the Alicycloc ring of morphine will

A. Give potent derivatives
B. Increase anti-tussive activity
C. Decrease mu-agonistic property
D. Enhance mu-agonistic property

3783. Which one of the following is more toxic than morphine but analgesic effect is twice of morphine

A. Methadone
B. Alphaprodine
C. Lofentanil
D. ketobemidone

3784. Placement of m-hydroxy group in phenyl ring of di-phenyl haptanone result in

A. Decrease in analgesic activity
B. Increase in analgesic activity
C. Increase in potency
D. Decrease in potency

3785. Pentazocine produces analgesia because of it's agonistic action on

A. Mu- receptors B. Delta receptors
C. Kappa receptors D. Sigma receptors

3786. In benzomorphanan derivatives, placement of methyl group in which position increase the activity

A. 5th B. 2nd
C. 9th D. 4th

3787. Which group decreases the activity when placed on 9th position in benzomorphanan derivatives

A. Methyl group B. -OH
C. N-allyl group D. CH2 -CH3

3788. 6-dimethylamino-4,4-diphenylheptan-3-one is

A. Dipanone B. Normethadone
C. Normethadone D. Methadone

3789. Which one of the following is the partial agonist of morphine type

A. Naloxone B. Naltrexone
C. Propiram D. Levallorphan

3790. Which of the following is partialagonist of nalorphine type

A. Naloxone B. Naltrexone
C. Profadol D. Levollorphan

3791. Which of the following is pure antagonistwith nomorphine like effect

A. Naloxone B. Propiram
C. Nalorphine D. Cyclazocin

3792. Precursor compound in the synthesis ofnaloxone

A. Thebaine B. Morphinan
C. Cyclohexanone D. Cyanoacetate

3793. Name the compound which are selective for kappa opioid receptors

A. Ethylketazocine B. Nor-binaltorphimine
C. +PD117302 D. All of the above

3794. Compound selective for Delta opioid receptors

A. Nor-OMI B. SNC-80
C. DADLE D. All of the above

3795. Que no. 24 and 25 are based on following structure-

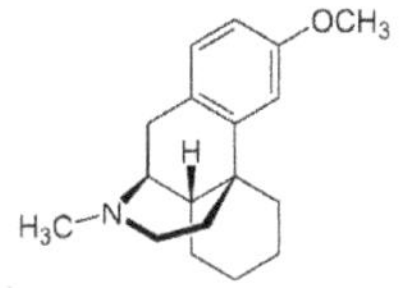

In above structure, ring C of pentacyclic opioids is forced into a pseudo boat conformation due to the presence of

A. 7,8- double bond

B. Restraining furan E- ring

C. Both A and B

D. OH-substitution on 6th position

3796. What will be the effect when C-ring assume the more stable chain conformation

A. Increase toxicity

B. Increase in activity

C. No effect

D. Decrease the activity

3797. Which moiety will be produced when inactive narcodine undergoes ortho-demethylation

A. Morphine B. Nor-morphine

C. Codeine D. None of the above

3798. Which of the following is an inactive prodrug

A. Codeine B. Morphine

C. Nor-morphine D. Norcodeine

3799. Wheninactive prodrug codeine undergoes ortho-demethylation in the presence of CYP-2D6 it produce

A. Active narcodeine

B. Inactive Norcodeine

C. Active morphine

D. Inactive morphine

3800. Name an opioid agonistwhich is only tertiary amines provide clinically significant opioids agonist and antagonist activity in the CNS

A. Oxymorphone B. Nubaine

C. Narcan D. Dezocine

3801. Which one of the following is the multicyclic kappa agonist

A. Talwin B. Nubaine

C. Stadol D. All of the above

3802. Which among the following is multicyclic-mu- agonist

A. Talwin B. Revex

C. Opana D. Nubaine

3803. Which among the following is the partial mu- agonist

A. Buprenex B. Relistor

C. Talwin D. All of the above

3804. which among the following multicyclic opioids the level of mu-antagonism will be lower than of cyclopropyl methyl

A. N-butyl methyl

B. Tert-butyl methyl

C. N-cyclobutyl methyl

D. None of the above

3805. When di-hydro codeine subjected to Oppenauer oxidation and treat with equimolar quantity of tartaric acid it result in

A. Hydromorphine HCl

B. Hydrocodone tartrate

C. Dihydro codeine phosphate

D. Diamorphine HCl

3806. Which one of the following is also known as fentanyls

A. Dezocine B. Bitartrate

C. Oxymorphone D. Anilinopiperidine

3807. 5,6,7,8-tetrahydro-2-methylisoquinolinium bromide and pera-methoxybenzyl magnesium bromide reacts to form

A. Levorphanol tartrate

B. Hydrocodone tartrate

C. Dextromethorphan hydrobromide

D. None of the above

3808. Identify the compound

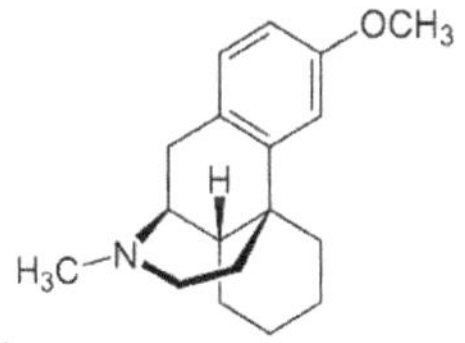

A. Levorphanol tartrate

B. Dextromethorphan

C. Butorphanol tartrate

D. Metazocine

3809. What is the value of R in following structure to produce the structure of dihydro codeine

A. R=CH3 B. R=CH3O
C. R=OH D. R=COOC2H5

3810. Name the structure, where

A. Meperidine B. Bemidone
C. Properidone D. Keto-bemidone

3811. Identify the compound where

R= CH3, R' = CH3

A. Pentazocine B. Ketazocine
C. Phenazocine D. Metazocine

3812. Following is the structure of

A. Sufentanic B. Tilidine
C. Tramadol D. Nixeridine

3813. What is the IUPAC name of the pethidine hydrochloride

A. 4-ethox-1-methyl-4-phenyl piperidine
B. 4-ethoxy-carbonyl-4,2-dimethy-piperidine
C. 4-ethoxy-carbonyl-1-methyl-4-phenyl piperidine
D. 1-ethoxy-carbonyl-4-methyl-4-phenylpiperidine

3814. Which of the following compound is formed when 3,4-epoxide bridge in morphine structure is removed

A. Morphinans B. Codeine
C. Tilidine D. Hydrocodeine

3815. When tertiary nitrogen in morphine is converted to the N-allyl, propyl then the compound formed will be

A. Less active than morphine
B. More active than morphine
C. Morphine antagonist
D. None of these

3816. N-phenyl-N-[1-(2-phenyl ethyl) -4-piperidinyl] propanamide is

A. Etorphine
B. Phenyl acetonitrile
C. Pethidine hydrochloride
D. fentanyl citrate

3817. Which method is used to synthesized anileridine

A. 4-phenylpiperidine-4-ethylcarboxylate
B. Bengal cyanide or 2-phenyl acetonitrile
C. Both A and B
D. Ethyl-4-phenyl piperidine-4- carboxylate

3818. Following is the structure of

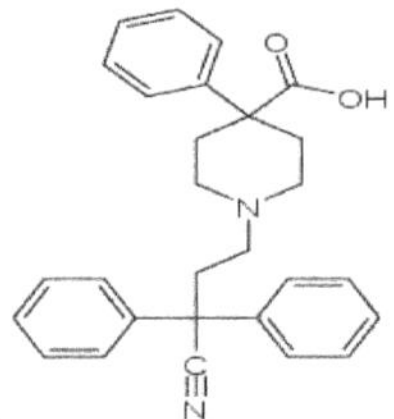

A. Dizocine B. Difenoxin
C. Sufentanil D. Naloxone

3819. Following is the structure of

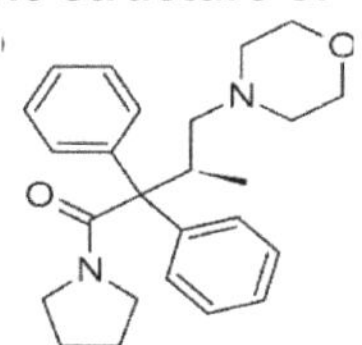

A. Dextromoramide B. Naloxone
C. Naltrexone D. Nalorphine

3820. Benzomorphan undergoes alkylation with phenyl ethyl chloride and form

A. Sufentanil B. Tramadol
C. Tilidine D. Phenazocine

3821. Following is the structure of

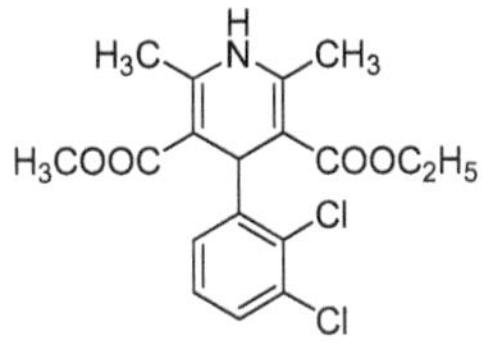

H
H_3C N CH_3
H_3COOC $COOC_2H_5$
Cl
Cl

A. Dipanone B. Normethadone
C. Isomethadone D. Methadone

3822. Which of the following isolated Acetylcholine from the ergot extract

A. Ewins
B. Hobnstedt
C. Kier and hall
D. November of the above

3823. Which of the following is the only muscarinic antagonist to block gastric acid secretion at concentration that did not block the effects of muscarinic agonist

A. Amphetamine B. Pirenzipine
C. Salmeterol D. None of these

3824. Which of the following posses GTPase activity?

A. Alpha-sub unit B. Beta-sub unit
C. Kappa-sub unit D. None of these

3825. Which of the following is involved with receptor operator K+ current?

A. Alpha B. Beta
C. Gamma D. Beta-gamma

3826. Which of the following drugs in predominantly block the muscarinic actions of Ach.?

A. Atropine B. Amphetamine
C. Propranolol D. All

3827. Which of the following are the naturally occurring alkaloid

A. Homoatropine B. Tiotropiun
C. Scopolamine D. All of the above

3828. Which of the following is the neuro muscular blocking agents

A. Tubocurarine B. Metocurine
C. Both A and B D. Hexamethonium

3829. Which among the following is the ganglionic blocking agent?

A. Hexamethonium
B. Curare alkaloids
C. Pancuronium bromide
D. All of the above

3830. Identify the compound

A. Atropine B. Hyoscine
C. Homoatropine D. Clidinium

3831. Which of the following is the tropine ester of racemic tropic acid?

A. Homoatropine B. Atropine
C. Hyoscine D. All

3832. What does *MR* represent in a QSAR equation?

A. Molar refractivity is a steric factor
B. Molar refractivity is an electronic factor
C. Molar refractivity is a hydrophobic factor
D. Molar refractivity is a stereo-electronic factor

3833. Which of the following produces brocho-dilation by competitive Inhibition of cholinergic receptors?

A. Ipratropium bromide
B. Atropine
C. Cyclo-pentolate Hydrochloride
D. None of these

3834. All are true about anti-muscarinics except

A. This agents do not have nocotinic receptor affinity
B. Mostly excreted unchanged into the urine
C. Agents biotransformed in the liver
D. Exerts both therapeutic and toxic actions in brain

3835. All of the following are amino alcohol esters except

A. Ipratropium bromide
B. Eucatropine HCl
C. Dicyclomine
D. Clidinium

3836. Homotropine synthesized by

A. Tropine
B. Tropine + tropic acid
C. Epoxytropine + tropic acid
D. Tropine + mandelic acid

3837. Epoxy tropine and tropic acid undergoes Esterification and gives

A. Atropine B. Homoatropine
C. Scopolamine D. Mandelic acid

3838. 3-OH-1-methylquinuclidium bromide benzilate is the

A. Glycopyrrolate bromide
B. Clidinium bromide
C. Diclidinium bromide HCl
D. Propanthelin bromide

3839. The drug illustrated below

1. White crystalline powder with bitter taste
2. Synthesized by 1,5-dibromo pentane
3. Spasmolytic effect on the various smooth muscle spasm
4. Usually used as eye drop to cause mydriasis

A. 1 and 2 and not true
B. 4 is not true
C. Only 3 and 4 are true
D. All are the true

3840. 8-methyl-8-aza-bicyclo(3.2.1) octane-3-yl-3-hydroxy-2-phenylpropanoate is the chemical name of

A. Tropicamide B. Atropine
C. Pirenzipine D. Scopolamine

3841. Following is the structure of

A. Trihexyl phenidyl B. Tropicamide
C. Ethopropazine HCl D. Pirenzipine

3842. When tropine and Mandelic acid reacts and undergoes Esterification it produce

A. Scopolamine B. Homoatropine
C. Atropine D. Dicyclomine

3843. IUPAC name of trihexyl- phenidyl is

A. 1-cyclohexyl-1-phenyl-4-piperidin-1-propan-3-ol
B. 4-cyclohexyl-1-phenyl-3-piperidin-1-ylpropan-1-ol
C. 1-cyclohexyl-1-phenyl-3-piperidin-1-ylpropan-1-ol
D. 1-cyclohexyl-1-phenyl-3-piperidin-1-ylpropan-1-one

3844. IUPAC name of dicyclomine HCl

A. 4-(diethylamino)ethyl 1-cyclohexylcyclohexane-1-carboxylatehydrochloride
B. 2-(diethylamino)ethyl 1-cyclohexylcyclohexane-1-carboxylatehydrochloride
C. 1-(diethylamino)ethyl 3-cyclohexylcyclohexane-1-carboxylate hydrochloride
D. 2-(diethylamino)ethyl 5-cyclohexylcyclohexanehydrochloride

3845. Following is the structure of

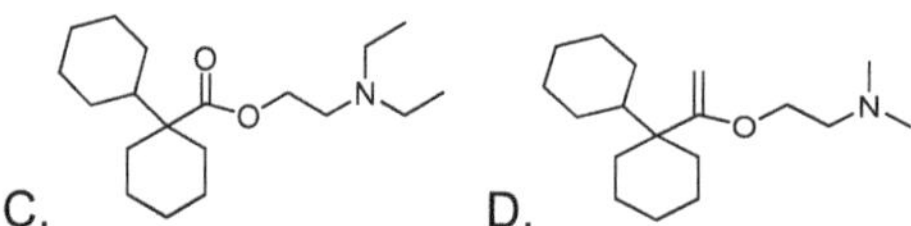

A. Tropicamide B. Atropine
C. Procyclidine D. Biperiden

3846. Identify the correct structure of dicyclomine

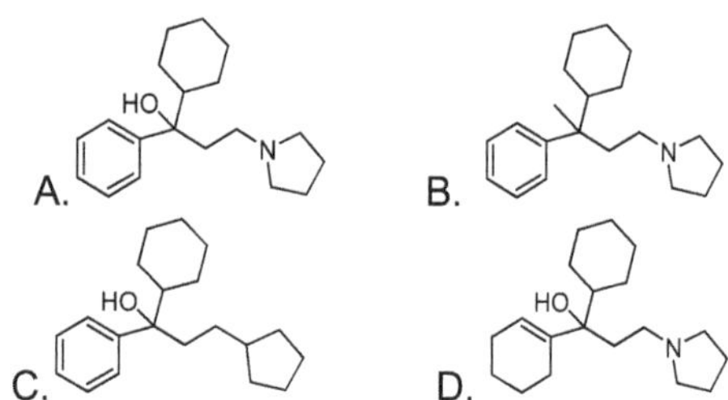

3847. Which one of the following is the correct structure of procyclidine HCl

A. B. C. D.

3848. 2-methyl benzhydrol reacts with 2-dimethyl amino ethanol to produce

A. Orphenadrine B. Biperiden
C. Procyclidine D. Trihexyl phenidyl

3849. Identify the compound

A. Propanthelin bromide
B. Glycopyrrolate bromide
C. Clidinium bromide
D. None of these

3850. 1-cyclohexyl-1-phenyl-3-pyrrolidin-1-yl-1-propanol HCL is the chemical name of

A. Dicyclomine HCl
B. Cyclo-pentolate HCl
C. Procyclidine HCl
D. Ethopropazine HCl

3851. IUPAC name of Acetylcholine chloride is

A. (2-acetoxyl ethyl) -trimethyl ammonium chloride
B. (2-acetoxylethyl)-triethylammoniumchloride
C. (3-acetoxyl ethyl) -dimethyl ammonium chloride
D. (2-acetoxylethyl)-dimethylammoniumchloride

3852. Choose the correct structure of VMA (vanillymandelic acid)

A. 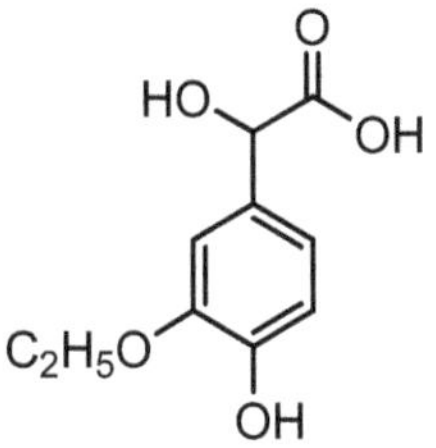 O, HO, OH, C_2H_5O, OH

B. 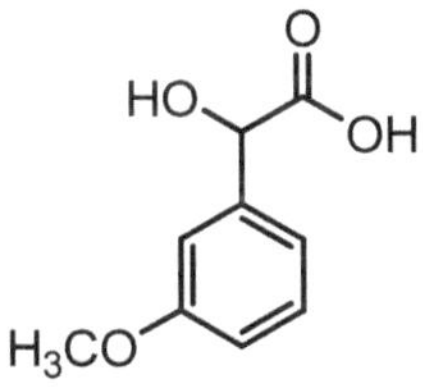 O, HO, OH, H_3CO

C. O, HO, OH, H_3CO, OH

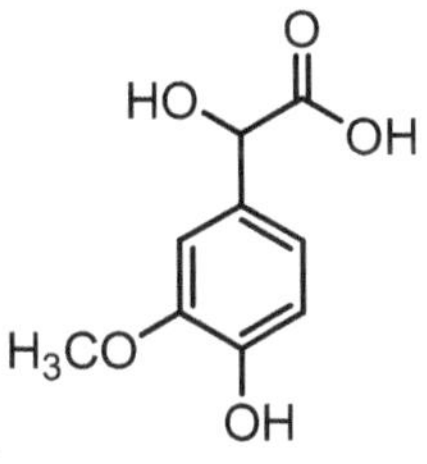

D. 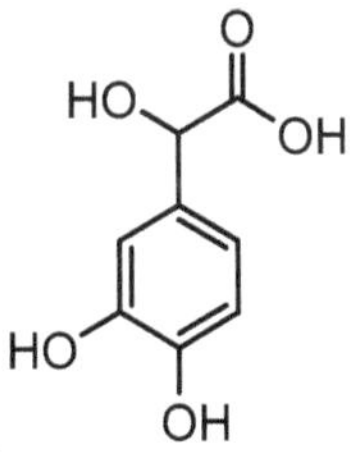 O, HO, OH, HO, OH

3853. Spasticity disorders can be characterized by the following:

A. Increase in tonic stretch reflexs.
B. Flexer muscle spasm together with muscle weakness.
C. Both a and b
D. None of the above

3854. Muscle spasticity mostly associated with

A. Multiple sclerosis
B. Spinal cord injury
C. Stroke and cerebral palsy
D. All of the above

3855. Parkinsons disease was 1st discovered by

A. James parkinsons
B. William gowers parkinsons
C. Charcot Parkinson
D. Corolus Linnaeus

3856. Which dopaminergic pathway degenerated in brain and cause parkinson's disease

A. Entorhinal cortex pathway
B. Corpus striatum pathway
C. Negostriated pathway
D. Frontal cortex pathway

3857. Analysis of brain tissue of Parkinson's disease patient has.

A. Increased level of glutathione
B. Increased lipid peroxidation
C. Increased oxidation of DNA and protein
D. All of the above.

3858. Rotenone is

A. Flavones.
B. Isoflavone.
C. Polyphenol.
D. Equol.

3859. Parkinsons disease is caused by the deficiency of which chemical in brain

A. GABA
B. Alpha synuclein
C. Dopamine
D. None of the above

3860. Average age of persons with parkinsons disease

A. Below 15
B. Between 15-25
C. Between 25-45
D. 50 or above

3861. Why dopamine is not used to treat parkinsons

A. Expensive
B. Have too many side effects
C. Cholinergic in nature
D. Does not cross BBB

3862. Parkinsons disease is

A. Movement disorder
B. Mental disorder
C. Psychological disorder
D. Personality disorder

3863. Nigrostriated neurodegenerative properties of MPTP are mediated by

A. MPDP+ B. MPPP
C. MPP+ D. Deprenyl

3864. PKa value of L-dopa is.

A. 10.6 B. 8.72
C. 11.6 D. 9.72

3865. Lewy bodies are.

A. Proteins deposits found in the brain
B. Clots of blood found in brain
C. Lipid deposits found in brain
D. A salt and crystalline matter

3866. What is the cause of parkinsons disease

A. Proteolytic stress B. Oxidative stress
C. Chronic stress D. Unknown

3867. Which one of the following is the co-factor for l-aromatic amino acids decarboxylase?

A. Riboflavin B. Pyridoxine
C. Cobalamine D. Niacin

3868. Which one of the following drugs shouldn't used in combination with levodopa

A. Droperidol B. Carbidopa
C. Pariopa D. Stavelo

3869. Parkinsons disease has how many stages

A. 3 stages B. 4 stages
C. 5 stages D. 7 stages

3870. Use of carbidopa-levodopa with MAOI's anti-depressants like isocarboxazid can result in

A. Severe elevations in blood pressure
B. Influenza
C. Anti-nausea treatments
D. Damage the cell

3871. Which one of the following known as "designer heroin" or :synthetic heroin"?

A. MPDP B. L-DOA
C. MPTP D. MPPP

3872. Which one of the following is the reverse ester of narcotic analgesics meperidine?

A. MPTP B. MPPP
C. L-DOPA D. MAO-B

3873. Levodopa is converted into the 3-orthomethyldopa in the presence of

A. Dopa decarboxylase B. COMT
C. MAO-B D. MAO-A

3874. Diphenhydramine is-

A. Phenothiazine analogue
B. Piperidine analogue
C. Pyrrolidine analogue
D. Piperazine analogue

3875. 3-(3,4-diphdroxyphenyl)-2-hydrazinyl-2-methylpropanoic acid is the IUPAC name of-

A. Levodopa B. Droxidopa
C. Carbidopa D. Benserazid

3876. Which one of the following drugs have both anti-parkinsonism and anti-viral activity

A. Procyclidine HCl
B. Trihexyphenidyl HCl
C. Ethopropazine HCl
D. Amantadine HCl

3877. Which drug is more effective than levodopa against parkinsons tremor

A. pramipexole B. Ropinirole
C. safinamide D. Trihexyphenidyl HCl

3878. Bromocryptine mesylate is-

A. Non- ergoline derivative
B. Glycoside derivative
C. Ergot derivative
D. Quercetin derivative

3879. Precursor compound for the synthesis of levadopa is

A. 4-methylbenzene-1,2-diol
B. 2-methylbenzene-1,2-diol
C. 4-methylbenzene-2,1-diol
D. 4,2-dimethylbenzene-2,1-diol

3880. Which one of the following atructure is the correct structure of biperiden

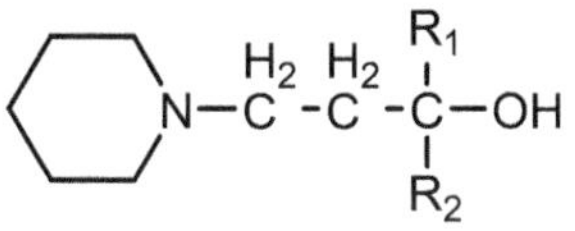

R_1
N–$\overset{H_2}{C}$–$\overset{H_2}{C}$–C–OH
R_2

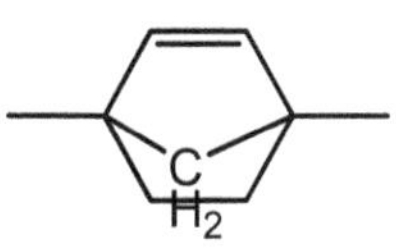

A. $R_1=R_2$

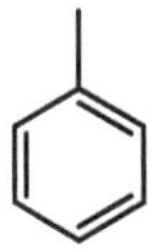

B. $R_1=$ C H_2 $R_{2=}$

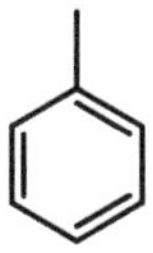

C. $R_1=$ 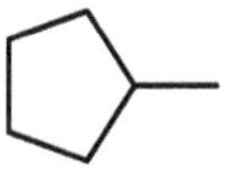 $R_{2=}$

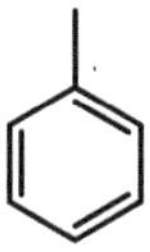

D. $R_1=$ 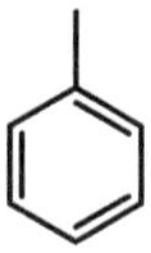 $R_{2=}$ C H_2

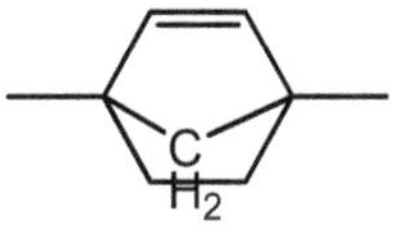

3881. IUPAC name of carbidopa

A. 3-(2,3,4-trihydroxyphenyl)-2-hydrazino-2-methylpropanoic acid

B. 3-(2,3-dihydroxyphenyl)-2-hydrazino-4-methylpropanoic acid

C. 3-(3,4-dihydroxyphenyl)-2-hydrazino-2-methylpropanoic acid

D. 3-(2,3-dihydroxyphenyl) propanoic acid

3882. Biperiden reduces all except

A. Tremor and akinesia

B. Drooling and sweating

C. Muscle rigidity

D. Muscle cramps

3883. IUPAC name of procyclidine

A. 1-cyclohexyl-1-phenyl-3-pyrrolidine-1-yl-propan-1-ol-hydrochloride

B. 1-cyclohexyl-3-phenyl-1-pyrrolidine-1-yl-propan-1-ol-hydrochloride

C. 1-cyclohexyl-1-phenyl-1-pyrrolidine-3-yl-propan-1-ol-hydrochloride

D. 1-cyclohexyl-1-phenyl-1-pyrrolidine-1-yl-propan-3-ol-hydrochloride

3884. All drugs are ergot derivatives except

A. Pergolide B. Bromocriptine

C. Apomorphine D. Lisuride

3885. Ethopropazine also used to control severe reactions of certain medicines except

A. chlorprothixene B. Reserpine

C. loxapine D. None of above

3886. Dopaminergic mediated physiological effects are dependent on

A. Affinity for DA receptors

B. Selectivity of ligand for DA receptors

C. Both a and b

D. Pattern for nerve impulse for DA receptors.

3887. Drugs used to treat spastic neuromuscular disorder have MOA that differ from those who used to treat

A. Alzheimer B. Parkinson's disease

C. Myopathy D. Myasthenia gravis

3888. Spasticity is characterized by

A. Skeletal muscle spasm

B. Increase in tonic stretch reflexes

C. Muscle weakness

D. All of the above

3889. Spasticity is frequently associated with

A. Cerebral palsy B. Multiple sclerosis

C. Spinal cord injury D. All of the above

3890. All of the following are glycerol monoethers and derivatives except

A. Mephenesin

B. Meprobamate

C. Methocarbamole

D. Chlorphenesin carbamate

3891. Correct structure of cyclobenzaprine

A. 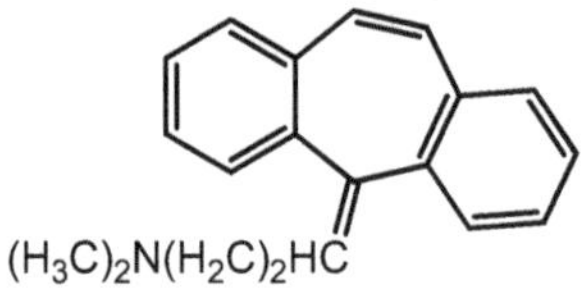 $(H_3C)_2N(H_2C)_2HC$

B. 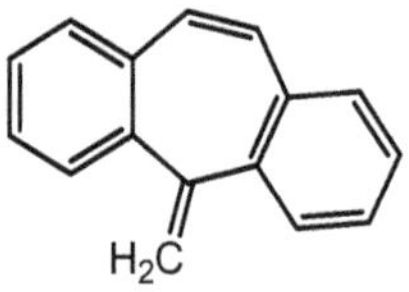 H_2C

C. 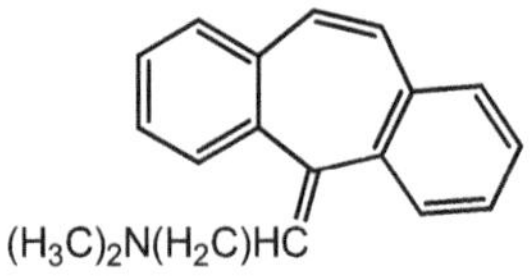 $(H_3C)_2N(H_2C)HC$

D. 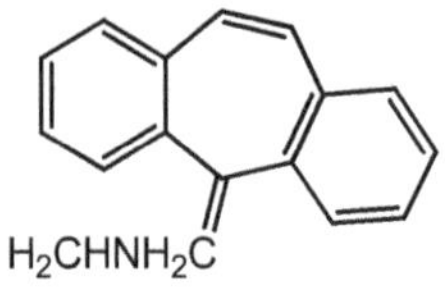 H_2CHNH_2C

3892. Dantrolene is

A. Adrenergic α2 receptor
B. Benzodiazepine derivative
C. Hydantoin derivative
D. GABAB receptor agonist

3893. Site of action of dantrolene

A. Sarcoplastic reticulum
B. Blood brain barrier
C. Adrenergic pathway
D. None of the above

3894. Mode of action of baclofen

A. Inhinit spinal cord monosynaptic and polysynaptic refelxes via GABAB receptor
B. Binds to calcium channel protein on the sarcoplasmic reticulum to close the channel
C. Bind as agonist at the benzodiazepine receptor at the GABAA receptor complex, increase chloride conductance
D. Inhibit release of excitatory amino acids in the spinal interneurons

3895. IUPAC name of diazepam

A. 7-chloro-1,3-dihydro-1-methyl-5-phenyl-2H-1, 4-benzodiazepine-2-one
B. 5-chloro-1,3-dihydro-1-methyl-7-phenyl-2H-1,4-benzodiazepine-6-one
C. 7-chloro-4,7-dihydro-1-methyl-3-phenyl-2H-1, 4-benzodiazepine-2-one
D. None of the above

3896. 3-(2-methylphenoxy) propane-1, 2-diol is chemical name of which one of skeletal muscle relaxants

A. Metaxolone B. Mephenesin
C. Chlorzoxazone D. Cyclobenzaprine

3897. First drug recognised to exhibit spasmolytic activity was

A. Mephenesin
B. Chlorphenesin carbamate
C. Antodyne
D. Methocarbamole

3898. Mode of action of dantrolene

A. Inhibit excitation- contraction coupling in muscle fibre
B. Inhibit multi-synaptic reflexes in the spinal cord
C. Inhibit interneuron action
D. Inhibit polysynaptic excitation of motor neurons

3899. Lioresal is

A. Zanaflex B. Baclofen
C. Dantrium D. Valium

3900. Which one of the following inhibit prolactin release from interior pituitary mammotrophic cells

A. Ropinrole B. Rotingotine
C. Bromocriptine D. Lisuride

3901. Which one of the following is the MAO-B inhibitor

A. Metaprolol B. Rasagiline
C. Imipramine D. 1-aminoindan

3902. Which one of the following are the drugs which are able to reduce unwanted spasm-without interfering the consciousness

A. Tubercurarine B. Nefopem
C. Bretylium tosylate D. Both A and B

3903. Which one of the following occur when there is a release of acetylcholine from presynaptic vesicles

A. Skeletal muscle relaxants
B. Skeletal muscle contraction
C. Adrenergic
D. Cholinergic

3904. Which one of the following is the auto immune disease associated with skeletal muscle relaxants

A. Parkinson's B. Myasthemia gravis
C. Schizophrenia D. None of the above

3905. The drug which contain two acetylcholine binding site

A. Gallamine triethiodide
B. Dobutamine
C. Aramine
D. None of the above

3906. Most of the non- depolarizing blockers have ____________ nitrogen atoms

A. Zero
B. One
C. Two
D. Two or more quaternary atom

3907. Which one of the following is the precursor of the succinyl choline chloride

A. CH_2COOH–CH_2COOH

B. H_2C–$C(H_2)$–COOH / H_2C–$C(H_2)$–COOH (the two H_2C carbons bonded together)

C. H_2C–$COCH_3$ / H_2C–$COCH_3$ (the two H_2C carbons bonded together)

D. CH_3–HC(–COOH)–CH_3

3908. Aliskiren belongs to which category of anti-hypertensive drugs?

A. Arteriolar dilator
B. Alpha-beta adrenergic blockers
C. Central sympatholytic
D. Direct renin inhibitor

3909. What are the drugs of choice for uncomplicated hypertension?

A. Indapamide
B. Furosemide
C. Hydrochlorthalidone
D. Chlorthalidone

3910. Tick the percent by which plasma 4 ecf. Volume is reduced by thiazide?

A. 5-15% B. 20-25%
C. 35-40% D. 15-30%

3911. Anti hypertensive action of thiazides is attenuated by which category of drugs?

A. Sedative and hypnotic
B. NSAIDs
C. Local anaesthetic
D. Adrenergic

3912. What is the major drawback of thiazide due to which it is withdrawn from market?

A. Gynacomastia
B. Sudden episodes of tausades de pointes
C. Congestive heart failure
D. Sexual dysfunction

3913. Precursor compound in the synthesis of captopril

A. 2-oxo-4-phenyl ethyl butyrate
B. 2-methyl-2-propenoic acid
C. 2-formyl benzoic acid
D. Guanidine

3914. When 2-oxo-4-phenyl ethyl butyrate and L-alanyl proline react together they lroduce

A. Lisinopril B. Ramipril
C. Enalapril D. Candesartan

3915. Mode of action of losartan

A. Inhibit the binding of angiotensin II to the AT 1 receptor
B. Decrease peripheral resistance
C. Increase vascular resistance and blood pressure
D. Increase action of angiotensin II

3916. 2,4- diamino-6-piperidino pyrimidine-3-oxide is the

A. Valsartan B. Losartan
C. Hydralazine D. Minoxidil

3917. Reaction of 2-amino-chlorobenzene sulfonamide and triethyl-o-acetate result in the
A. Diazoxide
B. Minoxidil
C. Sodium nitroprusside
D. Benazepril

3918. Which of the following high ceiling diuretic is a strong diuretic but weak hypertensive than thiazide?
A. Torsemide B. Bumetanide
C. Furosemide D. None of these

3919.Fall of blood pressure depends on
A. Reduction of plasma volume
B. Cardiac output
C. Natriuretic
D. All of the above

3920. Which one of this is a side effect of high ceiling diuretic?
A. Electolyte imbalance
B. Weakness
C. Skin rashes
D. Nausea

3921. Which of the category of drug causes erectile dysfunction in males?
A. Thiazide
B. Loop diuretics
C. High ceiling diuretic
D. Weak diuretic

3922. Which of the drug causes precipitation of diuretics?
A. Furosemide
B. Chlorthalidone
C. Hydrochlorothiazide
D. Indapamide

3923. Why precipitation of diuretics occurs?
A. Die to deposition of potassium
B. Hyponatremia
C. Hypocalcaemia
D. Due to inhibition of insulin release

3924. Which kind or category of drug increases atherogenic risk?
A. High ceiling diuretic
B. Moderate efficiency diuretic
C. Potassium diuretic
D. Thiazide

3925. Which category of drug causes increases incidence of gout?
A. Thiazide
B. Aldosterone antagonist
C. Potassium sparing
D. High ceiling diuretic

3926. Which of the drug is not contraindicated in dialutes?
A. Furosemide B. Hydrochlorothiazide
C. Indapamide D. Zipamide

3927. Which of the category of drug reduces left ventricular hypertrophy?
A. High ceiling B. Weak diuretic
C. Thiazide D. Case inhibitor

3928. Which of the following osmotic diuretic is non-hygroscopic and non carcinogenic
A. Manitol B. Isosorbide
C. Urea D. Glycerol

3929. Which of the drug treat moutain sickness?
A. Brinzolamide B. Acetazolamide
C. Dorzolamide D. Dolbutamide

3930. Which of the drug treat morning sickness?
A. Dolbutamine B. Amlodipine
C. Doxylamine D. Nifidipine

3931. Which of the drug causes bone marrow depression?
A. Acetazolamide B. Indapamide
C. Xipamide D. Brinzolamide

3932. Which of the drug is contraindicated to dialutes patient?
A. Xipamide B. Indapamide
C. Dorzilamide D. Acetazolamide

3933. Which of the drug is given in lithium induced dialutes insipidus
A. Trianturene B. Methotrexate
C. Amiloxide D. Spironolactone

3934. What is the metabolite of sodium nitropreside?
A. Prazocine B. Thiocyanate
C. Xipamide D. Amiloxide

3935. Plasma half life of prazosin hydrochloride is between
A. 7-8 hours B. 10-12 hours
C. 30 min-1 hour D. 2-3 hours

3936. Terazosin hydrochloride specifically inhibits which receptors?

A. alpha 1 adrenergic receptors
B. Alpha 2 adrenergic receptors
C. Beta 1 adrenergic receptors
D. Beta 2 adrenergic receptors

3937. What effect does p-hydroxy clonidine produces over body?

A. Increase blood pressure
B. Decrease blood pressure
C. Decrease pulse rate
D. No effect

3938. 1st line drug of choice for the patients younger than 55 in hypertension is

A. Calcium channel blockers
B. Thiazide type diuretic
C. Drugs acting on sympathetic system
D. ACE inhibitor

3939. As the anti-hypertensive agents, what is the efficacy of beta- adrenergic blockers in mild to moderate cases?

A. 10-20% B. 30-40%
C. 50-60% D. 90%

3940. 1st orally effective ACE inhibitor is

A. Lisinopril B. Ramipril
C. Captopril D. Enalapril

3941. which of the following drug is used to treat severe hypertension and baldness?

A. Minoxidil B. Diazoxide
C. Verapalmil D. Moxonidine

3942. Name the compound whose structure is shown below

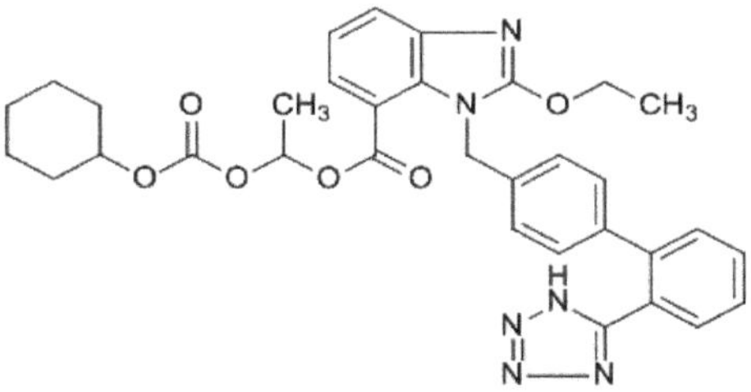

A. Losartan B. Irbesartan
C. Candesartan D. Valsartan

3943. Correct chemical structure of quinapril

A.

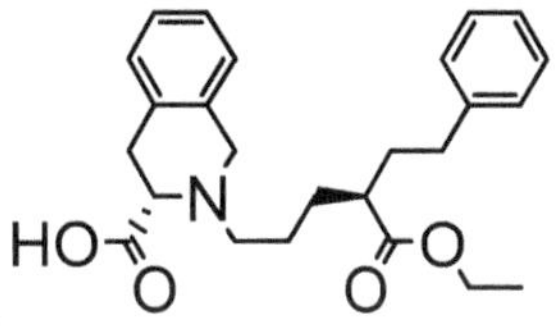

B.

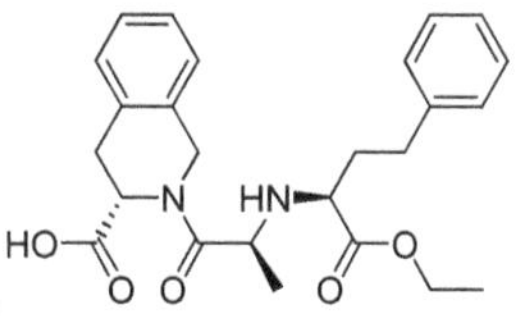

C.

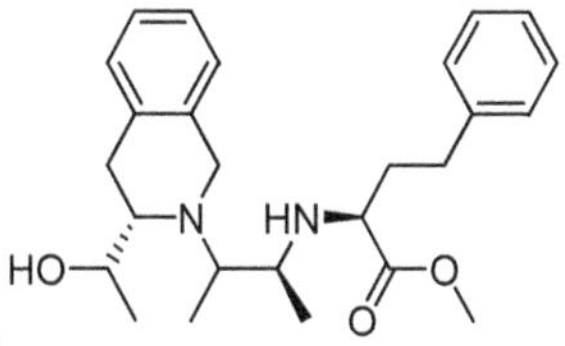

D.

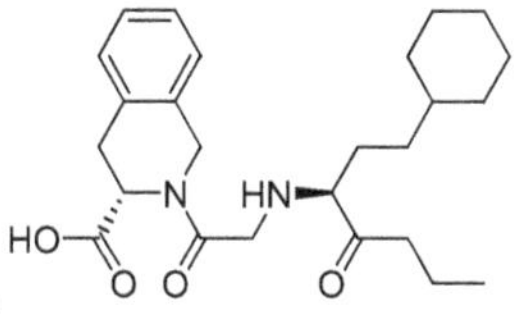

3944. 7-chloro-3methyl-H-1,2,4-benzothiadiazine-1, 1-dioxide is

A. Trietyl-o-acetate
B. L-alanyl proline dioxide
C. Hydralazide
D. Diazoxide

3945. Benazepril is produced by

A. 2,3--dihydro-1H- benzobazepin-1, (3H) – one
B. 1,5-dihydro-1H-benzo[b]azepin-2, (3H)-one
C. 4,5-dihydro-1H-benzo[b]azepin-2, (3H)-one
D. 2,3,5-trihydro-1H-benzo[b]azepin-2, (3H)-one

3946. Following is the structure of

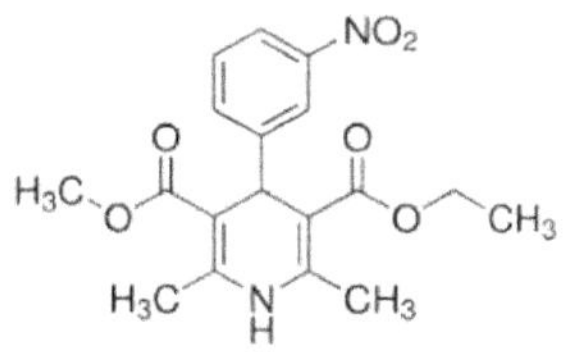

A. Nicardipine B. Amlodipine
C. Nitrendipine D. Felodipine

3947. Mode of action of verapalmil
- A. Increase vascular resistance
- B. Decrease peripheral resistance
- C. Dilate blood vessels
- D. Inhibit calcium influx

3948. Following is the structure of

- A. Guanabenz
- B. Alpha-methyl dopa
- C. Reserpine
- D. Atenolol

3949. 1-[N-(S)-1-carboxy-3-phenylpropyl]-L-alanyl]-1-proline-1'-ethyl ester is
- A. Captopril
- B. Enalapril
- C. Spirapril
- D. Moexipril

3950. What is the Name the structure

- A. Enalapril
- B. Lisinopril
- C. Enalaprilat
- D. Ramipril

3951. Correct structure of pempidine

A. 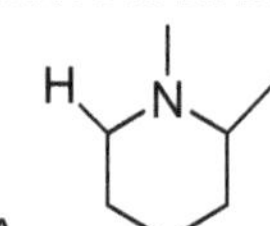

B.

C. 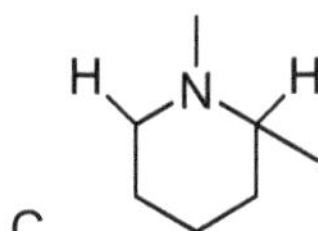

D.

3952. Correct structure of the debrisoquine

A.

B.

C.

D.

3953. Potassium Ferrocyanide is dissolved in 50% HNO3 boiled and then neutralized with sodium carbonate and later evaporate to form
- A. Diazoxide
- B. Methyl dopa
- C. Sodium nitroprusside
- D. Hydralazine

3954. When 2-amino-5-chlorobenzene sulphonamide is react with ethylorthoacetate they form
- A. Diazoxide
- B. Clonidine
- C. Methyldopa
- D. Minoxidil

3955. The given structure is of

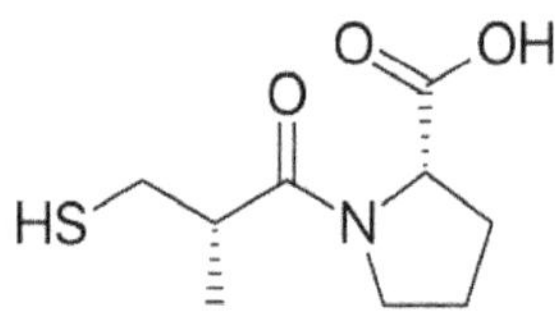

- A. Moexipril
- B. Ramipril
- C. Trandolapril
- D. Captopril

3956. 1-[(2S)-3-mercapto-2-methyl-1-oxopropionyl] pyrrolidine-2-carboxylic acid is the chemical name of the
- A. Pinacidil
- B. Captopril
- C. Pargyline
- D. Metyrosine

3957. Following is the structure of
- A. Diltiazem
- B. Amlodipine
- C. Felodipine
- D. Nicardipine

3958. Drugs used in Prinzmental angina is
- A. Verapalmil
- B. Propranolol
- C. Amlodipine
- D. Felodipine

3959. Nitrates are used for
- A. Increase venous return
- B. Increase myocardial O2 demand
- C. Esophageal spasm
- D. Increase preload and afterload

3960. Drugs used sublingually is
A. Amlodipine
B. Ergotamine tartate
C. Isosorbide-5-mononitrate
D. Methyl nocotinate

3961. Nitroglycerin can not be administered by
A. Oral B. Sublingual
C. Intramuscular D. Intravenous

3962. Which one of the following is the not the side effect of nitrates
A. Headache and dizziness
B. GI disturbance
C. Rapid heart beat
D. Nausea and vomiting

3963. All are true about organic nitrated except
A. Dominated the treatment of angina over the last 100 years
B. Esters of simple organic alcohols or polyols with nitric acid
C. Presence of nitrates receptor on vascular smooth muscles postulated by L. P. Needleman and K. Johnson
D. typically given sublingually and have a rapid onset of action

3964. Which type of angina is triggered by exertion or exercise
A. Hyberden angina
B. Variant angina
C. Classical angina
D. Microvascular angina

3965. Prinzmental angina may not be referred as
A. Angina inversa
B. Prinzmental-variant angina
C. Variant angina
D. Classical angina

3966. Which one the following is rare type of angina
A. Prinzmental angina
B. Classical angina
C. Heberden angina
D. Microvascular angina

3967. Class of drug which reduce and prevent ischaemic episodes in patient with variant angina is
A. Nitrites
B. Calcium channel blockers
C. Both of the above
D. β- blockers

3968. Which one of the following is the IUPAC name of the nitroglycerin
A. 1,2,3-trinitroxypropane
B. 1,2,3-trinitroxypropene
C. 1,2-dinitroxypropane
D. 2,3,6-trinitroxypropane

3969. Precursor compound in the synthesis of Pentaerythritol is
A. Acetaldehyde B. Formaldehyde
C. Both D. Erythritol

3970. What is the bioavailability of diltiazem
A. 45% B. 64%
C. 35% D. 40%

3971. IUPAC name of Felodipine
A. 4-(2,3-Dichlorophenyl)-2,6-dimethyl-1,4-dihydropyridine-3,5-dicarboxylic acid
B. 4-(2,3-Dichlorophenyl)-2,6-dimethyl-3,5-dihydropyridine-1,4-dicarboxylic acid
C. 4-(2,6-Dichlorophenyl)-2,3-dimethyl-1,5-dihydropyridine-3,4-dicarboxylic acid
D. 4-(2,6-Dichlorophenyl)-1,4-dimethyl-3,5-dihydropyridine-2,3-dicarboxylic acid

3972. Richest source of cardiac glycoside is
A. Digitalis B. Squill
C. Strophanthus D. Quabin

3973. Anti anginal agents prevent anginal attacks by
A. Dilating the coronary vein
B. Contracting the coronary vein
C. Dilating the coronary artery
D. Contracting the coronary artery

3974. All of the following drugs is organic nitrate esters except
A. Nitroglycerin
B. Amyl nitrite
C. Isosorbide dinitrate
D. Erythrityl tetranitrate

3975. How many classes of calcium channel blockers approved for use in prophylactic treatment of angina
A. 2 classes B. 1 class
C. 3 classes D. All of the above

3976. All are the side effects of calcium channel blockers except

A. Dizziness and headache
B. Hypotension
C. Rapid heart beat
D. Peripheral and pulmonary edema

3977. Duration of action of nicardipine and diltiazem

A. 4-8 hours B. 6-8 hours
C. 5-8 hours D. 4-9 hours

3978. Duration of action of amlodipine

A. 24 hours B. 28 hours
C. 12 hours D. 20 hours

3979. Myocardial workload will be decreased by

A. Decrease in preload and increase in after load
B. Increase in preload and decrease in after load
C. Decrease in both preload and after load
D. Increase in both preload and after load

3980. Placement of electron withdrawing substitution in dihydropyridines result in

A. Antagonistic activity
B. Agonistic activity
C. Increase the activity
D. Reduce the activity

3981. At which position phenyl substitution is optimum for activity in dihydropyridines

A. 4th B. 5th
C. 3rd D. 1st

3982. Precursor compound in the synthesis of nicorandil

A. Methyl nicotinate B. 2-aminoethanol
C. Both A and B D. Isopentyl alcohol

3983. Lacidipine is

A. β-adrenergic blocking agent
B. Diphenyl alkylamines
C. Diamino propanol ether
D. Calcium channel blockers

3984. Mode of action of isradipine is

A. relax the smooth muscle in the walls of arteries, resulting in them opening and allowing blood to flow more easily
B. Binds to calcium channels with high affinity and specificity and inhibits calcium flux into cardiac and smooth muscle.
C. inhibits the transmembrane influx of calcium ions into cardiac and vascular smooth muscle
D. None of the above

3985. 2,2',2'',2'''-(4,8-di(piperidin-1-yl)pyrimido[5,4-d]pyrimidine-2,6-diyl)bis(azanetriyl)tetraethanol is the iupac name of

A. Dipyridamole B. Quabain
C. Verapalmil D. Deslonoside

3986. Nifedipine synthesized by

A. M-chloro cyano benzene
B. 4-mercaptophenol
C. Hantzsch synthesis
D. 3-methyl pyridine

3987. Mode of action of beta- adrenergic blockers

A. Block specific channel and decrease the threshold for excitability
B. Slow the heart rate and decrease myocardial contractility
C. Decrease the conduction velocity in fast response tissue
D. Increase QRS duration

3988. Pentaerythritol is

A. Nitrate ester B. Amyl nitrite
C. Diacetyl derivative D. Nitroglycerin

3989. Drug used in emergency management of cyanide poisoning is

A. Nitroglycerin B. Amyl nitrite
C. Erythrityl tetranitrate D. Erythritol

3990. Following is the structure of

A. Nitroglycerin B. Bepridil
C. Isosorbide dinitrate D. Nicorandil

3991. All are true about organic nitrates except

A. They can activate Guanyly cyclase
B. Activate PKG
C. Decrease the cellular level of cyclic GMP
D. Modulate the activities of phosphodiesterases

3992. Which one of the following drug is nitric acid ester of the tetrahydric alcohol pentaerythritol

A. Erythritol tetranitrate
B. Pentaerythritol tetranitrate
C. Pentaerythritol nitrate
D. None of the above

3993. Which of the following cause the oxidation of haemoglobin toh the compound methemoglobin

A. Amylnitrite B. Nicorandil
C. Nitroglycerin D. Isosorbide dinitrate

3994. Drug which inhibit adenosine deaminase in erythrocytes is

A. Deslanoside B. Digoxit
C. Digitoxin D. Dipyridamole

3995. Angina will be cause by

A. Atherosclerotic plaque in the coronary artery
B. Coronary vasospasm
C. Imbalance between oxgen required in blood and oxygen supply to it by coronary artery
D. All of the above

3996. Angina may be corrected by

A. Increasing O2 delivery
B. Reducing O2 requirement
C. Efficiency of O2 utilization
D. All of the above

3997. In phenyl-dihydropyridine derivatives structural features which are essential for the activity are-

A. Dihydropyridine ring
B. Bulky substituent in 4th position of heterocycle
C. Secondary nitrogen in the ring
D. All of the above

3998. What is the name of following compound where:

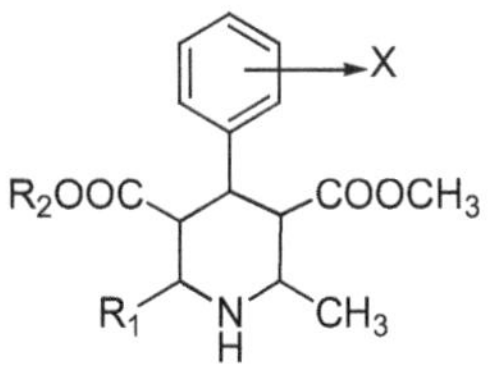

X
R_2OOC $COOCH_3$
R_1 N H CH_3

R1 = CH3
R2 = CH3
X = 2,3-Cl

A. Felodipine B. Nifidipine
C. Nicardipine D. Nimodipine

3999. Following is the structure of

O O O N S O

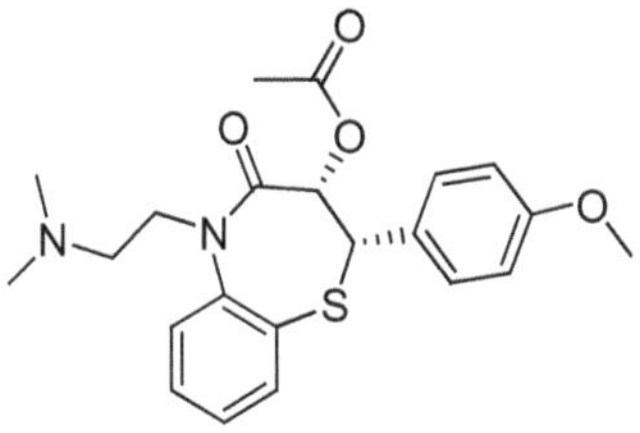

A. Aspirin B. Verapalmil
C. Diltiazem D. Bepridil

4000. 2,2-bis(hydroxymethyl) -1,3-propane diol tetranitrate is the

A. Pentaerythritol tetranitrate
B. Erythrityl tetranitrate
C. Nicorandil
D. Nitroglycerin

4001. Following is the structure of

HO O N H

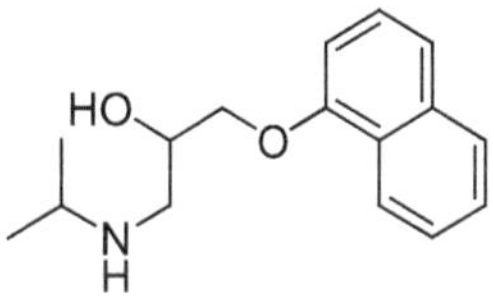

A. Sotalol B. Timolol
C. Propranolol D. None of these

4002. Which of the following is the Correct structure of cyclandelate

A. 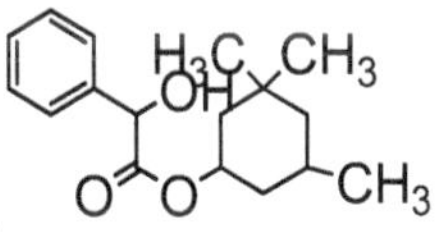 H_3C CH_3 OH O O CH_3

B. 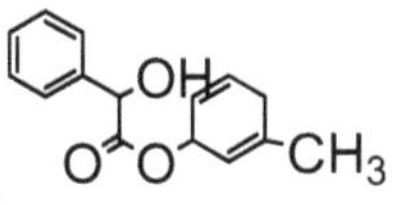 OH O O CH_3

C. 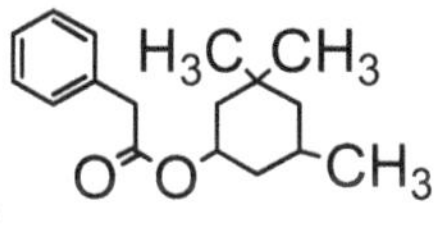 H_3C CH_3 O O CH_3

D. 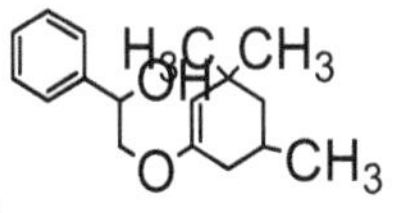 H_3C CH_3 OH O CH_3

4003. Identify the correct structure of isosorbide dinitrate

A.

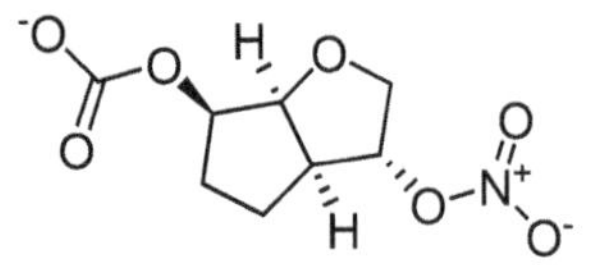

B.

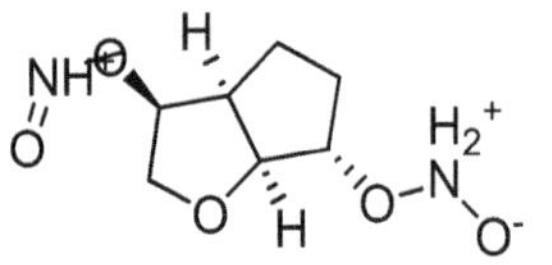

C.

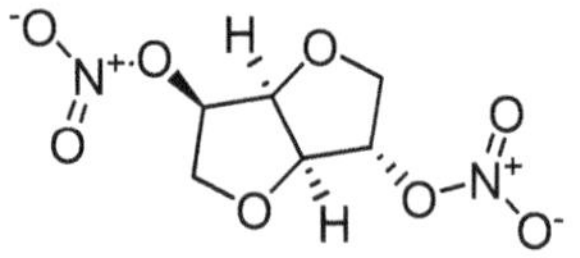

D.

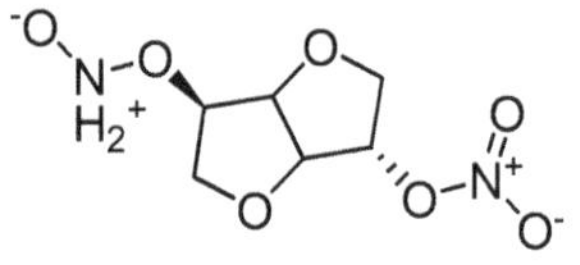

4004. Precursor compound in the synthesis of bepridil

A. Pyrrolidine B. Epichlorhydrine
C. Both A and B D. Ethyl acetoacetate

4005. 2,2-bis(diethanol amino) -4,8-dipiperidine pyrimido-(5, 4,d) -pyrimidine is the

A. Dipyridamole B. Pyrrolidine
C. Digoxin D. Digitoxin

4006. Following is the structure of

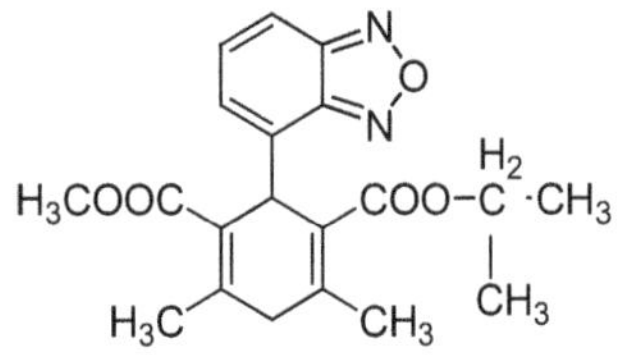

A. Amlodipine B. Nimodipine
C. Nisoldipine D. Isradipine

4007. What is the IUPAC name of the amlodipine

A. 3-ethyl 5-methyl-2-(2-aminoethoxymethyl)-4-(2-chlorophenyl)-6-methyl-1,4-dihydropyridine-3,5-dicarboxylate
B. 3-ethyl 5-methyl-2-(2-aminoethoxymethyl)-4-(2-chlorophenyl)-6-methyl-1,4-dihydropyridine-3,5-dicarboxylate
C. 3-ethyl-(2-aminoethoxymethyl)-4-(2-chlorophenyl)-5-methyl-1,4-dihydropyridine-3,5-dicarboxylate
D. 3-ethyl 5-methyl-2-(2-aminoethoxymethyl)-4-(2-chlorophenyl)-6-methyl3-carboxylate

4008. Diuretics are the chemical which

A. Increase the rate of urine formation
B. Increase the blood flow
C. Decrease the rate of urine formation
D. Decrease the blood flow

4009. Important functions of kidney

A. Maintain homeostatic balance of electrolytes and water
B. Excrete water-soluble end products of metabolism
C. Both
D. None of these

4010. Majority of filtered sodium is reabsorbed from which part of nephron?

A. Proximal straight tubule
B. proximal convulated tubule
C. Descending loop's of henle
D. Distal convulated tubule

4011. Which one of the following is the primary site for the bicarbonate reabsorbtion?

A. DCT B. PCT
C. Descending loop of henle
D. Ascending loop of henle

4012. In which segment of nephron, 20-25% of the filtered Na+ and Cl- are absorbed on the luminal membrane

A. PCT
B. DCT
C. Descending loop of henle
D. Ascending loop of henle

4013. Why calomel replaced by the organomercurials

A. Poor absorption from GIT
B. Toxicity C. Both
D. Tolerance

4014. Anti- diuretic hormomes (ADH) act on which part of nephron

A. Bowman's capsule
B. Collecting tubule
C. PCT D. DCT

4015. Site of action of thiazides and thiazide like drug
A. Distal tubule B. PCT
C. Collecting duct D. Bowman's capsule

4016. Site of action of osmotic
A. Proximal tubule B. Loop of henle
C. Collecting tubule D. All of the above

4017. Mechanics of action of osmotics involve all except
A. Decrease water and sodium reabsorbtion
B. Inhibition of Na+ Cl- symporter
C. Increase medullary blood flow to decrease medullary hypertonicity
D. Reduce medullary hypertonicity and elevated urinary flow rate

4018. The thiazide diuretics are
A. Strongly acidic B. Strongly basic
C. Weakly acidic D. Weakly basic

4019. Commonly used diuretics used in sport doping are, except
A. Hydrochlorothiazide
B. Triamterene
C. Furosemide
D.

4020. Diuretics used in sport doping because
A. Eliminate rapidly B.
C. D.

4021. Site of action of thiazide and thiazide like compound
A. DCT B. PCT
C. Collecting tubule D. Loop of henle

4022. Duration of action of acetazolamine
A. 2min-60 min B. 1-4hrs
C. 4-8 hrs D. 8-12 hrs

4023. Isosorbide is the basically
A. Bicyclic form of mannitol
B. Bicyclic form of sorbitol
C. Cyclic form of sorbitol
D. Cyclic form of mannitol

4024. Which of the following inhibits angiogenesis?
A. VEGF
B. FGF-2
C. Angiostatin
D. Interleukin-6

4025. Structure of acetazolamine

A. $H_2N-C(=O)-$ thiadiazole ring (S, N–N) $-NH-C(=O)-CH_3$

B. H_2N-SO_2- ring (N–N) $-NH-C(=O)-CH_3$

C. $H_2N-C(=O)-$ thiadiazole ring (S, N–N) $-NH-C(=O)-Cl$

D. H_2N-SO_2- thiadiazole ring (S, N–N) $-NH-C(=O)-CH_3$

4026. Structure of brinzolamine

A. H_2N-SO_2- thienothiazine dioxide, N-(CH$_2$)$_3$-OCH$_3$, HN-CH$_2$-

B. H_2N-SO_2- thienothiazine dioxide, N-(CH$_2$)$_3$-OCH$_3$, HN-CH$_2$-CH$_3$

C. CH_3-SO_2- thienothiazine dioxide, N-(CH$_2$)$_3$-OCH$_3$, HN-CH$_2$-CH$_3$

D. H_2N-SO_2- thienothiazine dioxide, N-(CH$_2$)$_3$-OCH$_3$, HN-CH$_3$

4027. Structure of dichlorphenamide

A. 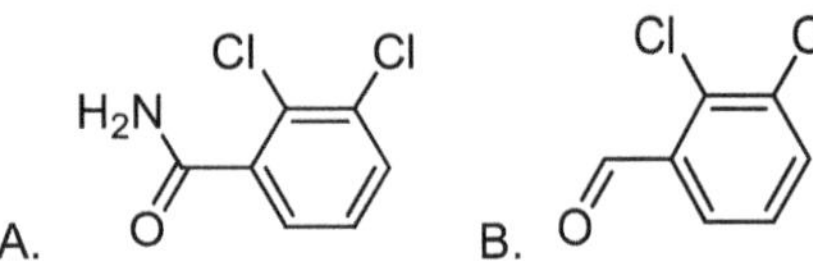

B. (Cl, Cl, O)

C. (Cl, Cl, H_2N, H)

D. (Cl, Cl, H_2N, H)

4028. Which one of the following is the first carbonic anhydrase inhibitors to be introduced as an orally effective diuretic

A. Ethoxzolamide B. Acetazolamide
C. Methazolamide D. Dorzolamide

4029. Methazolamide have a greater penetration into the ocular fluid because of

A. Thiazide ring replaced by methyl group
B.
C. D.

4030. Dichlorophenamide is

A. Phenoxyacetic acid derivative
B. Sulphonamide derivative
C. Disulfonamide derivative
D. Anthranilic acid derivative

4031. The drug which penetrate cornea are

A. Brinzolamide B. Dichlorphenamide
C. Ethoxzolamide D. Methazolamide

4032. In the structure, at which position an electron withdrawing group is necessary for diuretics activity

(N, NH, S, O, O)

A. 4 B. 5
C. 6 D. 7

4033. Following substitution increase lipid solubility of molecule with longer duration of action except

A. Haloalkyl B. Aralkyl
C. Thioether D. Methoxyl

4034. Tri-fluoromethyl substituted diuretics are

A. More lipid soluble and shorter duration of action
B. More lipid soluble and longer duration of action
C. Less lipid soluble and longer duration of action
D. Less lipid soluble and shorter duration of action

4035. Saturation of double bond to give 3,4-dihydro derivatives produces a diuretic that is ___________ fold more active than unsaturated diuretics

A. 10 fold B. 8 fold
C. 4 fold D. 2 fold

4036. Effect of alkyl substitution on the 2-N position on polarity and duration of diuretic action

A. Increase the polarity and increase the duration of diuretic action
B. Increase the polarity and decrease the duration of diuretic action
C. Decrease the polarity and increase the duration of diuretic action
D. Decrease the polarity and decrease the duration of diuretic action

4037. Duration of effect of benzthiazide

A. 01-04 hours B. 04-08 hours
C. 08-12 hours D. 12-16 hours

4038. Bioavailability of bendroflumethiazide

A. >75% B. >90%
C. >80% D. >60%

4039. Long term use of thiazide diuretics may result in

A. Decrease glucose tolerance
B. Increase blood lipid content
C. Both A and B
D. Electrolyte embalance

4040. Half life and duration of action of quinethazone

A. 14 hours and 12-24 hours
B. 6-15 hours and 18-24 hours
C. 35-50 hours and 48-72 hours
D. 14-18 hours and 8 weeks

4041. Replacement or removal of the sulfonamide group at position 7 yield compound have

A. Increase in potency
B. More lipid solubility

C. Little and no diuretic activity
D. High diuretic activity

4042. All of them are true about chlorthalidone except
A. Belongs to sulfamolbenzamide class
B. Long acting thiazide like diuretic
C. Increase calcium and uric acid secretion
D. Devoid of benzothiadiazine structure

4043. Indapamide contain
A. Polar chlorobenzamide moiety
B. Thiazide ring
C. Non-polar hydrophobic methyl indoline group
D. Polar lipophilic methylindoline group

4044. Correct structure of furosemide

A. 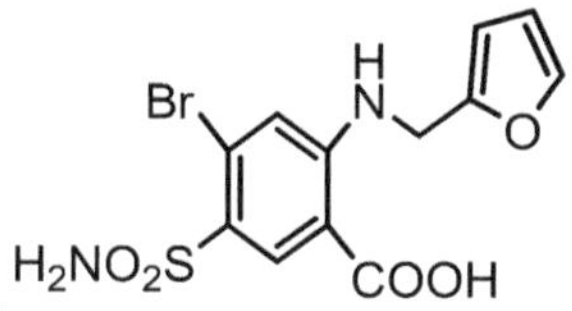 Br, H, N, O, H_2NO_2S, COOH

B. 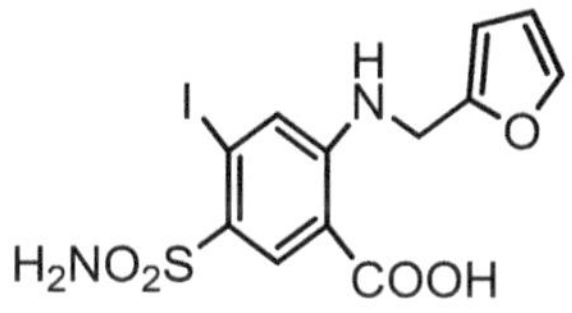 I, H, N, O, H_2NO_2S, COOH

C. 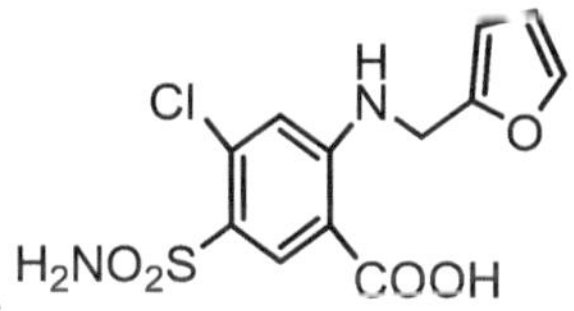 Cl, H, N, O, H_2NO_2S, COOH

D. 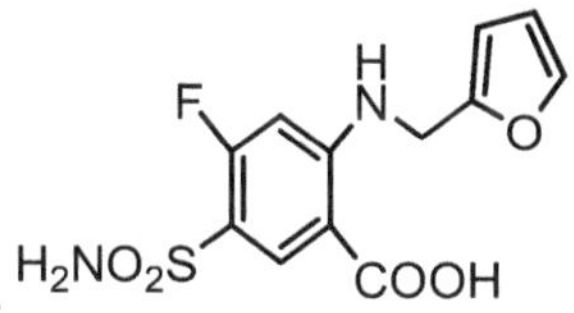 F, H, N, O, H_2NO_2S, COOH

4045. What happen when double bond of ethacrynic acid isreduce
A. Compound active, activity increase
B. Compound inactive, activity decrease
C. Compound active, activity decrease
D. Compound inactive, activity increase

4046. Which one of the following is loop diuretic, but not a sulphonamide derivative
A. Tripamide B. Azosemide
C. Piretamide D. Ethacrynic acid

4047. In spironolactone, MR-antagonist activity is dependent on the presence of
A. γ-lactone ring on C-7 and substituent on C-17
B. γ-lactone ring on C-3 and substituent on C-13
C. γ-lactone ring on C-13 and substituent on C-3
D. γ-lactone ring on C-17 and substituent on C-7

4048. Eplerenone is
A. Generic medicine
B. Potassium sparing diuretic
C. Sodium sparing diuretic
D. Calcium sparing diuretic

4049. In case of spironolactone which one of the following is essential for MR-antagonism
A. Lactone ring
B. Acetyl group(C-7)
C. 9α, 11α epoxy group
D. All of the above

4050. In triamterene structure, if we introduce para-methyl group on phenyl ring, what will happen
A. Activity decrease to 90%
B. Activity decrease to half
C. Activity decrease to 70%
D. Activity increase

4051. Derivative of anthranilic acid and ortho-amino benzoic
A. Bumetamide B. Torsemide
C. Furosemide D. Anthacrynic acid

4052. Eplerenone has limited or no inhibitory effects on
A. AR B. GR
C. PR D. All of the above

4053. Which one of the following used by paracelsus as a diuretic

A. Calomel B. Benzthiazide
C. Both A and B D. None of the above

4054. Which one of the following contain steroidal ring

A. Amphenone B B. Canrenoate
C. Disulfamide D. Metyrapone

4055. Which one of the following contain indole ring in its structure

A. Xipamide B. Canrenone
C. Clorexolone D. Canrenoate

4056. All of the following drugs have steroidal ring, except

A. Eplerenone B. Spironolactone
C. Canrenoate D. Amphenone B

4057. Which one of the following is acidic diuretic

A. Ammonium chloride
B. Indacrinone
C. Muzolimine
D. None of the above

4058. Precursor compound in the synthesis of marcaptomerin sodium

A. 3- chloroaniline
B. 3-fluromethylaniline
C. Acetaldehyde
D. Camphoric acid

4059. Mode of action of thiazide and hydrothiazide

A. Inhibit Na+ Cl- symport at the luminal membrane
B. Increase Na+ concentration at the luminal membrane
C. Inhibit the aldosterone action on mineralocorticoid receptor
D. None of the above

4060. 3-[(benzylthio) methyl]-6-chloro-2H-1, 2,4-benothiadiazine-7-sulphonamide-1,1-dioxide is the IUPAC name of

A. Chlorthiazide
B. benzthiazide
C. Hydrochlorthiazide
D. Cyclothiazide

4061. IUPAC name of hydrochlorthiazide

A. 6-chloro-3,4-dihydro-1,2,4-benothiadiazine-7-sulphonamide-1,1-dioxide
B. 6-chloro-1,4-dihydro-1,2,4-benothiadiazine-7-sulphonamide-1,1-dioxide
C. 6-chloro-1-hydro-1,2,4- benothiadiazine-7-sulphonamide-1,1-dioxide
D. 6-chloro-3,4-dihydro-4- benothiadiazine-7-sulphonamide-1,1-dioxide

4062. In thiazide diuretics which position tolerate the presence of small alkyl group

A. 1st B. 2nd
C. 3rd D. 4th

4063. Substitution of the 6th position on a thiazide ring with an activating group is essential for the diuretic activity. The substituent's include

A. Cl B. Br
C. CF3 D. All of the above

4064. In loop diuretics , at which position carbonyl group provide optimal diuretic activity

A. C-1 B. 5th
C. C-4 D. 2nd

4065. Precursor compound in the synthesis of elorexolone

A. 5-chloroisobenzofuran-1,3-dione
B. Ortho- phenylene diamine
C. Dihydroepiandrosterone
D. benzaldehyde

4066. Which one of the following group when substituent on position 4 in loop diuretic increase diuretic activity

A. Alkoxy B. aniline
C. Benzyl D. All of the above

4067. Antibiotics is wed to killing at :-

A. Fungi B. Beta dine
C. Bactria D. All microorganisms.

4068. Antibiotics Example are :-

A. Ciprofloxacin B. Beta dine
C. Ketoconazole D. cisplatin

4069. Ehrlich's Phase at dyes and organ metallic compounds these are : -

A. 1859-1902 B. 1889-1908

C. 1890-1835 D. 1900-1963

4070. The Period of empirical are wed at : -

A. Penicillin B. Griseofulvin

C. Pollens D. Mouldy curd

4071. Spectrum at activity of narrow spectrum

A. Penicillin G B. Penicillin C

C. Penicillin D D. Penicillin E

4072. Antibiotics are obtained from bacteria are:-

A. Cephalosporin B. Polyenes

C. Bacitracin D. Macrolides

4073. B- Lactam antibiotics are :-

A. Chloramphenicol B. Rifampin

C. Penicillin's D. Amikacin

4074. Antibiotic Nicotinic acid derivatives are :-

A. Isoniazid B. Clofazimine

C. Nystatine D. spectinomycin

4075. Antibiotic are interferes with DNA synthesis these are :-

A. Sulphonamides B. Acyclovir

C. Sulfones D. Penicillin

4076. The basis of selective microbial toxicity is the action of the drug on a component of the microbes examples are :-

A. Bacterial cell wall

B. Bacterial mitochondria's

C. Bacterial rhizomes

D. None of these

4077. Chloramphenicol acetyl transferase is acquired by resistant by :-

A. E. Coli B. H. influenza

C. S. typhi D. All of the above.

4078. In Drug tolerant loss of affinity at the target bio molecule at the microorganism for a particular AMA Exp. are :-

A. P. falciparum B. Staph. Aureus

C. H. influenza D. All of the above.

4079. Infection by organisms notorious for developed resistance exp. :-

A. Proteus B. Candida albicans

C. Pseudomonas D. None of these.

4080. Conditions predisposing to superinfections there are :-

A. Corticosteroid therapy

B. leukaemia's

C. ATDS

D. All of these.

4081. The Example at clinical diagnosis itself directs choice of the AMA is :-

A. Syphilis B. Emphysema

C. AIDS D. None of these

4082. The Conditions prevailing at the site at infection greatly affect the action of --------------------

A. BMB's B. AMAS

C. CMC's D. DMD.s

4083. Antimicrobials in liver disease dose reduction needed are :-

A. Talampicillin B. Pefloxacin

C. Metronidazole D. All of those

4084. Antimicrobials needing reduce dose even in mild failure :-

A. Cephalothin B. Nalidixicacid

C. Sulphuric acid D. Ethambutol

4085. Antimicrobial needing drug to be avoided are :-

A. Tetracycline B. Cotrimoxazole

C. Aztreonam D. All of these

4086. Patient factor of antibiotics are :-

A. Age

B. Renal & hepatic function

C. Pregnancy

D. All of these

4087. Use to combination of AMA's whenever prolonged therapy is undertaken. Examples are :-

A. Staph. Aureus B. M. tuberculosis

C. tuberculosis D. E. Coil

4088. Sulpha pyridine (M&B 693) was the first sulphonamide is marketed in ------------------------

A. 1933 B. 1954

C. 1939 D. 1938

4089. Which also inhibit micro organisms example are :-

A. Antifungal B. Antibodies

C. Antimicrobial D. C & b

4090. Antibiotics are obtained from fungi are :-
A. Tetracycline B. Griseofulvin
C. A and B D. bulitralin

4091. Type of organisms against which primarily active of antifungal are ;-
A. Ketoconazole B. Zidovudine
C. Chloroquine D. Diloxanide

4092. Sulphonamides are related drugs :-
A. Ciprofloxacin
B. trimethoprim
C. Metramine
D. Sulfones dapsone (DDS)

4093. The phenomenon of antibiosis was demonstrated by pusteur. In
A. 1856 B. 1877
C. 1885 D. 1867

4094. Antimicrobial drug azoles derivatives are:-
A. Hamycin B. Miconazole
C. Metronidazole D. bullatacin

4095. Choice to be based on bustriolog ices examination examples are :-
A. Tonsillitis B. Empyema
C. Vaginitis D. None or those

4096. Choice of an antimicrobial agent drug baitors relative toxicity example are
A. β. lactam B. α- lactam
C. α-βLactam D. None of those

4097. Ciprofloxacin and Rifampin have very good in :-
A. Extracellular penetration
B. Intracellular
C. Chloramphenicol
D. Cefuroxime

4098. Another special ex is the combination at :-
A. B- lactamase B. X- lactamase
C. Lactamase D. All of those

4099. Problem that arise with the use of AMA's in systemic toxicity are polymyxin B :-
A. Kidney toxicity
B. Anti anabolic tract
C. New logical 7 renal toxicity
D. Bone marrow

4100. Gene transfer from one organism toanother can occur by :-
A. Conjugation B. Transduction
C. Transformation D. All of those

4101. The resistant microbe elaborates and example which in actives the drug are
A. Drug tolerant B. drug destroying
C. Drug inperipherals D. None of those

4102. The example of antibacterial are :-
A. Cholorquine B. Amantadine
C. Erythromycin D. None of those

4103. In antibiotics types at action are in primarily bacteriostatic are :-
A. Polymyxin – B B. Codistin
C. Cephalosporin D. Sulphonamide

4104. Antimicrobial drugs can be inhibit cell wall synthesis are :-
A. Nystatin B. Vancomycin
C. Gentamicin D. Bacitracin

4105. Antimicrobial drug are chemically oxazolidinone are :-
A. Linezolid B. Bacitracin
C. Tyrothricin D. Furazolidone

4106. Spectrum at antimicrobial action treatment of mixed infection :-
A. Topically B. Bacitracin
C. Neomycin D. Bronchiectasis

4107. Practically all of them intercalate b/w those are :-
A. RNA B. DNA
C. RNA and DNA D. None of those

4108. Antibiotics are produced --------------- as a unique adverse effect :-
A. Cardio toxicity B. Sarcomas
C. Steatites D. All of those

4109. This highly toxic drug is used only in resistant cancer of stomach there are :-
A. Procarbazine B. Mitomycin c
C. Hydroxyurea D. All of those

4110. Intracellular to a form which acts as an alkylating agent and kills cells in :-
A. G1 M Phases B. G2 – M Phases
C. G2 N Phases D. G- M Phases

4111. Hydroxyurea primary therapeutic value is in chronic myeloid is :-

A. Carcinoma B. Sarcoma
C. Leukaemia D. None of those

4112. Procarbazine is a weak ------------------------------------

A. AMO Inhibitor B. OMA inhibitor
C. MAO Inhibitor D. None of those

4113. The leukemic cells are deficient in :-

A. L- asparagines syntheses
B. M- asparagines syntheses
C. N- - asparagines syntheses
D. o- asparagines syntheses

4114. The dose limiting toxicity is

A. Thrombocytopenia
B. Astrocytopenia
C. hemocytopenia
D. None of those

4115. Corticosteroids are also reliable for the control of complications like

A. Hypocalcaemia
B. Haemolysis
C. thrombocytopenia
D. All of those

4116. Hormones are not

A. ototoxic B. Edema
C. Myalgia D. None of those

4117. Drug acting directly on cell cytotoxic drug of alkylating agents are :-

A. Ifosfamide B. Triptorelin
C. Flutamide D. Examestane

4118. Gratifying results are obtained and life is prolonged by chemotherapy in breast cancer are :-

A. Non- Hodgkin lymphomas
B. Chronic myeloid leukaemia
C. Chronic lymphatic leukaemia
D. Head and neck cancers.

4119. Drug acting directly on cell metabolites in pyrimidine:-

A. Fosfestrol B. To remifene
C. Mitoxantrone D. S- fluorouracil (5-fu)

4120. Anticancer drug ultring hormonal Mineralo & glucocorticoids are :-

A. Fulvestrant B. Prednisolone
C. Cisplatin D. imatinib

4121. Emetogenic potential of cytotoxic drug mild are :-

A. Busulfan B. Vincristine
C. Etoposide D. All of those

4122. hyperuricemia in addition to these general toxicities individual drug may produce specific adverse effect example are :-

A. Purine B. Mustine
C. cisplatin D. Lystits

4123. Drug altering hormonal milieu estrogens are

A. fosfestrol B. fulvestrant
C. Flutamide D. Finasteride

4124. Anticancer drug acting directly on cellanti metabolites antagonist are :-

A. 6- thioguanine (6-TG)
B. 6- mercaptopurine (6-MP)
C. 5- thisguanin (5-TG)
D. 8- thioguanine (6- TG)

4125. Drug hormon altering hormonal miliele selective estrogens :-

A. Prednisolone B. tamoxifen
C. Fulvestrant D. Triptorelin

4126. Emetogenic potential of cytotoxic drug moderate are :-

A. Vinblastine B. fluorouracil
C. Lomustine D. Mustine

4127. General toxicity of cytotoxic drug are :-

A. Bone marrow B. Busulfan
C. Thio TEPA D. Ifosfamide

4128. Anticancer drug altering hormone milies anti androgen are :-

A. Flutamide B. ibrutinib
C. Fulvestrant D. Finasteride

4129. GIT drug that frequently cause mucositis are :-

A. toremifene B. Nafarelin
C. Doxorubicin D. busulfan

4130. Drug acting directly no cell vincaalkalodeare

A. irinotecan B. Fulvestrant
C. carboplatin D. Vinblastine

4131. Progestin drug are altering hormonal milieu :-
A. Carboplatin
B. Hydroxyprogesterone
C. Cytarabin
D. Toremifene

4132. Anticancer drug acting directly on cell selective estrogensrecptor down regulators :-
A. Fulvestrant B. Imatinib
C. Triptorelin D. Exemestane

4133. Drug are may be nitrosomonas are acting on the alkylating agents :-
A. Methotrexate (mtx)
B. Cytarabin
C. Dacarbazine (DTIC)
D. tamoxifen

4134. Drug acting directly on cell antibiotic are :-
A. Topotein B. Carboplatin
C. Triptorelin D. doxorubicin

4135. Garh analogues are may be the drug altering hormonal milieu are :-
A. Nafarelin B. Dutasteride
C. letrozole D. bicalutamide

4136. Depression at bone marrow result in :-
A. granulocytopenia B. Agranulocytosis
C. Aloyticaremia D. All of those

4137. Infection and blooding are the complication of :-
A. Bone marrow B. lymphoreticular issue
C. Oral cavity D. GIT

4138. Inhibition of gonadel cells caules
A. Gonads B. Foetus
C. Carcinogenicity D. All of those

4139. The vinca alkaloid is useful type at anticancer agents. Which of the following is true about these agents?
A. They all function by targeting that microtubule
B. Paclitatxel and docetaxel
C. A and B
D. None of those

4140. Humanized monoclonal antibodies (Unabe) haven caule immune :-
A. True B. False

4141. Cytotoxic and radiomimetic actions show are :-
A. Alkylating agents B. Fortus
C. Ganade D. None of those

4142. The position at guanine residues in:-
A. DNA B. RNA
C. DNA AND RNA D. None of those

4143. Cross linking of nucleic and with proteins can also takes place with :-
A. salicylic B. Hypesruricammia
C. Alkylating agents D. All of those

4144. Nausea and vomiting are prominent with many
A. Cytotoxic drugs B. ototoxin drug
C. Analgesic drug D. All of those

4145. Damage to the germinal cells may result in –
A. Mutagenesis B. Organises
C. Para genesis D. All of those

4146. Used to control mania and to break into cyclic affective disorders are :-
A. Antimanic B. Antidepressants
C. anti anxiety D. All of those

4147. Phenothiazines are aliphatic side chain at
A. Chlorpromazine B. tranquilizers
C. Analgesic D. None of those

4148. Pharmacology of chlorpromazine id described as
A. Prototypes B. Psychotic
C. A and B D. None of those

4149. The primarysymptoms is change in mood state at
A. Affective disorders
B. Defecticvedisoder
C. A and B
D. None of those

4150. Dramatic symptoms resembling serious physical illness in :-
A. Hysterical B. Reactive depreusion
C. Anxiety D. All of those

4151. Used in all types of functional psychosis :-
A. Antipsycholic B. Hysterical
C. Antxicty D. All of the above

4152. A drug which reduces mental tension and produce camnese without inducing sleep or dispersing mental faculties are :

A. tranquilizers B. Analgesic
C. Antibiotic D. Antacid

4153. Varied symptom following distressing experience like was riots

A. Post- traumatic stress disorder
B. Reactive depression
C. A & b both
D. None of those

4154. Used to control mania and to break into cyclic affective disorder in

A. Antimania B. Anticancer
C. diuretics D. All of those

4155. Sometimes as a least resort neurosurgery has become an intervention in OCD the most command procedine is :

A. neurobiotaxis
B. Habituation
C. emotional anaesthesia
D. Cinngulatory

4156. Which of the following is correspondent to be a symptom of post traumatic stress disorder CPID :

A. Increased arousal B. Decreased arousal
C. A and B D. None of those

4157. which of the following of this on is predominant evolutionary theory of phobias

A. Specific phobia acquisition
B. Learned bean responses
C. Biological preparedness
D. None of those

4158. Recent of evidence are suggested that at least some phobia are closely associates with the emotion of :

A. Disgust B. Anger
C. Distinction D. Conflagration

4159. It is the considered that successful CBt treatments of social phobia include elements of the following :

A. Exposuretherapy
B. Social skills training
C. Cognitive restructuring
D. All of the above

4160. Which are may be the following physical symptoms are associated with panic attacks

A. heart palpitations
B. Porspiring
C. Hyperventilating
D. All of the above

4161. They may be the following is a drug treatment for social phobia

A. Antibiotics
B. Anticancer
C. anti inflammatory drug
D. Serotonin reuptake inhibitors (SSRIS)

4162. __________ are used for anxiety and phobic state.

A. Antianxiety B. Anti hypertensive
C. Anticancer D. All of those

4163. Generalised anxiety discordant (GA) is a pervasive condition in which the sufferen experience

A. Continual apprehension and anxiety about future events
B. Fear of fear
C. A and b
D. None of those

4164. __________ used to control mania and to break into cyclic affective disorder

A. Antimania B. Anti anxiety
C. tranquilizer D. All of those

4165. Effects differ in normal and psychotic ______________ in

A. CNS B. PNS
C. A And B D. None of those

4166. The classification at thioxanthenes is

A. Flupenthixol B. Clozapine
C. aripiprazole D. None of those

4167. Classifications at aliphatic side chain is

A. Chlorpromazine B. Triflupromazine
C. A and B D. None of those

4168. This may be according to conditioning theory incubation is a phenomenon that should lead to

A. extinction B. Non- associative feas
C. Conflagration D. All of those

4169. Which of the following of this on is predominant evolutionary theory of phobias

A. Specific phobia acquisition

B. Learned bean responses

C. Biological preparedness

D. None of those

4170. Recent of evidence are suggested that at least some phobias are closely associated with the emotion of ;

A. Disgust B. Anger

C. Distinction D. Conflagration

4171. It is the considered that successful CBT treatments of social phobia include elements of the following.

A. Exposure therapy

B. Social skills training

C. Cognitive restructuring

D. All of the above

4172. Which are many of the following physical symptoms are associated with panic attacks

A. heart palpitations B. Porspriting

C. Hyperventilating D. All of the above

4173. They may be the following is a drug treatments for social phobia

A. Antibiotics

B. Anticancer

C. Anti- inflammatory drug

D. Serotonin reuptake inhibitor (SSRIs)

4174. An anxiety disorder is

A. Disordered thinking

B. An emotional state identified by panic attacks

C. An excessive or unused state uncategorized by feeling of apprehension uncertainty and fear

D. B And C

4175. Comparative properties of anti psychotic drug are :

A. Thioridazine B. Aripiprazole

C. Ziprasidone D. All of the above

4176. Distinctive features of neuroleptics are :

A. Triflupromazine B. Haloperidol

C. A and B D. None of those

4177. : it is the metabolized in liver mainly by ---------------- into a number of metabolites

A. Cyp 3 D 6 B. Cyp 2 D 6

C. Cyp 3 D 8 D. Cyp 2 D 5

4178. nonepileptic may develop seizures with nigh doses of some antipsychotics like clozapin and olanzapine are :-

A. Risperidone B. Quetiapine

C. A and B D. None of those

4179. Reversible inhibitors of MAO-S [RIMAs] drug are :

A. Trimipramine B. moclobemide

C. Venlafaxine D. None of those

4180. Selective serotonin reuptake inhibitors [SSRIS] drug are :

A. Sertraline B. Citalopram

C. A and B D. None of those

4181. There may be the atypical antidepressants drug are :

A. Reboxetine B. Nortriptyline

C. Duloxetine D. All of the above

4182. The choice of an antiepileptic drug are :

A. Lifestyle aspects B. Seizure control

C. Seizure type D. All of the above

4183. Barbiturate is which types drug :

A. Antiepileptic B. Antibiotic

C. antianxiety D. Anticancer

4184. These may be are adverse effects of antiepileptic :

A. Hyperactivity

B. CNC depression

C. Cardiovascular stimulation

D. None of those

4185. Carbamazepine is type of drug :

A. Anticancer B. Antiepileptic

C. PPI D. Analgesic

4186. Which category drug is diazepam

A. Barbiturate B. Benzodiazepines

C. Newer drugs D. hydantoin

4187. Phenobarbitone is used in :

A. Antibiotic B. CNS stimulants

C. Antiepileptic D. PPI

4188. Phenytoin was synthesized in :

A. 1920 B. 1995

C. 1908 D. 1927

4189. clobazam are used in :
A. Antidepressant B. Anti hypertension
C. Antiepileptic D. None of the above

4190. Zonisamide is which classified in Anti epileptic :
A. Barbiturate B. Iminostilbene
C. phenyltriazine D. Newer drugs

4191. lorazepam is used in :
A. PPI B. Analgesic
C. Antiepileptic D. None of the above

4192. divalproex is used in :
A. Anticancer B. Anti epileptic
C. A and B D. None of the above

4193. Carbamazepine was introduced in :
A. 1960 B. 1940
C. 1950 D. 1970

4194. Carbamazepine adverse effect is :
A. Sedation B. Dizziness
C. Vertigo D. All of the above

4195. clonazepam drugs adult dose are in TDS :
A. 0.2 – 2 mg B. 0.5 -5 mg
C. 0.6 -6 mg D. 0.8 -8 mg

4196. Valproic acid are also known by :
A. Sodium valproate
B. sodium hydroxide
C. Sodium Bi carbonate
D. None of the above

4197. neuroses depending on the predominant feature it may be labelled are :
A. Anxiety
B. Phobia state
C. Obsessive compulsive
D. All of those

4198. Anti psychoticusefull in all types of functional :
A. Psychosis B. Schizophrenia
C. A and B D. None of those

4199. Classification of butyrophenones are :
A. Haloperidol B. Trifluperidol
C. Penfluridol D. All of those

4200. Classification of thioxanthenes are :
A. Flupenthixol B. Clozapine
C. Penfluridol D. All of those

4201. Classification of other heterocylic are :
A. Pimozide B. Loxapine
C. A and B D. None of those

4202. Classification of phenothiazine are :
A. Aliphatic side chain
B. Piperidine side chain
C. Piperazine side chain
D. All of those

4203 Classification of aliphatic side chain is :
A. Chlorpromazine B. Triflupromazine
C. A and B D. None of those

4204. Classification of atypical neuroleptics these are :
A. Clozapine B. Risperidone
C. Olanzapin D. All of the above

4205. Classification of piperidine side chain is :
A. Thioridazine B. Chlorpromazine
C. Fluphenazine D. All of those

4206. In post traumatic stress disorder varied symptoms following distressing expressions like :
A. War B. Riots
C. Zanthqunalce D. All of those

4207. Ziprasidone are the sub classification of :
A. Atypical neuroleptics
B. Thioxanthenes
C. A and B
D. None of those

4208. Antipsychotic drugs are also known are :
A. Neuroleptics B.Transderimis
C. epidermis D. All of those

4209. In normal individuals CPZ produces in differones to :
A. Surroundings
B. emotional quietening
C. Psychomotor slowing
D. All of those

4210. ----------- Are used to control mania and to break into affective disorders are :
A. Anti manic B. Antihypertensive
C. Anti lipidemic D. All of the above

4211. ----------- Are used for anxiety and phobia states :
A. Anti anxiety B. Anti manic
C. A and B D. None of those

4212. ---------- are uaried symptoms following distressing experience like was :
A. Post traumatic stress disorder
B. Hysterical
C. Anxiety
D. None of those

4213. ------------- used for minor an well as major clopresive illness phobia states :
A. Anti depressants
B. Anti anxiety
C. A and B
D. None of those

4214. ------------- An aliphatic side chain phenothiazine same what more potent them CPZ :
A. triflupromazine B. Thioridazine
C. A and B D. None of those

4215. ------------------ It is similar to but silently more potent than haloperidol :
A. Trifluperidol B. Pen fluridone
C. A and B D. None of those

4216. -------------- a low potency phenothiazine having market central anti cholinergic action :
A. thioridazine B. Triflupromazine
C. Haloperidol D. All of those

4217. ------------- a dibenzoxazepine having CPZ like DA blocking and anti psychotic activity :
A. Loxapine B. pimozide
C. flupentixol D. All of those

4218. ------------------------- is save, more common with clozapine :
A. agranulocytosis B. myocarditis
C. cholestatic jaundice D. All of those

4219. ---------------- few cases have occurred with clozapine :
A. Myocarditis B. Cholestatic
C. A and B D. All of those

4220. _____________ are not drugs related :
A. hypersensitivity reactions
B. Skin rashes
C. A and B
D. None of the above

4221. Lithium has practically no acute effects in normal individuals are well as in MDI patients :
A. CNS B. PNS
C. ANS D. All of those

4222. -------------------- is symptomatic
A. Disease B. Treatment
C. A and B D. None of those

4223. Lithium is used are its :
A. Carbonate sell B. Hygroscopic
C. Neuroleptic D. All of those

4224. ------------- close relative of LSD but 10times lees potent :
A. Lysergic and amide B. Psilocybin
C. A and B D. None of those

4225. ------------ Isolated from skin of a toad :
A. Bufotenine B. mescalines
C. A and B D. None of those

4226. Phencyclidine is an :
A. Anticholinergic B. cholinergic
C. Anti hypertensive D. All of those

4227. Harmine is present in a :
A. Vine B. Beta
C. Sine d. All of those

4228. ------------- A reduction in muric relapses is noted when valproate is used in bipolar disorder :
A. Sodium valproate
B. Magnesium valproate
C. Potassium
D. All of those

4229. Tolerance to the sedative and hypotensive action develops within
A. Day B. Weakly
C. A and B D. None of those

4230. extrapyramidal side effects are :
A. Maximal B. Minimal
C. A and B D. None of those

4231. ------------- should not be used during pregnancy lactation and in children's :
A. Tetracyclines B. Tricyclines
C. Dicydeline D. All of those

4232. --------------- resolver in 2-3 weeks :
A. Lymphogranulomavenereum
B. granuloma
C. A and B
D. None of those

4233. -------------------- due to borreliarecurrentive response adequately :
A. Relapsing fever B. Plague
C. Cholera D. All of those

4234. ------------- is noted in some infants
A. inhaled intracranial pressure
B. Vestibulan toxicity
C. A and B
D. None of those

4235. ---------------- is tetracyclines reduces protein synthesis and have an overall catabolic effects :
A. Anti anabolic effects
B. diabetes insipidus
C. A and B
D. None of those

4236. Preparations should never be used beyond their :
A. MFY date B. Expiry date
C. A and B D. None of those

4237. ----------- due to borreliarecurrentis respond adequately :
A. Relapsing fever B. plague
C. A and B D. None of those

4238. ------------- chloramphenicol given systematically attainhigh cancer in ocular fluid :
A. Intraocular infections
B. Extra ocularinfections
C. A and B
D. None of those

4239. The classification of anticholinergics are :
A. hyoscine B. dicyclomine
C. A and B D. None of those

4240. Classification of neuroleptics are :
A. Chlorpromazine B. prochlorperazine
C. Donpenid one D. All of those

4241. There is no cross resistance with any other :
A. AMA B. BMA
C. CMA D. All of those

4242. ---------------- It is one at the earliest discovered antibiotics from a strain of bacillus subtilis :
A. Bacitracin B. Macitroacin
C. A and B D. None of those

4243. ---------------- are dependability in acute UTI has decreased : not used now as single drug :
A. Sulphonamides B. cotrimaxazole
C. quinolones D. None of those

4244. ---------------- it is a mixture at gramicidin and tyrocidine , obtained from bacillus bravais
A. tyrothricin B. nitrofurantoin
C. A and B D. None of those

4245. Adverse effect of comets is gastrointestinal intolerence is
A. Nausea B. epigastric pain
C. A and B D. None of those

4246. Polypeptide antibiotics are clinically used are :
A. Polymyxin B B. Bacitracin
C. Colistin D. None of those

4247. Penicillin was the first antibiotic to be used clinically as :
A. 1942 b. 1947
C. 1941 D. None of those

4248. The penicillin nucleus consists of fused are :
A. Thiazolidine B. b- lactam ring
C. A and B D. None of those

4249. They may be side chain of natural penicillin can be split off by an amides to produce are :
A. 8- amino-penicillamine acid
B. thiazolidine
C. 6- uminopenicillamine acid
D. All of the above

4250. All B- lactan antibiotics interfere with the synthesis of bacterial are :

A. Cell wall
B. Golgi apparatus
C. Endoplasmicreticulum
D. All of the above

4251. The bacterial synthesize UDp-N acetylmurarric acid pentapeptide called :

A. Pork nucleotide
B. Non park nucleotide
C. A and B
D. None of those

4252. These enzyme and related proteins constitute are the ;

A. Penicillin binding proteins
B. acetylglucosamine
C. A and B
D. None of those

4253. When susceptible bacteria divide in the presence of a B- lactam antibiotic produced are :

A. Anti psychotic B. Cell wall deficient
C. Beny penicillin D. All of the above

4254. The peptidoglycan cell wall is unique to a :

A. D- alanine B. l- lysine
C. Bacteria D. None of those

4255. In gram positive bacteria the cell wall is almost entirely made of :

A. Vancomycin B. Neighbouring
C. peptidoglycan D. All of those

4256. Gram negativecoci ________________ are susceptible to PnG

A. Neisseria B. n meningitidis
C. A and B D. None of those

4257. The primary mechanism of acquired resistance is production of :

A. Penicillinase B. pancreas
C. A and B D. None of those

4258. The gram negative bacteria have ------------ channels formed by a specific proteinslocated in their outer membrane :

A. PnG B. Leptospira
C. Porin D. None of those

4259. Penicillin is the drug of choice for infections are may be organising susceptible are :

A. Antiseptic B. Antibiotic
C. antifungal D. None of those

4260. The aim of producing semi– synthetic penicillins has bees to overcome the shortcoming of PnG which are :

A. Poor efficacy
B. Neuro spectrum of activity
C. Susceptibility to Penicillanse
D. All of the above

4261. These may be acid- resistant alternative to penicillin an drug are :

A. Penicillin V B. Sulbactam
C. tazobactam D. ampicillin

4262. Penicillinase resistant penicillin drug are :

A. Cloxacillin B. clavulanic acid
C. phenoxymethyl D. None of those

4263. These may be the B- lactamaseinhibitor are :

A. Penicillin V B. Methicillin
C. Tazobactam D. All of the above

4264. Extended spectrumpenicillin drug are :

A. Aminopenicillins B. ureidopenicillins
C. A and B D. None of those

4265. These may be the extended spectrumpenicillin of larboxypenicillin drug are :

A. Ticarcillin B. piperacillin
C. Cloxacillin D. All of the above

4266. Gram negative bacteria and anaerobes its cannot be depended upon to serious infections and used only for are :

A. Streptococcal B. sinusitis
C. otitis media D. All of the above

4267. This may be of systemicamino glycosides are :

A. Streptomycin B. Amikacin
C. Gentamicin D. All of the above

4268. This may be of topical amino glycosides are :

A. Neomycin B. Framycetin
C. A and B D. None of those

4269. Streptomycin was the first member discovered in :
A. Waksman B. S. aureofaciens
C. A and B D. None of those

4270. The tetracycline's still available in India for clinical use are :
A. Tetracycline B. Demeclocycline
C. oxytetracycline D. All of those

4271. Protein synthesizing apparatus of host cell is less sensitive to :
A. Penicillins B. Tetracyclines
C. A and B D. None of those

4272. Tetracyclines are not active against fall.
A. N. gonorrhoea B. N. meningitides
C. A and B D. None of those

4273. Most gram positive bacilli of example are :
A. Clostridia B. Listeria
C. anaerobes D. All of the above

4274. Which are sensitive gram negative bacilli of example are :
A. v. chodecrey B. Listeria
C. Corynenactria D. None of those

4275. Which notable bacilli that are not in inhibited are :
A. Pseudomonas aeruginosa B. Proteus
C. Klebsiella D. All of the above

4276. Which alcohols are hydroxyl derivatives of aliphatic by drocurbors when unqualibied alcohol refers are :
A. Ethyl alcohol B. Ethanol
C. A and B D. None of those

4277. Which may be of antipsychotic drug of phenothiazine aliphatic side chain drug are :
A. Chlorpromazine B. Fluphenorine
C. penfluridol D. None of those

4278. Which may be antiepileptic drug are aliphatic carboxylic acid are :
A. Valproic acid B. clobazam
C. Tiagabine D. None of those

4279. These may are benzodiazepines are drug are :
A. vigabatrin B. Diazepam
C. Topiramate D. phenytoin

4280. They may be cyclic GABA analogue drugs are :
A. Lorazepam B. Vigabation
C. Gabazam D. All of the above

4281. Which can antiepileptic drug of succinimide are :
A. Ethosuximide B. phenytoin
C. Primidone D. divalproex

4282. A ------------ converted by liver to phenobarbitone and phenylethylmultimedia (PEMA)
A. Epilepticus B. Deoxy barbiturate
C. A and B D. None of those

4283. Which its anticonvulsant activity was specificallylisted in :
A. 1931 B. 1936
C. 1938 D. 1939

4284. Commonest more in younger patients and is due to overgrowth of gingival collagen tibres are :
A. Gum hypertrophy B. Hirsutism
C. A and B D. None of those

4285. Which may be phenytoin desensities target tissues to vit D and interferes which calciummetabolism
A. Megaloblastic B. Osteomalacia
C. epigastric D. All of the above

4286. Which may be valproate increases are the phenobarbitone by inhibiting its metabolism :
A. Plasm levels B. Protein binding
C. A and B D. None of those

4287. Which are antiepileptic drug of newer drug are :
A. clobazam B. primidone
C. Tiagabine D. None of those

4288. These may be are the phenyltriazine drug are :
A. valproic acid B. Zonisamide
C. Diazepam D. Lamotrigine

4289. Febrile convulsions some children especially under year develop conversions during fever :
A. 5 year B. 10 year
C. 6 year D. None of those

4290. Those was obtained from micro monosporapurpurea un :

A. 1912 B. 1964
C. 1916 D. 1918

4291. Chloramphenicol was initially obtained from streptomycinVenezuelae un :

A. 1947 B. 1956
C. 1933 D. 1978

4292. Which has assumed special signification due to officiallyagainst MRSA are :

A. Strep viridians B. enterococcus
C. Cl. Difficile D. All of the above

4293. Which may to second choice of drug to metronidazole for antibiotic associate are used by :

A. C. difficile B. m. tuberculosis
C. VRSA D. Bact. fragilis

4294. It is active against most gram positive cocci including MRSA, some VRSA and Some VRF as:

A. Neisseria B. Leginonella
C. Chlamydia D. All of the above

4295. They exhibit synergism with many other AMA.s by improving their penetration into the :

A. Bacterial cell B. Cell wall
C. A and B D. None of those

4296. All are produced by bacteria clinically used are :

A. Colistin B. Tyro thricin
C. Bacterian D. All of the above

4297. Both have very similar rang of activity but colisitin in more potent are :

A. Pseudomonas B. Salmonella
C. Shigella D. All of the above

4298. How many number in tetracycline :

A. 10 B. 6
C. 5 D. 4

4299. Antimalarial drug of 4 am/quinolones are drug from :

A. amodiaquine B. Antovaquone
C. sulfadoxine D. None of those

4300. Which are first generation ceph also prions drug of parental are :

A. Cefazolin B. cephalothin
C. A and B D. None of those

4301. quinoline methanol Antimalarial drug of :

A. Dapsone B. Mefloquine
C. arteether D. None of these

4302. cephalosporins are second generation drug of oral are :

A. Cefaclor B. Cefoperazone
C. cefepime D. None of these

4303. These may be the anti malarial drug of naphthoquinone drug are :

A. Atovaquone B. Halofantrine
C. tetracycline . D. None of these

4304. Which may be are fast acting high efficacy drug are :

A. chloroquine B. Amodiaquine
C. Quinine D. All of the above

4305. Which may be the diaminopyrimidines drug are :

A. Atovaquone B. Artether
C. Pyrimethamine D. None of the these

4306. These may be the 8 – amino quinoline drug are :

A. Primaquine B. Bulaquine
C. A and B D. None of these

4307. Which may ne are third generation cephalosporins are parenteral drug are :

A. Cefotaxime B. Ceftizoxime
C. Ceftazidime D. All of the above

4308. Fourth generation of cephalosporin are darenteral drug are :

A. Cefepime B. Cefpirome
C. A and B D. None of these

4309. Third generation cephalosporin are oral drug are :

A. Cefdirinir B. Cefoxitin
C. Cefazolin D. None of these

4310. These enzymes including PNG and ampicillin resistant are :

A. H influeezane B. Staph. Aureus
C. A and B D. None of these

4311. Tetracyclines reduce protein of synthesis and have and overall catabolic effect are :

A. Antianabolic effect B. Vestibular toxicity
C. Diabetes insipidus D. None of these

4312. Tetracyclines are the first choice drug are:
A. Cholera B. Plague
C. Brucellosis D. All of the above

4313. Tetracyclines can cause epigastric pain, nausea, vomiting and diarrhoea by their are ;
A. Irritative effects B. Antianabolic effect
C. A and B D. None of these

4314. Enterobacteriaceae are now largely resistant notable bacilli that are not inhibited are :
A. Proteus B. Salmonella typhi
C. Bact. Fragilis D. All of the above

4315. Which may be are tetracycline drug are :
A. Doxycycline B. Atovaquone
C. A and B D. None of these

4316. Proguanil was introduced in --------------- by the british as a well toletrate clinical curative :
A. 1946 B. 1945
C. 1947 D. 1948

4317. The important additions of the recent yeane are :
A. Mefloquine B. Artemisinin
C. Pyronaridine D. All of the above

4318. Which may be sesquiterpene lactones are:
A. Artesunate B. Artemether
C. Arteether D. All of the above

4319. These may be the mannich base are :
A. Pyronaridine B. Atovaquone
C. Tetoucycline D. None of these

4320. Gentamicin was obtained from micromonosporepurpurea in :
A. 1961 B. 1962
C. 1964 D. 1965

4321. Macrolide antibiotics of Erythromycin is first member discover in the :
A. 1950 s B. 1960 s
C. 1940 s D. 1970 s

4322. Erthromycin base in a remarkably safe as:
A. gastrointestinal B. Hyper sensitivity
C. A and B D. None of these

4323. Which may be high activity in exerted on respiratory pathogens are :
A. Mycoplasma B. Legionella
C. Ch. Trachomatis D. All of the above

4324. What is a aminoglycoside :
A. Gram – negative
B. Gram – positive
C. Negative positive
D. None of these

4325. Which of the following amino glycosides is the amino glycoside which present the synthesis of :
A. Carbohydrate B. Fat
C. Vitamins D. Protein

4326. Which patients should not be given amino glycosides :
A. HIV B. Myasthenia grovis
C. Typhoid D. None of these

4327. Which of these produce amino glycoside :
A. Airbactinomyceted
B. Water actinomycetey
C. Soil actinomycetes
D. All of these

4328. Which of the following is the first class of amino glycosides :
A. Heomvcine B. Gentumycen
C. Streptomyces D. None of these

4320. Which of the following is most affected by the honest intake of amino glycosides :
A. Eyes B. Liver
C. Ear D. None of these

4330. How many parts of the following aminoglycosides are divided into ecosides:
A. 4 B. 6
C. 5 D. 10

4331. Which of the following are the main agents of amino glycosides
A. Tetracycline B. Betadine
C. Gentamycin D. All of the above

4332. Which of these amino glycosides is given to potent by :
A. IV B. Inversion
C. IM D. Oral

4333. Which of the following is the oldest agents used against tuberculosis :
A. Streptomyces B. Gentamycine
C. Neomycin D. Tobramycin

4334. Tetracycline is used to treat which of these interties :

A. AIDS B. Rickettsia
C. HIV D. None of these

4335. Who got the first tetracycline from

A. Streptomy B. Streptomyces
C. A and B D. None of these

4336. Tetracycline microbial RNA inhibits the synthesis of :

A. Fat B. Carbohydrate
C. Lipid D. Protein

4337. Which is used to treat respiratory tract infectionscausedmycorlasma pneumonia :

A. Tetracycline B. Penicillin
C. Gentonycine D. None of these

4338. Of these tetracycline has a brand name :

A. dynacin B. Adorca
C. Declomycin D. Ala-tat- tatrap

4339. Tetracycline mainly consist of -

A. Hydrostatic B. Bacteriostatic
C. A and B D. None of these

4340. Tetracycline is mainly find in which flax :

A. 1950 B. 1954
C. 1940 D. 1942

4341. Tetracycline drug prevents bacteria from which of the following :

A. RNA B. Ribosome
C. DNA D. Golgibody

4342. How many numbers in tetracycline :

A. 10 B. 6
C. 5 D. 4

4343. Tetracycline is most soluble in :

A. Water B. Hydro chloride
C. Salt solution D. All of the above

4344. Haw many type of tetracycline are found in America :

A. 3 B. 4
C. 2 D. 6

4345. Which of the following are two type of tetracycline :

A. Doxcycyline B. Gentamycine
C. minocycline D. A and C both

4346. The classification of barbiturates :

A. Phenobarbitone B. Primidone
C. A and B D. None of these

4347. Classification of benzodiazepines are :

A. Clonazepam B. Diazepam
C. Lorazepam D. All of these

4348. Classification of succinimide are :

A. Ethosuccinimide B. Diazepam
C. Phenytoin D. All of these

4349. ------------------- is the drug of choice for absence seizures :

A. Valproic acid B. Citric acid
C. Oviric acid D. All of these

4350. Adverse effect of the toxicity at valproate is :

A. High B. Medium
C. Low D. All of these

4351. ------------ increase each athensmetabolism:

A. carbamazepine B. chloramphenicol
C. A and B D. None of these

4352. Phenobarbitone is one of the cheapest and least toxic :

A. Antiepileptics B. Antiallergic
C. Anticancer D. All of these

4353. ------------------- are produced by application of alumina gram on the motor cortex of monkey :

A. Chronic local seizures
B. Pentylenterazol
C. A and B
D. None of these

4354. Presence of a phenyl substitution confers activity against -----------------------

A. Tonic – clonic seizures
B. phenobarbitone
C. A and B
D. None of these

4355. The adverse effect is safe and well tolerated --------------------------

A. Flumazenil B. Epilepsies
C. A and B D. None of these

4356. ------------------- are shock – like momentary contraction of muscles at a limb or the whole body

A. Myoclonic B. Absence seizure
C. A and B D. None of these

4357. Classification of ACE inhibitors :

A. captopril B. Enalapril
C. Lisinopril D. All of these

4358. Classification of calcium channel blocker

A. Verapamil B. Dittiazem
C. Atenol D. All of these

4359. Desirable properties at diuretics as antihypertensive are :

A. Low cost B. High cost
C. Welium cost D. All of these

4360. Do not compromise haemodunamicsnoimpairment of ------------

A. Physical work capacity
B. Chemical WORK CAPACITY
C. A and B
D. None of these

4361. Tricyclic antidepressants reverse its action by blocking its active transport into the :

A. Adrenergic neurones
B. Antihypertensive neurones
C. A and B
D. None of these

4362. Cardiovascular risk factors are :

A. Smoking B. Diabetes mellitus
C. Hypertensions D. All of these

4363. The contamination of the ppt by substance which are normally soluble in mother liquor is called

A. Precipitation B. Both A and B
C. Co precipitation D. Post precipitation

4364. are sulphonamide and sulfone drug are :

A. Dapsone B. proguanil
C. chloroquine D. All of the above

4365. These may be the amino alcohols drug are:

A. Amodiaquine B. Tetracycline
C. Pyronaridine D. Lumefantrine

4366. Antimalarial of cinchona alkaloid drug are:

A. Piperaquine B. quinine
C. Proguanil D. All of the aboe

4367. Which may be are sesquiterpene lactones drug are :

A. Arteether B. Artesunate
C. Artemether D. All of the above

4368. They may be the first generation of oral cephalosporin :

A. Cefadroxil B. cephalexin
C. Cephradine D. All of the above

4369. primaquine was the first amino quinoline to be tested in Germany in the :

A. 1921 s B. 1920 s
C. 1925 s D. 1926 s

4370. Pyrimethamine was produced in ------------------------ under a planned post was research programme for Antimalarial drug:

A. 1955 B. 1956
C. 1952 D. 1951

4371. Antimalarial drug of biguanides drug are :

A. Sulfadoxine B. Depsone
C. proguanil D. None of these

CHAPTER 3A

Pharmacognosy and Phytochemistry

1. **Which one is the high molecular which carbohydrates**
   A. Glucose B. Pectins
   C. Sucrose D. Fructose

2. **Which may be obtained by the hydrolysis of polysaccharides**
   A. Heptonses B. Hexoses
   C Bioses D. Pentoses

3. **Which cannot be further hydrolysed to simple sugars is known as?**
   A. Disaccharides B. Polysaccharides
   C. Monosaccharides D. Proteoglycan

4. **Which sugars differs form each other only around single carbon atom is called**
   A. Epimer B. Momomer
   C. Both A & B D.

5. **Amino sugar are present in which bacterial cell was ?**
   A. Sialic acid
   B. N-acetylmuramic acid
   C. Azide
   D. Aminoglycoside

6. **Invert sugar is also known as_____?**
   A. Fructose B. Dextrose
   C. Sucrose D. Glucose

7. **Anti diarrhoeal are use in th______?**
   A. Inulin B. Locust bean
   C. Manna D. Carrageenan

8. **What is the general formula of carbohydrate**
   A. (C4H2O)n B. (CH2O)n
   C. (C6H2O)n D. (C2H20)nCOOH

9. **What is the synonyms of BAEL**
   A. Bael fruits B. Beagal Quince
   C. Both A & B D. None

10. **The chitr constituent of the drug Bael is ?**
    A. Echinacoside B. Arabin
    C. Arabinogalactan D. Marmelosin

11. **The two alkaloids O-methylhalfordinol and isopentylhalfordinol have be isolated which part of the beal**
    A. Burk B. Seeds
    C. Fruits D. Leaves

12. **Bael are used in which treatment**
    A. Diarrhoea B. Dysentery
    C. Both A&B D. None

13. **In the bael the pulp 0 which type of vitamin contain good amount**
    A. Vitamin C B. Vitamin A
    C. Both A&B D. None

14. **How much pairs of side veins of bael which are joined at the margin**
    A. 12-20 B. 1-5
    C. 4-12 D. 0-3

15. **The young leaves of bale are which colour?**
    A. Pale green B. Pinkish
    C. Both A&B D. None

16. **Which is the size of Bael flowers ?**
    A. 1.5 to 2 cm B. 3 to 4.5 cm
    C. 5 to 7 cm D. 7.5 to 9 cm

17. **In the bael flower which one usually appear ?**
    A. Shirf leaves B. Mature leaves
    C. Young leaves D. Immature leaves

18. **The bael fruit typically has which diameter?**
    A. 5 and 12 B. 1 and 5
    C. 0 and 5 D. 6 and 12

19. The fruits of bael can be eaten in which from

A. Fresh from trees
B. After being dried and produced into candy
C. Both
D. None

20. One large bael fruit may yield how many liters of sharbat ?

A. 1 or 2 B. 3 or 4
C. 5 or 6 D. 7 or 8

21. The vale left are consumed as a..........?

A. Disease control
B. Food
C. Dietary supplement
D. None

22. How many species of plantago are available in india ?

A. 5 B. 10
C. 15 D. 20

23. Size of plantago seeds are.......?

A. Large
B. Very large
C. Small
D. Very small

24. Isapgol consists of dried seeds of the plant known as ....?

A. Plantago psyllium
B. PlantagoOvata
C. Both A and B
D. None

25. The plant are cultivated in which state ?

A. Gujarat
B. M.p
C. U.P
D. Udisa

26. In the india how many hectares of area is said to be under cultivation for the drugs.

A. About 50 thousand
B. About 70 thousand
C. About 60 thousand
D. About 80 thousand

27. How much seeds are needed per hectare ?

A. 1-10 B. 6-12
C. 10-15 D. 13-18

28. Ammonium sulphate is found to be which fertilizer for the plant

A. Satisfactory
B. Non satisfactory
C. Both A and B
D. None

29. This crop is harvested in which month

A. January/ February
B. March/April
C. May/June
D. August/September

30. India producing how much tonnes of seed annually at present ?

A. 50,000
B. 48,000
C. 45,000
D. 40,000

31. What is the order of isapgol ?

A. Sweet
B. Astringent
C. Aromatic
D. None

32. The shape of isapgol are .....?

A. Cylindrical
B. Irregular
C. Ovate cymbiform
D. Flattened

33. Isapgol seeds are processed to take out seed coats, commercially known as______?

A. Flea seeds
B. Ispaghula
C. Husk
D. Iabgul

34. The crushed material is then winnowed to separate, which of them

A. Kernels
B. Husk
C. Both A and B
D. None

35. Indian psyllium seeds are available in which price ?

A. Higher
B. Lower
C. Middle
D. None

36. In the isapgol which species content are more ?

A. Cartilage B. Mucilage
C. Both D. None

37. What would be yields practically

A. Colourful mucilage
B. Colourless mucilage
C. Odour less mucilage
D. Testless mucilage

38. Isapgol husk and seeds contain mucilage, In which part of the seeds are present

A. Cork
B. Cortex
C. Epidermis
D. Medullary

39. The products of hydrolysis is____?

A. Xylose
B. Glucose
C. Lactose
D. Glucoroic acid

40. Fixed oil and proteins are which big the other important constituents

A. Isapgoal seeds
B. Isapgol husk
C. Flea seeds
D. Isapgolovala

41. In isapgol, Which swelling factor of the drug is swelling due to mucilage present in the drug

A. Quantitative
B. Qualitative
C. Both A and B
D. None

42. Swelling factor for seeds Is _____?

A. 1to 10
B. 10 to 14
C. 15 to 20
D. 20 to 25

43. Being the mucilage chemically isapgol which colour is give with the solution of ruthenium red ?

A. Red
B. Yellow
C. Pale brown
D. Pink

44. Isapgol are used in which treatment ?

A. Chronic constipation
B. Appetizer
C. Diarrhea
D. Viral infection

45. In whiCh preparation the isapgol are used?

A. Capsule
B. Tablets
C. Liquid orals
D. Suspension

46. The mucilage of isapgol has a property of______?

A. Slairiness
B. Stringiness
C. Both A and B
D. None

47. Which are substitutes of official drug with good mucilage forming capacity

A. Plantagopurshii
B. Plantagoaristata
C. Both A and B
D. None

48. In which state plantago Asiatics are found

A. Andhra pradesh
B. M.P
C. U.P
D. Maharashtra

49. The oil was prescribed for leprosy as a mixture of which suspended ?

A. Gum
B. Emulsion
C. Both A and B
D. None

50. What is thahindi name of chaulmoogra

A. Suranti
B. Kodi
C. Marotti
D. Chalmogra

51. Except india in which other countries chaulmoogra are found

A. America
B. South East Asia
C. South West Asia
D. None

52. Which deciduous tree grows up to 10 m tall

A. Semi deciduous
B. Auto deciduous
C. Both A and B
D. None

53. Which type of chulmoogra Branch let's.

A. Round
B. Minutely velvet hairy
C. Both A and B
D. None

54. In which month chaulmoogra flowering takes place ?

A. January to April
B. May to july
C. August to October
D. November to December

55. In India trees bear fruits in______?

A. January and March
B. April and may
C. August and September
D. October and November

56. Biological source of neem _____?

A. Rolts and rhizomes
B. Aerial part of azadiracta indica
C. Schoenoeauionoffioinale
D. None of the above

57. Azadirechtinnimbinnimbidin is active constituents of_____?

A. Ryania
B. Sabadilla
C. Derris
D. Neem

58. Margosa is synonym of____?

A. Pyrethrum
B. Neem
C. Tabacco
D. Derris

59. Uses of neem oil is___?

A. Insecticide
B. Antifeedant
C. Both A and B
D. None of the above

60. What is the family of neem

A. Composital
B. Leguminase
C. Meliaceal
D. None

61. Commercial product of neem in india is ____?

A. Vepaside
B. Margo–o
C. Both A and B
D. None

62. Anti –nematodes is_____?

A. Neem oil
B. Neem cake
C. Both A&B
D. None

63. In tamil neem oil is also known as ____?

A. Veppennai
B. Margosan
C. Both A &B
D. None

64. Neem oil is composed of ____?

A. Triglycerides
B. Triterpenoids
C. Both A & B
D. None

65. What is the nature of neem ?

A. Hydrophilic
B. Hydrophobic
C. Both A & B
D. None

66. Which are the active constituent present in the neem

A. Maliantriol
B. Allethrin
C. Cinerin
D. Pyrethrosin

67. In neem azadirachtin is act as a_____?

A. Anti feedant
B. Ativiral
C. Insect repellant
D. Both A &B

68. In neem nimbin and nimbidin are used for_____?

A. Anti viral activity
B. Anti feedant activity
C Insect repellant activity
D. All of the above

69. Which are the flavonol glycosides are present in neem ?

A. Nimaton B. Quercetin
C. Myrecentin D. All of the above

70. Oleum selachoids are the synonym of____?

A. Cod liver oil B. Coca butter
C. Shark liver oil D. None of above

71. Biological source of shark liver oil

A. Hypoprionbrevirostris
B. Galeorhinuszyopterus
C. Both A&B
D. None of the above

72. Shark liver oil is extracted from which species_____?

A. Scoliodon B. Carcharias
C. Sphyna D. All of the above

73. Shark liver oil is soluble in which solvent

A. Ethyl alcohol B. Water
C. Light petroleum D. All of the above

74. Shark liver oil is insoluble in which solvent

A. Water B. Chlorofeom
C. Ester D. Ether

75. Acid value of oleum selachoids is not more then_______?

A. 1 B. 0.5
C. 2 D. 3.1

76. Iodine value of shark liver oil is not less the

A. 10 B. 120
C. 50 D. 90

77. Which vitamin are present in oleum selachoids

A. Vitamin c B. Vitamin D
C. Vitamin A D. All of the above

78. The test of oleum selachoids ?

A. Fiahy B. Bland
C. Both A & B D. None

79. In volume selachoids 1gm of oil should contain not less than ______ International units of vitamin activity

A. 5000
B. 6000
C. 7000
D. 8000

80. In shark liver oil dissolve 1 ml shark oil in 10 ml chloroform and treat with saturated solution of antimony trichloride in chloroform then Blue colour is developed due to the presence of_______?

A. Vitamin C B. Vitamin D
C. Vitamin A D. Vitamin B

81. In which temperature shark liver are stared at_______?

A. Hight temperature
B. Moderate temperature
C. Low temperature
D. Very low temperature

82. Shark liver oil is preserved in which containers to protected from light

A. Well filled B. Well closed
C. Airtight D. Both A & B

83. Shark liver oil is used in deficiency of which vitamin

A. Vitamin D B. Vitamin A
C. Vitamin C D. Vitamin B

84. Shark liver oil is not a genuine substitute for cod liver oil due to the absence of which vitamin

A. Vitamin A B. Vitamin E
C. Vitamin C D. Vitamin D

85. Oleum more hi are the synonym of____???

A. Shark liver oil B. COD liver oil
C. Hydrous wool fat D. Cocoa butter

86. Biological source of cod liver oil

A. Gadusmorrhua
B. Hypoprionbrevirostris
C. Galeorhinuszyopterus
D. None

87. Large quantities of oil consingnmenst are prepared in which coastal regions

A. Narway B. Scotland
C. Iceland D. All of the above

88. The healthy livers of cod are free from

A. Gall bladder B. Microorganisms
C. Both A & B D. None

89. Cod liver oil are soluble in which solvent

A. Chlorofrom B. Ether
C. Petroleum ether D. All of the above

90. Which major steps involved in refining of medicinal cod liver oil

A. Removal of impurities
B. Winterization
C. Deodorisation
D. All of the above

91. Spectrophotometrically in cod liver oil determind which content of the oil ?

A. Vitamin A B. Vitamin C
C. Vitamin D D. Vitamin B

92. Acid value of cod liver oil is less than ______?

A. 1 B. 2
C. 5 D. 8

93. Iodine value of cod liver oil is____?

A. 180 - 190 B. 145- 180
C. 180 -220 D. 200-250

94. The medicinal value of cod liver oil is due to which vitamin

A. Vitamin A B. Vitamin D
C. Both A & B D. None

95. In cod liver oil glycery esters contains of____?

A. Oleic acid B. Palmitic acid
C. Linoleic D. All of the above

96. In Cod liver oil contains how many percent (%) of eicosapentalnoic acid

A. 6.5 % B. 5.5%
C. 7% D. 7.5%

97. Omega-3 Fatty acid are ____?

A. Eicosapentaenoic acid
B. Docosahexaboic acid
C. Both A & B
D. None

98. Cod liver oil are used as a source of_____?

A. Vitamins
B. Nutritive
C. Treatment of rickets
D. All of the above

99. Which oil resulting from in nutritional requirements for polyunsaturates in diet

A. Shark liver oil B. Cocoa butter
C. Cod liver oil D. All of the above

100. Scented Bdellium are the synonym of_____?

A. Storax B. Tar
C. Guggul D. Mxrrh

101. What is the family of Guggul

A. Hamamelidaceae
B. Pinaceae
C. Leguminosae
D. Burseraceae

102. Guggul is which one of the noted drugs

A. Ayurveda system
B. Unani System
C. Both A & B
D. None

103. In recent time it's demand in therapeutics has been substantially _________?

A. Increased B. Decresed
C. Both A & B D. None

104. In india guggul plant is mainly found in which states

A. Rajasthan B. Gujarat
C. Ajmer D. Both A &B

105. In guggul who are natural mode of propagation

A. Seed B. Stem
C. Bark D. Root

106. In which month the seeds are collected from matured red berries

A. July - September B. January- March
C. August - October D. October- December

107. The gum resin portion of guggul contains_____?

A. Steroids B. Diterpenoids
C. Carbohydrates D. All of the above

108. Guggul are used as ______?

A. Anti inflammatory
B. Anti rheumatic hypolipidemic
C. Both A & B
D. None

109. In the C3 cycle how many ATP and NADPH molecules are required to synthesized on molecule of glucose

A. 12 ATP & 12 NADPH
B. 18 ATP & 12 NADPH
C. 12 ATP & 14 NADPH
D. 18ATP & 14 NADPH

110. In the VE cycle all steps are involves except

A. Co2 fixation
B. ATP synthesis
C. Reduction
D. Regeneration of RUBP

111. In cow fixation of C3 cycle the enzyme involved are ?

A. RUBIS CO
B. RUBIS O
C. PEP carboxylase
D. Phosphoglycerokinase

112. To synthesize one glucose molecule to required HoW many glyceraldehyde-3-phosphate

A. 3 B. 6
C. 2 D. 12

113. Calvin cycle is involved in the ?

A. Hydrolysis of water
B. Synthesis of NADPH
C. Synthesis of glucose
D. Synthesis of ATP

114. In the C3 cycle who is the initial CO2 acceptor

A. Phosphoenolyrubate
B. Phosphoglycolate
C. RUBP
D. Citric acid

115. In TCA cycle how many molecules of CO2 are produced per mole of acetyl CoA

A. 1 B. 3
C. 2 D. 4

116. Gluconeogenesis can not be utilized of which of the following intermediates

A. Malate
B. Acetyl COA
C. Alpha - keto glutarate
D. Succinate

117. In the TCA malonate is an inhibitor of ?

A. Succinate dehydrogenase
B. Aconitase
C. Isocitrate dehydrogenase
D. Malate dehydrogenase

118. In the TCA cycle what form does the product of glycolysis enter ?

A. Pyruvate B. Glucose
C. Acetyl COA D. NADH

119. Oxidation of a molecule involves by __________ electron ?

A. Loss of electron B. Gain of electron
C. Both A & B D. None

120. Which chemical is generally used to stop ATP Synthesis

A. DDT B. DNSA
C. 2,4 dinitrophenol D. None of this

121. In the TCA cycle which of the following enzyme does not take part of this

A. Citrate synthase
B. Pyruvate dehydrogenase
C. Malate dehydrogenase
D. Iso-citrate dehydrogenase

122. In TCA cycle who is the first intermediate

A. Succinate B. Citrate
C. Molate D. Fumerate

123. Molate aspartate shuttle operates in which part of the body

A. Heart B. Liver
C. Both D. None

124. In the kreb`s cycle which one of the following is not the intermediate

A. Fumerate B. Stearate
C. Succinate D. Isocitrate

125. Which enzyme is used for formation of anthranilic acid

A. Lipase B. Synthetase
C. Carboxylase D. DeCarboxylase

126. Pimary substrate used in shikmic acid pathway

A. Erythrose -4-po4
B. Erythrose-2-po4
C. 3-hydroquinic acid
D. Dehydroshikmic acid

127. Two isoforms of choresmatemutase has been isolated from which species

A. Rauwolfia B. Poppy
C. Belladonna D. Vinca

128. Which one of the following is used as precursor for formation tryptophan

A. Anthranilic acid B. Phenyl pyruvic acid
C. Tyrosine D. Phenlalanine

129. Choresmicmutase converts choresmic acid to give

A. 3-dehydroquinic acid
B. Shikmic acid
C. Shikmic acid -3-phosphate
D. Prephenic acid

130. Enzyme used to convert glucose-6-phosphate to fuctose-6- phosphate

A. Aap hexokinase
B. Phosphogluco isomerase
C. Phosphofructokinase
D. Aldolase

131. The end product forward after glycolysis ?

A. Pyruvic acid
B. Acetylcoenzyme A
C. Phosphonolpyruvic acid
D. Glyceraldehyde -3-phophate for

132. For embedded -meyerhoff pathway the substrate used in ?

A. D-glucose
B. Fructose-6-phosphate
C. Fructose-1:6-dip
D. Acetylcoenzyme

133. Anthocyanin pigments occur in which vacuoles of

A. Bactaria cell B. Plant cell
C. Animal cell D. None of them

134. Which of these antho-cyanidins are converted to their glucose ?

A. Pelphinidin -3-glucoside
B. Cyanidin-3-glucosid
C. Both A & B
D. None

135. The free energy released in this process is used in this process is used in which form

A. Very high energy molecules
B. Very low molecule
C. High energy molecule
D. Low energy molecules

136. Glycolysis is a sequence of How much enzyme catalyzed reaction ?

A. One B. Five
C. Eight D. Ten

137. Glycolysis is an which metabolic pathway

A. Carbon independent
B. Oxygen dependent
C. Oxygen independent
D. None

138. Charges are balanced by the difference between of ?

A. ADT and NADP B. NADH and ATP
C. ADP and ATP D. NAD and ADP

139. In embden -meyerhoff pathway glucose generate

A. NADH and NAD B. ADP and ATP
C. ATP and NADH D. NAD-N and NAD

141. The mevalonate pathway is also known as the

A. Dimethylallyl pathway
B. Acetate pathway
C. Isoprenoidpatheay
D. None

142. A diverse class of over 30000 biomolecules such as

A. Heme B. Vitamin k
C. Cholesterol D. All of the above

143. In the mevalonate pathway which one in the same way

A. Eukaryotes B. Eubacteria
C. Archaea D. All of the above

144. In upper mevalonate pathway which one is the enzymatic step

A. Acetyl CoA B. HMG-CoA
C. Mevalonate D. All of the above

145. In mevalonate pathway which are the terpanoids

A. Phytol B. Abletic acid
C. Cembrene D. All of the above

146. Isopentenyl diphosphate is the central intermediate in the biosynthesis of ?

A. Mevalonate B. Acetyl- COA
C. HMG - COA D. Isoprenoids

147. Although isoprenoid are synthesis ubiquitously among______?
A. Eubacteria B. Archaebacteria
C. Eukaryotes D. All of the above

148. Translated amino acid sequenles were aligned by using
A. PILEUP OF GCG B. GAPPED
C. Both A & B D. None

149. The skin of animal(animal hide)are treated with tannin to prevent...
A. Puterfaction
B. Crystalline substance
C. Non crystalline substance
D. None of the above

150. Tannins form which type of solution with water and non crystalline substance.
A. Colloidal B. Non colloidal
C. Both a&b D. None of the above

151. Tannins are hydrolyzed by
A. Acids B. Enzymes
C. Both a&b D. None of the above

152. Condensed tannins are also known as
A. Non hydrolysable
B. Phlobatannins
C. Pronthrocyanifins
D. All of the above

153. Condensed tannins are related with
A. Flavanoid pigment
B. Plant
C. Tissue
D. Enzymes

154. Which tannin does not obey to goldbrater's skin test
A. Condensed tannins
B. Hydrolysable tannins
C. Pseudotannins
D. Non hydrolysable tannins

155. Biological source of pale catechu
A. Uncaria gambier roxburgh
B. Gambier
C. Roxburgh
D. Pterocarpous

156. The cultivation is carried out in fields upto
A. 170 B. 160
C. 150 D. 180

157. Propogation is done by which type of seed in damp soil
A. Sowing B. Damp soil
C. Both a &b D. None of the above

158. How many months the seedling are transplanted in open fields
A. 9 B. 10
C. 11 D. 5

159. Geographical source of pale catechu
A. Malaysia B. Singapore
C. Indonesia D. Bangalore

160. Pale catechu is also cultivated in which countries
A. Singapore B. Indonesia
C. Both a&b D. Japan

161. The first harvesting is done when the plant reaches a which height
A. 2m B. 3m
C. 4m D. 10m

162. The plant gives how much amounts of yields the dry upto
A. 20y B. 40y
C. 10y D. 14y

163. Pale catechu occurs which colour
A. Reddish brown B. Black
C. Green D. Yellow

164. Synonyms of pale catechu
A. Gambier B. Catechin
C. Catechu D. All of the above

165. What is the nature of pale Catechu
A. Porous B. Crystalline
C. Non crystalline D. Amorphous

166. Synonyms of black catechu
A. Martha or cutch B. Catechu
C. Khadir-catechu D. All of the above

167. Which family belongs to black catechu
A. Leguminosae B. Piparaceae
C. Barbaraceae D. Rowlfia

168. Biological source of black catechu
A. Acacia catechu B. Acacia chundra
C. Both a&b D. None

169. What's is the taste of black catechu
A. Non astringent B. Astringent
C. Very astringent D. Pungent

170. By the presence of catechin, black catechu gives which colour with vanillin or hcl acid

A. Pink B. Red
C. Both a&b D. Green

171. In black catechu presence of ferric ammonium sulfate gives which colour

A. Green B. Red
C. Yellow D. Pink

172. Plant used for preparation of catechu are grown in

A. Japan B. Myanmar
C. India D. Bothb&c

173. Synonyms of terminaliaarjuna

A. Arjuna bark B. Arjun
C. Both a&b D. None

174. What is the biological source of arjuna

A. Terminaliaarjuna rob
B. Terminalia
C. Both a&b
D. None

175. Geographical source of arjuna

A. Indian peninsula B. Jammu
C. U.p. D. Japan

176. Arjun is common in which region

A. Chottanagpur B. Delhi
C. Both D. None

177. What is the shape of arjuna

A. Flat B. Bottom
C. Curve D. Cylindrical

178. What is the size of arjuna

A. 15×10×1cm B. 10×23×3cm
C. Both D. None

179. Synonyms of bahera (terminaliabelerica)

A. Beleric myrobalan
B. Bahera
C. Bibhitak
D. All of the above

180. Biological source of bahera

A. Terminaliabelerica linn
B. Bahera
C. Both
D. None

181. Bahera belongs to which family

A. Leguminosae B. Combretaceae
C. Paparaceae D. None

182. How many days bahera takes time for germination of seed

A. 15-30 B. 12-13
C. 10-20 D. 12-20

183. What is the maximum height of bahera

A. 40m B. 14m
C. 10m D. 37m

184. What is the taste of bahera

A. Astringent B. Pungent
C. Spicy D. Non astringent

185. Terminaliachebula is also known as

A. Chebula B. Myrobalan
C. Both D. None

186. Synonyms of terminaliachebula

A. Chebulic myrobalan
B. Haritak
C. Harde
D. All of the above

187. Biological source of terminaliachebula

A. Chebula B. Terminalia
C. Terminaliaretzr D. None

188. Terminaliachebula belongs to which family

A. Combretaceae B. Piparaceae
C. Leguminosae D. None

189. What is the altitude contains in growing of plant

A. 1800m B. 1200m
C. 3550 D. 1300m

190. What is the colour of flower in the terminal spikes

A. Yellowish white B. Black
C. Pink D. Green

191. What is the size of terminaliachebula

A. 20-25mm long & 15-25mm wide
B. 14 mm
C. Both
D. None

192. Myrobalan or terminaliachebula are the important source of

A. Tannins B. Glycol
C. Terpenes D. Flavanoid

193. What is the taste of terminaliachebula
A. Astringent B. Slightly bitter
C. Sweetish D. All of the above

194. Myrobalan contains how much amounts of tannins
A. 25-67% B. 25-32%
C. 57-67% D. 56-50%

195. Coriander should contain volatile oil :
A. Less than 0.3 %
B. Between 55 - 70 %
C. Not less than 0.3 %
D. All of the above

196. Biological source of coriander is
A. Dried pulp of Coriandrumsativum
B. Dried ripe fruit of Coriandrumsativum
C. Dried fruit of Coriandrumsativaous
D. None of them

197. Coriander leaves are rich in
A. Minerals B. Vitamin d and c
C. Vitamin A D. Both A and B

198. 90% Chemical constituent of coriander consists
A. Coriandrol (D-linalool)
B. piperine
C. Alcohol
D. Beta- santalol

199. The main use of coriander is
A. Carminative, expectorant and stimulant
B. Counter irritant
C. Laxative
D. Expectorant and counter irritant

200. Citronella oil biological source is
A. Obtained by Steam distillation from fresh leaves of Cymbopogon Narudus, Graminae
B. Obtained by steam distillation of fresh leaves of CymbopogonNidrum, Graminae
C. Obtained by cold maceration of leves of CymbopogonNigrum, Graminae
D. Obtained by cold maceration of leaves of CymbopogonNarudus, Graminae

201. Main chemical constituent of citronella is
A. Citral
B. Citral acid
C. 1 – citral acetic acid
D. Citronellal and geraniol

202. Citronella is soluble in
A. Water B. 20% acetic acid
C. 80% Alcohol D. chloroform

203. Citronella is used as
A. Perfume for soup and mosquito repellent creams and sprays
B. Brilliantine and flavouring agent
C. Both A& B
D. None of the above

204. Biological source of Fennel is
A. Dried ripe fruit of FoeniculumVulgare, Umbellifarae
B. Dried rip fruit of Foeniculum Selenium, Umbellifarae
C. Fresh fresh of Foeniculumvukgare, Umbellifarae
D. None of them

205. The sweet taste of fennel is due to
A. Fenchone B. Fencholine
C. Anethole D. Both A and B

206. Fennel fruit contain the ketone with
A. Anethole and Fenchone
B. Only Fenchone
C. Only Anethole
D. None of them

207. Use of Fennel fruit is
A. Carminative Expectorant
B. Only Carminative
C. Stimulant
D. Both A and B

208. Synonyms of fennel is
A. Sweet fennel and large fennel
B. Fennel fruit and Foeniculli
C. Foenum
D. Both A and B

209. Nature if primary ridges in coriander is
A. Straight B. Both A and C
C. Wavy D. None of them

210. Adulterants of fennel, Exhausted fennel contain
A. 6-8% volatile oil
B. 15-16 % volatile oil
C. 1-2 % volatile oil
D. None of them

211. Black pepper belongs to which family
A. Piperaceae B. Pipaver
C. Umbellifarae D. Apocynacae

212. The characteristic flavor of black pepper is due to
A. Chavicine B. piperine
C. Piperidine D. Piperettine

213. The main use of black pepper
A. Carminative and bioavibility enhancer
B. Tranquilizer
C. Laxative
D. expectorant

214. The alkaloid in black pepper is
A. Piperine B. pipridine
C. 1 phellandrene D. caryophyllene

215. The biological source of black pepper is
A. Dried ripe fruit of Piper Nigrum, piperaceae
B. Dried unripe fruit of Piper Nigrum, piperaceae
C. Fresh leave of pepper Nigrum, piperaceae
D. None of them

216. The main chemical consistuent of Mentha is
A. Isoprnoid
B. 1- menthol
C. 1,3 dialkeyl menthol
D. Both A and B

217. Mentha belongs to family
A. Metracae B. Labiatae
C. Umbellifarae D. papeaveraceae

218. Which of the fallowing is not a use of Mentha
A. Caa+ channel blocking activity
B. vasodilation
C. Nasal decongestant
D. Carminative and stimulant

219. The shape of menthe leaves is
A. Obloged B. Longitudinal
C. lanceolate D. Both A and C

220. Synonym of cinnamon is
A. Kalmi – dalchini B. Cinnamon bark
C. Cinnamon tork D. Both A and B

221. The biological source of turpentine is
A. From oleoresin of pinusroxburghi, pinaceae
B. From oleoresin of pinocucus, pinaceace
C. From oleoresin of pinuspalustris, Pinaceae
D. Both A and C

222. Which of the fallowing is not the chemical constituent of turpentine oil
A. Beta carolene B. Beta pipene
C. Limonene
D. Beta phenllandreane

223. Which of the fallowing is one of the use of turpentine oil
A. Rubefecient B. Cardio tonic
C. Carminative D. Purgative

224. The synonym of turpentine oil is
A. Oleum terbenthae
B. Alivium terpenoid
C. Turpentine exoses
D. None of them

225. Which of the fallowing is the common adulterant of turpentine
A. Oiliveterpin B. Rosemaryil
C. Resin oil D. None of them

226. Mentha is soluble in
A. 70% ethyl acetate B. 70% Alcohol
C. Water D. 40% Ether

227. Cardamom belongs to which family
A. Papervaracae B. Zingiberaceae
C. Umbellifarae D. Rosacea

228. The shape of cardamom is
A. Ovoid or oblong B. Both A and C
C. Straight D. None of them

229. The seeds of cardamom is derived from
A. Bytrophous ovules
B. Both A and D
C. Unitrophous ovules
D. Anatropous ovules

230. Cardamom seed contain volatile oil content extent to
A. 1-2 % B. 2-8%
C. 9-12 % D. 14-17%

231. The active constituent of volatile oil in cardamom is
A. Starch and protein
B. Turpentine
C. Cineole
D. Borneol

232. Cardamom is used as
A. Carminative and stimulant
B. Flavouring agent
C. Positive inotropic
D. Antiseptic

233. Citronella belongs to which family
A. Myrtaceae B. Umbellifarae
C. Graminae D. Laguminoceae

234. Cinnamon belongs to which family
A. Lauraceae B. piperaceae
C. Myrtaceae D. laguminoceae

235. Cinnamon consist of dried inner bark of shoot of copied trees of
A. Cinnamumzylanicum
B. Cinnamomumzeylanicum
C. Cinamomumzylanicus
D. all of them

236. Which of the fallowing is true about cinnamon
A. Cork and primary cortex is present
B. Cork and primary cortex is absent
C. Rarely, primary cortex may be present
D. Both B and C

237. The sweet substance in cinnamon is
A. mannitol B. Eugenol
C. carbohydrate D. None of them

238. Cinnamon oil consists 60-70 % of
A. Benzaldehyde B. Eugenol
C. cymene D. cinnamaldehyde

239. Which of the fallowing is not a substituent or adulterant of cinnamon
A. Java cinnamon
B. Cinnamon chip
C. Cinnamon slogs
D. Cultivated Saigon cinnamon

240. Synonym of bitter orange peel is
A. Orange valour B. Orange buncher
C. Orange cortex D. None of them

241. The amount of volatile oil in the Orange peel should be
A. Not more than 3%
B. Not less than 2.5 %
C. Between 5-9%
D. between 10-14 %

242. Orange peel belongs to which of the following family
A. Apocynacae B. Umbellifarae
C. Rutaceae D. None of them

243. Volatile oil in bitter orange peel contain
A. Citral B. limonene
C. Both A and B D. None of them

244. The medicinal use of bitter orange peel is
A. Stomachic and carminative
B. antibiotic
C. purgative
D. antiaging

245. Which of the fallowing is not synonym of Lemon grass oil
A. Indian mellissa oil
B. Grass cascaria oil
C. Grass oil
D. Both A and B

246. Amount of aldehyde calculated as citral in Lemon Grass oil should be
A. Not less than 0.9 %
B. Not less than 20%
C. Not less than 75%
D. Not less than 30-80 %

247. Lemon grass is entirely soluble in
A. 5 parts of 40% ether
B. Water
C. 3 parts of 70% alcohol
D. 30% ethyl acetate

248. Which of the following is a chemical constitute of Lemon Grass Oil
A. Citral B. Citric acid
C. Aldehyde D. Gallic acid

249. The common use of Lemon Grass Oil is
A. antioxidant
B. Cleaning agent
C. Flavouring agent in perfumery
D. None o them

250. Synonym of lemon peel is
A. Lemon limonis B. Lemon fressis
C. Lemon Jessie D. All of the above

251. Which of the fallowing is not the chemical constituent of lemon peel other thanvolatile oil

A. Bitter substance and calcium oxalate
B. hesperidin
C. Pectin
D. Ascorbic acid

252. The volatile oil Lemon peel contain limonene about

A. 20% B. 78.3 %
C. 90% D. 54%

253. Which of following is not the Synonym of chinopoduim oil

A. Chenoposan
B. chinomustein
C. chenopodiol
D. American wormeed oil

254. Biological source of chinopoduim is oil of steam distillation fresh aerial part of

A. Chinopoduimamborosisoids
B. Chinopoduimanthlmenticum
C. Both A and B
D. None of the above

255. The major component of oil of chinopoduim are:

A. Ascaridole (60-80)% and limonene
B. Isosascaridol and p-cymene
C. Both A& B
D. Archedoicchinopoduim acid

256. Main use of chinopoduim is

A. To treat internal parasites
B. To treat microbial bites
C. To treat bacterial infection
D. None of them

257. The biological source of eucalyptus oil is; Distillation of fresh leaves of

A. Eucalyptus globulus
B. Eucalyptus globuie
C. Eucalyptus traceaseas
D. None of these

258. Main chemical constituent of Eucalyptus is

A. Cineole 80% (Eucalyptol)
B. Crinoline
C. Acetic acid 50%
D. Both A and C

259. Which of the following is not use of Eucalyptus oil

A. Counter irritant and antiseptic
B. Chronic bronchitis
C. Expectorant
D. Anti-allergic

260. Synonym of Eucalyptus is

A. Eucalipulus B. Eucalyptus
C. Dinkum oil D. Both B and C

261. Eucalyptus belongs to family

A. Umbellifarae B. Apocynacae
C. Myrtaceae D. Roseceae

262. Spearmint belongs to which family

A. Graminae B. Labiatae
C. Myrtaceae D. None of them

263. Use of spearmint is

A. Flavouring agent and carminative
B. Pupil dilator
C. Positive inotropic
D. Nome of them

264. The main chemical constituent of spearmint is

A. anetholene B. 1 deoxyriboxydiose
C. 1- Carvone D. 1-4 Thiolidiine

265. Biological source of Ajowan is ; Dried ripe fruit of

A. Trycuscarauginia
B. Trychyspermumammi
C. Trychaspermumnigrasia
D. Trycuspermumgingorba

266. Ajowan belongs to family

A. Apocynacae B. scaramaceae
C. Umbellifarae D. None of them

267. Which of the fallowing is main chemical constituent of Ajowan

A. vincristine
B. P cymene and pinene
C. thymol
D. Both B and C

268. Which of the following is use of Ajowan

A. Anti-spasmodic B. antiaging
C. antibacterial D. carminative

269. Biological source of Anise is ; Dried ripen fruit of
A. Pimpinellaanisum
B. Driginellaanisum
C. Pimpinelllaaniscusion
D. None of them

270. Main chemical constituent of Anise is
A. Methylcharvical B. Anisaldehide
C. Anethole D. All of the above

271. Use of anise is
A. Stimulant and carminative
B. Favouring agent
C. Expectorant
D. All of the above

272. Main chemical constituent of Jira is
A. Cumin ketone B. Cumin aldehyde
C. Qunollic aldehyde
D. None of them

273. The common use of Jira is
A. Diarrhoea
B. Carminative and stimulant
C. Dyspepsia
D. All of the above

274. Which family Jira does belongs too
A. Umbellifarae B. piperaceae
C. Lauraceae D. None of them

275. The biological source of Jira is; dried ripe fruit of
A. Cuminumcyminum
B. Both A and B
C. Cuminumanthecean
D. None of them

276. Caraway biological source; dried ripe fruit of
A. Caraway curculine
B. Carumcarvi
C. Caraway carvium
D. None of these

277. Caraway belongs to which family
A. Rosacea B. Myrtaceae
C. Rutaceae D. None of Them

278. Carvone present in caraway as chemical constituent is in amount of
A. 90-92 % B. 50-60%
C. 60-80% D. 20-26%

279. The medical use of caraway is
A. stimulant B. Carminative
C. expectorant D. All of the above

280. Biological source of Indian Dill is
A. Dried ripe fruit of anilium
B. Dried ripe fruit of Anethum
C. None of these
D. Both A and B

281. Biological source of European Dill is
A. Dried ripe fruit of Anethumribulavium
B. Dried ripe fruit of Anethumgraveoulens
C. Dried ripe fruit of aniliumAnethum
D. All of these

282. The main chemical Toxic constituent in the Indian Dill is
A. Dill apiole B. Dill apinoline
C. Dill quniole D. None of these

283. The main chemical constituent of European dill is
A. Dill apiole B. Carvone
C. d- limonene D. Both B and C

284. The Indian dill is used in
A. Clinical practice B. Vetinary practice
C. antibiotic D. antimicrobial

285. The main use of European Dill is
A. Aromatic
B. Gripe water
C. Gastric disturbance of infants
D. All of the above

286. Nutmeg belongs to family
A. Myrtaceae B. liilaceae
C. Myristicaceae D. lagimusoseae

287. The biological source of nutmeg is; dried kernels of seeds of
A. Myristicafalunum
B. Myristicfragrans
C. Myristicaallicivam
D. All of the above

288. The nutmeg fat and volatile oil is used in
A. Arthritis B. Rheumatism
C. gout D. None of the above

289. Which of the following is not chemical consistuent of nutmeg
A. Eugenol B. elimicin
C. myristicin D. saffrole

290. Biological source of clove is dried flower buds of
A. Szyoguimaromaticim
B. SzyoguimMyrtaceae
C. Eugenia caryophyllus
D. None of the above

291. Main chemical constituent of clove is
A. Eugenol B. Citral
C. Citronella D. Gallic acid

292. The main use of clove is
A. Dental analgesic
B. Manufacture of vanillin
C. carminative
D. All of the above

293. Synonym of clove is
A. Clove flower
B. Caryophyllum
C. Clove bud
D. All of the above

294. Clove belongs to family
A. Myrtaceae B. Umbellifarae
C. Apocynacae D. None of the above

295. The volatile content of clove should
A. Not less than 15% V/W
B. Between 30-40% V/W
C. Not less than 5% V/W
D. Both C and B

296. Adulterants of clove is
A. Exhausted clove, blown clove and mother clove
B. Blown clove only
C. Exhausted clove only
D. None of them

297. Sandalwood belongs to family
A. Santalaceae B. laguminoceae
C. solenaceae D. Both A and C

298. Main chemical constituents of sandalwood is
A. Qurcitine B. Beta santalol
C. Alpha santalol D. Both B and C

299. Sandalwood is used in Treatment of
A. Dysuria and diminishing frequency of micturition in TB
B. Incense sticks
C. Perfume and cosmetics
D. All of the above

300. Cassia bark used as
A. Carminative, stimulant
B. Aromatic and as spice
C. Flavouring agent
D. All of the above

301. Biological source of Cassia bark is; dried stem bark of
A. Cinnamomum cassia
B. Cinnamomumangustifirica
C. Cassia cinnamum
D. Both A and B

302. The volatile oil (cinnamic aldehyde) content in Cassia Bark is
A. 56%
B. 26%
C. Not less than 85%
D. 90%

303. biological source of Star anise is ; dried ripe fruit of
A. Iiluvanisvercum B. Alive sativum
C. Illiciumverum D. None of these

304. Star anise belongs to family
A. solenaceae B. schisandraceae
C. Umbellifarae D. None of them

305. Chemical constituent of star anise
A. Anethole B. pepeverine
C. quinine D. All of them

306. The percentage of fixed oil in coriander is
A. 66 % B. 44 %
C. 13% D. 10%

307. No of primary ridges in one mericarp fennel are
A. 5-6 B. 9-10
C. 3-4 D. None of them

308. No of stylopode in one fennel fruit
A. 3% B. 3%
C. 1% D. 5%

309. In cinnamon the percentage of volatile oil contain should not less then
A. 30% B. 0.1 %
C. 2.0 % D. 5.4%

310. Types of quill found in cinnamon bark are
A. compound B. single
C. Multifractured D. Both A and B

311. Shape of coriander fruit is
A. Sub globular B. Sub longitudinal
C. Sub glandular D. None of them

312. Father of medicine.
A. Hippocrates B. Sushrutha
C. Aristotle D. None

313. What reagent used in Molisch's test
A. Alpha napthol and sulphuric acid
B. Alpha napthol and HCl
C. Both
D. None

314. Acacia belong to which category:
A. Alkaloid B. Carbohydrates
C. Glycosides D. Flavanoid

315. Which drug come under in Leguminosae family:
A. Gum acacia and tragacanth
B. Indian senna and aloes
C. Agar and guar gum
D. Both A and B

316. Biological source of Indian gum:
A. Acacia arabica
B. Aeglemarmelos
C. Echinacea augustifolia
D. Gelidiumamansi

317. Which part is used to obtained Indian gum:
A. Leaf
B. Flower
C. Stem and branches
D. Root

318. Arabin is main constituent of:
A. Gum acacia B. Guar gum
C. Tragacanth D. Agar

319. Which reagent used for identification of acacia:
A. Benzyl alcohol and potassium hydroxide
B. Ferric ammonium sulphate and NaOH
C. Alpha napthol and sulphuric acid
D. Hydrogen peroxide and benzidine

320. Function of carbohydrates:
A. Energy source
B. Structural framework
C. Both A and B
D. none

321. Carbohydrates are:
A. Polyhydoxy aldehydes and phenols
B. Polyhydroxy aldehydes and ketones
C. Polyhydroxy ketones and phenols
D. Polyhydroxy phenols and alcohol

322. Monosaccharide unit joined by which bond in polysaccharide unit:
A. Ionic bond B. Peptide bond
C. Glucose bond D. Glycosidic bond

323. Starch consist of:
A. Brancedamyolse and branced amylopectin
B. Unbranced amylase and branced amylopectin
C. Both
D. None

324. Amylum is a synonym of:
A. Starch B. Dextrin
C. Xanthin Gum D. None

325. Starch consist of:
A. Monosaccharide
B. disaccharide
C. polysaccharide
D. trisaccharides

326. Biologica source of starch is :
A. Zea mays linn
B. oryza sativa linn
C. triticumaestivum linn
D. all

327. Family of starch is
A. Solanaceae B. gramineae
C. leguminaceae D. both A and B

328. On hydrolysis of starch it is converted into glucose, which base is used for hydrolysis
A. Acidic base B. Neutral base
C. Alkalin base D. Salty base

329. Storage form of starch is :
A. Fats B. Amino acid
C. Lipids D. Carbohydrates

330. Identification test for starch is :
A. Iodine test B. Biuret test
C. Bendict test D. Bromine test

331. Which two different polysaccharide are starch contain:
A. Amylose B. Amylopectin
C. Amylum D. Both A and B

332. Which color are obtained when amylase react with iodine.
A. Yellow B. Blue
C. Green D. Purplish green

333. Antidote for iodine poisoning
A. Starch B. Dextrin
C. Caramel D. None

334. In what percentage starch is used for binder:
A. 1% B. 3-5%
C. 5-10% D. 15-20%

335. Which variety of starch is used as asubstituent of starch:
A. Tapioca starch B. Cassava
C. Brazillian root D. All

336. Synonymn of tragacanth
A. Gum tragacanth B. Indian tragacanth
C. Karaya gum D. all

337. Astragalus gummifer is a biological source of :
A. Indian tragacanth
B. gum tragacanth
C. Both
D. None

338. Which part of plant is used for tragacanth:
A. Stem and branches
B. Only branches
C. Root
D. None of these

339. Leguminosae is family of :
A. Indian tragacanth B. Tragacanth
C. Both D. none

340. Taste of tragacanth
A. Bitter B. Mucilaginous
C. Sweet D. Characterst

341. Chemical constituent of tragacanth
A. tragacathin B. Arabinogalactan
C. marmelosin D. none

342. Which chemical moiety is present in tragacanth :
A. o-methylhalfordinol
B. Metoxy group
C. Aldobionic acid
D. Both A and B

343. What is the HLB value of tragacanth .
A. 11 B. 13
C. 16 D. 10

344. Which chemical constituent of tragacanth is water insoluble.
A. tragacathin B. Bassorin
C. Both D. None

345. Which product is obtained from tragacanth on hydrolysis:
A. Galactouronic acid
B. D-galactopyranose
C. L- arbino-ehamnose
D. All of the above

346. Which colour ppt is obtained,whenboiled tragacanth react with aqueous ferric chloride :
A. Green precipitate
B. Yellow precipitate
C. Deep blue precipitate
D. Bluish red

347. Which colour is obtained ,when boiled tragacanth react with iodine solution:
A. Green colour B. Purplish blue
C. Yellow colour D. Orange colour

348. Tragacanth is which type of binder:
A. wet binder
B. Dry binder
C. Available in both type
D. None

349. Which of the following non ionic agent is used as a synthetic emulsifiers,choose the correct one :
A. Tragacanth
B. Sodium lauryl sulphate
C. Gelatine
D. All

350. Biological source of pectin :
A. Citrus simon B. Citrus aurantium
C. Both D. None

351. Which drug belong in the family of rutaceae:

A. Pectin B. jaborandi
C. Both D. None

352. On hydrolysis of pectin which chemical moiety is obtained from pectin :

A. D-galacturonic acid
B. Galactose
C. Arabinose
D. All

353. Pectin is a polysaccharide, while on fruit ripening it is break down by certain enzyme. What is the name of that enzyme.

A. pectinase B. lipase
C. Pectinestrase D. Both A and C

354. Pectin is use as:

A. Repair DNA of seed
B. As a demulcent
C. In cosmetic product
D. All

355. Ricinus oil is synonymn of :

A. Arachis oil
B. Castor oil
C. Hydrogenated castor oil
D. Olice oil

356. Castor oil is obtained by the cold expression of which seeds:

A. Ricinuscommunis
B. Oleaeuropoea
C. Taraktogenouskurjii
D. None

357. Which oil is obtained by cold expression method :

A. Chaulmoogra oil B. Sesame oil
C. Castor oil D. Both A and C

358. Which enzyme is contain by castor seed

A. Lipase B. Maltase
C. Invertase D. All

359. The complex mixtures of volatile oil:

A. Mono and diterpens alcohol and ethers
B. Sesquiterpines and other aromatic compounds
C. Monoterpene ethers and aldehydes
D. Mono and sesquiterpenes and phenylprrpane derivatives

360. Which of the following contain a fixed oil rich in gamma –linolic acid:

A. Zea mays
B. Oenotherabiennis
C. sesamumindicum
D. Ricinuscommunis

361. Castor oil is a fixed oil, which one acid is contain by castor oil:

A. Ricinoleic acid B. Linolic acid
C. Stearic acid D. All

362. Sebacic acid and undecenoic acid is contain by which oil:

A. Castor oil B. Olive oil
C. Linseed oil D. Chaulmoogra oil

363. Which of the following is a use of castor oil:

A. Cathartic B. Lubricant
C. Enamel D. All

364. Cathartic property of castor oil is due to which acid:

A. Ricinoleic acid B. Stearic acid
C. Sebacic acid D. None

365. What is the other name of teel oil:

A. Sesame oil B. Benne oil
C. Both of the above D. Kokum oil

366. Sesame oil is a fixed oil it is obtained from:

A. Seeds of sesamumindicum
B. Leaf of sesamumindicum
C. Seed of garcinia indica
D. None

367. The main constitutent of sesame oil:

A. Sesamolin B. Sasamin
C. Both D. None

368. Which test is used for identification of sesame oil and which color is obtained :

A. Benedict test and red colour
B. Keller killani and reddish brown
C. Legal test and pink to red colour
D. Bodouin's test and pink or red colour

369. Which oil is uses as a vehicle for intramuscular injection and also used in prepration of liniments:

A. Sesame oil B. Chaulmoogra oil
C. Linseed oil D. All

370. Cottonseed oil is a fixed oil obtained from the dried seeds of:
A. Gossypiumherbaceum
B. Theobroma cacao
C. Galeorhinuszyopterus
D. None

371. Gossypiumherbaceum is the biological source of :
A. Gossypol B. Cottonseed oil
C. Both D. None

372. What is the family of Cotton seed oil and gossypol which is obtained from gossypiumherbaceum:
A. Malvacae B. Sterculiaceae
C. Meliaceae D. Both A and C

373. What is the chemical constituent of cotton seed oil:
A. Palmitic acid B. Oleic acid
C. Linoleic acid D. All

374. Oleum olivae is the synonymn of :
A. Oleaeuropoea
B. Hydnocarpus anthelmintic
C. Sesamumindicum
D. None

375. Olive oil if the fixed oil obtained from the ripe fruit of :
A. Sesamumindicum
B. Oleaeurpoea
C. Carthamustinctorius
D. none

376. Oleaeurpoea obtained from the ripe fruit and belonging to the family:
A. Oleaceae B. Lilaceae
C. Linaceae D. Pedaliaceae

377. Which triglycerides is contain by olive oil:
A. Olein B. Palmitin
C. linolein D. All

378. Which color is given by olive oil under ultra violet radiaton :
A. Deep golden-yellow color
B. Green color
C. Deep brown-yellow color
D. None

379. What is the use of oleaeurpoea:
A. Emollient agent B. Mild laxative
C. Both of the above D. none

380. What is the synonymn of arachis oil:
A. Ground nut oil B. Peanut oil
C. Ricinus oil D. Both A and B

381. Arachis oil is a fixed oil which is obtained from the seed of :
A. Arachishypogaea
B. Ricinuscommunis
C. Both
D. None

382. What is the family of peanut oil :
A. Leguminosae B. Lilaceae
C. Flacourtriaceae D. None

383. Oleic acid palmitic acid, linoleicacid, arachidic acid all are the main constituent of which oil:
A. Arachishypgaea B. Ricinuscommunis
C. Oleaeuropoea D. None

384. Which color is show by peanut oil in presence of ultra violet radiation:
A. Blue
B. Green
C. Does not show color
D. Bluish green

385. What is the synonymn of shellac:
A. Lac B. Catkins
C. Embelia D. None

386. What is the biological source of shellac:
A. Lacciferlacca B. Piper longum
C. Both D. None

387. What is the main constituent of shellac:
A. Aleuritic acid B. Shellolic acid
C. Both D. None

388. On adding ammonium molybolate and sulphuric acid into shellac which color is produced by shellac:
A. Green color
B. Blue color
C. Yellow color
D. Clear solution is obtained

389. Hydrous wool fat is obtained from the wool of the sheep another name of wool fat is :
A. Lanolin B. Adepslanae
C. Both D. None

390. Lanolin is fat like subsatance which secreted by sebaceous gland of sheep then biological source of lanolin wil be:
A. Ovisaries
B. Apis mellifeca
C. Caperniciaprunifera
D. Both A and C

391. Wool fat is secreted by sebaceous gland belong to which family :
A. Bovidae B. Palmae
C. Suidae D. Physeterdae

392. What is the main constituent of wool fat:
A. Cholesterol B. Lanoceric acid
C. Caranubic acid D. All

393. On adding chloroform and acetic anhydride with 2 drop of sulphuric acid then which color is indicated the presence of cholesterol:
A. Green colour
B. Blue colour
C. Does not appear
D. Orange colour

394. Choose the correct one :
A. Wool fat is used as ointment base
B. Wool fat is used as cosmetic prepration
C. Wool fat is used as water soluble cream
D. All

395. What is the synonymn of madhu :
A. Honey B. Mel
C. Honey pourified D. All

396. Honey is deposited by honey comb by the bees, what is the biological source of honey:
A. Apis mellifera
B. Xanthomonascompestris
C. Both
D. None

397. Which constituent is present in madhu:
A. Fructose B. Succinic acid
C. Acetic acid D. All

398. Fiehe's test is used to determination of :
A. Honey B. Caramel
C. Dextram D. Xanthan gum

399. Honey is used as a sweetening agent also it is used in:
A. Creams B. Lotions
C. Candies D. All

400. Bees wax is also known as yellow bees wax what is the other name of yellow bees wax:
A. Ceraflava B. Brazil wax
C. Adeps D. None

401. Ceraflaves is collected from the comb which is made by bees, what is the biological source of ceraflaves :
A. Apis mellifera
B. Cooperniciaprunifera
C. Both
D. None

402. Which drug come in cateogory of apidae family:
A. Honey B. Ceraflaves
C. Carnauba wax D. Both A and B

403. Ceraflaves contain esters of monohydric alcohol, the main constituent of ceraflaves is:
A. Myricyl B. Cerotic acid
C. Palmitin D. None

404. Saponification claud test is used to determination of
A. Bees wax B. Carnauba wax
C. Suet D. Lard

405. Ceraflava is used in prepration of ointments along with it is also used in prepration of :
A. Face cream B. Lipsticks
C. Polishes D. All

406. The name of coccus cacti is cochineal, what is the another name of cochineal:
A. Coccus B. Red scale insect
C. Foxglove D. Both A and B

407. Coccidae is the family of cochineal then what is the biological source of cochineal:
A. Coccus cacti B. Cape aloe
C. Both D. None

408. What is the family of coccus :
A. Coccidae B. Apocynaceae
C. Lilaceae D. Scrophulariaceae

409. Cochineal contain fat and wax along with it also contain which main constituent:
A. Carminic acid B. Cerberin
C. Neriifolin D. Peruvosidic acid

410. Cochineal is FDA Approval drug it is used as a :
A. Colouring agent
B. Sweetening agent
C. Cosmetic purpose
D. Both A and C

411. Kasturi is obtained from moschusmoschiferus, its another name is moschus but it is also knowm as other name which is :
A. Musk B. Zibeth
C. Thyme D. None

412. Kasturi is occur from which source :
A. Cymbopogennardus
B. Moschusmoscuiferus
C. Viverrazibetha
D. Both A and B

413. Musk belong to the which family:
A. Graminae B. Cervidea
C. Viverridea D. castoridae

414. Kasturi is a terpenoids it contain fat ,wax along with it also contain one of the drug which given below:
A. Muskone B. Albuminoids
C. Both D. None

415. Lard is a lipid it is also known by another name which is :
A. Adeps B. Sevum
C. Cetaceum D. Both Aand B

416. Adeps is a fat which family is suidae and it is obtained from :
A. Susscrofa
B. Ovisaries
C. Coperniciacerifera
D. Coperniciaprunifera

417. What si the family of lard:
A. Bovidae B. Suidae
C. Physeteridae D. None

418. Benzoinated lard contain benzoin it is used as a:
A. Preservative B. Ointment base
C. Formulation D. All

419. Lard is a lipid which contain following chemical constituent which is :
A. Palmitin B. Olein
C. Stearin D. All

420. Silk is fibre which is occur form which source:
A. Bombyxmori
B. Ovisaries
C. Corchoruscapsularis
D. None

421. Bombyxmori is the fibre what is the family of bombyxmori:
A. Bovidae B. Bombyxmori
C. Both D. None

422. A special protein is contain by silk which give glycine on hydrolysis:
A. Fibroin B. Keratin
C. Both D. Only B

423. Sulphur moiety is contain by which animal product :
A. Silk B. Wool
C. Jute D. None

424. Wool fibre is occur from:
A. Ovisaries
B. All
C. Gossypiumherbaceurre
D. All

425. Which drug belong to the family of bovidae:
A. Wool B. Wool fat
C. Silk D. Both A and B

426. The highest amount of cystine is present in keratin, kerain is contain by which animal product:
A. Wool B. Flax
C. Jute D. Rayon

427. Which colour is obtained when wool is react with solution of caustic soda with lead aceate:
A. Black precipitate
B. Blue precipitate
C. Orange precipitate
D. Green precipitate

428. What is the synonymn of gossypiumherbaceurre:
A. Raw cotton B. Absorbent cotton
C. Surgical cotton D. All

429. Gossypiumherbaceurre is the biological source of whch plant fibres:

A. Surgical cotton B. Purified cotton
C. Cotton wool D. All

430. Raw cotton belong to the which family :

A. Bovidae B. Malvaceae
C. Lilacae D. Palmae

431. Which cotton contain trichomes :

A. Purified cotton B. Absorbent cotton
C. Raw cotton D. bothA and B

432. Raw cotton contain fat,wax,cellulose and others, what is the percentage criteria of all this chemical:

A. 90% cellulose and 7% other fat wax and remain protoplasm
B. 95%cellulose and 2% fat, wax, other and remin protoplasm
C. 89% cellulose and 7% other, fat, wax and remain protoplasm
D. None

433. Add sulphuric acid in cotton which previously contain iodine water, which colour is produced:

A. Purplish blue
B. Purplish green
C. Cleat solution is obtained
D. Bluish yellow

434. Raw cotton is used as :

A. Surgical dressing
B. Filtering medium
C. Prevent wound from infection
D. All

435. What is the another name of asbestos:

A. Amianthus B. Floridin
C. Armenian bole D. None

436. Amianthus is a mineral silicates which found in two form which is :

A. Serpentine B. Amphibole
C. Both D. None

437. Which elements is present is asbestos

A. Iron B. Calcium
C. Magnesium D. All

438. Amianthus is used as a :

A. Bacterial filters B. Insulaters
C. Fire proof gloves D. All

439. Kaolin is also known as kaolinumprodeesum, it is also known by another name which is :

A. China clay B. Amianthus
C. Floridin D. Armenian bole

440. China clay contain one of the following moiety:

A. Aluminium silicate
B. Aluminium hydroxide
C. Magnesium silicate
D. None

441. Various type of kaolin is available in different variety, choose the correct one:

A. Heavy kaolin
B. Light kaolin
C. Natura light kaolin
D. All

442. Which colour is obtained when china clay is treated with charcoal and with cobalt nitrate:

A. Blue mass B. Greem mass
C. Orange D. Bluish yellow

443. Prepared chalk is known by name chalk ,what is the other name prepared chalk:

A. Creta B. Whiting
C. Industrial earth D. Both A and B

444. Chalk contain calcium carbonate ,what is the percentage criteria :

A. NLT97% B. NLT 95%
C. NLT 80% D. NLT 85%

445. Prepared chalk contain calcium carbonate along with it also contain more chemical moiety, choose the coorect one:

A. Magnesium carbonate
B. Iron traces
C. Aluminium oxides
D. All of the above

446. Prepared chalk is used in pharmaceutical industry, choose the correct use of prepared chalk:

A. Antibiotics B. Antacid
C. Anti diarrhoeal D. All

447. Industrial earth is also known by name kieselguhr, it is also known by another name which is :

A. Celite super cel
B. Diatomaceous earth
C. Both A and B
D. English white

448. What is the family of kieselguhr :

A. Bacillariceae B. Liliaceae
C. Apidae D. None

449. Kieselghur contain calcium oxide along with it also contain :

A. Aluminium oxide
B. Iron oxide
C. Magnesium oxide
D. All

450. Agar is also known as agar agar, what is another name of agar :

A. Japanese isinglass
B. Vegetable gelatine
C. Both
D. None

451. Agar agar is gelatin substance which is taken form algae species like gracilaria, what is the other source of agar:

A. Gelidiumamansii
B. Chondruscrispus
C. Both
D. None

452. Vegetable gelatin is obtained froemspeices algae like pterocladia, then what is the family of pterocladia :

A. Gelidaceae B. Gracilariaceae
C. Rhodophyceae D. Both A and B

453. The two main constituent which is polysaccharide is contain by agar which is:

A. Agarose B. Agaropectin
C. Both D. Only A

454. Which constituent of agar gives Gel strength property :

A. Agarose B. Agaropectin
C. Only A D. Both

455. Boil agar with water and cool at 25 to 30.c it shows which property or colour

A. Formation of jelly B. Pink colour
C. Precipitate D. Red ppt

456. The use of agar as a laxative along with it also used as a :

A. Binder
B. Emulsifying agent
C. Prepration for jellies
D. All

457. What is the another name of sodium alginate :

A. Algin
B. Sodium polumannuronate
C. Both
D. None

458. Polyuronic form is algnic acid which is taken from algae , then it belong to which family :

A. Phaeophyceae B. Leguminosae
C. Combretacae D. Only B

459. On reaction with calcium chloride with sodium alginate it gives:

A. Brown ppt B. Red ppt
C. Jelly D. Copious ppt

460. What is other name of rectified oil of turpentine:

A. Turpentine oil B. Oleum terbinthae
C. Both D. None

461. On distillation of oleo resin a volatile oil which is turpentine oil is obtained then what is the biological source of turpentine oil ;

A. Pinusroxnurghii B. Pinuspalustris
C. Both D. None

462. What is the family of pinusroxnurghii ,it is a volatile oil obtained by distillation :

A. Pinaceae B. Liliceae
C. Graminae D. None

463. About around 40 terpens are reported, following are the main constituent which is contain by turpentine oil which is ;

A. Pinene B. Careen
C. Limonene D. All

464. Turpentine is a volatile liquid it is uses as a:

A. Cunter irritant B. Antiseptic
C. Expectorant D. All

465. Colophony is known by various name like resin, then it is also known by another name which is :

A. Amber resin B. Gum rosin
C. Colophonium D. All

466. Amber resin is obtained from ditillation process of oleo resin, what is the biloogica source of colophony:

A. Pinus B. Laccifer
C. Piper longum D. All

467. Colophony belong to which family :

A. Pinaceae B. Leguminaceae
C. Solancae D. Only A

468. The main active cotituentwhich act as stimulant is present in colopony which is :

A. Abietic acid B. Cinnamein
C. Both D. None

469. Heated acetic anhydride solution with a sulphuric acid treated with colophony which color is obtained:

A. Bright red to violet
B. Bright red to pink
C. Bright red to black
D. Bright red to orange

470. Gnetaceae is the family of ephedra ,what is the synonym of Ephedra :

A. Ma hung B. Cancer tree
C. Cork tree D. None

471. Ma hung is the synonymn of ephedra, dried stems used to obtained ephedra, from which source it is obtained:

A. Ephedra gerardiana
B. Ephedra nebrodensis
C. Both
D. None

472. The two main alkaloid is contain by ephedra which show sympathomimetic effect, choose the correct one:

A. Nor ephedrine B. Ephedrine
C. Both D. None

473. Which macrocyclic alkaloid is present in root :

A. Ephedradines B. n-methyl ephedrine
C. Only b D. None

474. To detect presence, ephedrineaqu.. solution dissolve in hydrochloric acid along with copper sulphate and sodium hydroxide, on shaking which colour is give by organic layer:

A. Purple colour B. Blue colour
C. Orange colour D. Green

475. The onset of action of ephedra is slow than adrenaline, it used in condition of hay fever, along with is also use in :

A. Bronchodilater
B. Bronchoconstricter
C. Use in low blood pressure
D. Both A and C

476. The amolytic enzymes diastase which is present in saliva is also known by name :

A. Amylase B. Pancreatic diastase
C. Amylopsin D. All

477. Choose the correct amylotic enzyme :

A. Zymase B. Invertase
C. Sucrose D. All

478. Diastase enzyme is thermolabile its activity is good at which temperature:

A. 35-40 B. 55-60
C. 15-20 D. 20-25

479. At what pH dlastase enzyme is work

A. 6-7 B. 3-4
C. 4-5 D. None

480. Papin enzyme is which type of enzyme

A. Amolytic enzyme
B. Transferase
C. Proteolytic enzyme
D. All

481. It is obtained from unripe fruit of which tree :

A. Carica papaya B. Ananas cosmosus1
C. Both D. None

482. Papain is belong to the family of :

A. Caricaceae B. Bromeliacae
C. Suidae D. None

483. Papain is a proteolytic enzyme ,proteolytic enzyme act as a:

A. Poplpeptide B. Amide
C. Both D. None

484. The use of prteolytic enzyme papain in silk industry along with is also use in:

A. Cheese manufacturing
B. Leather industry
C. Clarification of beverages
D. All

485. Pancreatin is obtained from animal like hog or ox, which part is used for extraction:

A. Intenstine A B. Stomach
C. Pancreas D. none of the above

486. Pancreatin contain several enzyme which is :

A. Amylase B. Lipase
C. Protease D. All

487. Pancreatin enzyme give better activity in which medium:

A. Alkaline B. Acidic
C. Both D. None

488. Pancreatin enzyme used in which disease of pancreas :

A. Pancreatitis B. Fibrocystic disease
C. Both D. Only A

489. About 1 gm of pancreatin contain not less than :

A. 12000 units of amylase
B. 1000units of protease
C. 15000 units of lipase
D. All are correct

490. Enzyme urokinase is secreted by kidney and it is obtained from:

A. Human urine
B. Kidney tissue culture
C. Both
D. Only A

491. Urokinase enzyme is activate endogenous chemical which convert plasminogen into_and fibrinogen into_____

A. Plasmin B. Fibrin
C. Protein D. Both A and B

492. Urokinase is a lyophilised white powder, it is soluble in :

A. Organic solvent
B. Water
C. Choloroform and ethane
D. All

493. Pepsin is obtained form stomach fluid of animals then pepsin is which type of enzyme :

A. Hydrolase B. isomerases
C. Lyses D. Proteolytic enzyme

494. What is the function of pepsin:

A. Conversion of protein into proteose
B. Digestion of starch
C. To enhance absorption
D. All

495. Which part of animal (hog)is used to extracted pepsin:

A. Intestine B. Stomach
C. Pancreas D. None of the above

496. Susscrofa belong to which family :

A. Suidae B. Bovidae
C. Caricaceae D. None

497. Many enzyme source belong to family of bovidae, choose the correct enzyme:

A. Rennin B. pancreatin
C. Chymotrypsin D. All

498. Alkali is mixed with pepsin and provide heat then what will be the effect if shown:

A. Activiy is lost B. Activity is increases
C. No effect D. Activity is decrease

499. Pepsin show its good activity at which pH:

A. 6.0 B. 8.2
C. 1.8 D. 7.0

500. The efficiency of pepsin to digest _______times to its weight of coagulated egg albumin:

A. 2500 B. 3000
C. 1000 D. 10000

501. Which class of antisecretary drug have effect on acid and pepsin content and along with it show reduce gastric motility:

A. PG'S B. Anticholinergic
C. 5HT3 Antagonist D. None

502. Trypsin in an enzyme ,it is a proteolytic enzyme which is occur from aqu.acid extraction .which part of animal is used to extraction :

A. Pancreas
B. Stomach
C. Obtained from ox pancreas
D. Both A and C

503. Identify the correct proteolytic enzyme :

A. Trypsin B. Pepsin
C. Diastase D. Both A and B

504. Which enzyme work at 7.6-8 pH, choose the correct one :

A. Trypsin B. Rennin
C. Pepsin D. none

505. When we use the solution of trypsin, which condition is maintained :

A. Use fresh solution B. Store at pH3.0
C. Both D. None

506. What is the effect of stability of trypsin in presence of calcium ion:

A. Stability increases B. Stability decreases
C. No effect D. It loss its activity

507. How much units of trypsin is conatin in 1 mg of trypsin :

A. NLT2000 B. NLT2500
C. NLT1500 D. NLT2300

508. Which proteolytic enzyme occur from ananas comosus:

A. Bromelain B. Prolein
C. Both D. None

509. Which part of plant of ananas comous is used to occur proteolytic enzyme :

A. Stem B. Bark
C. Root D. Leaves

510. Bromelain belong to which family :

A. Bromeliaceae B. Palmae
C. Suidae D. Bovidae

511. What is the function of bromelain :

A. Anti inflamatery B. Oedema
C. Analgesic D. Both A and B

512. Streptokinase is an enzyme which convert:

A. Plasminogen into plasmin
B. Fibrinogen into fibrin
C. Both
D. None

513. Streptokinase show its activity at which pH:

A. 3 B. 5
C. 7 D. 10

514. Streptokinase enzyme store at high concentration, but at which temperature this solution keep stable :

A. 10 degree B. 4degree
C. 25 degree D. 20 degree

515. Dilute solution of streptokinase is:

A. Stable B. Unstable
C. Both D. Only B

516. At which purpose streptokinase is used :

A. Thromboembolic disorder
B. Deep vein thrombus
C. Acute coronary artery disorder
D. All

517. Which fibrinolytic drug are antigenic:

A. Urokinase B. Streoptokinase
C. Both D. None

518. What is diffuclty occur in streptokinase therapy:

A. Bleeding B. Hypertension
C. Clotting D. No effect

519. What is the route of administration of streptokinase in condition of acute myocardial infraction:

A. I.V. B. Intracoronory
C. I.M D. Intracardiac

520. The absorption of drug is increased by using:

A. Hyaluronidase
B. Vasoconstrictor substance
C. Combination of drug
D. None of the above

521. What is the use of lycopodium spore method :

A. Defined particle size for powdered drug
B. Uniform thickness
C. both
D. None

522. Pencillinase is obtained form the which source:

A. Bacillus cereus B. E.coli
C. Streptocooci D. Hog organ

523. Which enzyme is used in treatment of advese reaction to pencilline:

A. Pencillinase B. Streptokinase
C. Pepsin D. Hyaluronidase

524. The activity of hyaluronidase is mycolytic , form which source it is obtained:

A. Human kidney B. Human testes
C. Hog pancreas D. None

525. What is the other name of yeast:

A. Brewer yeast B. Baker yeast
C. Both D. None

526. From which family saccharmycescerevisiae is belong :

A. Saccharmycetaceae
B. Fabaceae
C. Leguminosae
D. None

527. Yeast are use as various purpose, following are the example of various type of yeast. choose the correct one:

A. Wine yeast B. Baker yeast
C. Distiller yeast D. All

528. What is the percentage of moisture, glycogen, fat in yeast:

A. 65 to 85% B. 25 to 35%
C. 90 to 95% D. None of the above

529. What is the potency for nonprescription antifungal agent fo vaginal yeast infection:

A. 40% B. 70%
C. 80% D. 90%

530. What is the choice to treat vulvur pruritus in a women with a vaginal yeast infection :

A. External miconazole
B. Intravaginallybutoconazole
C. Both
D. none

531. Cyanocobalamine is occur in all except:

A. Yeast B. Liver
C. Kidney D. Meat

532. Yeast is convert into dried yeast by apply heat, but the temperatre not exceeding :

A. 30 degree B. 40 degree
C. 20 degree D. 50 degree

533. Torula yeast is the type of yeast it is derived form

A. Candida utilis
B. Saccharomysescervisiae
C. Both
D. None

534. Which enzyme is present in yeast, choose the correct one:

A. Diastase B. invertase
C. Zymase D. All

535. Glutathione and invertase enzyme is obtained form which source:

A. Yeast B. Thaumatin
C. Lectins D. None of the above

536. For manufaturing purpose yeast is use as various prepration, choosr the correct one:

A. Manufacturing of alcohol
B. Manufacturing of wine
C. Bread industry
D. All

537. Which is correct one for adulteration :

A. Deterioration B. spoilage
C. admixture D. All the above

538. Which statement is true for adulteration :

A. Deterioration: adding one article into another sue to ignorance
B. Sophistication: intentionally add adulterant
C. Substitution: impairment in the quality of drug
D. Inferiority: attack of microbes

539. What is the example of substitution with substandaed commercial variety:

A. Capsicum minimum replcaced by capsisum annum
B. Belladonna leaves substitute by ailanthus leaves
C. Strychnaausnuxblanda replaced by S.nucvomica
D. Both A and C

540. Adulterants use substance resemble original crude drug by:
A. Morphological character
B. Chemical character
C. Therapeutic character
D. All

541. Aging of the skin is cumulative phenomenon and influenced by which factor:
A. Temperature fluctuation
B. Exposure to sunlight
C. Exposure to chemical gases
D. All

542. Which of the following has morphological resemblance to aunthentic drug:
A. Belladonna leaves and ailanthus leaves
B. Capsicum minimum and capsicum annum
C. S.potatoum and S.nucvomica
D. All

543. Which of the following are example of harmful adulterants:
A. Piece of amber coloured glass in colophony
B. Lead shot in opium
C. White oil in coconut oil
D. All

544. Following statement is realted to lycopodium method, which statement is correct:
A. This techniques is for powdered drug
B. It not measure accurate of quantiy
C. Expensive technique
D. All of the above

545. What is the size of lycopodium sopre method:
A. 2.5micro meter
B. 0.25 micrometer
C. 25 micrometer
D. 25nanometer

546. Which one is not correct for lycopodium sopre method:
A. It is used for well defined particles
B. For multi layered cell or tissue
C. The object of uniform thickness
D. None of theabove

547. Whch formula is useful to calculate percentage purity of drug:
A. N*W*94000*100/SMP
B. N*W*9400*1000/SMP
C. N*M*94000*100/SWP
D. S*P*N*94000*100/WM

548. In the formula of percentage purity of drug: N*W*94000*100/SMP, where S is?
A. No.of spore in same 26 field
B. No. Of charecterstic structure in 26 field
C. No.of sopres in the same 25 field
D. No.ofcharacterstic structure in 25 field

549. Chemical evaluation include ______of active constitutent:
A. Isolation
B. Purification
C. Identification
D. All

550. Chemical evaluation are not usesful for
A. Resins
B. Balsams
C. Cardamon
D. Volatile oil

551. Hulphen' test is used for :
A. Ergot
B. Copper acetate
C. Cotton seed
D. Tropane

552. Van- urk's reagent is used for :
A. Troane alkaloid
B. Ergot
C. Cotton seed
D. Purine bases

553. The method useful fo fluiding pressure of signal active constituent or the group of related constituent present in the same drug:
A. Chemical evalution
B. Morphological evalution
C. Physical evalution
D. None

554. Which is correct about structure of spirulina:
A. Cell wall is single layer
B. Contain chloroplast
C. Chlorophyll A is present but chlorophyll B is absent
D. Nucleus is eukroyotic

555. Chemical assay are not carried out or perfomed for :
A. Aldehyde in lemon oil
B. Carvone in caraway oil
C. Aldehyde in caraway oil
D. None

556. Evaluation of drug defines:
A. Congirmation of drug identify
B. Determination of drug quality
C. Detection of nature and adulteration
D. All

556. What is the biological source of tobacco:
A. Nicotiana tobacum
B. Schoenocaulonofficinale
C. nicotinafabilia
D. none

557. Which part of nicotinatobacum is used to obtained tobacco:
A. Root B. Leaves
C. Flower D. Bark

558. Whic type of alkalois is present in tobacco:
A. Pyridine
B. Indole
C. Imidazole derivatives
D. Purine

559. Which alkaloid moiety is present in nicotiana tobacum:
A. Nicotine B. Nor nicotine
C. Anabasine D. All of the above

560. Nicotine is a :
A. Poison B. Stimulant
C. Both D. None

561. Which purpose nicotinic is used:
A. Manufacturing of nicotinic acid
B. Insecticides
C. Nicotinamide
D. All

562. The evalution of crude drug is necessary because of :
A. Biochemical variation in the drug
B. Deterioration due to treatment and storage
C. Substitution and adulteration
D. All of the above

563. The moisture comtent is determined by heating at drug at:
A. 10 degree celesius
B. 105 degree celesius
C. 105 F
D. 150degree celesius

564. Microscopic evaluation is used to identify organised drug by their :
A. Histological character
B. Morphological character
C. Anatomical character
D. None

565. Which chemical mixture gives red stain:
A. Pharoglucinal +con.HCl
B. Mucilage +rhuthenium red
C. Iodine +hemiucellulose
D. Sodium carbonate +carolling soda

566. The diameter of starch glain in cinnamomum cassia is :
A. 10microns B. 100microns
C. .1micons D. 1microns

567. Important function of stomata:
A. Primary: gaseous exchange, Secondary: transpiration
B. Primary: transpiration, Secondary:gaseous exchange
C. Only A
D. None

568. Kidney shaped cell containing chorplast known:
A. Guard cell B. Subsidiary cell
C. Trichome D. Water pore

569. Type of stomata:
A. Moss type B. Gramineaus type
C. GymnospermansD. All the above

570. Paracyclic stomata is also known:
A. Rubiaceaus B. Both A and B
C. Parallel celled D. None

571. Optical rotation can be derermined by:
A. Sodium lamp at 25 degree
B. Sodium lamp at 50 degree
C. Nitrogen lamp 250 degree
D. Nitrogen lamp 25 degree

572. Stomatal index can be find out by :
A. S/E+S*100 B. S+E/S*100
C. E/E+S*100 D. None

573. Glycine wax is the biological source of:
A. Royal jelly B. Soya beans
C. Garlic D. Spirulina

574. The name 'rhamnose' is a carbohydrate which present in :
A. Garlic B. Omega fatty acid
C. Soya beans D. Spirulina

575. The antibiotic activity of garlic is show by which form of garlic :
A. Allicin B. Allium sativium
C. Both D. None

576. Which type of L.aadophillus species are include in neutrceuticals :
A. Prebiotics B. Probiotics
C. PUFA D. Dietryfibres

577. Which neutaceuticals are used as bone protectives:
A. Osteogenetic B. Curcumess
C. Lycopene D. None

578. Which neutraceuticals are derived from microbial source:
A. Laclobacllus acidophilus
B. Spinogolipids
C. Mylobacterium
D. None

579. Which herbal drug show property of anti acne :
A. Vetiver B. Apricol
C. Hazel D. Fenugreek

580. What is the another name of ergot:
A. Ergota B. St.antomyfire
C. Both D. None

581. In which stage of ergot cycle ,the ergot alkaloid is obtained :
A. Sclerotinum stage B. Sphacelial stage
C. Both D. None

582. Which type of reproduction happen in sphacelial stage:
A. Asexual B. Sexual
C. Both D. None

583. Which fungus is going to asexual reproduction:
A. Conidospose B. Ascospose
C. Only b D. Both

584. Calvicepspurpurea is belong to which family :
A. Clavicipitaceae B. Hypocreaceae
C. Both D. Only A

585. Which chemical moiety is present in ergot:
A. Ergometrin B. Ergocriprin
C. Ergometrinine D. All

586. Following which chemical moiety is water insoluble:
A. Ergocripin B. Ergocroptin
C. Ergometrin D. Both A and B

587. Which form of ergot is livo form :
A. Ergometrin B. Ergometrnine
C. Ergocriptinine D. None

588. Which form of ergot is dextro form of ergot :
A. Ergometrinine B. Ergocriptinine
C. Ergometrin D. Both A and B

589. Which colour is obtained when ergot is react with elrich reagent:
A. Blue B. Green
C. Orange D. Brown

590. Choose the coorect test for ergot:
A. Van_urk' s test B. Vitali morin
C. Meconic acid D. Legal test

591. What is the elrich reagent :
A. Para dimethyl amino benzaldehyde
B. Para di ethyl amino benzaldehyde
C. Ortho di methyl amino benzaldehyde
D. None

592. Which of the following is absent in ergot:
A. Calcium oxalate B. Stomata
C. Trichome D. All

593. Choose the correct shape of ergot tissue seed:
A. Fusiform B. Oval
C. Circle D. None

594. In which drug calcium oxalate crustal is absent :
A. Digitalis B. Ergot
C. Opium D. All

595. Which is true about neutraceuticals:
A. Addition to normal nutritional value
B. Provide health benefit
C. Prevent disease
D. All

596. Which disease is controlled by neutraceuticals:

A. Heart disease

B. Cancer

C. Neural tube defect

D. All of the above

597. Neutraceuticals are classified on the basis of

A. Food source

B. Action of mechanism

C. Chemical nature

D. All of the above

598. Which neutraceutical obtained from plants:

A. Choline B. Lecithine

C. Beta carotene D. None

599. All of the following, which neutraceutical show anti inflammatory action:

A. Beta carotene B. Daidzein

C. Lycopene D. Curcumin

600. On the basis of chemical nature of neutraceuticalsisoprenoids does not include:

A. Corotenoides B. Tacotrienols

C. Eocopherls D. Flavonols

602. Which of the following is not present in fruits and vegetable:

A. Antioxidants B. Probiotics

C. Prebiotics D. Omega 3 fatty acid

603. Which antioxidant is contain by neutraceuticals:

A. Vitamin E B. VitaminA

C. Vitamin B D. Both A and B

604. Which are the following drug show anti acne properties:

A. Arjuna B. Cucumber

C. Aloe vera D. Both A and B

605. Aloe vera show which type of action:

A. Anti inflammatory B. Anti aging

C. Anti wrinkle D. All

606. Which are the following statement is correct about PUFA:

A. Help to lowert cholesterol level

B. Belong to linoleic group

C. Prevent atherosclerosis

D. All of the above

607. Prebiotics also promote the selective growth of :

A. Colonic probiotics bacteria

B. Gastric probiotics bacteria

C. Renal probiotics bacteria

D. Liver pro biotics bacteria

608. According to FDA of united state of America soyabean reduce the risk of :

A. Coronary heart disease

B. Cancer

C. Diabetes

D. Both A and B

609. Spirulina belong to following which algae:

A. Red algae B. Blue green algae

C. Brown algae D. Green algae

610. Choose the correct one about spirulina:

A. Belong to spirulinamnaxima family oscillatoriaceae

B. Grows in fresh water

C. It is a link between green plant and bacteria

D. All of the above

611. Which is true about omega 3 fatty acid activites:

A. Increase in HDL level

B. Reduce in HDL level

C. Increase in LDL level

D. None

612. What is the mean of rasa

A. Lymph B. Blood

C. Tissue D. Body

613. Which term are related with tridoshaconsept

A. Vata B. Guna

C. Prabhava D. Meda

614. Which physician and chemist developed homeopathic system of medicine

A. Edward bach

B. Samuel Hahnemann

C. Hardy

D. Aristole golden

615. Which one is the source of occurance of homeopathic medicine

A. Haikalli B. Neriumindicum

C. Aloe barbadensis D. Vegetable drug

616. Which one is the not merely a system of treatment
A. Naturopathy
B. Austerity
C. Sidhha
D. Bach flower remedies

617. Which physician discovered bach flower remedies
A. Edward bach
B. Samuel Hahnemann
C. Hardy
D. Aristotle

618. Which type of classification related the crud drug.
A. Taxonomical B. Pharmalogical
C. Both A and B D. Morphological

619. Which drug are acting on autonomic nervous system
A. Ephedra B. Dill
C. Squill D. Morphine

620. Which drug are used in sidhha system of medicine
A. Cantharis
B. Alari [neriumindicum]
C. Colchium
D. Nuxvomica

621. Which one is unani medicine
A. Kulthi
B. Qust
C. Ethi
D. Both [kulth and qust]

622. Glycosides are under which classification of crude drug
A. Chemical classification
B. Morphological classification
C. Pharmacological classification
D. Taxonomical classification

623. Which term is related with aayurveda
A. Kampoh medicine
B. Bhaishajyavigyan
C. Ginseng
D. Schizonepeta

624. What is abini
A. Papaversomniferum
B. Neriumindicum
C. Euphoribianerifolia
D. Aloe barbadensis

625. The system of yoga is as old as
A. Unanai B. Ayurveda
C. Homeopathic D. Elopethic

626. Whivh method of classification is based on the consideration pf natural relationship
A. Alphabetical B. Toxonomical
C. Chemical D. Morphological

627. Pharmacological classification are also known as ?
A. Chemical classification
B. Biological classification
C. Therapeutic classification
D. Morphological classification

628. Which classification established a relationship between position of the plant and attempts to utilize chemical
A. Chemotaxonomic
B. Morphological
C. Toxonomical
D. Alphabetical

629. Which book are write by charak
A. Sushrutsamhita
B. Analecta pharmacognostica
C. Charaksamhita
D. Non of these

630. What is the meaning of pharmakon
A. Knowledge B. A drug
C. Gignosco D. Contraceptives

631. Pharmacognosy is drived from which two words
A. Pharmakon and gignosco
B. Gignosco and pharma
C. Pharmakon and knowledge
D. Pharmakon and cognosy

632. The anatomical atlas of crud drug was published by
A. Bentham B. Berg
C. Voehl D. Collin

633. Which one is the type of plant tissue
A. Embryonic tissue B. Connective tissue
C. Edipose tissue D. Meristestatic

634. Which one is lipid
A. Clove B. Peppermint
C. Bees wax D. Agar

635. Sub- aerial modification of stems includes
A. Stolon B. Tuber
C. Bulb D. Corm

636. Hoe much water is in fresh leaves
A. About 50-60% B. About 70-80%
C. About 10-20% D. About 30-40%

637. Which is related with bark
A. External tissue
B. Pericycle
C. Belladonna's
D. Both[external tissue and pericycle]

638. The seeds is derived from
A. Antharacene B. External tissue
C. Pollen D. Feetilized ovule

639. What is the opening of the apex called
A. Pollen B. Micropyle
C. Embryo D. Sac

640. What is embryo sac
A. Tissue B. Cell
C. Root D. Micropyle

641. What are albuminous or endospermic and exalbuminaus or non endospermic
A. Seeds B. Root
C. Bark D. Leaves

642. What is exalbuminaus
A. Type of root B. Type of bark
C. Type of seeds D. Type of leaves

643. In which type of seeds embryo and endosperm are formed as a result of daule fertilization
A. Albuminous
B. Endospermic
C. Perispermcantaining
D. Exalbuminaus

644. Cardamom and nutmeg seeds have
A. Raphe B. Perisperm
C. Hilum D. Stone

645. Which one isthe type of ovules
A. Anatropous B. Raphe
C. Perisperm D. Chalaza

646. In which ovule nucellus is in straight line and micropyle
A. Amphitropous B. Campylotropous
C. Anatropous D. Atropous

647. Some seeds like nuxvomica cell wall are thick walled because of
A. Protein
B. Reserve carbohydrates
C. Hilum
D. Apocynaceae

648. Which one ovule is inverted at an angle of 180° over funicle
A. Antropous ovule
B. Atropous ovule
C. Campylotropous ovule
D. Antronipous ovule

649. Which type of ovules nucellus is straight and funicle
A. Amphitropous B. Atropous
C. Anatropous D. Campylotropous

650. What is a fleshly covering originated from
A. Caruncle B. Arie
C. Strophiole D. Micropyle

651. Which grains hive yellow colour with iodine solution and they are present only in seeds
A. Pericarp B. Aleurone
C. Caprel D. Olive

652. Ovarian wall develops into a case know as
A. Ovule B. Pericarp
C. Grains D. Olive

653. If the pericarp is hard the fruit is called
A. Olive fruit
B. Aggregate fruit
C. Dry fruit as fennal
D. Syncarpous fruit

654. Aggregate fruit is formed from
A. Apocarpous gynaecium
B. Mesocarp
C. Pyrethrum
D. Santonica

655. Glycyrrhiza mostly consists of
A. Stolons B. Minopodial
C. Hypodarmal D. Epicarp

656. Pericarp is differentiated into how many parts
A. 3 B. 4
C. 5 D. 6

657. Epicarp is the part of
A. Endocarp B. Pericarp
C. Mesocarp D. Exocarp

658. What is endocarp
A. Uper layer B. Surface layer
C. Innermost layer D. Upermost layer

659. What is the reproductive part of the plant
A. Seeds B. Roots
C. Flower's D. Fruits

660. Which part of rhizome is runs near and under the soil
A. Stolon B. Scars
C. Bud D. Minopodial

661. Rhizome may be
A. Sonopodail B. Monopodail
C. Tanopodail D. Misopodail

662. Encircling scars of aerial leaves as seen in
A. Adventitious roots
B. Orris rhizome
C. Leaf scars
D. Stolons

663. What is the mesocarp cantain
A. Oil-cell B. Oil-roots
C. Oil-tissue D. Vessels

664. Which vessele present in the phloem of the vascular bundles of the poppy capsule
A. Stony B. Laticiferous
C. Sclereids D. Spongy

665. Colchicum seeds belongs to
A. Anatropous ovule
B. Atropous ovule
C. Amphitropous ovule
D. Compylotropous ovule

666. In which seed AWn is present
A. Strophanthus B. Aril
C. Aleurone D. Globaids

667. What is the biological origin of guarana
A. Linne B. Paulliniacupana
C. Theaceae D. Rubiaceaae

668. What is the use of plantago seed
A. Cathartic
B. Motion sickness
C. Anticholinergic
D. Antineoplastic agents

669. What is the specific gravity of honey
A. 1.35-1.36 B. 2.11-2.12
C. 1.42- 1.43 D. 1.32-1.33

670. What is the synonym of honey
A. Meta B. Mel
C. Amylum D. Apis

671. What is the taste of starch
A. Bland and mucilaginous
B. Sweet
C. Slightly
D. Bitter

672. Inulin is quickly hydrolized by
A. Base B. Acid
C. Both A & B D. Non of these

673. What is the synonym of inulin
A. Alantin B. Amylum
C. Mel D. Madhu

674. What is the geographical source of lappa
A. Western Himalayas
B. Eastern Himalayas
C. Europe
D. Nilgiri hills

675. What is the use of insulin
A. Cosmetic pripration
B. Culture media
C. Prevention
D. Laxative

676. Cellulose treatment with sodium bisulphite are known as
A. Soda process
B. Sulphate process
C. Sulphonate process
D. Cellulose process

677. The long - lint hairs of cotton are known as
A. Staple B. Fibers
C. Loculus D. Fragment

678. Short -fuzz hairs of cotton are called
A. Linters B. Fibers
C. Fragment D. Loculus

679. The cotton plant after flowering bears fruit which are also called
A. Pyrometris B. Floss
C. Delintering D. Capsules

680. What is the synonym of dextrin
A. Pyrometris B. Starch gum
C. Collodian D. Wool

681. Which one is not the synonym of acacia
A. Indian gum B. Gum acacia
C. Gun arabic D. Starch gum

682. What is the biological source of tragacanth
A. Astragalus gummifer
B. Senegal
C. G.herbaccum
D. Malevaceae

683. What is the colour of tragacanth
A. Red B. Pale green
C. White D. Ydark yellow

684. What is the taste of tragacanth
A. Solty B. Bitter
C. Tasteless D. Sweet

685. Tragacanth comprises of two vital fraction term know as
A. Tragacanth &bassorin
B. Bassorin& gum
C. Tragacanth & acetate
D. Bassorin&methoxyl

686. Which one is not the synonym of karaya gum
A. Kadaya B. Katilo
C. Kuteera D. Gossypium

687. What is the use of karaya gum in the paper industry
A. Binder B. Adhesive
C. Emulsifier D. Theckner

688. Pactin is naturally found in which plant
A. emon peel B. Apple peel
C. Orange pomace D. Amblica peel

689. In general pectin is a group of
A. Polymers B. Polypeptide
C. Polysaccharides D. Mineral

690. Pactin is a fairly incompatible with
A. Ca2+ B. Cl2+
C. SN^4 D. Mg2+

691. What is the synonym of locust bean gum
A. Linn B. Ceretonia
C. Carob flour D. Siliqua

692. Locust bean gum comprises of
A. Protein B. Polysaccharides
C. Meneral D. Polymers

693. What is the family of guar gum
A. Leguminosease B. Rubiaceacea
C. Laminaria D. Gelidiam

694. Which one is not the synonym of algin
A. Sodium alginate B. Numis
C. Kelgin D. Alginic acid sodium

695. A variety of algae and seaweeds comprise of
A. Algin B. Marine gum
C. Lamour D. Indian gum

696. Algin is insoluble in
A. Water B. Ethanol
C. Ether D. Aqueous solution

697. What is the colour of laraya gum
A. Pink B. Red
C. Green D. Black

698. What is the meaning of pantago [letin word
A. Sale of the foot B. Shape of the foot
C. Sale of the leaf D. Shap of the root

699. What is the synonym of plantago seed
A. Pellium seed B. Psyllium seed
C. Gum seed D. Plantin seed

700. Plantago seeds belongs to which family
A. Gintianceae B. Rutaceae
C. Plantaginaceae D. Papaveraceae

701. The term kibbling machine is related to
A. Preparation of locust bean gum
B. Preparation of acacia
C. Preparation of pactin
D. Preparation of guar

702. The cotyledons are separated from the endosperm by which process
A. Grinding B. Gramular
C. Winnowing D. Splitter

703. In which solution guar gum is insoluble
A. Alcohol B. Water
C. Ether D. Ethanol

704. Chinese- isinglass are commonly known as

A. Agar B. Mel
C. Gum D. Guar gum

705. What is the family of agar

A. Gracilariaceae B. Papaveraceae
C. Rutaceae D. Gintianceae

706. Chinese - isinglass is largely produced in which country

A. England B. Japan
C. Shri-lanka D. Indonesia

707. The name "layorcarang" is related to

A. Agar B. Acacia
C. Gum D. Guar

708. How many persentage (%) w/v solution of agar when boiled and cooled produced stiff jelly

A. 1.5 to 2% (w/v) B. 2 to 3 %(w/v)
C. 1 to 2 % (w/v) D. 3.5 to 4 % (w/v)

709. What is usually used as substituents for agar

A. Gum B. Gelatin
C. Guar gum D. Dextrin

710. What is the synonym of irish moss

A. Carrageenan B. Xanthan gum
C. Kelzan D. Gelose

711. What is the synonym of irish moss

A. Carrageenan B. Xanthan gum
C. Kelzan D. Gelose

712. What is the biological source of keltrol F;

A. Gigartina
B. Xanthomonascampestris
C. Hydrocolloid
D. Mamillosa

713. What is the synonym of kelzan

A. Xanthan gum B. Carrageenan
C. Chitin D. Crustacean

714. What is the synonym of chondrus

A. Gigartina B. Irish moss
C. Crispus D. Malillosa

715. What is obtained as an amorphous solid substance

A. Gum B. Chondrus
C. Xanthan D. Chitin

716. Which one is the type of glycosides

A. O- glycosides B. B- glycosides
C. D- glycosides D. M- glycosides

717. Sinigrin is obtain from

A. Blackmustard seed
B. Red mustard seed
C. Yellow mustard seed
D. Brown mustard seed

718. Rhein-8-glucoside is obtained from

A. Rhubarb B. Frangula
C. Mustard seed D. Brassica

719. What is the family of brassica compestris

A. Cruciferae B. Ericaceae
C. Lythreaceae D. Leguminosease

720. What is the biological source of aloe

A. Curacao aloe B. Capee aloe
C. Sopel aloe D. Curasao aloe

721. What is the colour of zinzibar aloe

A. Red B. Liver brown
C. Brownish yellow D. Greenish

722. What is the colour of socotrine aloe

A. Brownish yellow B. Red
C. Greenish D. Liver black

723. What is the colour of cape aloe

A. Greenish B. Brown
C. Dark brown D. Yellow

724. What is the colour of curacao aloe

A. Red B. Greenish
C. Dark brown D. Brownish black

725. Whatt is the taste of curacao aloe

A. Intense bitter B. Nauseating
C. Sweet D. Slightly

726. What is the taste of cape aloe

A. Sweet
B. Slightly
C. Nouseating& bitter
D. Intense bitter

727. What is the taste of socotrine aloe

A. Extremely bitter & nauseous
B. Sweet
C. Intense bitter
D. Slightly

728. What is the taste of Zanzibar aloe
A. Bitter B. Sweet
C. Slightly D. Nauseous

729. What is the meaning of rheum
A. Rhubarb B. Cape
C. Distinct D. Waxy

730. Piperidine alkaloid is found in
A. Aloe gililandii B. Anthraquinone
C. Barbaloin D. Volatile oil

731. Due to the isobarbaloin which colour produced by cape aloe
A. Faint pink B. Faint yellow
C. Fait brown D. Faint black

732. What is the synonym of radix rhei
A. Rhubarb B. Webbianum
C. Bail D. Balsam

733. What is the geographical source of rheum
A. Indonesia B. Sikkim
C. Nilgiri hills D. Misoram

734. Rhubarb gives a blood red coloration with
A. 5% potassium chloride
B. 5% potassium hydroxide
C. 5% sodium chloride
D. 5% potassium sulphate

735. Rhubarb is also used as a
A. Cathartic B. Purgative
C. Antibiotics D. Antiemetic

736. What is the synonym of cortex
A. Chitten bark B. Redixrhei
C. Rheum D. Curacao aloe

737. What is the family of cascara Sagrada
A. Rhamnaceae B. Cruciferae
C. Ericaceae D. Lythreaceae

738. What is the biological source of sacred bark
A. Rhamanuspurshiana Dc
B. Rhamnusfrangulalinne
C. Rootbark
D. Frangulins

739. What is the taste of Bearwood
A. Persistently bitter B .Sweet
C. Slightly D. Nauseous

740. Which one is the C-glycosides
A. Barbaloin B. Epicatechin
C. Adenosine D. Sinigrin

741. Wich one name is not related to cascara Sagrada
A. Sacred bark B. Cascara bark
C. Searwood bark D. Chittin bark

742. What is the synonym of black dogwood
A. Frangula B. Tinnevelley
C. Sacred bark D. Bearwood

743. What is the family of buckthorn bark
A. Rhamnaceae B. Cruciferae
C. Ericaceae D. Lythreaceae

744. Berry alder is drived from which bark
A. Rhamanusalnifolia
B. Frangula
C. Rootbark
D. Rhamanusfrangulalinne

745. Frangula bark cantains which acid
A. Chrysophanic acid
B. Franguline
C. Hydrofluoric acid
D. Hydrobromic acid

746. What is the use of arrow wood
A. Cathartic B. Laxative
C. Antibiotics D. Antiemetic

747. Senna was first used in the
A. European medicine
B. Indian medicine
C. Mecca medicine
D. Judaeus medicine

748. What is the synonym of senna
A. Sennae folium B. Senna leaf
C. Indian senna D. All of these

749. What is the biological source of senna
A. Cassia senna L. B. Cassia semna c.
C. Senna frangula D. Senna linne

750. What is the family of tinnevelley senna
A. Cruciferae B. Lythreaceae
C. Leguminosease D. Legitimately

751. What is the colour of alexandria senna
A. Pale greyish green
B. Yellowish brown
C. Pale yellow
D. Brownish

752. What is the shape of tinnevelley senna
A. Lanceolate B. Ovate
C. Neanceolate D. Ovate- lanceolate

753. The term alkaloid was first ans foremost proposed by which pharmacist
A. W.meissner B. H.a. ibrahim
C. Harborne D. Mobry T.N

754. Naturally occurring plant compounds having a basic character and cintaining at least one nitrogen in a heterocyclic ring which scientist gives this dafination
A. W.meissner B. Landenburg
C. Mobry T.J D. Harborne

755. Piperidine is obtained from
A. Piper nigrum B. Ephedrine
C. Plant origin D. Cholines

756. What is the botanical name of nicotine
A. Tabacum nicotiana
B. Nicotiana tabacum
C. Solanum tuberosum
D. Chillies

757. What is the family of capsaicin
A. Solanaceae B. Lythreaceae
C. Cricease D. Leguminosease

758. What is the botanical name of capsaicin
A. Capsicums annum linn
B. Capsicums linne
C. Capsicums var
D. Capsicums linne var

759. What is the N.rustica
A. Nicotinine B. Nicotine
C. Niger L. D. Stramonium

760. What is the botanical name of solanine
A. Solanum tuberosum L.
B. Annum linn L.
C. Solamiumtuberosum
D. Tuberosum L.

761. What is the synonym of datura stramonium L
A. Hyoscyamine B. Capsaicin
C. Solanine D. Nicotine

762. General characteristics of alkaloid may be grouped together in how much categories
A. Two B. Four
C. Five D. Three

763. What is the melting point of ajmaline
A. 150-160 °c B. 90-100 °c
C. 120-130 °c D. 180-190°c

764. What is vinblastine
A. Carbohydrates B. Lipids
C. Alkaloids D. Polymers

765. What is the pKa value of morphine
A. 9.98 B. 9.85
C. 8.87 D. 9.51

766. What is the pKa value of reserpine
A. 6.6 B. 9.4
C. 7.1 D. 5.71

767. What is the pKa value of papaverine at 25°C
A. 8.07 B. 8.9
C 9.1 D. 5.56

768. What is the melting point of morphine
A. 197 °C B. 200 °C
C. 175 °C D. 140 °C

769. What is the pharmacological action of brucine
A. CNS stimulants B. Narcotics analgesic
C. Mydriatics D. Myotics

770. What is the example of pyrrolidine alkaloid
A. Atropine B. Hygrine
C. Lupanin D. Aconitine

771. What is the exam of purin alkaloid
A. Pilocarpine B. Caffeine
C. Ephedrine D. Aconitine

772. Aconitine used as a
A. Neuralgia B. Laxative
C. Antimicrobial D. Oxytocic

773. What is the family of hygrine
A. Labitatae B. Erythroxylaceae
C. Rutaceae D. Rubiaceacea

774. What is the botanical name of lobeline
A. Punicagranatum
B. Lobelia inflata
C. Atropine
D. Uragogasolida

775. What is the family of emetine
A. Rubiaceacea B. Fumariaceae
C. Rutaceae D. Solanaceae

776. What is the family of hordenine
A. Graminae B. Gnetaceae
C. Cactaceae D. Palmaceae

777. Conhydrine is obtained from
A. Coniummaculatum L.
B. Coniine
C. Coniummaculatum B.
D. Conium seed

778. What is the synonym of katine
A. Norpseudoephedrin
B. Minusin
C. Amorphan
D. Norpseudo

779. What is the family of gelatin
A. Bovidae B. Rutaceae
C. Solanaceae D. Lebiatae

780. Yeast is obtained from
A. Minusin
B. Saccharomycescerevisae
C. Pilocarpine
D. Pepernegirum

781. What is the melting point of behenic
A. 85°C B. 80 °C
C. 95 °C D. 65 °C

782. What is the saponification value of corn
A. 187-193 B. 168-180
C. 188-196 D. 188-194

783. What is the synonym of oleum ricini
A. Castor oil B. Olive oil
C. Mustard oil D. Peanut oil

784. What is the family of castor oil
A. Rutaceae B. Euphorbiaceae
C. Solaceae D. Leguminosease

785. What is the family of teel oil
A. Pedaliaceae B. Euphorbiaceae
C. Rutaceae D. Leguminosease

786. What is the synonym of kunjid
A. Gingely oil B. Oleum ricini
C. Castor oil D. Zait al- kharwaa

787. What is copaiba
A. Resins B. Lipid
C. Wax D. Oil

788. Resins in association with volatile oil and gum are called
A. Gum- resins B. Oleo-gum-resins
C. Asafoetida D. Oleo resins

789. Resins associated with volatile oil are called
A. Gum resins B. Oleo-resins
C. Myrrh D. Balsams

790. If the resins cantain benzoic acid they are called
A. Balsams B. Copaida
C. Gamboge D. Oleo-gum

791. Which one is the example of balsams
A. Tolu B. Capaida
C. Strorax D. Benzoin

792. Which one is the oleo-gum-resins
A. Myrrh B. Gamboge
C. Copaiba D. Tolu balsam

793. Which one is the oleo-resins
A. Tolu B. Myrrh
C. Copaiba D. Colophony

794. Which one is the gum resin
A. Gamboge B. Colophony
C. Asafoetida D. Myrrh

795. Which one is the acid resin
A. Gamboge B. Amber resin
C. Colophony D. Myrrh

796. What is the synonym of rosin
A. Colophony B. Balsam
C. Myhhr D. Copaiba

797. What is the family of amber resin
A. Pinaceae B. Leguminosease
C. Rutaceae D. Solanaceae

798. Which one is not a synonym of peru balsam
A. Balsamumperuvianum
B. Peruvian balsam
C. Balsam of peru
D. Peruviam

799. What is the biological source of peru balsam
A. Myroxylonpereirae
B. Nlotzsch
C. Visicid
D. Cinnamate bark

800. What is the family of peru balsam
A. Rutaceae B. Leguminosease
C. Solanaceae D. Rubiaceacea

801. What is the synonym of benzoin
A. Sumatra benzoin B. Benzoin fungus
C. Benzoin resin D. Benzoimum

802. What is the family of loban (guj.)
A. Leguminosease B. Rutaceae
C. Styaceae D. Solanaceae

803. What is the biological source of sumatra benzin
A. Sorched B. Klotzsch
C. Dryander D. Styrax benzoin

804. What is the use of peru balsam
A. Laxative B. Antiseptic
C. Antiemetic D. Antimicrobial

805. What is the botanical name of siam benzoin
A. Styrax tonkinesis B. Sorched
C. Styrax benzoin D. Klotzsch

806. What is the family of shilaras (guj.)
A. Leguminosease B. Rutaceae
C. Solanaceae D. Hamamelidaceae

807. What is the biographical source storax
A. India B. South -west turkey
C. Japan D. South Africa

808. What is the synonym of Levant storax
A. Styrax B. Nyrax
C. Mtyrax D. Levinate storax

809. What is the taste of crude storax
A. Bitter B. Sweet
C. Shilghty D. Solty

810. What is use of storax
A. Laxative B. Antiseptic
C. Antiemetic D. Antibiotics

811. What is the family of copaiva
A. Rutaceae B. Solanaceae
C. Leguminosease D. Rubiaceacea

812. Which type of alkaloids are derived from lysine
A. Atropine B. Ephedrine
C. Colchicine D. Lupinine

813. Isopelletierine alkaloid is derived from
A. Lysine B. Atropine
C. Scopolamine D. Ephedrine

814. What is the synonym of filix mass
A. Asafoetida B. Male fern
C. Copaiba D. Ferulic

815. What is the family of aspidium
A. Polypodiaceae B. Rutaceae
C. LaGuardia D. Leguminosease

816. What is the botanical source of male fern
A. Aspiditris mass
B. Oblique
C. Dryopterisfilix mass
D. Malo fern rhizome

817. What is the family of mallotusphilippinesis
A. Euphorbiaceae
B. Rutaceae
C. Leguminosease
D. Polypodiaceae

818. What is the family of black vidang
A. Myrsinaceae B. Euphorbiaceae
C. Polypodiaceae D. Convolvulaceae

819. What is the family of Indian podophyllum
A. Myrsinaceae B. Euphorbiaceae
C. Berberidiaceae D. Convolvulaceae

820. What is the synoynm of Indian podophyllum
A. Rhizome podophyliiindicii
B. Podophyllumemodi
C. Rhizome indicii
D. Podophyliiindicum

821. The plant of perennial hurb found at which hight
A. 1000 meters B. 1500 meters
C. 2000 meters D. 3000 meters

822. What is the colour of rhizome podophyliiindicii
A. Earthy brown B. Greenish
C. Pale yellow D. Dark brown

823. What is the taste of Indian podophyllum
A. Bitter B. Salty
C. Slightly D. Sweeties

824. The Indian podophyllumcantain which persentage (%) of resin
A. 8-16% B. 20-30%
C. 9-15% D. 25-30%

825. The American podophyllum contain which percentage of resin
A. 8% B. 15%
C. 6% D. 20%

826. What is the family of cannabis
A. Cannabinaceae B. Polypodiaceae
C. Myrsinaceae D. Euphorbiaceae

827. What is the synonym of Indian hemp
A. Cannabis Indica B. Caustic
C. Cystaliths D. Narihuana

828. What is the synonym of Nilpushpi (marathi)
A. Tropicas B. Kaladana
C. Convolvul D. Merihuana

829. What is the family of Mirchi (hindi)
A. Cennabinaceae B. Convolvulaceae
C. Myrsinaceae D. Berberidiaceae

830. What is the botanical source of Kaladana
A. Ipomoea hederacea
B. Weraceuz
C. Purgahayne
D. Exogoniumpurga

831. What is the geographical source of KalaDana
A. India B. Japan
C. Africa D. Europe

832. What is the shape of plant of kaladana
A. Triangular B. Rounded
C. Surcular D. Longlen

833. What is the use of KalaDana
A. Laxative B. Purgative
C. Antibiotics D. Antiemetic

834. What is the synonym of radix jalapae
A. Jalap B. Veraciuzjelder
C. Maxicunjelder D. Jala-tolu

835. What is the botanical source of jalap
A. Weracurz
B. Ipomoea purgahayne
C. Ipomoea purge
D. Exominiunpurga

836. What is the family of jalap
A. Convolvulaceae B. Polypodiaceae
C. Myrsinaceae D. Berberidiaceae

837. What is the synonym of turpeth
A. Brazilian jalap B. Moshotar
C. Indian jalap D. Surpetham

838. What is the family of ipomoea
A. Convolvulaceae B. Euphorbiaceae
C. Polypodiaceae D. Myrsinaceae

839. What is the synonym of ipomoea
A. Scmmony root
B. Orizabensis
C. Radix jalap
D. Maxican scammony root

840. What is the synonym of digitalis leaves
A. Folia digitalis
B. Foxlia digitalis
C. Digitalis Purpureae
D. Folia purpureae

841. What is the botanical source of foxglove leaves
A. Digitalis purpurea B. Purpurea
C. Folialpurpurea D. Digoxigenin

842. What is the family of digitalis leaves
A. Scrophulariaceae B. Apocynaceae
C. Myrsinaceae D. Berberidiaceae

843. Which type of lanatoside are not contain by digitalis lonata
A. A lanatoside B. C lanataside
C. F lanatoside D. E lanataside

844. Mullelin leaves are leaves of ?
A. Verbascum thapsus
B. Officinale
C. Primulavulgaris
D. Valgaristhapsus

845. What is the synonym of strophanthus
A. Semen strophanthi
B. Strophanthuscuvns
C. Havitalstrophanthi
D. Senemstophanthi

846. What is the family of strophanthus
A. Apocynaceae B. Berberidiaceae
C. Myrsiceae D. Euphorbiaceae

847. What is the shape of strophanthus
A. Lanceolate B. Sessile
C. Triangular D. Biennial

848. What is the taste of strophanthus
A. Sweeties B. Salty
C. Bitter D. Slightly bitter

849. S.kombe seeds cantain how many percent of cardiac glycoside
A. 9-16% B. 8-10%
C. 5-10% D. 15-20%

850. Strophanthusgratus seeds cantain which type of crystalline glycosides
A. A-strophanthin B. B-strophanthin
C. C-strophanthin D. G-strophanthin

851. What is the synonym of squill
A. Scilla bulb B. Indian scilla
C. Scilla D. Cillae

852. What is the family of white squill
A. Liliaceae B. Berberidiaceae
C. Myrsinaceae D. Polypodiaceae

853. What is the colour of white squill
A. Brown B. Dark brown
C. Pale yellow D. Greenish

854. What is the family of Indian squill
A. Liliaceae B. Rutaceae
C. Solenoceae D. Legumunacese

855. What is the synonym of Indian squill
A. Urginea B. Scilla
C. Scilla bulb D. Indian scilla

856. What is the biological source of critoxin
A. Digitalis lonata B. Digitalis cariensis
C. Digitalis species D. Digitalis ferruginea

857. What is the biological source of scillaren A
A. Digitalis lonata
B. Digataliscariensis
C. Digitalis burkei
D. Strophanthuskombe

858. What is the aglycone of cymarin
A. Strophanthidin B. Scillaridin
C. Ouabagenim D. Gitoxigenin

859. Which sugar moieties present in cymarin
A. Rhamnose B. Cymarose
C. Glucose D. L-Rhamnose

860. What is the Agycone of eritoxin
A. Digitoxigenin B. Gitoxigenin
C. Scillaridin D. Strophanthidin

861. What is the biological source of digoxin
A. Digitalis lonata B. Digitalis obscura
C. Digitalis Purpuria D. Digitalis Thapsi

862. What is the biological source ouabain
A. Adonis vernalis
B. Strophanthusgratus
C. Strophanthuskombe
D. Adonis murensis

863. Which type of alkaloids are derived from lysine
A. Lupinine B. Atropine
C. Colchicine D. Ephedrine

864. What is the botanical source of opium
A. Papeversomniferum Linn
B. Purpuriatulas
C. Clavicepspurpuria
D. Papavarclaviceps

865. What is the family of A fim
A. Papaveraceae B. Polypodiaceae
C. Euphorbiaceae D. Myrsinaceae

866. What is the synonym of calumbae radix
A. Columba B. Kalambhu
C. Ipecac rio D. Cephealis

867. What is the family of columba root
A. Papaveraceae B. Manispermaceae
C. Rutaceae D. Polypodiaceae

868. Which one is the example of Indole Alkalodis drugs
A. Opium B. Ergot
C. Columba D. Ipecacuahha

869. Ergotamine is obtained from
A. Swiss ergot
B. Iberiam ergot
C. American wild grasses
D. Japanese ergot

870. Ergot are cantains how many percent (%) of fixed oil
A. .50-60% B. 10-20%
C. 30-40% D. 25-30%

871. What is the family of aconite
A. Ranunculaceae B. Apocaynaceae
C. Palmae D. Labiatae

872. What is the synonym of aconitumnopellus
A. Acomite B. Hapellus
C. Aconite D. None of them

873. What is the biological sources of Aconite
A. Aconite root B. Wolfsbane root
C. Both (A) and (B) D. Aconite leaf

874. What is the family of rauwolfia vomitoriaAfz.
A. Apocynaceae B. Cruciferae
C. Solanaceae D. Rutaceae

875. What is the synonym of rauwolfia vomitoria Afz.
A. American rauwolfia
B. Indian rauwolfia
C. African rauwolfia
D. Japanese rauwolfia

876. The isodiametric sclereids occasionally
A. Phelloderm
B. Fairly abundant
C. Prisms of calcium oxalate
D. Pericyclicfibres

877. A group of sclereids from the mesocarp with which adjacent
A. Trichomes
B. Unlignified parenchyma
C. Fibro vascular tissue
D. Striated cuticle

878. Endospermcontainingmicrorosette crystals of
A. Calcium oxalate
B. Magnesium oxalate
C. Sodium bicarbonate
D. Calcium carbonate

879. What is the family of areca catechu L.
A. Palmae B. Rurosaceae
C. Phytolaccaceae D. Labiatae

880. What is the biological source of areca
A. Areca nuts B. Betel nuts
C. Both (A) and (B) D. None of them

881. The abundant of endosperm composed of
A. Mast cell
B. Parenchymatous cell
C. Polygonal cell
D. Pigment

882. What is the synonym of ocimumbasilicum L.
A. Basilimum B. Basil
C. Sweet basil D. Basil L.

883. What is the family of basilicum L.
A. Labiatae B. Lythraceae
C. Cannabaceae D. Solanaceae

884. The vescular tissue contain
A. Lignified vessels B. Papillose
C. Trichomes D. Longitudinal

885. A thik walled ofbasil fruit
A. Parenchyma
B. Phoem
C. Elongated sclereids
D. Isodiametric sclereids

886. What is the family of trachyspermum
A. Solanaceae B. Umbelliferae
C. Ericcacea D. Apocynaceae

887. What is the synonym of ajowam
A. Trachyspermumcopticum L.
B. Trachyspermum Ajowan
C. Trachyspermumvittae
D. Trachyspermumcoptimum

888. What is the synonym of pimpinellaAnisum L.
A. Aniseed B. Anisum
C. Anise D. Anisem

889. What is the family of anise
A. Ranunculaceae B. Piperaceae
C. Solanaceae D. Umbelliferae

890. What is the biological source of pimpinellaanisumL.
A. Aniseed
B. Anise fruit
C. Both (A) and (B)
D. None of them

891. What is the family of atropaBelladonna L.
A. Lauraceae B. Liliaceae
C. Turneraceae D. Solanaceae

892. What is the synonym of Belladonna herb
A. Atropa belladonna L.
B. Atropus belladonna
C. Atropine Belladonna
D. None of them

893. Which taste are contain by atropa belladonna
A. Sweet B. Salty
C. Slightly bitter D. Bitter

894. What is the biological source of Belladonna herb
A. Belladonna root
B. Belladonna leaf
C. Belladonna flower
D. Belladonna fruit

895. What is the colour of Belladonna root
A. Yellow B. Palefawnish brown
C. Brown D. Greemnish

896. What is the family of laurusnobilis L.
A. Lauraceae B. Fagaceae
C. Leguminosae D. Liliaceae

897. What is the synonym of BAY
A. Laurusnobalis B.
B. Laurusnobilis L.
C. Laumumnobilis L.
D. Laurusmobilis L.

898. What is the color of BAY
A. Brown B. Greenish brown
C. Yellow D. Both (A) and (B)

899. What is the biological source of laurusnobilis L.
A. Bay Laurel leaf B. Bay Laurel fruit
C. Bay Laurel Root D. Bay Laurel flower

900. What is the family of Arctostaphylos UVA-URSI (L.) Spreng
A. Berberidaceae B. Ericaceae
C. Araceae D. Labiatae

901. What is the color of bearberry
A. Greenish - fawn B. Brown
C. Yellow D. Red

902. What is the biological source of bearberry
A. Bearberry fruit B. Bearberry leaves
C. Bearberry root D. Bearberry flower

903. What is the family of brassica nigra (L.)
A. Cruciferae B. Simarubaceae
C. Rosaceae D. Umbelliferae

904. What is the biological source of black mustard
A. Mustard root B. Mastard flower
C. Mustard fruit D. Musterd seed

905. What is the family of Piper nigurm L.
A. Piperaceae B. Lobeliaceae
C. Compositae D. Apocynaceae

906. What is the colour of buchu
A. Brown B. Greenish brown
C. Yellowish D. Greenish – yellow

907. What is the family of agathosmabetulina (Berg.) Pillans
A. Rutaceae B. Lytheaceae
C. Fagaceae D. Convolvulaceae

908. What is the synonym of calamus
A. Acorus calamus B.
B. Acomus calamus
C. Acorus calamus L.
D. Across calamus L.

909. What is the biological source of calumba
A. Calumba root B. Colombo root
C. Calumba leaf D. Both (A) and (B)

910. What is the colour of jate orhizapalmatamiers
A. Yellowish brown B. Reddish
C. Greenish D. Brown

911. What is the family of veratrumvirideaiton
A. Lythraceae B. Liliaceae
C. Convolvulaceae D. Lobeliaceae

912. Herbal dosage form can be categorised into?
A. Ayurvedic or modern dosage form
B. Unani dosage form
C. Homoeopathic dosage form
C. Both a& b

913. Ayurvedic dosage form include ?
A. Churna B. Asava/ arista
C. Cream D. Both a & b

914. Modern dosage form include?
A. Pill /Gulika/Bati
B. Ark
C. Bhasma
D. Powder/Tablet /Capsule

915. What is the selection of Herb/Herb part depends upon ?
A. Leaves containing aromatic principle
B. Separation of medicinally active principle from plant
C. The pharmacological action required or by reference to traditional literature
D. Both a & b

916. How can herbs be produced ?
A. From reliable botanical source & get it authenticated by treatment
B. From industrial suppliers
C. From vegetable suppliers
D. Natural source

917. Herb should not have been stored in clear glass jar or in direct sunlight , as it causes
A. Reduction B. Oxidation
C. Per oxidation D. Evaporation

918. Herbs should be stored in
A. Sterilised, dark glass containers with air-tight lids
B. Plastic containers
C. Bottles
D. Boxes or metals containers

919. For how many months after harvesting herbs can be kept ?
A. 10 B. 8
C. 12 D. 6

920. When herbs can be collected ?
A. Autumn
B. Clean dry weather
C. Morning after the dew has disappeared
D. Time of maturity

921. When flowers can be collected ?
A. In autumn
B. Before leaves decay
C. Before fade in dry weather
D After opens completely in dry weather in morning

922. When leaves (herbs) can be collected ?
A. After vegetation ends
B. Collected in autumn
C. In summer
D. Full development just before it fades

923. When Biennial leaves must be collected ?
A. In autumn
B. During second year
C. At temperature 65c
D. Spring or early summer

924. When Barks can be collected ?
A. During second year
B. Dry weather after the due has disappeared
C. In autumn by incision on stem and root
D. Spring or early summer by making suitable longitudinal & transverse incision

925. When do seeds can be collected?
A. Time of full maturity B. In summer
C. During 2nd year D. In autumn

926. Bulbs can be collected?
A. Dug out from soil just before leaves decay
B. In autumn
C. Just before fads
D. In early summer

927. When stalks can be collected?
A. Spring or early summer
B. Monsoon
C. Autumn
D. Before the dew disappeared

928. When twings can be collected?
A. After dew disappeared
B. Spring or early summer
C. Later winter
D. Autumn

929. When roots & rhizome can be collected?
A. Before autumn
B. After late summer
C. Before leaves fades
D. Just before flowering

930. Biennials roots are collected after vegetation of
A. First year has ended
B. Beginning of second year
C. End of second year
D. None of the above

931. When Perennials are collected ?

A. Autumn
B. Late summer
C. In spring or before vegetation begins
D. None of above

932. Leaves containing aromatic principle must be dried

A. In shade but must be placed in sunlight for short time
B. In dry room
C. Hot air oven
D. Dried directly to sun

933. When flowers can be dried ?

A. Dried in sun B. Air drying
C. In shade D. None of above

934. Roots can be dried at temperature

A. 65 to 80 f B. 70 to 90 f
C. 50 to 60 D. 80 to 100 f

935. When bulb can be dried ?

A. Before cutting transverse slices dried in air drying
B. Peeled & bulb cut into transverse slice dried in sunlight
C. In shade
D. Both a & b

936. Herbal parts or herbs can be dried by

A. De – humidifying B. Freeze drying
C. Microwaving D. All of the above

937. Size reduction of plant material is kept between mesh.

A. 20-30 B. 10-20
C. 30-40 D. 40 -60

938. The selected plant material is dried and subjected to powdering with help of

A. Hamermill B. Disc pulveriser
C. Motor pestle D. Both a & b

939. Size reduction provides surface area of the particle which in turn gives mass transfer between the material in contact with solvent.

A. Minimum B. Intermediate
C. Maximum D. None

940. Size reduction between mesh is optimal.

A. 30-40 B. 20-30
C. 10-20 C. 40-50

941. A size reduction of plant material beyond 30-40 mesh may make the material which creates difficulty during filtration.

A. Sticky with surface
B. Sling with the solvent
C. Adhere to the surface
D. Filtered out

942. The process of separation of medically active principle from the plant material with help of suitable solvent, is called

A. Percolation B. Maceration
C. Extraction D. None of the above

943. The material or ingredient in the hot aqueous extraction is allowed to boil till the volume of water is reduced to of its original volume.

A. One –fourth B. Two-third
C. One- third D. Two- fourth

944. Which apparatus is used for the solvent extracton process ?

A. Percolator
B. Soxhlet extractor
C. Haverhill
D. Clevanger apparatus

945. Soxhlet extractor consist of

A. An extractor
B. A distillation still
C. Tubular condenser
D. All of the above

946. In the solvent extraction solvent is added till it reduces the siphon point of the extractor and then the extractor and then the extract get siphoned out into

A. Distillation still
B. Extractor
C. Tubular condenser
D. None of above

947. The extract obtained is separated out from the exhausted plant material by allowing it to take into hold tank through the boil in fuse bottom of extractor, which is covered with filter cloth is called

A. Menstrum B. Filtrate
C. Marc D. Distillate

948. Marc is retained on

A. Hold tank B. Spray drier
C. Receiver D. False bottom

949. During filtration of extract from the hold tank, the extract is fed into a with the help of a pump to remove any fine or colloidal particle present in the extract .

A. Fine filter B. Cloth filter
C. Sparked filter D. Rapa filter

950. The concentrated extract is subjected to spray drier with the help of at a controller feed rate to get dry powder.

A. Wiped film evaporator
B. Distillation still
C. Rota meter
D. High pressure pump

951. The dilute solution of readily soluble constituent of crude drug are called

A. Diluents B. Infusion
C. Diffusion D. None of the above

952. Which types of infusion are there in preparation of pharmaceutical dosage from?

A. Cold B. Hot
C. Pot D. All of the above

953. When the active principle of drug are volatile in nature or sensitive to heat treatment Infusion is preferred.

A. Hot B. Cold
C. Pot D. Both a &b

954. These are prepared by pouring boiling water over the herb or herbal part and keeping the infusion in covered container for 5-10 min.

A. Cold B. Hot
C. Pot C. All of above

955. What among following is an example of hot infusion ?

A. Herbal tea B. Herbal drink
C. Herbal serum D. Herbal cream

956. Solvent used for extraction is called

A. Menstrum B. Marc
C. Extract solvent D. Extract solute

957. Crude drug is boiled in a specified volume of water for a defined time, it is often cooled & strained or filtered is called

A. Digestion B. Infusion
C. Decoction D. Maceration

958. Solution of medicinal substance in alcohol or diluted alcohol is called as

A. Medicated solution
B. Non medicated solution
C. Tinctures
D. None of above

959. According to Indian mythology there are

A. 1 B. 2
C. 3 D. 4

960. The father of surgery as claimed by traditional medicine lived and practiced surgery in Varanasi.

A. Bugbahtta B. Sushrata
C. Arya Bhatt D. Bhavamishra

961. In which century AD Bugbahtta of Sind work Astanga Hridaya is considered unrivalled for the principle and practice of medicine?

A. 15th B. 17th
C. 16th D. 18th

962. Which writer of Magadha is the best writer on the Hindu medicine where treatise bhavaprakasha, written around 1550 is held in high extremely modern practitioner forits description of approximately 470 medicinal plants ?

A. Arya Bhatt B. Bagbagtta
C. Bhavamishra D. Bhavaprakasha

963. Charaksumhita classified plant drug into group based on its Sanskrit name.

A. 30 B. 40
C. 20 D. 50

964. After full development of ayurveda, it has branched into wings, which are called Ashtanga Ayurveda.

A. 1 B. 5
C. 8 D. 6

965. Kayachiktsa comprises of treatment related to

A. Sareera Agni B. Surgery
C. Genetics
D. Rejuvenation and aphrodisiacs

966. Ayurvedic science deals with its pre – emblem of
A. Swasthasyaswasthyarakshanam
B. rtorasyarognath
C. Swasthasyarjaskaram
D. Both a &b

967. The second aspect of ayurveda is AturasyaRoganath that deals with
A. Cure of disease B. Surgery
C. Toxicology D. None of the above

968. Tridoshas deals with
A. Purosha, mootra, sweda
B. Rassa, rakta, meda
C. Vata, pitta, kapha
C. None of the above

969. Maintenance of balance in Ayurveda called as
A. Swasthyaraksha B. Aturasyarognat
C. Ritucharya D. Vajikarana

970. The theory of Rasa –guna-veerya-vipaka was established for formulation made in the form of
A. Panchavidhakashayakalpana
B. Kayachiksta
C. Swasthyarakshanam
D. Purusha, mootra, sweda

971. Basic concept of diagnosis & drug development in ayurveda is based on which theory
A. Trimalas B. Tridosha
C. Chikitsa D. Raktasdusti

972. Vaya (vata) explain the entire biological phenomenon, which are controlled by function of system
A. Central & autonomous
B. Respiratory
C. Digestive
D. Cardiovascular

973. Pitta is the manifestation of in the living organism that help digestion, assimilation, tissue building, heat production etc.
A. Agni B. Tejas
C. Chikitsa D. Asthi

974. Kapha implies function of
A. Thermotaxu or heat regulation
B. Formation of various preservative fluid
C. Nutrition to body
D. All of the above

975. The presence of treatment in Ayurveda consist of
A. Shodhana B. Shaman
C. Karmas D. All of the above

976. Shodhana karma is called as
A. Panchakarmas B. Tejas
C. Trimala D. None of the above

977. Panchakarma, i.e are important procedure to eliminate the morbid factors such as vikriodoshas, dustadhatu, mulas.
A. Vamama, nasya B. Vichchan, vasti
C. Raktamokshama D. All of the above

978. The principal of plays a vital role in maintaining internal environment, buffer system &homeostasis.
A. Shodhana karmas
B. Rasayanvajikarana
C. Swasthasyorjaskaran
D. Atorasyarognath

979. The term siddha comes from "siddhi" which means
A. Treatment for entire body
B. Homeostasis maintenance
C. Manifestation of energy
D. Attainment of perfection

980. The siddha medicine consist of psychosomatic system where attention is given to
A. Minerals & metals
B. Plant constituents
C. Animal constituents
D. Genetic medicine

981. Chindrooran refers to
A. Medicament prepared by calcinations
B. Reddish powdered medicine
C. Brown powder medicine
D. Powdered drug

982. Choornam refers to
A. Powdered drug
B. Medicament prepared by calcinations
C. Reddish powdered drug
D. Brown powdered medicine

983. Siddha system is similar to

A. Homoeopathic system

B. Ayurvedic system

C. Unani system

D. Allopathic system

984. Like ayurvedic completely based on the theory of panchamahabhuta ; siddha also constitute

A. Raktadushti

B. Chikitsa

C. Rosa –guna –veerya –vipaka

D. Panchaboothaspanjeekaranam

985. In siddha system, detoxification is a common phenomenon for any given drug to increase their therapeutic potency thereby minimizing the toxicity popularly known as

A. Suddhiseithavai B. Dhatuvargam

C. Jeevavargam D. Suddhisethai

986. As per siddha terminology, substance of plant origin are known as

A. Dhathuvargam B. Thavravargam

C. Jeevavargam D. Suddhisethai

987. As per siddha terminology, substance of animal origin are known as

A. Suddhisethai B. Jeevavargam

C. Dhatuvargam D. Thavravargam

988. As per sidhha system, substance of mineral origin called as

A. Suddhisethai B. Thavavargam

C. Jeevavargam D. Dhatuvargam

989. Formulary of siddha medicine was established in which year ?

A. 1993 B. 1994

C. 1995 D. 1996

990. According to sushruta the medication which is prepared by mixing together different kinds of medicated juice, decoction, jaggery & flower of dhataki in earthen vessel buried deep into a heap of grains for flavouring and to initiate fermentation is called as

A. Asava B. Arishta

C. Ghutika D. Avaleha

991. What among the following are example of Asava ?

A. Kumariasva B. Punarnavasava

C. Both a & b D. Ashokarsava

992. According to Bhavprakashsamhita the formulation which are prepared with the use of pakvavshadha siddha; earlier prepared by medication like herbal infusion& decoction is called as

A. Asava B. Ghutika

C. Bhasma D. Arishta

993. What among the following are example of Arishta ?

A. Ashokarishta

B. Dashmularishta

C. Ashwagandaarishta

D. All of the above

994. What is the other name of Ghrita ?

A. Medicated clarified butter

B. Non medicated clarified butter

C. Standard clarified butter

D. Sample mediated butter

995. Ghrita are preparation for consumption & are stable for about 16 months.

A. External B. Internal

C. Both a & b D. Mixed

996. What among the following are example of Ghrita ?

A. Ashokaghrita B. Brahmighrita

C. Lasunadighrita D. Both a & b

997. Fine powder of drug or drugs known as

A. Churna B. Powder

C. Bhasma D. Asava

998. What among the following are an example of churna ?

A. Trikatachurna B. Suadarshanchurna

C. Triphalachurna D. All of the above

999. Taila (medicated oil) are also called as

A. Snehakalpa / pakka

B. Drava

C. Bhasma

D. Arishta

1000. What among the following is an example of taila ?

A. BhrinrajTaila B. MahanarayanTaila
C. Shankpushpi D. Both a & b

1001. Gutika are one of the form of

A. Pills B. Powder
C. Oil D. Churna

1002. What among the following is an example of Gutika ?

A. LasunadiGutika B. PrandaGutika
C. KhadiradiGutika D. All of the above

1003. is semi solid preparation of drug prepared by addition of sugar candy & boiled with prescribed drug juice or decoction .

A. Avaleha B. Arishta
C. Ghutika D. Kalmegh

1004. Which among the following is an example of Avaleha?

A. Chawanprash B. Drakshavaleha
C. Both a & b D. None of the above

1005. Who credited with the discovery of safoof?

A. Aristole
B. Hippocrates
C. Bhavprakashmishra
D. Arya bhatt

1006. May be defined as solid material in a fully divided state which is ment for internal and external use.

A. Safoofs B. Majoon
C. Kushta D. Khameera

1007. Which among the following is an example of Snoofs?

A. Sanoon&manjan B. Barood
C. Kohal D. All of the above

1008. Are semisolid which have been prepared from the Qiwan of white sugar or honey & medicinal sufuf .

A. Majoon B. Kushta
C. Khameera D. Itrifal

1009. Are ayurvedic preparation that contain self generated alcohol content and herbal extracts soluable in both water as well as alcohol.

A. Asava B. Majoon
C. Arishta D. Gutika

1010. Alcohol content of Asava and Arishta can be determined by two methods ?

A. Distillation & chromatographic method
B. Extractive value & acid value
C. Ash value & total ash value
D. Both a & b

1011. Asava and Arishta have of alcohol content.

A. 10-15% B. 5-10%
C. 15-20% D. 20-25%

1012. The word cosmetic is derived from the Greek work 'kosmtikos' meaning ?

A. Having the power arrange
B. Skill in decorating
C. Both a & b
D. None

1013. The term cosmeticals was first used by founding member of US society of cosmetic chemist in 1961

A. Dr Albert klingman
B. Raymond Reed
C. Bhavprakashmishra
D. Sushruta

1014. The term cosmeceuticals was first used by Raymond Reed founding member of US society of the cosmetics chemist in year

A. 1961 B. 1960
C. 1959 D. 1958

1015. The term cosmeceuticals referred that the substance that have both cosmetic and therapeutic benefits was used by in year 1984.

A. Raymond reed
B. Bhavprakashmishra
C. Aristole
D. Dr Albert klingman

1016. An article intended to be rubbed , poured , sprinkled ,or sprayed on , introduced into or otherwise applied to the human body or beautifying , promoting attractiveness , or altering the appearance without affinity structure function called as

A. Powder B. Cream
C. cosmetic D. Lotion

1017. The variety of ingredient which have been incorporated in cosmeceuticals include

A. Vitamins , minerals
B. Herb , hormone
C. Antioxidant, anti inflammatory
D. All of above

1018. The concept that orally ingestible dietary products may support healthier and thus more beautiful skin called as

A. Skin cosmetics B. Nutri cosmetics
C. Herbal cosmetics D. Both a& b

1019. Skin is most extensive organ of our body.

A. Largest B. Smooth
C. Smallest D. Biggest

1020. The average adult has about cm2 of skin

A. 120-150 B. 150-170
C. 170-200 D. 200-230

1021. The average weight of skin in adult is

A. 10kg to 12kg B. 15kg to 17kg
C. 18kg to 20kg D. 21kg to 22kg

1022. Which is the outermost layer of skin?

A. Stratum coreneum
B. Stratum granulosm
C. Epidermis
D. Dermis

1023. The thickness of epidermis of skin is about mm in the thinnest area to at thickest point

A. 0.5mm to 5-6mm B. 0.6mm to 5-7mm
C. 0.3mm to 8-9mm D. 0.1mm to 7-8mm

1024. The play as a nutritional structure whose function also particularly important for the maintenance, coherence, elasticity.

A. Epidermis B. Dermis
C. Hypodermis D. None

1025. Which part of skin has protective & reserve function ?

A. Epidermis B. Dermis
C. Hypodermis D. None

1026. Which is the most external layer in contact with the environment?

A. Dermis B. Epidermis
C. Hypodermis D. Keratinocytes

1027. Below the epidermis is the structural component of skin and underlying organ

A. Dermis B. Epidermis
C. Hypodermis D. Melanocytes

1028. The layer of adipose cells and representing a "cohesion" of fat between the skin and the organ underneath called as

A. Dermis B. Epidermis
C. Hypodermis D. Melonocytes

1029. Which is the prominent cell type which produce protein keratin responsible for specific, important skin function?

A. Melanocytes B. Langerhan cell
C. Merkel cells D. Keratinocytes

1030. Which pigment responsible for skin colour?

A. keratin B. Melanin
C. Collagen D. None

1031. Melanin pigment contained in the structure called

A. Melanin B. Keratinosme
C. melanosome D. None

1032. The blood pigment in human being is

A. Carotene
B. Chlorophyll
C. Hemoglobin
D. Melanin

1033. Which cell are considered as "tactile receptor" responsible for sense of touch?

A. Langerhan cell B. Merkel cell
C. lymphocytes D. None of the above

1034. Most abundant cell production site of dermal component.

A. Lymphocytes B. Mastocytes
C. Histiocytes D. Fibroblast

1035. Skin mainly correspond to structural and function modification of the components of the epidermis.

A. Dry B. Soft
C. oily D. Hard

1036. Skin result from an excessive production , involving skin surface and possibly hair .

A. Hard B. Soft
C. Oily D. Dry

1037. Which layer of epidermis contains melanocytes?
A. Stratum basale
B. Stratum lucidum
C. Stratum spinosum
D. Stratum corneum

1038. By which gland most body odour is the result of bacterial metabolism of secretion?
A. Sebaceous B. Apocrine sweat
C. Misocrine sweat D. Eccrine sweat

1039. The fibrous protein that is responsible for the strength and water resistance of the skin surface is
A. keratohylin B. Collagen
C. Elastin D. Keratin

1040. Which layer of skin provides protection against bacteria as well as chemical & mechanical injuries ?
A. Dermis B. Sebum layer
C. Epidermis D. Subcutaneous layer

1041. At what temperature body temperature rises above normal?
A. Blood flow to skin increases
B. Blood flow to the skin decreases
C. Vasoconstriction occur
D. Sweat gland activity decreases

1042. Macrophages found in the epidermis are
A. Merkel cell B. Langerhan cell
C. Squamous cell D. Basal cell

1043. Into hair follicles which gland discharge an oil secretion ?
A. Apocrine sweat B. Sebaceous
C. Mesocrine sweat D. Mammary

1044. Which of the following function include in the integumentory system?
A. Maintenance of body temperature
B. Synthesis of vitamin c
C. Protection of underlying tissue
D. Excretion of salt and waste

1045. Contains the cells that are undergoing mitosis
A. Stratum spinosum
B. Stratum lucidum
C. Stratum corneum
D. Stratum grnaulosum

1046. Hair follicles & finger nails originate in the
A. Subcutaneous layer
B. Epidermis
C. Dermis
D. Hypodermis

1047. Body heat is produced by
A. Blood vessels
B. Hypothalamus
C. Contraction of skeletal muscle
D. Contraction of cardiac muscle

1048. To maintain its health, elasticity skin requires
A. pallor B. Colour
C. dryness D. Dullness

1049. Which layer of skin does not contain blood vessel
A. Corium B. Cuties
C. Epidermis D. Dermis

1050. What is the other name of stratum germinativum
A. Basal layer or stratum basale
B. Epidermis
C. Stratum lucidum
D. Dermal layer

1051. Where does mitosis of skin takes place
A. Stratum lucidum
B. Stratum germinatium
C. Stratum corneum
D. Stratum granulosum

1052. What is the synonym of olive oil?
A. Oleum olivae B. Oleum sipa
C. Allium sipa D. Allium stiva

1053. What is the biological source of olive oil?
A. Azadirachta indica
B. Papaversomniferum
C. Oleo europoealinne
D. Linumusitatissimum

1054. Which type of technique is used to generate olive oil?
A. Cold pressing B. Hot pressing
C. Dry pressing D. Wet pressing

1055. What is the color of olive oil?
A. Brownish B. Reddish
C. Greenish yellow D. Yellow

1056. What is the odour of olive oil?
A. sweet
B. Slight & characteristic
C. Pungent
D. Acrid

1057. What is the taste of olive oil?
A. sweet B. Bitter
C. salty D. Faintly acrid

1058. What is the specific gravity of olive oil?
A. 0.910 B. 0.810
C. 0.710 D. 0.610

1059. What is the iodine value of olive oil?
A. 69-78 B. 99-108
C. 79-88 D. 88-98

1060. What is the chemical constituent of olive oil ?
A. Olein, linolein B. Palmatic
C. Arachidic D. Oleic

1061. In the chemical test of olive oil under ultra-violet radiation it give colour
A. Dark golden yellow
B. Deep golden yellow
C. Light golden yellow
D. Golden green

1062. Olive oil is used as
A. Demollient B. Emollient
C. Ear wax D.

1063. What is the family of olive oil is ?
A. Oleaceae B. Liliaceae
C. Papaveracy D. Liquorice

1064. What is the biological source of sunflower?
A. Carthamustineturius
B. Oryza sativa
C. Helianthus Annus
D. Truticumaestium

1065. What is the family of sunflower ?
A. Pedaliaceae B. Gramincae
C. Compositae D. Papilionaceae

1066. What is the sunflower oil is generally?
A. Monoglyceride B. Triglyceride
C. Diglyceride D.

1067. What is the colour of sunflower oil is ?
A. Amber-coloured B. Faint-yellowish
C. Greenish-yellow D. Yellowish-green

1068. Density of sunflower oil is
A. 918.8kg/m3 B. 812.7kg/m3
C. 572.6kg/m3 D. 415.7kg/m3

1069. What is the iodine value of sunflower oil?
A. 130-155 B. 120-145
C. 110-135 D. 150-175

1070. Viscosity of sunflower oil?
A. 0.04914 B. 0.0391
C. 0.0291 D. 0.0254

1071. What is the biological source of coconut oil ?
A. Cocus sativa B. Cocusnucifera
C. Cocusastivum D. Cocuslucidum

1072. Cocusnucifera belongs to family
A. Graminceae B. Compositae
C. Pedaliaceae D. Palmae

1073. Which part of cocusnucifera is used?
A. Dreid solid part of edosperm
B. Liquid part of endosperm
C. Dried part of leaves
D. Dried part of root

1074. Colour of coconut oil is
A. Pale reddish yellow
B. Light yellowish green
C. Pale brownish yellow
D. Pale greenish yellow

1075. What is the melting point of coconut oil ?
A. 20 to 22 c B. 23 to 26 c
C. 26 to 29 c D. 21 to 17 c

1076. What is the other name of turmeric ?
A. Indian saffron B. Haridra
C. Curcuma D. All of the above

1077. What is the biological source of turmeric ?
A. Ipomoea orizabersis
B. Commipheramolmol
C. Curcuma longa
D. None

1078. What is the family of curcuma
A. Zingiberaceae B. Convolvulaceae
C. Berberidaceae D. Leguminaceae

1079. What is the colour of haridra?
A. Yellowish green B. Yellowish brown
C. Greenish yellow D. Reddish brown

1080. Haridra taste like
A. Slightly alkaline B. Slightly sweet
C. Slightly bitter D. None

1081. Abundant zingiberaceous starch grains & yellow colouring substance known as
A. Curcuminoids
B. Zingiberone
C. Dimethoxycurcumin
D. Bis dimethoxycurcumin

1082. What is the ash value of haridra?
A. Not more than2.0%
B. Not more than 4.0%
C. Not more than 6.0%
D. Not more than 8.0%

1083. What is the moisture content of curcuma ?
A. Not more than 10.0%
B. Not more than 9.0%
C. Not more than 8.0%
D. Not more than 7.0%

1084. When powdered drug of curcuma reacts with sulphuric acid it produces colour
A. Reddish B. Brown
C. Black D. Crimson

1085. When aqueous solution of curcuma reacts with boric acid it gives reddish-brown colour which on addition of an alkali changes into
A. Bluish green B. Yellowish green
C. Greenish yellow D. Brownish yellow

1086. What is the substitute for turmeric ?
A. Curcuma longa B. Curcuma amada
C. Curcuma D. None

1087. What is the synonym of aloe ?
A. Musabbar B. Rheum
C. Brahmi D. Yasti

1088. Aloe is the dried juice of the leaves of
A. Aloe spicata B. Aloe barbedinsis
C. Aloe perrgi D. All of above

1089. Henna consist of fresh and dried leaves of plant
A. Law Sonia innermis
B. Law barbedinsis
C. Law indica
D. Law Sonia linn.

1090. Henna has colour
A. Greenish red B. Greenish brown
C. Yellowish green D. Reddish green

1091. Odour of henna
A. Characteristic B. Alkaline
C. Acidic D. Slight

1092. What is the chemical constituent of heena ?
A. Oxalic acid B. Lawsone
C. Glycerol D. Palmatic acid

1093. What is the Moisture content of heena ?
A. 10.0% B. 8.0%
C. 9.0% D. 5.0%

1094. What is the ash value of henna ?
A. 9% B. 10%
C. 15% D. 12%

1095. Henna is used for
A. Hair dye B. Colouring agent
C. Flavouring agent D. None

1096. What is the other Name for Amla ?
A. Emblica B. Indian goose berry
C. Amalki D. All of the above

1097. What is the biological source of amla ?
A. Emblicaofficinalis
B. Termmaliaofficinalis
C. Termmaliaselerica
D. Mangifera indica

1098. Amla is generally a
A. Brick red B. Green colour
C. Light yellow D. All of the above

1099. What is the taste of amla ?
A. Sore and bitter B. Astringent &sore
C. Characteristic D. Sweet

1100. What is the chemical constituent of amla ?
A. Vitamin C B. Vitamin A
C. Vitamin B D. Vitamin D

1101. What is the other name of tea ?
A. Camellia indica B. Camellia officinalis
C. Camellia Thea D. Camellia sinensis

1102. Tea contain the prepared leaves &leaf bed of
A. Thea sinensis B. Thea officinalis
C. Thea beleria D. Thea indica

1103. Tea belongs to which family ?
A. Zingiberacae B. Leguminoseae
C. Theaceae D. None

1104. What is the chemical constituent of tea includes ?
A. Caffeine B. Pilocarpine
C. Isopilocarpine D. Kolacatechin

1105. Caffeine produces white ppt with acid solution ?
A. Hydrochloric acid B. Sulphuric acid
C. Tannic acid D. Boric acid

1106. What is the biological source of pumpkin
A. Curcurbita pepo B. Vitisuiniferd
C. Matricariarecutita D. Helianthus annus

1107. What is the family of pumpkin?
A. Liliaceae B. Vitaceae
C. Zingiberaceae D. Cucurbitaceae

1108. What chemical constituent does pumpkin contains ?
A. Palmitolic acid B. Stearic acid
C. Linolic acid D. All of the above

1109. What is the biological source of onion?
A. Allium cepa B. Vitisunifera
C. Cammeliathea D. Helianthus annus

1110. Onion belongs to which family?
A. Liliaceae B. Zingerberaceae
C. Leguminose D. Compositae

1111. What is the biological source of cucumber?
A. Tamarendis indica
B. Cucumis sativa
C. Curcuma longa
D. Lignum rhodium

1112. Allium sativum is the biological source of?
A. Onion B. Garlic
C. Galonga D. Vasca

1113. What is the biological source of hibiscus ?
A. Hibiscus rasa-sinensis
B. Hibiscus rosa –damascena
C. Hibiscus rubiacardifolia
D. Hibiscus sweritacherayita

1114. What is the family of hibiscus ?
A. Leguminosae B. Mawaceae
C. Liliacea D. Compositae

1115. Vetiver is perennial bunchgrass belongs to
A. Chrysopogenzizanioides
B. Callicarpamacrophylla
C. Eclipta alba
D. Withaniasomnifera

1116. Vetiver belongs to family of
A. Compositae B. Liliacae
C. Poaceae D. Leguminacae

1117. Biological source of lemon is
A. Citrun lemon B. Cassia tora
C. Cocuminssativs C. Eclipta alba

1118. What is the family of lemon ?
A. Leuminose B. Compositae
C. Berbidensis D. Rutaceae

1119. What is the biological source of Punarnava ?
A. Boerhaviadiffusa
B. Convolvulus pluricaulis
C. Bacapamonnieri
D. Convolvulus microphyllus

1120. What is punarnava used for ?
A. Anti –inflammatory
B. Expectorant
C. Reduce swelling & Faull smell in skin disease
D. All of the above

1121. What is the English name of punarnava ?
A. Spreading hogweed
B. Red hogweed
C. Horse purslane
D. All of the above

1122. What is the family of punarnava?
A. Nyctaginaceae B. Combritaceae
C. Scrophulariaceae D. Leguminoseae

1123. What are the chemical constituent of punarnava?
A. Hentriacontane
B. B-sitosterol
C. Boeravinones G & H
D. All of the above

1124. What is the synonym of Shankhpushpi ?
A. Shankhapushpi B. Aparajit
C. Shankavila D. All of the above

1125. What is the biological source of shankhpushpi?
A. Convolvulus pluricaulis
B. Convolvulus microphyllus
C. Bacopamonnieri
D. Both a & b

1126. What is the family of shankhpushpi ?
A. Scrophulariaceae
B. Leguminoseae
C. Convolvulaceae
D. Combretaceae

1127. What is the use of Shankhpushpi ?
A. Prominent memory improving
B. Psychostimulant& tranquilize
C. Reduce mental tension
D. All of the above

1128. Which among the following are marketed prepration of shankpushpi ?
A. Brahma B. Agastyaharitaki
C. Mustakarishta D. Both a & b

1129. What is the synonym of Ashoka ?
A. Asogam B. Koha
C. Arusa D. Sadada

1130. What is the biological source of Ashoka ?
A. Saraca indica B. Trigonellafoenum
C. Adhatadovasica D. Terminaliaashoka

1131. What is the family of ashoka
A. Leguminoseae B. Fabaceae
C. Liliaceae D. Compositae

1132. What is the chemical constituent of ashoka ?
A. leucoanthoinidin
B. Pelargonidin-3
C. Leucopelargonidin
D. All of the above

1133. What is Ashoka used for ?
A. Phenolic glycoside show oxytocic activity
B. Menorrhagia treatment
C. Leucorrhoea
D. All of the above

1134. What among the following is the marketed preparation of ashoka ?
A. Ashokarishta B. Nagarjunanhra rasa
C. Parthadyarishta D. Mustakarishta

1135. What is the other name for lahsun ?
A. Garlic B. Moql
C. Tesu D. Palash

1136. What is the biological source of lahsun ?
A. Buteamonosperma
B. Allium sativum
C. Commiphorawightti
D. Saraca indica

1137. What is the family of lahsun?
A. Liliaceae B. Fabaceae
C. Burseraceae D. Leguminoseae

1138. What is the chemical constituent of lahsun?
A. Ajoene B. Allylproyl
C. Vinyldithinines D. All of the above

1139. What are the marketed product of lahsun ?
A. Garlic pill B. Garlic powder
C. Lasunadivati D. All of the above

1140. What is the synonym of Guggul?
A. Salaitreeguggulipid
B. Mesashringi
C. Asphatt
D. Margosa

1141. What is the biological source of Guggul?
A. Gymnemasyvestre
B. Commiphorawightti
C. Cypercusrotundus
D. Azadiracta indica

1142. What is the family of guggul ?
A. Leguminoseae B. Burseraceae
C. Asclepiadaceae D. Cyperaceae

1143. What is guggul used for ?
A. Anti –inflammatory
B. Antidiabetic
C. Antisweetner
D. Aphrodisiac

1144. What among the following is marketed product of guggul?
A. Lakasminarayan rasa
B. Rodhrasava
C. Musakrishta
D. Both a & b

1145. What is the synonym of kalmegh?
A. King of bitter B. Bitter stick
C. Bitter root D. Felwart

1146. What is the biological source of kalmegh?
A. Commipherawightti
B. Swerticachirata
C. Andrographispaniculata
D. Gentianalutea

1147. What is the family of kalmegh?
A. Acanthaceae B. Gentianceae
C. Scrophulariaceae D. Compositae

1148. What is the chemical constituent of kalmegh?
A. Kalmeghin B. Andrographolide
C. Oxalic acid D. Both a& b

1149. What is the use of kalmegh?
A. Febrifuge B. Astringent
C. Antitytphoid D. All of the above

1150. What is the synonym of chirata ?
A. Indian gentian or bitter stick
B. German gentian
C. European gentian
D. African gentian

1151. What is the biological source of chirata?
A. Azaracta indica B. Swertiachirata
C. Allium sativum D. None

1152. What is the family of chirata?
A. Leguminoseae B. Compositae
C. Gentianceae D. Liliaceae

1153. What is the chemical constituent of chirata?
A. Chiritin B. Gentiopicrin
C. Ophelic acid D. All of the above

1154. What is the use of chirata?
A. Digestive B. Stimulant
C. Dyspepsia D. All of the above

1155. What is the biological source of valerian?
A. Valerian officianalis
B. Valerian sativum
C. Valerian barbedensis
D. None

1156. What is the family of chirata?
A. Caprifoliaceae B. Leguminoseae
C. Compositae D. Liliaceae

1157. What is the use of chirata?
A. Treat insomnia
B. Restless leg syndrome
C. Anti-inflammatory
D. Both a & b

1158. What is the synonym of Artemisia ?
A. Sweet warm wood
B. Bitter warm wood
C. Pungent warm wood
D. Both a & b

1159. What is the family of Artemisia?
A. Asteraceae B. Leguminoseae
C. Compositae D. Liliaceae

1160. What is the chemical constituent of Artemisia?
A. Artemisinin B. Coumarin
C. Quinic acid D. All of the above

1161. Artemisia is used for
A. Treatment of malaria
B. Anti-hypertensive
C. Anti-inflammatory
D. Treatment of anemia

1162. Which of these comes under intellectual property rights?
A. Patent B. Copyright
C. Trademark D. All of the above

1163. Which of the following intellectual property right is not published?
A. Trademark B. Patent
C. Trade secret D. Copyright

1164. Trademark is oriented by?
A. Product B. Consumer
C. Customer D. All of the above

1165. When was Patent act Amended by government in India?
A. 1986 B. 1999
C. 1996 D. 2001

1166. Which of the following is not affected by the changes which are Amended in Patent Act?
A. Biodiversity
B. Farmer rights
C. Traditional knowledge
D. All of the above

1167. Which of the following has been made a basis for the challenges of patent under Patent Act?
A. New uses of known substance
B. Duplication of traditional knowledge
C. Nondisclosure of source of origin of traditional material.
D. All of the above

1168. Biological diversity act can into force in?
A. 2001 B. 2003
C. 2004 D. 2002

1169. What is the Aim of biological diversity act?
A. Conserve biodiversity
B. Suitable use of biological resources
C. Equitable sharing of benefit of resources
D. All of the above

1170. Plant varieties protection and Farmer Right Act, 2001 which is TRIPS which mandates the :
A. Protection of land
B. Protection of plant
C. Protection of source of water
D. All of the above

1171. When was Plant varieties protection and farmer right act Amended?
A. 2001 B. 2004
C. 2002 D. 2000

1172. Plant varieties protection legislation protect the Right of?
A. Breeders B. Farmers
C. Both a & b D. None of the above

1173. Which of the following provide strongest IP Protection?
A. Trademarks B. Copyrights
C. Patent D. Trade secret

1174. For which of these patent is most difficult to obtained?
A. Herbal medicine B. Allopathic medicine
C. Laboratory test D. All of the above

1175. Which of the following is a objective of patent?
A. Economic benefit
B. Legal monopoly
C. Develop new idea
D. All of the above

1176. Patent satisfy the requirement of?
A. Novelty B. Utility
C. Both a & b D. Obviousness

1177. Which of these Intellectual Property Right is restricted to a country, region or territory where protection is sought and is not valid in other Region ?
A. Patent B. Copyright
C. Trademark D. Trade secret

1178. Which of the steps is not included in the procedure of patent?
A. Revocation of granted Patent
B. Opposition
C. Examination of Patentee by officer
D. Filling an application

1179. Which of the following is taken in consideration during examination of application of patent?
A. Novelty
B. Usefulness
C. Nature of claims
D. All of the above

1180. How much time period is given to opposition to fill contrary claims during procedure of potency?
A. 4 months B. 6 months
C. 3 months D. 2 months

1181. Which of the following cannot qualify for patent?
A. A method of agriculture
B. An invention related to atomic energy
C. A discovery or scientific theory
D. All of the above

1182. Which of these countries is first in the world to evolved an IPR legislation simultaneously granting rights to both breeder & farmer?
A. India B. Russia
C. USA D. South Africa

1183. On which of the principle breeder's Rights Act is based?

A. Protection of plant varieties
B. Consideration of plant & biodiversity
C. Distributing ownership right in fair manner
D. All of the above

1184. The tragedy of Anti- commons that is under use of resource arising from?

A. Growing needs
B. Multiple ownership
C. Competition in market
D. None of the above

1185. Which of the Aspect is adopted & expanded in definitive of Farmer's Right in the Act?

A. Farmer's privilege B. Benefit sharing
C. Ownership D. All of the above

1186. Which of the following is not included in farmer's privilege under farmer's right?

A. Right to serve material of seed
B. Sale of branded seed
C. Exchange of seed
D. Sell propagating of seed

1187. Which of these legislation enacted by parliament to honour India's obligation in TRIP'S?

A. Sui seed B. Sui generis
C. Sui plants D. None of the above

1188. Sui generis law enacted by parliament with respect of plant variety & family right?

A. Plant variety & family right
B. Breeder's right
C. Both a & b
D. None of the above

1189. Plant variety and Farmer's Right Act Recognize concept of which of these between provider & recipient of the plant genetics resource?

A. Farmer's privilege
B. Benefit sharing
C. Traditional knowledge
D. Ownership

1190. Applicant seeking registration of variety must disclose which of these whole evolving new variety?

A. Genetic material
B. Nature of variety
C. Geographical location
D. Life span

1191. PBR Law only apply to which of the following?

A. Plant B. Biodiversity
C . Seeds D. All of the above

1192. Which of these union or association responsible for protection of new varieties of plant?

A. SAI B. WTD
C. UPOV D. None

1193. Which of these act is opened presently by UPOV to new members?

A. 1972 B. 1978
C. 1961 D. 1991

1194. Which of these is a Indigenous heritage & customary heritage Right ?

A. Plant breeder right
B. Traditional knowledge
C. Biopiracy
D. Patent

1195. According to which of these traditional knowledge is an Indigenous heritage?

A. WIPO B. SIA
C. UPOV D. WTD

1196. Traditional knowledge cannot be patented because of?

A. Lack of source B. Lack of inventive
C. Lack of novelty D. Both a & c

1197. Which of these reason is Responsible for the threat to natural population of 6000 species of medicinal plant?

A. Lack of cultivation
B. Degradation
C. Loss of habitat
D. All of the above

1198. Which of these should taken in consideration by international cooperation in exploration of traditional health system?

A. Strategic research collaboration
B. Establishing wellness centre
C. Increase market of herbal medicine
D. Both a & b

1199. Which of the following is the biggest threat to biodiversity?

A. Biopiracy B. Bio prospecting
C. Encroachment D. All of the above

1200. Which of these filed nowadays highly provide usefulness of traditional knowledge for the development of new product of commercial knowledge?

A. Medical science
B. Pharmaceutical science
C. Biotechnology
D. Radiology

1201. The name ayurveda derived from two words ayur and Veda, which means?

A. Medicine of life B. Science of life
C. Life to cure D. Cure the cause

1202. According to German physician Samuel Hahnemann, homeopathy is based on which principle?

A. Like cure like
B. Similar cure similar
C. Medicine gives life
D. Science of life

1203. Which system of medicine depends on the interaction of panchmahabhutas?

A. Unani system
B. Siddha system
C. Homeopathic system
D. Ayurvedic system

1204. In ayurvedic system, what are the three principal humours in the body called as doshas?

A. Body, bile ,spirit
B. Wind ,bile, phlegm
C. Wind ,kapha, phlegm
D.Vata , pitta , kapha

1205. Unani system is based on whose teachings ?

A. Teachings of Hippocrates
B. Teachings of Dhanwantri
C. Teachings of SushrutaSamhita
D. Teachings of Avicenna

1206. Which of the following is not under the law and principles of Homeopathy ?

A. Law of similar
B. Law of immediate action
C. Law of minimum
D. Law of single remedy

1207. Which theory was developed by Hippocrates under the unani system of medicine ?

A. Medicinal theory
B. Remedial theory
C. Humoral theory
D. Dosage theory

1208. Which of the following is not the type of humours present in unani system ?

A. Blood B. Kapha
C. Yellow bile D. Black bile

1209. Out of this following comprises 70% of ayurveda

A. Vishachiktsa
B. Bala chiktsa
C. Rasayanachiktsa
D. Kayachiktsa

1210. Treatment of chemicals comes under which branch of astanga ayurveda ?

A. Kayachiktsa B. Graham chiktsa
C. Rasayanachiktsa D. Bala chiktsa

1211. What are the three main tridosha in ayurvedic system of medicine ?

A. Vata , Pitta , Kapha
B.Vata ,Kapha, Medo
C. Kapha , Vayu , Agni
D. Pitta , Kapha , Rasa

1212.In which year central council for research in Indian medicine and homeopathy was established ?

A. 1979 B. 1969
C. 1989 D. 1959

1213. Where are the headquarters of central council for research in yoga and neuropath(CCRYN)

A. Bangalore B. Delhi
C. Chennai D. Lucknow

1214. According to siddha terminology what is the term given to

A. Jeevavarganm B. Thavravargam
C. Dhatuvargum D. Bhasmavargam

1215. In which medicine system combination of minerals such as calcium and phosphorous are given and known as "Bhasmas"?

A. Siddha system
B. Homeopathy system
C. Unani system
D. Ayurveda system

1216. Which of the following system consist of following number such as blood, phlegm, yellow bile?

A. Unani system
B. Ayurveda system
C. Homeopathy system
D. Siddha system

1217. What is term used for stability of the chemical composition and physiochemical properties of internal environment?

A. Homeodynamics
B. Homeostasis
C. Homeostability
D. Homeokinetics

1218. What is the term used for palatative treatment in Ayurveda system of medicine?

A. Shodhana
B. Vamama
C. Shaman
D. virchana

1219. Which of the following system of council have 51 research centres around the country?

A. CCRAS
B. CCRH
C. CCRUM
D. CSIR

1220. According to Hippocrates , which of the following components help to keep body and mind healthy ?

A. Arkhan, safra , soada
B. Arkhan ,bhalgam , soada
C. Akhlat, arkhan, mijaz
D. Mijaz, akhlat, safra

1221. In which of the following system, treatment such as dietotheraphy, pharmacotherapy is done ?

A. Unani system
B. Ayurvedic system
C. Siddha system
D. Homeopathy system

1222. What is the basic philosophy theory of Ayurvedic which deals with Tridosha ?

A. "DashaDhatuMala"
B. "NaphaVayaMala"
C. "Pitta maua"
D. "Rasa- Guna –veerya"

1223. What was the major emphasis of Sushrutasamhita?

A. Medicine
B. One time dosage form
C. Surgery
D. Dose

1224. As per Charaksamhita , what was the main use of kasahar in ayurvedic system ?

A. Promoting strength
B. Promoting longivity
C. Emetic
D. Antitussive

1225. Who was the father of surgery in Ayurvedic medicinal system?

A. Sushruta
B. Hippocartes
C. Mukherjee
D. Magadha

1226. What is the common phenomenon of siddha system which increases therapeutic potency of drug and minimize toxicity?

A. Dehydration
B. Detoxification
C. Homeostasis
D. Positive feedback mechanism

1227. What is the basic terminology used for the "purification" in Siddha system?

A. Suddhiseithal
B. Parpams
C. Bhasmas
D. Suddhiseithavai

1228. In "Astanga ayurvedia" what is the basic terminology used for the treatment with rejuvenation and aphrodisiac?

A. Graham chikitsa
B. Vajikaramachikitsa
C. Tara chikitsa
D. Kayachikitsa

1229. How many group of plant drug are divided in CharakSamhita of Ayurvedic system?

A. 25
B. 50
C. 55
C. 75

1230. In which of the following system , the main emphasis was given on the plant material and its collection?
A. Ayurvedic system
B. Homeopathy system
C. Siddha system
D. Unani system

1231. Which of the following element is not present in sanchamahabhutas of ayurvedic system ?
A. Water B. Fire
C. Soil D. Air

1232. In which of the following system , drug treatment is not specified , but the choice of drug depends on symptoms and clinical condition ?
A. Allopathic system
B. Homeopathy system
C. Unani system
D. Ayurvedic system

1233. Who was the founder of homeopathy ?
A. Hippocrates
B. Christian fedrich Samuel Hahnemann
C. Avicenna
D. Rhazes

1234. In which of the following treatment of Ayurvedic , the main emphasis on re – adoption of rehabilitation ?
A. Poorva karma B. Pashata karma
C. Pradhana karma D. Anuvasa karma

1235. What is the term " siddha "mean in siddha system of medicine ?
A. Achievement B. Discovery
C. Invention D. Medicine

1236. According to Chinese medical system , on which condition , there is the imbalance in the body and caused disease?
A. Due to excess or deficiency
B. Due to deficiency
C. Due to imbalance in homeostasis
D. Due to toxicity

1237. The "yin"and "yang" theory based on which traditional system of medicine?
A. Unani system B. Ayurvedic System
C. Siddha system D. Chiense system

1238. Which system apart from ayurvedic believes in the role of three numors i.e. vata, pitta and kapha ?
A. Unani system
B. Homeopathy system
C. Siddha system
D. Chinese system

1239. From which country unani system of medicine serves its origin?
A. Nepal B. India
C. Greece D. Bangladesh

1240. "Pachana " "Snehana " and Swedana are the types of which stage of treatment in ayurveda ?
A. Pradhana karma
B. Poorva karma
C. Vtara karma
D. Paschata karma

1241. What is the basic terminology used for excretion of doshas from the mouth in the treatment therapy of pradhana karma ?
A. Virechana B. Nasya
C. Vamana D. Basti

1242. "Law of Similar" is the basic principle of which of the following medicinal system?
A. Homeopathy system
B. Ayurvedic system
C. Unani system
D. Siddha system

1243. How many monograph on single herb was contained by Ayurvedic Pharmacopeia of India?
A. 85 B. 90
C. 75 D. 80

1244. Which was the oldest repositories of human knowledge which mention 67 plant for therapeutic use ?
A. Yajurveda B. Rigveda
C. Atharveda D. Charaksamhita

1245. Which of the following plant valued in Ayurvedic for treatment of hypertension and Insomnia?
A. Rauwolfia serpentine
B. Papaver somniferous
C. Nuxvomica
D. Dhatura

1246. In which of the traditional system healthy individuals are given doses of undiluted substance called "proving"?

A. Ayurvedic system
B. Homeopathic system
C. Siddha system
D. Unani system

1247. What is the term Homeopathy means?

A. Homeo-similar , Pathy-disease
B. Homeo-like, Pathy-medicine
C. Homeo-same, Pathy-disease
D. Homeo-similar , Pathy- disease

1248. Which aspect of Ayurveda deals with the cure of disease?

A. AturasyaRognath
B. Ritucharya
C. Rasayana , vajikarana
D. Vishachikitsa

1249. How many regional research institute comes under CCRAS?

A. 18 B. 28
C. 8 D. 15

1250. According to which system, disease can cause because of internal factors or intrinsic causes ?

A. Siddha system
B. Ayurvedic system
C. Homeopathy system
D.Unani system

1251. The father of surgery as claimed by traditional medicine lived and practiced surgery in Varanasi.

A. Bugbahtta B. Sushrata
C. Arya Bhatt D. Bhavamishra

1252. In which century AD Bugbahtta of Sind work Astanga Hridaya is considered unrivalled for the principle and practice of medicine?

A. 15th B. 17th
C. 16th D. 18th

1253. Which writer of Magadha is the best writer on the Hindu medicine where treatise bhavaprakasha, written around 1550 is held in high extremely modern practitioner forits description of approximately 470 medicinal plants?

A. Arya Bhatt B. Bagbagtta
C. Bhavamishra D. Bhavaprakasha

1254. Charaksumhita classified plant drug into group based on its Sanskrit name.

A. 30 B. 40
C. 20 D. 50

1255. After full development of ayurveda , it has branched into wings , which are called Ashtanga Ayurveda .

A. 1 B. 5
C. 8 D. 6

1256. Kayachiktsa comprises of treatment related to

A. Sareera Agni
B. Surgery
C. Genetics
D. Rejuvenation and aphrodisiacs

1257. Ayurvedic science deals with its pre – emblem of

A. Swasthasyaswasthyarakshanam
B. rtorasyarognath
C. Swasthasyarjaskaram
D. Both a &b

1258. The second aspect of ayurveda is AturasyaRoganath that deals with

A. Cure of disease B. Surgery
C. Toxicology D. None of the above

1259. Tridoshas deals with

A. Purosha , mootra, sweda
B. Rassa, rakta ,meda
C. Vata, pitta, kapha
D. None of the above

1260. Maintenance of balance in Ayurveda called as

A. Swasthyaraksha
B. Aturasyarognath
C. Ritucharya
D. Vajikarana

1261. The theory of Rasa –guna-veerya-vipaka was established for formulation made in the formof

A. Panchavidhakashayakalpana
B. Kayachiksta
C. Swasthyarakshanam
D. Purusha, mootra, sweda

1262. Basic concept of diagnosis & drug development in ayurveda is based on which theory

A. Trimalas B. Tridosha
C. Chikitsa D. Raktasdusti

1263. Vaya (vata) explain the entire biological phenomenon, which are controlled by function of system

A. Central & autonomous
B. Respiratory
C. Digestive
D. Cardiovascular

1264. Pitta is the manifestation of in the living organism that help digestion, assimilation, tissue building, heat production etc.

A. Agni B. Tejas
C. Chikitsa D. Asthi

1265. Kapha implies function of

A. Thermotaxu or heat regulation
B. Formation of various preservative fluid
C. Nutrition to body
D. All of the above

1266. The presence of treatment in Ayurveda consist of

A. Shodhana B. Shaman
C. Karmas D. All of the above

1267. Shodhana karma is called as

A. Panchakarmas B. Tejas
C. Trimala D. None of the above

1268. Panchakarma, i.e are important procedure to eliminate the morbid factors such as vikriodoshas, dustadhatu, mulas.

A. Vamama, nasya
B. Vichchan, vasti
C. Raktamokshama
D. All of the above

1269. Theprincipal of plays a vital role in maintaining internal environment, buffer system &homeostasis.

A. Shodhana karmas
B. Rasayanvajikarana
C. Swasthasyorjaskaran
D. Atorasyarognath

1270. The term siddha comes from "siddhi" which means

A. Treatment for entire body
B. Homeostasis maintenance
C. Manifestation of energy
D. Attainment of perfection

1271. The siddha medicine consist of psychosomatic system where attention is given to

A. Minerals & metals
B. Plant constituents
C. Animal constituents
D. Genetic medicine

1272. Chindrooran refers to

A. Medicament prepared by calcinations
B. Reddish powdered medicine
C. Brown powder medicine
D. Powdered drug

1273. Choornam refers to

A. Powdered drug
B. Medicament prepared by calcinations
C. Reddish powdered drug
D. Brown powdered medicine

1274. Siddha system is similar to

A. Homoeopathic system
B. Ayurvedic system
C. Unani system
D. Allopathic system

1275. Like ayurvedic completely based on the theory of panchamahabhuta; siddha also constitute

A. Raktadushti
B. Chikitsa
C. Rosa –guna –veerya –vipaka
D. Panchaboothaspanjeekaranam

1276. In siddha system, detoxification is a common phenomenon for any given drug to increase their therapeutic potency thereby minimizing the toxicity popularly known as

A. Suddhiseithavai
B. Dhatuvargam
C. Jeeva vargam
D. Suddhisethai

1277. As per siddha terminology , substance of plant origin are known as

A. Dhathuvargam B. Thavravargam
C. Jeeva vargam D. Suddhisethai

1278. As per siddha terminology , substance of animal origin are known as

A. Suddhisethai B. Jeeva vargam
C. Dhatuvargam D. Thavravargam

1279. As per sidhha system, substance of mineral origin called as

A. Suddhisethai B. Thavavargam
C. Jeeva vargam D. Dhatuvargam

1280. Formulary of siddha medicine was established in which year ?

A. 1993 B. 1994
C. 1995 D. 1996

1281. According to sushruta the medication which is prepared by mixing together different kinds of medicated juice, decoction, jaggery & flower of dhataki in earthen vessel buried deep into a heap of grains for flavouring and to initiate fermentation is called as

A. Asava B. Arishta
C. Ghutika D. Avaleha

1282. What among the following are example of Asava?

A. Kumariasva B. Punarnavasava
C. Both a & b D. Ashokarsava

1283. According to Bhavprakashsamhita the formulation which are prepared with the use of pakvavshadha siddha; earlier prepared by medication like herbal infusion& decoction is called as

A. Asava B. Ghutika
C. Bhasma D. Arishta

1284. What among the following are example of Arishta ?

A. Ashokarishta
B. Dashmularishta
C. Ashwagandaarishta
D. All of the above

1285. What is the synonym of olive oil?

A. Oleum olivae B. Oleum sipa
C. Allium sipa D. Allium stiva

1286. What is the biological source of olive oil?

A. Azadirachta indica
B. Papaversomniferum
C. Oleo europoealinne
D. Linumusitatissimum

1287. Which type of technique is used to generate olive oil?

A. Cold pressing B. Hot pressing
C. Dry pressing D. Wet pressing

1288. What is the color of olive oil?

A. Brownish B. Reddish
C. Greenish yellow D. Yellow

1289. What is the odour of olive oil?

A. Sweet
B. Slight & characteristic
C. Pungent
D. Acrid

1290. What is the taste of olive oil?

A. Sweet B. Bitter
C. Salty D. Faintly acrid

1291. What is the specific gravity of olive oil?

A. 0.910 B. 0.810
C. 0.710 D. 0.610

1292. What is the iodine value of olive oil?

A. 69-78 B. 99-108
C. 79-88 D. 88-98

1293. What is the chemical constituent of olive oil ?

A. Olein, linolein B. Palmatic
C. Arachidic D. Oleic

1294. In the chemical test of olive oil under ultra-violet radiation it give colour

A. Dark golden yellow
B. Deep golden yellow
C. Light golden yellow
D. Golden green

1295. Olive oil is used as

A. Demollient B. Emollient
C. Ear wax D. Lubricant

1296. What is the family of olive oil is ?

A. Oleaceae B. Liliaceae
C. Papaveracy D. Liquorice

1297. What is the biological source of sunflower?

A. Carthamustineturius
B. Oryza sativa
C. Helianthus Annus
D. Truticumaestium

1298. What is the family of sunflower ?
A. Pedaliaceae B. Gramincae
C. Compositae D. Papilionaceae

1299. What is the sunflower oil is generally?
A. Monoglyceride B. Triglyceride
C. Diglyceride D. biglyceride

1300. What is the colour of sunflower oil is ?
A. Amber-coloured
B. Faint-yellowish
C. Greenish-yellow
D. Yellowish-green

1301. Density of sunflower oil is
A. 918.8kg/m3 B. 812.7kg/m3
C. 572.6kg/m3 D. 415.7kg/m3

1302. What is the iodine value of sunflower oil?
A. 130-155 B. 120-145
C. 110-135 D. 150-175

1303. Viscosity of sunflower oil?
A. 0.04914 B. 0.0391
C. 0.0291 D. 0.0254

1304. What is the biological source of coconut oil ?
A. Cocus sativa B. Cocusnucifera
C. Cocusastivum D. Cocuslucidum

1305. Cocusnucifera belongs to family
A. Graminceae B. Compositae
C. Pedaliaceae D. Palmae

1306. Which part of cocusnucifera is used?
A. Dreid solid part of edosperm
B. Liquid part of endosperm
C. Dried part of leaves
D. Dried part of root

1307. Colour of coconut oil is
A. Pale reddish yellow
B. Light yellowish green
C. Pale brownish yellow
D. Pale greenish yellow

1308. What is the melting point of coconut oil ?
A. 20 to 22 c B. 23 to 26 c
C. 26 to 29 c D. 21 to 17 c

1309. What is the other name of turmeric ?
A. Indian saffron B. Haridra
C. Curcuma D. All of the above

1310. What is the biological source of turmeric ?
A. Ipomoea orizabersis
B. Commipheramolmol
C. Curcuma longa
D. None

1311. What is the family of curcuma
A. Zingiberaceae B. Convolvulaceae
C. Berberidaceae D. Leguminaceae

1312. What is the colour of haridra?
A. Yellowish green B. Yellowish brown
C. Greenish yellow D. Reddish brown

1313. Haridra taste like
A. Slightly alkaline B. Slightly sweet
C. Slightly bitter D. None

1314. Abundant zingiberaceous starch grains & yellow colouring substance known as
A. Curcuminoids
B. Zingiberone
C. Dimethoxycurcumin
D. Bis di methoxycurcumin

1315. What is the ash value of haridra?
A. Not more than2.0%
B. Not more than 4.0%
C. Not more than 6.0%
D. Not more than 8.0%

1316. What is the moisture content of curcuma ?
A. Not more than 10.0%
B. Not more than 9.0%
C. Not more than 8.0%
D. Not more than 7.0%

1317. When powdered drug of curcuma reacts with sulphuric acid it produces colour
A. Reddish B. Brown
C. Black D. Crimson

1318. When aqueous solution of curcuma reacts with boric acid it gives reddish-brown colour which on addition of an alkali changes into
A. Bluish green B. Yellowish green
C. Greenish yellow D. Brownish yellow

1319. What is the substitute for turmeric ?
A. Curcuma longa B. Curcuma amada
C. Curcuma D. None

1320. What is the synonym of aloe ?
A. Musabbar B. Rheum
C. Brahmi D. Yasti

1321. Aloe is the dried juice of the leaves of
A. Aloe spicata B. Aloe barbedinsis
C. Aloe perrgi D. All of above

1322. Henna consist of fresh and dried leaves of plant
A. Law Sonia innermis
B. Law barbedinsis
C. Law indica
D. Law Sonia linn.

1323. Henna has colour
A. Greenish red B. Greenish brown
C. Yellowish green D. Reddish green

1324. Odour of henna
A. Characteristic B. Alkaline
C. Acidic D. Slight

1325. What is the chemical constituent of heena?
A. Oxalic acid B. Lawsone
C. Glycerol D. Palmatic acid

1326. What is the Moisture content of heena ?
A. 10.0% B. 8.0%
C. 9.0% D. 5.0%

1327. What is the ash value of henna ?
A. 9% B. 10%
C. 15% D. 12%

1328. Henna is used for
A. Hair dye B. Colouring agent
C. Flavouring agent D. None

1329. What is the other Name for Amla ?
A. Emblica B. Indian goose berry
C. Amalki D. All of the above

1330. What is the biological source of amla ?
A. Emblicaofficinalis
B. Termmaliaofficinalis
C. Termmaliaselerica
D. Mangifera indica

1331. Amla is generally a
A. Brick red B. Green colour
C. Light yellow D. All of the above

1332. What is the taste of amla ?
A. Sore and bitter B. Astringent &sore
C. Characteristic D. Sweet

1333. What is the chemical constituent of amla ?
A. Vitamin C B. Vitamin A
C. Vitamin B D. Vitamin D

1334. What is the other name of tea ?
A. Camellia indica B. Camellia officinalis
C. Camellia Thea D. Camellia sinensis

1335. Tea contain the prepared leaves &leaf bed of
A. Thea sinensis B. Thea officinalis
C. Thea beleria D. Thea indica

1336. Tea belongs to which family?
A. Zingiberacae B. Leguminoseae
C. Theaceae D. None

1337. What is the chemical constituent of tea includes ?
A. Caffeine B. Pilocarpine
C. Isopilocarpine D. Kolacatechin

1338. Caffeine produces white ppt with acid solution ?
A. Hydrochloric acid
B. Sulphuric acid
C. Tannic acid
D. Boric acid

1339. What is the biological source of pumpkin
A. Curcurbita pepo
B. Vitisuiniferd
C. Matricariarecutita
D. Helianthus annus

1340. What is the family of pumpkin?
A. Liliaceae B. Vitaceae
C. Zingiberaceae D. Cucurbitaceae

1341. What chemical constituent does pumpkin contains ?
A. Palmitolic acid B. Stearic acid
C. Linolic acid D. All of the above

1342. What is the biological source of onion?
A. Allium cepa B. Vitisunifera
C. Cammeliathea D. Helianthus annus

1343. Onion belongs to which family?
A. Liliaceae B. Zingerberaceae
C. Leguminose D. Compositae

1344. What is the biological source of cucumber?
A. Tamarendis indica
B. Cucumis sativa
C. Curcuma longa
D. Lignum rhodium

1345. Allium sativum is the biological source of?
A. Onion B. Garlic
C. Galonga D. Vasca

1346. What is the biological source of hibiscus ?
A. Hibiscus rasa-sinensis
B. Hibiscus rosa –damascena
C. Hibiscus rubiacardifolia
D. Hibiscus sweritacherayita

1347. What is the family of hibiscus ?
A. Leguminosae B. Mawaceae
C. Liliacea D. Compositae

1348. Vetiver is perennial bunchgrass belongs to
A. Chrysopogenzizanioides
B. Callicarpamacrophylla
C. Eclipta alba
D. Withaniasomnifera

1349. Vetiver belongs to family of
A. Compositae B. Liliacae
C. Poaceae D. Leguminacae

1350. Biological source of lemon is
A. Citrun lemon B. Cassia tora
C. Cocuminssativs C. Eclipta alba

1351. What is the family of lemon ?
A. Leuminose B. Compositae
C. Berbidensis D. Rutaceae

1352. What is the biological source of Punarnava ?
A. Boerhaviadiffusa
B. Convolvulus pluricaulis
C. Bacapamonnieri
D. Convolvulus microphyllus

1353. What is punarnava used for ?
A. Anti –inflammatory
B. Expectorant
C. Reduce swelling &Faull smell in skin disease
D. All of the above

1354. What is the English name of punarnava ?
A. Spreading hogweed
B. Red hogweed
C. Horse purslane
D. All of the above

1355. What is the family of punarnava?
A. Nyctaginaceae B. Combritaceae
C. Scrophulariaceae D. Leguminoseae

1356. What are the chemical constituent of punarnava?
A. Hentriacontane
B. B-sitosterol
C. Boeravinones G & H
D.All of the above

1357. What is the synonym of Shankhpushpi ?
A. Shankhapushpi B. Aparajit
C. Shankavila D. All of the above

1358. What is the biological source of shankhpushpi?
A. Convolvulus pluricaulis
B. Convolvulus microphyllus
C. Bacopamonnieri
D. Both a & b

1359. What is the family of shankhpushpi
A. Scrophulariaceae
B. Leguminoseae
C. Convolvulaceae
D. Combretaceae

1360. What is the use of Shankhpushpi ?
A. Prominent memory improving
B. Psychostimulant&tranquilize
C. Reduce mental tension
D. All of the above

1361. Which among the following are marketed prepration of shankpushpi ?
A. Brahma B. Agastyaharitaki
C. Mustakarishta D. Both a & b

1362. What is the synonym of Ashoka ?
A. Asogam B. Koha
C. Arusa D. Sadada

1363. What is the biological source of Ashoka ?
A. Saraca indica B. Trigonellafoenum
C. Adhatadovasica D. Terminaliaashoka

1364. What is the family of ashoka

A. Leguminoseae B. Fabaceae
C. Liliaceae D. Compositae

1365. What is the chemical constituent of ashoka ?

A. leucoanthoinidin
B. Pelargonidin-3
C. Leucopelargonidin
D. All of the above

1366. What is Ashoka used for?

A. Phenolic glycoside show oxytocic activity
B. Menorrhagia treatment
C. Leucorrhoea
D. All of the above

1367. What among the following is the marketed preparation of ashoka ?

A. Ashokarishta B.Nagarjunanhra rasa
C. Parthadyarishta D. Mustakarishta

1368. What is the other name for lahsun ?

A. Garlic B. Moql
C. Tesu D. Palash

1369. What is the biological source of lahsun ?

A. Buteamonosperma
B. Allium sativum
C. Commiphorawightti
D. Saraca indica

1370. What is the family of lahsun?

A. Liliaceae B. Fabaceae
C. Burseraceae D. Leguminoseae

1371. What is the chemical constituent of lahsun?

A. Ajoene B. Allylproyl
C. Vinyldithinines D. All of the above

1372. What are the marketed product of lahsun ?

A. Garlic pill B. Garlic powder
C. Lasunadivati D. All of the above

1373. What is the synonym of Guggul?

A. Salaitreeguggulipid
B. Mesashringi
C. Asphatt
D. Margosa

1374. What is the biological source of Guggul?

A. Gymnemasyvestre
B. Commiphorawightti
C. Cypercusrotundus
D. Azadiracta indica

1375. What is the family of guggul ?

A. Leguminoseae B. Burseraceae
C. Asclepiadaceae D. Cyperaceae

1376. What is guggul used for ?

A. Anti –inflammatory
B. Antidiabetic
C. Antisweetner
D. Aphrodisiac

1377. What among the following is marketed product of guggul?

A. Lakasminarayan rasa
B. Rodhrasava
C. Musakrishta
D. Both a & b

1378. When was Patent act Amended by government in India?

A. 1986 B. 1999
C. 1996 D. 2001

1379. Which of the following is a objective of patent?

A. Economic benefit
B. Legal monopoly
C. Develop new idea
D. All of the above

1380. Patent satisfy the requirement of?

A. Novelty B. Utility
C. Both a & b D. Obviousness

1381. Which of these Intellectual Property Right is restricted to a country, region or territory where protection is sought and is not valid in other Region ?

A. Patent B. Copyright
C. Trademark D. Trade secret

1382. Which of the steps is not included in the procedure of patent?

A. Revocation of granted Patent
B. Opposition
C. Examination of Patentee by officer
D. Filling an application

1383. Which of the following is taken in consideration during examination of application of patent?

A. Novelty B. Usefulness
C. Nature of claims D. All of the above

1384. How much time period is given to opposition to fill contrary claims during procedure of potency?

A. 4 months B. 6 months
C. 3 months D. 2 months

1385. Which of the following cannot qualify for patent?

A. A method of agriculture
B. An invention related to atomic energy
C. A discovery or scientific theory
D. All of the above

1386. Which of these countries is first in the world to evolved an IPR legislation simultaneously granting rights to both breeder & farmer?

A. India B. Russia
C. USA D. South Africa

1387. On which of the principle breeder's Rights Act is based?

A. Protection of plant varieties
B. Consideration of plant & biodiversity
C. Distributing ownership right in fair manner
D. All of the above

1388. The tragedy of Anti- commons that is under use of resource arising from?

A. Growing needs
B. Multiple ownership
C. Competition in markot
D.None of theabove

1389. Which of the Aspect is adopted & expanded in definitive of Farmer's Right in the Act?

A. Farmer's privilege
B. Benefit sharing
C. Ownership
D. All of the above

1390. Which of the factor government the Indians policy on IPR Protection in Agriculture?

A. Common human heritage
B. Economic development
C. Resource at high prices to avoid
D. Both a & b

1391. Which of the following is not included in farmer's privilege under farmer's right?

A. Right to serve material of seed
B. Sale of branded seed
C. Exchange of seed
D. Sell propagating of seed

1392. Which of these legislation enacted by parliament to honour India's obligation in TRIP'S?

A. Sui seed B. Sui generis
C. Sui plants D. None of the above

1393. Sui generis law enacted by parliament with respect of plant variety & family right?

A . Plant variety & family right
B. Breeder's right
C. Both a & b
D. None of the above

1394. Plant variety and Farmer's Right Act Recognize concept of which of these between provider & recipient of the plant genetics resource?

A. Farmer's privilege
B. Benefit sharing
C. Traditional knowledge
D. Ownership

1395. Applicant seeking registration of variety must disclose which of these whole evolving new variety?

A. Genetic material
B. Nature of variety
C. Geographical location
D. Life span

1396. Which system of medicine depends on the interaction of panchmahabhutas?

A. Unani system
B. Siddha system
C. Homeopathic system
D. Ayurvedic system

1397. In ayurvedic system, what are the three principal humours in the body called as doshas?

A. Body, bile ,spirit
B. Wind ,bile, phlegm
C. Wind ,kapha, phlegm
D. Vata , pitta , kapha

1398. Unani system is based on whose teachings ?

A. Teachings of Hippocrates
B. Teachings of Dhanwantri

C. Teachings of Sushruta Samhita
D. Teachings of Avicenna

1399. Which of the following is not under the law and principles of Homeopathy ?
A. Law of similar
B. Law of immediate action
C. Law of minimum
D. Law of single remedy

1400. Which theory was developed by Hippocrates under the unani system of medicine ?
A. Medicinal theory
B. Remedial theory
C. Humoral theory
D. Dosage theory

1401. Which of the following is not the type of humours present in unani system ?
A. Blood B. Kapha
C. Yellow bile D. Black bile

1402. Out of this following comprises 70% of ayurveda ?
A. Vishachiktsa
B. Bala chiktsa
C. Rasayanachiktsa
D. Kayachiktsa

1403. Treatment of chemicals comes under which branch of astanga ayurveda ?
A. Kayachiktsa B. Graham chiktsa
C. Rasayanachiktsa D. Bala chiktsa

1404. What are the three main tridosha in ayurvedic system of medicine ?
A. Vata , Pitta , Kapha
B. Vata ,Kapha, Medo
C. Kapha , Vayu , Agni
D. Pitta , Kapha , Rasa

1405. In which year central council for research in Indian medicine and homeopathy was established ?
A. 1979 B. 1969
C. 1989 D. 1959

1406. Where are the headquarters of central council for research in yoga and neuropath (CCRYN)
A. Bangalore B. Delhi
C. Chennai D. Lucknow

1407. According to siddha terminology what is the term given to
A. Jeeva varganm
B. Thavravargam
C. Dhatuvargum
D. Bhasmavargam

1408. In which medicine system combination of minerals such as calcium and phosphorous are given and known as "Bhasmas"?
A. Siddha system
B. Homeopathy system
C. Unani system
D. Ayurveda system

1409. Which of the following system consist of following number such as blood, phlegm, yellow bile?
A. Unani system
B. Ayurveda system
C. Homeopathy system
D. Siddha system

1410. What is term used for stability of the chemical composition and physiochemical properties of internal environment?
A. Homeodynamics
B. Homeostasis
C. Homeostability
D. Homeokinetics

1411. What is the term used for palatative treatment in Ayurveda system of medicine?
A. Shodhana B. Vamama
C. Shaman D. virchana

1412. Which of the following system of council have 51 research centres around the country?
A. CCRAS B. CCRH
C. CCRUM D. CSIR

1413. According to Hippocrates, which of the following components help to keep body and mind healthy ?
A. Arkhan, safra , soada
B. Arkhan ,bhalgam , soada
C. Akhlat, arkhan, mijaz
D. Mijaz, akhlat, safra

1414. In which of the following system, treatment such as dietotheraphy, pharmacotherapy is done ?

A. Unani system
B. Ayurvedic system
C. Siddha system
D. Homeopathy system

1415. What is the basic philosophy theory of Ayurvedic which deals with Tridosha ?

A. "DashaDhatu Mala"
B. "NaphaVaya Mala"
C. "Pitta maua"
D. "Rasa- Guna –veerya"

1416. What was the major emphasis of Sushruta samhita?

A. Medicine
B. One time dosage form
C. Surgery
D. Dose

1417. As per Charaksamhita, what was the main use of kasahar in ayurvedic system ?

A. Promoting strength
B. Promoting longitivity
C. Emetic
D. Antitussive

1418. Who was the father of surgery in Ayurvedic medicinal system?

A. Sushruta B. Hippocartes
C. Mukherjee D. Magadha

1419. What is the common phenomenon of siddha system which increases therapeutic potency of drug and minimize toxicity?

A. Dehydration
B. Detoxification
C. Homeostasis
D. Positive feedback mechanism

1420. What is the basic terminology used for the "purification" in Siddha system?

A. Suddhiseithal B. Parpams
C. Bhasmas D. Suddhiseithavai

1421. In "Astanga ayurvedia" what is the basic terminology used for the treatment with rejuvenation and aphrodisiac?

A. Graham chikitsa
B. Vajikaramachikitsa
C. Tara chikitsa
D. Kayachikitsa

1422. How many group of plant drug are divided in Charak Samhita of Ayurvedic system?

A. 25 B. 50
C. 55 C. 75

1423. In which of the following system, the main emphasis was given on the plant material and its collection?

A. Ayurvedic system
B. Homeopathy system
C. Siddha system
D. Unani system

1424. Which of the following element is not present in sanchamahabhutas of ayurvedic system ?

A. Water B. Fire
C. Soil D. Air

1425. In which of the following system, drug treatment is not specified, but the choice of drug depends on symptoms and clinical condition ?

A. Allopathic system
B. Homeopathy system
C. Unani system
D. Ayurvedic system

1426. Who was the founder of homeopathy ?

A. Hippocrates
B. Christian fedrich Samuel Hahnemann
C. Avicenna
D. Rhazes

1427. In which of the following treatment of Ayurvedic, the main emphasis on re – adoption of rehabilitation ?

A. Poorva karma B. Pashata karma
C. Pradhana karma D. Anuvasa karma

1428. What is the term "siddha "mean in siddha system of medicine?

A. Achievement B. Discovery
C. Invention D. Medicine

1429. According to Chinese medical system, on which condition, there is the imbalance in the body and caused disease?

A. Due to excess or deficiency
B. Due to deficiency
C. Due to imbalance in homeostasis
D. Due to toxicity

1430. The "yin" and "yang" theory based on which traditional system of medicine?

A. Unani system B. Ayurvedic System
C. Siddha system D. Chiense system

1431. Which system apart from ayurvedic believes in the role of three numors i.e. vata, pitta and kapha ?

A. Unani system
B. Homeopathy system
C. Siddha system
D. Chinese system

1432. From which country unani system of medicine serves its origin?

A. Nepal B. India
C. Greece D. Bangladesh

1433. "Pachana " "Snehana " and Swedana are the types of which stage of treatment in ayurveda ?

A. Pradhana karma
B. Poorva karma
C. Vtara karma
D. Paschata karma

1434. What is the basic terminology used for excretion of doshas from the mouth in the treatment therapy of pradhana karma ?

A. Virechana B. Nasya
C. Vamana D. Basti

1435. "Law of Similar" is the basic principle of which of the following medicinal system?

A. Homeopathy system
B. Ayurvedic system
C. Unani system
D. Siddha system

1436. How many monograph on single herb was contained by Ayurvedic Pharmacopeia of India?

A. 85 B. 90
C. 75 D. 80

1437. Which was the oldest repositories of human knowledge which mention 67 plant for therapeutic use ?

A. Yajurveda B. Rigveda
C. Atharveda D. Charaksamhita

1438. Which of the following plant valued in Ayurvedic for treatment of hypertension and Insomnia?

A. Rauwolfia serpentine
B. Papaver somniferous
C. Nuxvomica
D. Dhatura

1439. In which of the traditional system healthy individuals are given doses of undiluted substance called "proving"?

A. Ayurvedic system
B. Homeopathic system
C. Siddha system
D. Unani system

1440. What is the term Homeopathy means?

A. Homeo-similar , Pathy-disease
B. Homeo-like, Pathy-medicine
C. Homeo-same, Pathy-disease
D. Homeo-similar , Pathy- disease

1441. Which of the factor government the Indians policy on IPR Protection in Agriculture?

A. Common human heritage
B. Economic development
C. Resource at high prices to avoid
D. Both a & b

1442. When is World intellectual Property Day celebrated?

A. April 23 B. April 24
C. April 25 D. April 26

1443. What is synonym of Loban?

A. Sumatra Benzoin B. Asafoetida
C. Capsicum D. Guggul

1444. What is Loban commercially known as?

A. Styrax benzoin
B. Sumatra benzoin
C. Stam benzoin
D. Styrax paralleleneurus

1445. Trees of Siam Benzoin are grown in which South Asian country?

A. Thailand B. Vietnam
C. Both a) and b) D. None

1446. How much of a material a 100 trees of Benzoin produce approximately ?

A. 10,000 kg B. 10 kg
C. 1,000 kg D. 100 kg

1447. When ether and sulphuric acid are mixed with Benzoin,then which colours are produced In the case of Sumatra Benzoin and Stam Benzoin respectively?

A. Yellow and deep Orange
B. Deep purple and deep red
C. Purple and Red
D. Deep brown and deep purplish red

1448. Benzoin has various uses one of the purposes for which it's not used is?

A. Expectorant B. Carminative
C. Treatment of UTI D. Diuretic

1449. What does alcoholic solution of Benzoin with water give ?

A. Clear liquid
B. Dark grey solution
C. Milky white solution
D. None

1450. Why is Benzoin used in Pharmaceutical industry ?

A. To mask the taste of pharmaceutical preparations
B. As a diluent
C. Suspending agent
D. Bulking agent

1451. The major constituent of Siam Benzoin is

A. Styrol
B. Vanillin
C. Siaresiudic acid
D. Coniferous benzoate

1452. When 4ml of KMnO4 is added to 1g Benzoin and warmed, which odour is produced ?

A. Cinnamic acid B. Benzaldehyde
C. Ammonia D. Sulphuric acid

1454. What is the geographical source of Peruvian Balsam ?

A. Central America B. Honduras
C. Guatemala D. All of the above

1455. In alcoholic and non alcoholic beverages , Peru Balsam can be used to the extent of?

A. 20ppm B. 18ppm
C. 15ppm D. 24ppm

1456. Balsam of Peru is partly soluble in ?

A. Water B. Alcohol
C. Petroleum ether D. Acetic acid

1457. The process of collection of Peru Balsam starts in which season ?

A. Winter season B. Spring season
C. Autumn season D. Summer season

1458. The taste of MyroxylonBalsamum is?

A. Bitter acrid B. Sweet
C. Sour D. Camphoraceous

1459. In which of the following preparation Balsum is not needed ?

A. Cosmetics
B. Treatment of bedsores
C. Expectorant
D. Flavouring agent

1460. What is the degree of compactness of Indian Black Balsam ?

A. 2.650-2.700 B. 0.01-0.02
C. 1.150-1.170 D. 1.6-1.9

1461. What odour or essence can be highlighted in Balsam ?

A. Cocoa nutty aroma
B. Vanilla aroma
C. Citric lime aroma
D. Camphoraceous

1462. Trees of what cannot be found in MyroxylonBalsamum?

A. Styrene B. Vanillin
C. Coumarrin D. Citric acid

1463. How is Balsam obtained from the rags ?

A. Rags are beaten
B. Rags are torched
C. Rags are boiled water
D. Rags are squeezed

1464. What is the approximate length of Balsam of Peru ?

A. 82 feet B. 94 feet
C. 101 feet D. 75 feet

1465. Colophon is a residue left after ?

A. Distillation of linseed
B. Percolating zinger rhizomes
C. Both a) and b)
D. Distillation of turpentine oil

1466. The angular, translucent masses of Amber resins are reactive because

A. Saturated

B. Contains Benzene ring

C. Unsaturated

D. Has free electrow in Structure

1467. Industrially, colophony is not used as ?

A. Preparation of varnishes

B. Printing inks

C. Preparation of insulating compounds

D. Production of fibres

1468. According to geographical source , in which Asian country is Colophony found?

A. Sri Lanka and Bhutan

B. Burma and China

C. India and Pakistan

D. Iran and Iraq

1469. In which does Colophony get oxidised quickly?

A. Powder form B. Liquid form

C. Resin form D. Gum form

1470. Adulteration of Colophony is done by ?

A. Apic resin B. Amber resin

C. Both a) and b) D. Black resin

1471. Rosins is insoluble in ——————

A. Carbon disulphide B. Ether

C. Alcohol D. Water

1472. Which chemical constituent is present in maximum quantity in gum rosin ?

A. Oleic acid

B. Abietic acid Resin acid

C. Resin acid

D. Sapinic acid

1473. After incineration of Pine resin, what is ash value obtained?

A. Not more than 0.125%

B. Not more than 0.625%

C. Not more than 1.25%

D. Not more than 5.12%

1474. Collection of commiphora mol mol herb is done as coagulated mass in the skins of which animal.

A. Goat B. Buffalo

C. Sheep D. Cow

1475. Myrrh is astringent to the mucous membrane, therefore it is used as -

A. Gargles B. Nail polish remover

C. Cleanser for skin D. Demulcent

1476. Substitution of Myrrh in India is done by?

A. Arabian Myrrh

B. Yemen Myrrh

C. BalsamodendronMukul

D. Israeli Myrrh

1477. What is the percentage of gum present in Myrrh ?

A. 90 % B. 50 %

C. 30 % D, 60 %

1478. On trituration with water, Myrrh forms ?

A. Dark brown emulsion

B. Yellowish - brown emulsion

C. Brownish - purple emulsion

D. Pinkish - red emulsion

1479. On dried state what is the minimum content of total gingrols?

A. Not less than 0.8%

B. Less then 0.08%

C, Not less than 1.8%

D. Not less than 6%

1480. Which is the leading country for production of Sunthi?

A. Nepal B. China

C. Japan D. India

1481. What are the suitable conditions for growth favourable growth of ginger ?

A. Sandy B. Red loamy soil

C. Clay D. All of the above

1482. What are the ideal climate conditions for cultivation of zingiber?

A. Dry, arid and climate

B. Warm and humid

C. Cool and humid

D. Dry and warm

1483. In transverse section of zingiber which layer contains no starch or is free of starch?

A. Endodermis B. Vascular bundle

C. Ground tissue D. Cortex

1484. How can Ginger be distinguished from exhausted Ginger?

A. Determination of acid- insoluble
B. Determination of aroma
C. Determination of water soluble ash
D. Determination of alcohol soluble ash

1485. Name the inert maternal zingiber is coated with after drying

A. Calcium sulphate
B. Calcium carbonate
C. Calcium sulphide
D. Calcium carbide

1486. How much yield of green ginger can be produced if a person has 2 hectare of land?

A. 1,500 kg B. 4,500 kg
C. 3,000 kg D. 6,000 kg

1487. What are the most common type of fertiliser used in sunthi as it is a soil exhausting crop ?

A. Urea
B. Diammenium phosphate
C, Calcium nitrate
D. Ammonium sulphate

1488. While storing ginger , how can we improve its colour and quality ?

A. It is coated with lime
B. It is coated with potash
C. It is coated with calcium carbonate
D. It is coated with NH3 so4

1489. Name the family of Indian hemp's seeds sown in which month ?

A. June - July B. Nov - Dec
C. March - April D. Oct- Nov

1490. When 4ml of KMnO4 is added to 1g Benzoin and warmed, which odour is produced ?

A. Cinnamic acid B. Benzaldehyde
C. Ammonia D. Sulphuric acid

1491. What is the average yield of ganja per hectare ?

A. 375 kg B. 275 kg
C. 475 kg D. 350/kg

1492. Which part of cannabis is used to make a narcotic substances and why ?

A. Male parts because of resinous material
B. Female parts because of resinous material
C. Male parts because of volatile oil
D. Female parts because of volatile oil

1493. There are two varieties of ganja available in the market , one of them is :

A. Flat or Bombay ganja
B. Flat or Bengal ganja
C. Round or Bombay ganja
D. Round or Bangalore ganja

1494. The glandular trichomes of bhang contains –

A. Volatile oils
B. Fixed oils
C. Glycosidal compounds
D. Hallucinogenic matter

1495. The flat ganja coming from ________ district of Maharashtra is well known in commerce

A. Aurangabad B. Nashik
C. Ahmednagar D. Solapur

1496. Name the state of India, where cannabis is produced commercially ?

A. Gujarat B. Maharashtra
C. Madhya Pradesh D. West Bengal

1497. Which cannaboid is responsible for psychotropic properties of ganja ?

A. Cannabigerd
B. Cannabidiol
C. Tetra hydrocannabivarin
D. Tetra hydrocannabinol

1498. Which products / narcotic substances is stored in earthenware vessels ?

A. Ganja B. Siddhi
C. Both a) and b) D. Chars

1499. Which is not the adverse effects of marijuana?

A. Intoxication B. Euphoria
C. Dermatitis D. Hyperglycemia

1500. Which crop is grown in India both as Kharif crop as well as Rabi crop commonly known as 'Chillies'?

A. Cayenne pepper B. Bitter apple
C. Sunthi D. Gingerin

1501. Which constituent of capsicum is volatile above 65 degree C ?

A.Capsinine B. Capcin

C. Captained D. Capsaicin

1502. Pungency of cayenne pepper can be destroyed by oxidising agent like ?

A. Potassium hydroxide

B. Potassium permanganate

C. Potassium chloride

D. Potassium sulphate

1503. Capsicum is not used for which purpose ?

A. Rheumatism B. Lumbargo

C. Dermatitis D. Neuralgia

1504. Pigments responsible for dull orang red to brownish red of capsicum .

A. Capsanthin B. Carotene

C. Chlorophyll D. Both a) and b)

1505. What is the percent of non- volatile ether soluble extractines present in Chillies?

A. 12 percent B. 7 percent

C. 17 percent D. 22 percent

1506. What is the biological source of bitter cucumber ?

A. CitrulluscolocynthisisSchrador

B. Citricuscolocyntusshrador

C. Colophyllusshrador

D. Itrulluscucurbitaceae

1507. The fruits of bitter apples are collected in which season ?

A. Summer B. Autumn

C. Winter D. Spring

1508. Bitter cucumber is marketed in which form?

A. Liquid solution

B. Big masses

C. Suspension form

D. Broken pieces

1509. Alkaloids and resin colocynth is responsible for its -

A. Laxative action

B. Cathartic action

C. Purgative action

D. Intensely bitter taste

1510. The dried pulp of colocynth contains Cucurbibitacin E also known as

A. X-cucurterin B. X-Elaterin

C. X-resin D. X-alkaloids

1511. The entire fruit of better Apple measures around

A. 10 mm B. 1000 mm

C. 1 mm D. 100 mm

1512. Name the deo - gum resin obtained by incision from the roots of the ferula foetidaregel?

A. Podophyllum B. Devil's dung

C. Jalap D. Ipomoea

1513. For identification of asafoetida, when he drug is treated with the H2SO4, what colour is produced?

A. Red B. Black

C. Yellow D. Blue

1514. One of the adulterants of asofietida is not -

A. Apic resin B. Red clay

C. Gum Arabic D. Gypsum

1515. What does resin of Devil's dung consists of chiefly ?

A. Filicic acid B. Aleuritic acid

C. AsaresinotannolD. Cinnamic acid

1516. What is the geographical source of Asafoetida?

A. Iran B. Sri lanka

C. America D. U.K

1517. What is the biological source of jalap?

A. Ipomoea hederaceae

B. Ipomoea orizabensis

C. Ipomoea hexandrumd

D. Ipomoea purga

1518. Jalap is a powerful Cathartic because it acts in presence of?

A. Pepsin B. Water

C. Bile D. Hydrochloride acid

1519. What is ether soluble partition of jalap called?

A. Jalapin B. Convolvulin

C. Exogenic acid D. Tiglic acid

1520. When cut transversly tubercles of jalap shows:
A. Vascular strands
B. Concentric cambium zones
C. Translucent surface
D. Cup shaped scars

1521. How are the nodes of jalap categorised?
A. Formation of lenticel
B. Formation of nodules
C. Formation of longitudinal groove
D. Formation of adventitious roots

1522. The Most common substitute of turmeric is
A. Curcuma Amanda roxbby
B. Curcuma longra
C. Curcuma molmol
D. Curcuma domestica

1523. Which part of Haridra is used most widely and its cultivation is done mainly for which part?
A. Leaf B. Flower
C. Rhizomes D. Stem

1524. Which species of curcuma is used as a substitute for arrow root?
A. C. Caesia B. C. Amada
C. C. Aromatica D. C. Caulina

1525. Aromatica is used for which purpose?
A. Cervical cancer B. Nausea
C. Indigestion D. Diarrhoea

1526. When cut in transverse section, what does rhizome of turmeric show?
A. Suberised cell wall
B. Parenchymatous cork
C. Endodermis
D. Starch grains

1527. Which one of them is not a synonym of Podophyllum?
A. PodophyllumBerberi
B. Indian Podophyllum
C. Podophyllum radix
D. Himalayan may - apple

1528. Which chemical constituent is present in American Podophyllum but absent in P. Hexandric ?
A. Quercetin B. Asiragalin
C. Astragalin D. Alpha Beta peltatins

1529. Podophylum is used in semi synthetic production of?
A. Cytoxan B. Carboplatin
C. Etoposide D. Cisplatin

1530. Rhizomes and roots of Podophyllum are cultivated at approximate altitude of?
A. 3km - 4km B. 6km-8km
C. 10km-12km D. 11km-17km

1531. Cortex of podophylum is similar to the rhizome but there is absence of?
A. Calcium phosphate crystals
B. Calcium Sulphate crystals
C. Calcium oxalate crystals
D. None

1532. From which tree of Leguminosae family is Tolu balsam obtained from?
A. MyroxylonBalsamum
B. Pinussylvestris
C. TolyxlinBalsamum
D. Liquidambar orientali miller

1533. When examined under a microscope crystals of Tolu Balsam exhibit which acid?
A. Citric acid B. Cinnamic acid
C. Magic acid D. Vanillin acid

1534. From where is the word "Tolu" derived from in Balsam of Tolu?
A. Name of monument
B. A plant found in India
C. Name of famous personality
D. A place in Columbia

1535. When warmed with KMnO4, odour of which chemical is produced?
A. Nitric acid B. Benzaldehyde
C. Chloroform D. Sulphuric acid

1536. What is the range of Saponification value of Balsam of Tolu?
A. 170-230 B. 130-170
C. 230-270 D. 200-270

1537. Which among is the following synonym of musabbar ?
A. Millepertius B. Foxglove
C. Urgine D. Kumari

1538. Which species of aloe is used with alum to treat sore eyes?

A. Aloe barbedensis
B. Aloe freon
C. Aloe perryi
D. Aloe socotrine

1540. Aloes is indigenous to which of these African region?

A. Northern Africa
B. Central Africa
C. Sub- Saharan Africa
D. Southern Africa

1541. How the natives of Congo region of Africa used the aloe for?

A. For improving digestion
B. For reducing perspiration
C. For improving muscle strength
D. For improving immunity

1542. Why is drug of cascara accepted only after storing for at least one year?

A. Shows nauseating effects
B. Shows indigestion
C. Shows emetic effects
D. Shows es sore eyes

1543. Outer bark of cascara sagar shows the presence of ?

A. Lenticels B. Lichens
C. Cork D. All of them

1544. The shape of Chittem Bark occurs in

A. Quills
B. Flat oval shape
C. Rings
D. Concave - convex slices

1545. When is drug of rhubarb considered high quality product?

A. When drug has pink fracture
B. when there are no fracture
C. When drug has purple fracture
D. When drug has yellow fracture

1546. What is the permissible minimum altitude required for growth of radix rhei?

A. More than 1 km
B. More than 3000 meter
C. More than 7 km
D. More than 5000 meter

1547. How is Indian rhubarb different from rhapontic rhubarb?

A. It doesn't contain tannins
B. It doesn't contain Rhaponticin
C. It contains rhaponticins
D. It doesn't contain Antheraquinoe

1548. For which of these infection is urgenia used?

A. Beritosis B. Pneumonia
C. Bronchitis D. Encephalitis

1549. What is the percentage of water Indian squill contains after it is sun dried

A. 20% B. 50%
C. 70% D. 80%

1550. Which Chemical constituent does sea onion not have?

A. Alcohol
B. Mucilage
C. Cardiac glycoside
D. Cinnamic acid

1551. When the Thivetia seeds are chewed they produce a certain certain reaction in mouth which is

A. Rashes in the mouth
B. Blisters in mouth
C. Numbness in mouth
D. Cavity in mouth

1552. Thevetia kernels are very rich in which particular constituent of cardiac glycoside?

A. Thevetin B. Thevetin A
C. Cereberoside D. Neriifolin

1553. Other than Cardiac related in which of these is thevetia plant used for ?

A. Rheumatism
B. Immunity improvement
C. Malaria
D. Indigestion

1554. Why are Bitter almonds used as sedative ?

A. Amygdalin
B. Hydrochloride acid
C. Hydrocyonic acid
D. Benzaldehyde

1555. Due to absence of which particular chemical constituent amygdala Amara does not produce volatile oil on hydrolysis?

A. Benzaldehyde B. Protiens
C. Emulsion D. Amygdalin

1557. The biological source of amygdala Amara comes from which family?

A. Liliaceae B. Rosaceae
C. Polygalaceae D. Leguminosae

1558. Which one of the following is not a synonym of wild cherry?

A. Cortex prunier B. Wild black cherry
C. Marian thistle D. Virginia prune

1559. Cortex pruni contains which of these Mandelonitrite glycoside ?

A. Prunasin B. Amygdalin
C. Taxyphillin D. Linamarin

1560. What is the amount of hydrocanic acid found in virgina prune bark when collected in Autumn ?

A. 0.12 to 0.50 B. 0.20 to 0.30
C. 0.9 to 0.11 D. 0.12 to 0.16

1561. Gentiopicroside a glycoside found in radix gentians is water soluble with a bitter value of -

A. 11,000 B. 12,000
C. 10,000 D. 9,500

1562. Under UV radiation what particular colour pattern is emitted from genital extract?

A. Light green fluorescence
B. Violet
C. Black
D. Light blue fluorescence

1563. In which season does collection of Radix gentianae takes place?

A. Rainy B. Autumn
C. Winter D. Spring

1564. Ginseng has various uses, for which type of patient is most suited for?

A. Patient suffering from stress
B. Patient suffering from dermatitis
C. Patient suffering from dehydration
D. Patient suffering from conjunctivitis

1565. From which two Chinese words is Ginseng derived from?

A. Gouji B. Gin xo
C. Shen sang D. Niu xi

1566. Where in India can one find cultivation of Ginseng?

A. Nagaland B. West bengal
C. Andhra Pradesh D. Bihar

1567. Which chemical test does quillaia responds to ?

A. Frothing B. Flame test
C. Acid test D. Spot analysis

1568. If ingested in higher dose what can Panama would cause?

A. Haemolysis B. Dehydration
C. Schizophrenia D. Rheumatitis

1569. What does cork cells of quillaia represent?

A. Pholem
B. Medullary rays
C. Parenchymatous tissue
D. Cork cells

1570. Bormatragers test for Sena leaves is employed for which chemical constituent?

A. Sucrose B. Flavonoid
C. Anthraquinone D. Rhsmnose

1571. The grappling effect caused by Senai- ki-Patti is due to which content ?

A. Salicyclic acid B. Emodin
C. Calcium oxalate D. Phytosterol

1572. During chemical assay of cassia Sena which method is not employed?

A. Spectrophotometer
B. Spectrocolorimetric
C. Thin layer chromatography
D. Gravimetric

1573. During biological assay, which dosage form of drug of Senna is administered to group of mice?

A. Suspension B. Emulsion
C. Syrup D. Pill

1574. What is the amount of starch present in Diascorea rhizomes? (In %)

A. 90% B. 75%
C. 50% D. 57%

1575. Name the potential source of Diosgenin which can be used as a substitute for genuine drug?

A. P. Japonica B. Costusspeciosus
C. CentellaAsiatica D. Tribulusterresteris

1576. Approximately how many days does it take for sprouting of tuber of Diascorea?

A. 70-80 days B. 10-20 days
C. 90-100 days D. 30-40 days

1577. On addition of sulphuric acid, Yasti powder shows which colour?

A. Deep brown color
B. Deep pink color
C. Deep Yellow color
D. Deep orange color

1578. What does glcyrrhizinic ā yield on hydrogen ?

A. Glycyrrhetic ā B. Glycyrrhetone
C. Glycyrrhitinoid D. None

1579. What is the ash value of unpeeled drug of mulethi?

A. NMT 30% B. NMT 10%
C. NMT 70% D. NMT 40%

1580. What is the route of administration of arrow poison ?

A. Optic route
B. Nasal route
C. Otic route
D. Parented always route

1581. On reaction of which ā does Seminole stropanthi shows emerald green colour ?

A. Lactic ā B. H2SO4
C. HCL ā D. Nitric ā

1582. Which part of strophantus is used by tribals as arrow poison ?

A. Seeds B. Root
C. Flower pod D. Stem

1583. Above what temperature, do leaves of foxglove lose their potency due to chemical degradation?

A. 100°C B. 70°C
C. 50°C D. 60°C

1584. Name the dehydrating agent which are used while storing digitalis powder?

A. calcium chloride B. None
C. Silica gel D. Both a) and c)

1585. The most frequent use of digitalis is in the treatment of?

A. Verbascum thapsus
B. Primula vulgaris
C. Symphytumofficinale
D. Psorelea

1586. Quassia has no stringent activity because of absence of?

A. Tannins B. Anthocyanins
C. Quercetin D. Catechins

1587. When cut and longitudinal section, the parenchyma of Quassia appears as what ?

A. Thickened pitted walls
B. Thick - walled cells
C. Irregular concentric rings
D. Long elongated walls

1588. The biological source of bitter wood comes from which family ?

A. Meloidae B. Simaroubaceae
C. Asterceae D. Scropholariaceae

1589. The chief constituent of winter cherry is

A. Tropine B. Somnine
C. Withananine D. Withanine

1590. In which state of India is Ashwagandha found?

A. Madhya Pradesh B. Sikkim
C. Assam D. Karnataka

1591. The smell of fresh roots of Ashwagandha is like that of?

A.Urine of horse
B. Urine of buffalo
C. Urine of pig
D. Urine of goat

1592. Habit of chewing Areca causes which oral problem?

A. Periodontitis B. Leukoplakia
C. Canker sore D. Cold Sore

1593. Which chemical constituent present in betel nut contains physiological activity?

A. Arecoline B. Arecaidine
C. Guvacine D. Guvacoline

1594. What is the Foreign organic matter value and acid insoluble Ash value of Betel nut?
A. Not more than 6 percent
B. Not more than 10 percent
C. Not more than 2 percent
D. Not more than 5 percent

1595. In which year was Belladonna first introduced in London Pharmacopoeia?
A. 1709 B. 1809
C. 1907 D. 1908

1596. Belladonna leaf is used as an antidote for which type of poisoning?
A. Potassium poisoning
B. Hydrogen Sulphide poisoning
C. Hydrogen peroxide poisoning
D. Chloral Hydrate poisoning

1597. Which fertiliser is not used in case of Deadly Night shade leaf?
A. Urea
B. Potash
C. Superphosphate
D. Phosphorous

1598. At what altitude is cultivation of Hyoscyamus done?
A. 2400 to 3300 m B. 2600-3600 m
C. 3300 to 3400 m D. 4000-4600 m

1599. Which one of the following sentence is true for leaves of Hyoscyamus?
A. Lamina is 25 cm
B. Presence of long petiole
C. Leaves have parallel venation
D. Leaves are dark reddish in color

1600. Time for germination of seeds of Henbane is for about?
A. 1 week B. 2 weeks
C. 4 weeks D. 3 weeks

1601. What is the length of solitary flowers of Stramonium?
A. 9.5 cm B. 5.7 cm
C. 7.5 cm D. 5.9 cm

1602. Due to the sedative property, Stramonium leaves are used to control?
A. Asthma B. Tremors
C. Motion sickness D. Salivation

1603. The seeds of Thorn Apple leaf contains about what percentage of fixed oil?
A. 25 % B. 52 %
C. 50 % D. 5 %

1604. The synthetic process for chemical constituent Atropine of Duboisia is of less reliance because
A. Process is tedious
B. Process gives inaccurate results
C. Process is lengthy
D. Process is costly

1605. Duboisia is used in ophthalmic practice because?
A. Dilatory effects on pupil
B. Photophobia
C. Contracting effects on pupil
D. Dry eye syndrome

1606. Name the family of Cork Wood?
A. Solanaceae B. Leukoplakia
C. Cornaceae D. Rubiaceae

1607. What is Coca commercially called?
A. Indian Coca B. Bolivian Coca
C. Truxillo Coca D. Huanuco Coca

1608. What smell does chemical test of Coca with sulphuric acid produce?
A. Nitric acid
B. Methyl Benzoate
C. Ammonium Sulphate
D. Chloroform

1609. In commerce price of Coca leaves is determined on the basis of which content?
A. Benzoyltropine B. Ecgonine
C. Tropocaine D. Truxilline

1610. The agreeable smell of coffee is due to which chemical constituent?
A. Caffeol B. Caffeine
C. Dextrin D. Glucose

1611. 'Qahuah', a popular beverage in different parts of the world comes from which family?
A. Theaceae B. Rubiaceae
C. Rutaceae D. Sterculiaceae

1612. What is the amount of coffee seeds produced by each plant?
A. 2-3kg B. 7-8kg
C. 9-10kg D. 5-6 kg

1613. Thea Sinensis belongs to which family?
A. Sterculiaceae
B. Rutaceae
C. Ternstroemiaceae
D. Solanaceae

1614. What is produced when Caffeine reacts with tannin acid solution?
A. White precipitate
B. White fumes
C. Clear solution
D. Deep Brown precipitate

1615. Besides being a CNS stimulant, Camellia Thea is also used as a __________.
A. Bronchodilator
B. Analgesic
C. Cardiac depressant
D. Diuretic

1616. How many alkaloids Cinchona bark contains which belong to Quinoline group?
A. 25 B. 35
C. 55 D. 45

1617. In Thalleoquin test, which color does powdered drug of Peruvian bark gives?
A. Ruby red B. Turquoise blue
C. Emerald green D. Amber yellow

1618. Quinine is a protoplasmic poison, especially for which type of protozoa?
A. Plasmodium vivax
B. Plasmodium falciparum
C. All of them
D. Plasmodium malarie

1619. Why is opium preserved in well closed container?
A. To prevent loss of morphine
B. To prevent loss of Narcotine
C. To prevent loss of codein
D. To prevent loss of Papaverine

1620. Which variety of opium is considered as only legal source of opium in Britain
A. American Opium
B. Israeli opium
C. Indian Opium
D. Pakistani opium

1621. Which one of them is not a condition required for cultivation of opium poppy?
A. Ph= 7 for soil
B. Distance between plants should be 25cm
C. Highly fertile, loamy soil
D. Extreme cold conditions

1622. What does Ipecac act as in high doses?
A. Expectorant B. Emetic
C. Purgative D. Cathartic

1623. Harvesting of roots of Ipecac is done after how many years of vegetative growth?
A. 3 years B. 1 year
C. 2 years D. 4 years

1624. What is the biological source of Ipecacuanha?
A. Cephaelisacuminata
B. Cephaelis rio
C. Cephaelisrubiac
D. Cephaelisbrazilian

1625. How are unripened reeds of Semen strychni separated?
A. Floating test B. Handpicking
C. Winnowing D. Filteration

1626. Which is better alkaloid is present in Nuxvonica is 1.5 - 5 % ?
A. Diterpene alkaloids
B. Quinoline alkaloids
C. Steroidal alkaloids
D. Indole alkaloids

1627. Chief chemical constituent present in NuxVonica is ?
A. Loganin B. Strychnine
C. Novacine D. Beta colubrine

1628. What is the sexual stage of Ergot called as?
A. Sclerotial stage B. Sulerotium stage
C. Sphacelial stage D. None

1629. What colour does Ergot powder produce with van-urk's reagent ?
A. Blue colour B. Red colour
C. Black colour D. Orange colour

1630. What is the amount of dosage of prepared Ergot taken by oral route ?
A. 0.15 - 0.5 g B. 0.55 - 1.5 g
C. 1.5 - 5.5 g D. 5.1 - 5.5 g

1631. Because of its snake like shape, Rauwolfia has been known as ?
A. Rasavanti B. Chottachand
C. Sarpgandha D. Serpentine

1632. The most significant alkaloid found in serpentine is
A. Yohimbine B. Reserpine
C. Serpentine D. Ajmalime

1633. Which family does the drug chottachand belongs to ?
A. Apocynaceae B. Loganiaceae
C. Berberideaceae D. Rubiaceae

1634. What is the biological source of periwinkle
A. Ferula foetida B. Catharantusroseus
C. Curcuma longa D. Pinussylvestris

1635. Vinca was first scientifically investigated by Canadian workers named ?
A. Beer and cult
B. Walter and Pedro
C. Alexander and rolls
D. Roberts and Morgan

1636. Vinca is not used to extract which one of the following ?
A. Vincristine B. Vinblastine
C. Ajmalicine D. Lochnerine

1637. Kurchi is the dried stem bark of ?
A. Veratrumviride
B. Aconitumnapellius
C. Holarrhenaantidysenterica
D. Eclipta Alba
Answer: C (Holarrhenaantidysenterica)

1638. One of the uses of Holarrhena is?
A. Diuretic B. Antiprotozoal
C. Expectorant D. Bronchodilator

1639. What is the alcohol solubility of Kurchi?
A. 4-6% B. 7-9%
C. 6-8% D. 9-11%

1640. Where was Ephedra explored first time chemically?
A. Sri Lanka B. China
C. Japan D. India

1641. In which season, the alkaloidal content of Ephedra is found to be maximum?
A. Autumn B. Spring
C. Summer D. Winter

1642. Other than seeds, how can Ephedra be propagated?
A. By divisions of root stock
B. By internodes of stem
C. By apex of leaves
D. By regeneration of branch

1643. What is the Meadow Saffron seeds popularly known as?
A. Stramonium B. Duboisia
C. Camptotheca D. Colchicum

1644. How does Colchicum reacts on exposure to air?
A. De-oxides B. Darkens
C. Degrades D. Disintegrates

1645. On reaction with which acid does Colchicine gives yellow colour?
A. Malic acid B. Nitric acid
C. Sulphuric acid D. Tannic acid

1646. Shape of leaves of Vasaka is?
A. Pinnate B. Acuminate
C. Cordate D. Lanceolate

1647. The stomatal index of Adhatoda leaves starts from about?
A. 28.1 B. 10.8
C. 18.2 D. 12.8

1648. Adulsa is indigenous to which country?
A. India B. Myanmar
C. Malaya D. Sri Lanka

1649. Which type of Venetian does leaflet of jaborandi has ?
A. Arcuate B. Pinnate
C. Reticulate D. Palmate

1650. Name the most important alkaloid present in leaflets of Jaborandi?
A. Pilocarpidine B. Pilocarpine
C. Isopilosine D. Pilosine

1651. On hydrolysis, pilocarpine results into which acid ?
A. Pilosinic acid B. Isopilosinic acid
C. Pilocarpic acid D. Isopilocarpic acid

1652. Which is the ether soluble not having poisonous reaction disterpene alkaloid present in monkshood ?
A. Aconitine B. Neoline
C. Sparteine D. Ephedrine

1653. Due to highly poisonous nature, use of aconite is restricted to which medicine system ?

A. Allopathy B. Ayurveda

C. Yunani D. Homeopathy

1654. What is true acid - insoluble ash value of a bachnag?

A. NMT 2 % B. NMT 1 %

C. NMT 3 % D. NMT 5 %

1655. What is the principle of limit test for heavy metals?

A. Precipitation of metal sulfides

B. Filtration of metal sulfides

C. Decantation of metal sulfides

D. Crystallisation of metal sulfides

1656. Out of the following metals, which metals gives black ppt on limit test for heavy metals?

A. Iron B. Arsenic

C. Zinc D. Gold

1657. In limit test for Arsenic which type of color-complex is formed with N-N diethylmethyldithiocarbamate?

A. Red-orange complex

B. Red-purple complex

C. Red-yellow complex

D. Purple-yellow complex

1658. B1, B2, G1, G2 are highly toxic components known as

A. Heavy metals B. Plant proteins

C. Aflatoxins D. Plant enzyme

1659. One of the bodies assesses the activity of concentration of isotopes of herbs called IAEA, state full form?

A. International Atomic Environmental Agency

B. International Atomic Energy Agency

C. Indian Atomic Energy Agency

D. None

1660. Find which of them is not typical source for finding markers?

A. Monographs

B. Experience, transfer from other plants

C. Scientific research

D. Study of adverse effects of drug

1661. Which term is invalid for determination of ash value?

A. Total ash

B. Acid insoluble ash

C. Water insoluble ash

D. Water soluble ash

1662. Name the inert material used for TLC plates?

A. Calcium Sulphate B. Calcium oxalate

C. Calcium acetate D. Calcium Nitrate

1663. TLC plates are heated at what temperatures and for time limit?

A. 110°C, 30 minutes

B. 100°C, 20 minutes

C. 100°C, 30 minutes

D. 110°C, 20 minutes

1664. Which of the following methods is not used to determine TVC of herbal material?

A. Membrane filtration

B. Serial dilation

C. Plate count

D. Plate pour

1665. Which of these microorganisms is determined by TVC?

A. Anaerobic bacteria

B. Algae

C. Protozoa

D. Fungi

1666. Which of the following acid is used to determine acid insoluble ash?

A. HNO3 B. Tannic acid

C. HCL D. H2SO4

1667. Which of the following is measured while determining acid insoluble ash?

A. Cellulose B. Silica

C. Clay D. None

1668. In alcohol soluble extractive, drug is macerated with?

A. Ethanol B. Acetone

C. Methanol D. Iso- propyl alcohol

1669. TLC works on principe of ?

A. Adsorption B. Partition

C. Both A and B D. None

1670. Separation of components in TLC is not dependent on ?
A. Nature of adsorbing
B. Nature of solvent system
C. Nature of plate
D. Nature of temperature

1671. What is the minimum distance for application of sample solution spot from base?
A. 30mm B. 10mm
C. 20mm D. 100mm

1672. Due to which reason different compound in sample mixture travel at different rate?
A. Difference in solubility of solvent
B. Difference in polarity of compund
C. Difference in attraction to stationary phase
D. All of the above

1673. Which of the following is not used for preparation of carrier sheet in TLC?
A. Glass B. Plastic
C. Aluminium foil D. Copper

1674. In TLC, thickness of adsorbent layer for analytical purpose is?
A. 3-4.2 mm B. 0.5-0.6mm
C. 0.3-0.5mm D. 0.1-0.25mm

1675. In TLC, thickness of adsorbent layer for preparative purpose is ?
A. 1-2 mm B. 3-4mm
C. 0-1mm D. 2-3mm

1676. In HPLC, temperature is __________ to analysis time for mobile phase.
A. Inversely proportional
B. Directly proportional
C. 140℃
D. None

1677. The mobile phase is what type of mixture?
A. Immiscible solvent
B. Miscible solvent
C. Miscible solution
D. Immiscible solution

1678. HPLC works best for compounds falling in which type of EM spectrum?
A. Ultraviolet B. Near infrared
C. X-rays D. Far infrared

1679. For which classes of compounds, HPLC is mainly used for?
A. Volatile B. Sesquiterpene
C. Non volatile D. Fatty acids

1680. What is the synonym of HPTLC?
A. Exclusion chromatography
B. Superior chromatography
C. Sorbent chromatography
D. Planar chromatography

1681. HPTLC is applied to obtain what type of print pattern of herbal formulation?
A. Matrix print B. Stomatal print
C. Cortex print D. Finger print

1682. Which of the following is a technique for spotting samples?
A. Reverse phase chromatography
B. Exclusion chromatography
C. Self loading capillaries
D. Gel chromatography

1683. One of the similarity of HPTLC and TLC is?
A. Average particle size
B. Precoated plates are employed
C. Separation power
D. Layer thickness

1684. HPTLC is better and dissimilar to TLC because?
A. Separation power
B. Pure aqueous eluents are used
C. Chromatogram
D. Easy to perform evaluation

1685. Name the sorbent used in HPTLC?
A. Silica B. Clay
C. Bentonite D. Cellulose

1686. What is the average particle size used in HPTLC?
A. 2 B. 10
C. 5 D. 3

1687. For isolation of caffeine, what color does Murexide test forms?
A. Purple B. Red
C. Yellow D. Green

1688. What is the concentration of Sulphuric acid used for washing the containers for isolation of caffeine of tea?

A. 0.5% B. 5%
C. 2% D. 0.2%

1689. Name the method used for extraction of Eugenol?

A. Vacuum Distillation
B. Steam Distillation
C. Ecuelle method
D. Enfleurage method

1690. Digoxin is obtained from which part of the plant?

A. Roots B. Stem
C. Leaves D. Flowers

1691. Which of the following method is used for extraction and isolation of Digoxin?

A. Stass-Otto method
B. USP assay method
C. Keller Kilani method
D. Dragondroff method

1692. Which extraction method is used for isolation of Piperine?

A. Maceration
B. Continuous Hot Extraction
C. Infusion
D. Counter Current Extraction

1693. What is the shape of crystal of Piperine obtained after isolation from black Pepper?

A. Spherical B. Prism
C. Rhombic D. Needle

1694. Which of the following drug is used for extraction of Tannic Acid?

A. Orange Peel B. Myrobalan
C. NuxVomica D. Nutmeg

1695. Which solvent is used for extraction of Tannic acid?

A. Denatured spirit
B. Liquid Paraffin
C. Petroleum Ether
D. Ethanol

1696. Which method is used for extraction of Diosgenin?

A. Alcoholic extraction of glycoside
B. Fermentation cum acid hydrolysis
C. Acid hydrolysis of total plant
D. All of the above

1697. Which acid is used for hydrolysis during extraction of Diosgenin?

A. H2SO4 B. HNO3
C. HCL D. Formic acid

1698. Orange peel is refluxed with which solvent for extraction of Hesperidine?

A. Carboxylate acid B. Ethanol
C. Pyridine D. Petroleum ether

1699. In which fruit was Hesperidine first detected?

A. Orange B. Grapefruit
C. Lemon D. Limes

1700. Which method is used for extraction of Berberine?

A. Ultrasonic assist extraction
B. Maceration
C. Freeze dried decoction
D. Percolation

1701. Berberine belongs to which category?

A. Flavanoid B. Glycoside
C. Alkaloid D. Tannins

1702. During estimation of calcium sennosides, what is the ratio of n-propanol-ethyl acetate-water-glacial acetic acid?

A. 1:29:40:40 B. 1:40:29:40
C. 40:40:29:1 D. 29:1:40:40

1703. In isolation of calcium sennosides, non ionic surfactants and polyethylene glycol is used with?

A. 70% ethanol B. 10% methanol
C. 50% ethanol D. 70% methanol

1704. What is the biological source of Rutin?

A. Menthapiperita
B. Cymbopogonflexuousus
C. Clavicepspurpurea
D. Fagopyrumesculentum

1705. What does Rutin yields on hydrolysis?

A. Quercetin B. Rhamnose
C. Glucose D. All of the above

1706. Name the method used for isolation of Glycyrrhizin?
A. Beer's method
B. Acid precipitation method
C. Svoboda's method
D. Soxhlation method

1707. What is the ratio of mobile phase (Toluene:Ethyl acetate:Glacial acetic Acid) for analysis of Glycyrrhizin in HPTLC?
A. 0.5:7.5:12.5 B. 7.5:12.5:0.5
C. 12.5:7.5:0.5 D. 0.5:12.5:7.5

1708. Natural Menthol is _________ in nature?
A. Levorotatory B. Racemic
C. Dextrorotatory D. None

1709. Menthol consists of three chiral centres, what are their positions?
A. 2,5,6 B. 1,3,4
C. 1,3,5 D. 2,4,6

1710. For isolation of Ephedrine, the drug is first defatted with?
A. Petroleum ether B. n-hexane
C. Methyl ether D. Ethyl ether

1711. Name the family of the drug through which Ephedrine is extracted?
A. Gnetaceae
B. Dioscoreaceae
C. Scrophulariaceae
D. Solanaceae

1712. One of them is not used for estimation of Quinine?
A. TLC Method
B. Non Aqueous Titration Method
C. Fluorimetry method
D. BP-1998 Method

1713. In Fluorimetry method, Quinine shows maximum intensity at ?
A. 150nm B. 350nm
C. 50nm D. 250nm

1714. Guggul is a dry gum resin obtained from incision of?
A. Commiphoramolmol
B. Commiphoraburseraceae
C. Commiphoraabyssinica
D. All of the following

1715. Guggul should be avoided in people with?
A. Haemophilia B. Anemia
C. Lymphoma D. Myeloma

1716. The most simplest method for extraction of andrographolides involves?
A. Distillation B. Cold maceration
C. Sublimation D. Hot percolation

1717. Andrographolide is the major ________ present for the therapeutic activities in the plant?
A. Sesquiterpenoids
B. Monoterpinoids
C. Hemiterpenoids
D. Triterpenoids

1718. One of the precipitation reaction of Alkaloid is?
A. Dragendorff's reagent
B. Frolide's reagent
C. Murexide test
D. Vitali reagent

1719. What is the synonym of Scheibler's Reagent used for general chemical test of alkaloid?
A. Phosphomolybdic acid
B. Marme's reagent
C. Phosphotungstic acid
D. Hager's reagent

1720. What is Mayer's reagent?
A. Saturated Picric acid solution
B. Bismuth+Nitric Acid+KI
C. KI+I
D. KI+Mercuric chloride

1721. Which chemical test can be applied for Ergot alkaloids?
A. Marqui's reagent
B. Van Urk Reagent
C. Picric Acid test
D. Frolides reagent

1722. Volatile oil is also known as_____ due to their 'Evaporation' on exposure to air?
A. Essential oils B. Crucial oils
C. Ethereal oils D. Key oils

1723. Which one of the following drug has the oil containing Cineole?
A. Eucalyptus B. Cloves
C. Rosemary D. Ajowan

1724. Turpentine comes under the category of?
A. Oil containing alcohol
B. Oil containing ketones
C. Oil containing esters
D. Oil containing Hydrocarbons

1725. What is the similarity between Lavender, Rose, Coriander and Sandalwood?
A. Oil containing esters
B. Oil containing ketones
C. Oil containing alcohols
D. Oil containing hydrocarbons

1726. Which one of them is not a character of Resins?
A. Non crystallizable
B. Transparent
C. Translucent
D. Hard masses

1727. What type of Resin does Podophyllum contain?
A. Glycoresins B. Balsams
C. Oleo-gum resin D. Oleo resins

1728. ______ are complex neutral inert substances which are insoluble and are not hydrolysed by alkalis?
A. Resenes B. Balsams
C. Resin acids D. Resin esters

1729. The resinotannols because of phenolic group gives color reaction with which salts?
A. Calcium salts B. Chloride salts
C. Iron salts D. Sulfides salts

1730. The non sugar moiety of glycosides is known as?
A. Glycone B. Oxyribose
C. Deoxyribose D. Genin

1731. In Baljet test of Glycoside, what color is obtained?
A. Pink B. Purple
C. Orange D. White

1732. Glycosides are colorless except which one?
A. Flavone B. Anthraquinone
C. Anthracene D. Anthranols

1733. For which type of water soluble plant constituent is paper chromatography used?
A. Sugars B. Proteins
C. Amino acids D. Lipids

1734. Name the mobile phase used in Adsorption Column Chromatography?
A. CHCl3 B. Pyridine
C. Acetone D. Option A, B and C

1735. Which one of the following is not a synonym of Gel chromatography?
A. Gel permeation chromatography
B. Partition chromatography
C. Size exclusion chromatography
D. Molecular sieve chromatography

1736. Chromatography means in Greek: khromatos= colour, graphos=?
A. Separation B. Partition
C. Written D. Scribble

1737. Which form of matter is the stationary phase in Adsorption chromatography?
A. Solid B. Gas
C. Liquid D. Plasma

1738. Name the inert porous solid used in Partition chromatography?
A. Silica gel B. Sephadex gel
C. Cellulose D. Polyamide gel

1739. Which chromatographic process can be used for liquid-liquid phase?
A. Counter current separation
B. Adsorption
C. Fractional Distillation
D. Ion-exchange

1740. Which detecting agent can be used for Resorcinol in TLC?
A. Antimony chloride
B. Concentrated H2SO4
C. Ninhydrin
D. Vanillin

1741. Main variable of Gas liquid chromatography is?
A. Temperature of operation
B. Detecting reagent
C. Mobile phase of column
D. Time of operation

1742. What is stationary phase in the process of chromatography?
A. Gas which moves over surface
B. Fluid which moves over surface
C. Both A and B
D. Fixed bed of large surface area

1743. Which one of them is not a standard size of chromatoplates?
A. 20x5cm B. 20x20cm
C. 20x25cm D. 20x10cm

1744. What is pH of inorganic adsorbent, Kieselguhr?
A. 2 B. 9
C. 3 D. 7

1745. Active Magnesia is obtained by?
A. Hydration of hydroxide
B. Hydration of Peroxides
C. Dehydration of hydroxide
D. Dehydration of Peroxides

1746. The chief constituent of winter cherry is
A. Tropine B. Somnine
C. Withananine D. Withanine

1747. In which state of India is Ashwagandha found?
A. Madhya Pradesh B. Sikkim
C. Assam D. Karnataka

1748. The smell of fresh roots of Ashwagandha is like that of?
A. Urine of horse B. Urine of buffalo
C. Urine of pig D. Urine of goat

1749. Habit of chewing Areca causes which oral problem?
A. Periodontitis B. Leukoplakia
C. Canker sore D. Cold Sore

1750. Which chemical constituent present in betel nut contains physiological activity?
A. Arecoline B. Arecaidine
C. Guvacine D. Guvacoline

1751. What is the Foreign organic matter value and acid insoluble Ash value of Betel nut?
A. Not more than 6 percent
B. Not more than 10 percent
C. Not more than 2 percent
D. Not more than 5 percent

1752. In which year was Belladonna first introduced in London Pharmacopoeia?
A. 1709 B. 1809
C. 1907 D. 1908

1753. Belladonna leaf is used as an antidote for which type of poisoning?
A. Potassium poisoning
B. Hydrogen Sulphide poisoning
C. Hydrogen peroxide poisoning
D. Chloral Hydrate poisoning

1754. Which fertiliser is not used in case of Deadly Night shade leaf?
A. Urea
B. Potash
C. Superphosphate
D. Phosphorous

1755. At what altitude is cultivation of Hyoscyamus done?
A. 2400 to 3300 m B. 2600-3600 m
C. 3300 to 3400 m D. 4000-4600 m

1756. Which one of the following sentence is true for leaves of Hyoscyamus?
A. Lamina is 25 cm
B. Presence of long petiole
C. Leaves have parallel venation
D. Leaves are dark reddish in color

1757. Time for germination of seeds of Henbane is for about?
A. 1 week B. 2 weeks
C. 4 weeks D. 3 weeks

1758. What is the length of solitary flowers of Stramonium?
A. 9.5 cm B. 5.7 cm
C. 7.5 cm D. 5.9 cm

1759. Due to the sedative property, Stramonium leaves are used to control?
A. Asthma B. Tremors
C. Motion sickness D. Salivation

1760. The seeds of Thorn Apple leaf contains about what percentage of fixed oil?
A. 25 % B. 52 %
C. 50 % D. 5 %

1761. The synthetic process for chemical constituent Atropine of Duboisia is of less reliance because

A. Process is tedious
B. Process gives inaccurate results
C. Process is lengthy
D. Process is costly

1762. Duboisia is used in ophthalmic practice because?

A. Dilatory effects on pupil
B. Photophobia
C. Contracting effects on pupil
D. Dry eye syndrome

1763. Name the family of Cork Wood?

A. Solanaceae B. Leukoplakia
C. Cornaceae D. Rubiaceae

1764. What is Coca commercially called?

A. Indian Coca B. Bolivian Coca
C. Truxillo Coca D. Huanuco Coca

1765. What smell does chemical test of Coca with sulphuric acid produce?

A. Nitric acid
B. Methyl Benzoate
C. Ammonium Sulphate
D. Chloroform

1766. In commerce price of Coca leaves is determined on the basis of which content?

A. Benzoyltropine B. Ecgonine
C. Tropocaine D. Truxilline

1767. The agreeable smell of coffee is due to which chemical constituent?

A. Caffeol B. Caffeine
C. Dextrin D. Glucose

1768. 'Qahuah', a popular beverage in different parts of the world comes from which family?

A. Theaceae B. Rubiaceae
C. Rutaceae D. Sterculiaceae

1769. What is the amount of coffee seeds produced by each plant?

A. 2-3kg B. 7-8kg
C. 9-10kg D. 5-6 kg

1770. Thea Sinensis belongs to which family?

A. Sterculiaceae
B. Rutaceae
C. Ternstroemiaceae
D. Solanaceae

1771. What is produced when Caffeine reacts with tannin acid solution?

A. White precipitate
B. White fumes
C. Clear solution
D. Deep Brown precipitate

1772. Besides being a CNS stimulant, Camellia Thea is also used as a __________.

A. Bronchodilator
B. Analgesic
C. Cardiac depressant
D. Diuretic

1773. How many alkaloids Cinchona bark contains which belong to Quinoline group?

A. 25 B. 35
C. 55 D. 45

1774. In Thalleoquin test, which color does powdered drug of Peruvian bark gives?

A. Ruby red B. Turquoise blue
C. Emerald green D. Amber yellow

1775. Quinine is a protoplasmic poison, especially for which type of protozoa?

A. Plasmodium vivax
B. Plasmodium falciparum
C. All of them
D. Plasmodium malarie

1776. Why is opium preserved in well closed container?

A. To prevent loss of morphine
B. To prevent loss of Narcotine
C. To prevent loss of codein
D. To prevent loss of Papaverine

1777. Which variety of opium is considered as only legal source of opium in Britain

A. American Opium
B. Israeli opium
C. Indian Opium
D. Pakistani opium

1778. Which one of them is not a condition required for cultivation of opium poppy?
A. Ph= 7 for soil
B. Distance between plants should be 25cm
C. Highly fertile, loamy soil
D. Extreme cold conditions

1779. What does Ipecac act as in high doses?
A. Expectorant B. Emetic
C. Purgative D. Cathartic

1780. Harvesting of roots of Ipecac is done after how many years of vegetative growth?
A. 3 years B. 1 year
C. 2 years D. 4 years

1781. What is the biological source of Ipecacuanha?
A. Cephaelisacuminata
B. Cephaelis rio
C. Cephaelisrubiac
D. Cephaelisbrazilian

1782. How are unripened reeds of Semen strychni separated?
A. Floating test B. Handpicking
C. Winnowing D. Filteration

1783. Which is better alkaloid is present in Nuxvonica is 1.5 - 5 % ?
A. Diterpene alkaloids
B. Quinoline alkaloids
C. Steroidal alkaloids
D. Indole alkaloids

1784. Chief chemical constituent present in NuxVonica is ?
A. Loganin B. Strychnine
C. Novacine D. Beta colubrine

1785. What is the sexual stage of Ergot called as?
A. Sclerotial stage B. Sulerotium stage
C. Sphacelial stage D. None

1786. What colour does Ergot powder produce with van-urk's reagent ?
A. Blue colour B. Red colour
C. Black colour D. Orange colour

1787. What is the amount of dosage of prepared Ergot taken by oral route ?
A. 0.15 - 0.5 g B. 0.55 - 1.5 g
C. 1.5 - 5.5 g D. 5.1 - 5.5 g

1788. Because of its snake like shape, Rauwolfia has been known as ?
A. Rasavanti B. Chottachand
C. Sarpgandha D. Serpentine

1789. The most significant alkaloid found in serpentine is
A. Yohimbine B. Reserpine
C. Serpentine D. Ajmalime

1790. Which family does the drug chottachand belongs to ?
A. Apocynaceae B. Loganiaceae
C. Berberideaceae D. Rubiaceae

1791. What is the biological source of periwinkle
A. Ferula foetida B. Catharantusroseus
C. Curcuma longa D. Pinussylvestris

1792. Vinca was first scientifically investigated by Canadian workers named ?
A. Beer and cult
B. Walter and Pedro
C. Alexander and rolls
D. Roberts and Morgan

1793. Vinca is not used to extract which one of the following ?
A. Vincristine B. Vinblastine
C. Ajmalicine D. Lochnerine

1794. Kurchi is the dried stem bark of ?
A. Veratrumviride
B. Aconitumnapellius
C. Holarrhenaantidysenterica
D. Eclipta Alba

1795. One of the uses of Holarrhena is?
A. Diuretic B. Antiprotozoal
C. Expectorant D. Bronchodilator

1796. What is the alcohol solubility of Kurchi?
A. 4-6% B. 7-9%
C. 6-8% D. 9-11%

1797. Where was Ephedra explored first time chemically?
A. Sri Lanka B. China
C. Japan D. India

1798. In which season, the alkaloidal content of Ephedra is found to be maximum?
A. Autumn B. Spring
C. Summer D. Winter

1799. Other than seeds, how can Ephedra be propagated?

A. By divisions of root stock
B. By internodes of stem
C. By apex of leaves
D. By regeneration of branch

1800. What is the Meadow Saffron seeds popularly known as?

A. Stramonium B. Duboisia
C. Camptotheca D. Colchicum

1801. How does Colchicum reacts on exposure to air?

A. De-oxides B. Darkens
C. Degrades D. Disintegrates

1802. On reaction with which acid does Colchicine gives yellow colour?

A. Malic acid B. Nitric acid
C. Sulphuric acid D. Tannic acid

1803. Shape of leaves of Vasaka is?

A. Pinnate B. Acuminate
C. Cordate D. Lanceolate

1804. The stomatal index of Adhatoda leaves starts from about?

A. 28.1 B. 10.8
C. 18.2 D. 12.8

1805. Adulsa is indigenous to which country?

A. India B. Myanmar
C. Malaya D. Sri Lanka

1806. Which type of Venetian does leaflet of jaborandi has ?

A. Arcuate B. Pinnate
C. Reticulate D. Palmate

1807. Name the most important alkaloid present in leaflets of Jaborandi?

A. Pilocarpidine B. Pilocarpine
C. Isopilosine D. Pilosine

1808. On hydrolysis, pilocarpine results into which acid ?

A. Pilosinic acid
B. Isopilosinic acid
C. Pilocarpic acid
D. Isopilocarpic acid

1809. Which is the ether soluble not having poisonous reaction disterpene alkaloid present in monkshood ?

A. Aconitine B. Neoline
C. Sparteine D. Ephedrine

1810. Due to highly poisonous nature , use of aconite is restricted to which medicine system ?

A. Allopathy B. Ayurveda
C. Yunani D. Homeopathy

1811. What is true acid - insoluble ash value of a bachnag?

A. NMT 2 % B. NMT 1 %
C. NMT 3 % D. NMT 5 %

1812. What is the principle of limit test for heavy metals?

A. Precipitation of metal sulfides
B. Filtration of metal sulfides
C. Decantation of metal sulfides
D. Crystallisation of metal sulfides

1813. Out of the following metals, which metals gives black ppt on limit test for heavy metals?

A. Iron B. Arsenic
C. Zinc D. Gold

1814. In limit test for Arsenic which type of color-complex is formed with N-N diethyl methyldithiocarbamate?

A. Red-orange complex
B. Red-purple complex
C. Red-yellow complex
D. Purple-yellow complex

1815. B1, B2, G1, G2 are highly toxic components known as

A. Heavy metals B. Plant proteins
C. Aflatoxins D. Plant enzyme

CHAPTER 3B

Biotechnology and Microbiology

1. **Which type of media generally used in callus culture?**
   A. Semisolid media B. Liquid media
   C. Solid media D. None of above
2. **The process of formation callus from meristmatic state is known as.....**
   A. Rediffentiation B. Dedifferentiation
   C. Cell division D. Botha a and b
3. **Culture can be maintained for extended periods via which process**
   A. Subculturing
   B. Totipotency
   C. Proliferating media
   D. Primary culture
4. **In vivo callus culture can be occurred by**
   A. Incorporating growth regulators
   B. Incorporating cells in media
   C. Result of wounding or cut
   D. All of the above
5. **In vivo callus culture can be done by.....**
   A. Endogenous auxin
   B. Exogenous auxin
   C. Both 1and 2
   D. By incorporating cells ongrowth media
6. **In vitroscllus formation can be induced by**
   A. Incorporating auxin
   B. Endogenous auxin
   C. Endogenous cytokinen
   D. Totipotency
7. **High ratio of cytokinen result in formation of**
   A. Root B. Shoot
   C. Leaves D. None of the above
8. **High ration auxin to cytokinen results in formation of.......**
   A. Root B. Shoot
   C. Leave D. None of the above
9. **Which type of media is used in suspension culture?**
   A. Broth media B. Agar media
   C. Semi solid media D. Solid media
10. **Which type if culture vessels are used in suspension culture?**
    A. Petridish
    B. Test tube
    C. Erlenmeyer flask
    D. None of the above
11. **Suspension culture is same as callus culture except addition of**
    A. Agar B. Tragacanth
    C. Gum acacia D. None of the above
12. **Which type of callus formed in callus culture?**
    A. Hard callus B. Semisolid callus
    C. Soft callus D. Stiff callus
13. **The suspension culture are incubated at**
    A. 50-55 C B. 20 C
    C. 25C D. 35-40C
14. **The culture are usually sealed with**
    A. Double aluminium foil
    B. Parafilms
    C. Both a and B
    D. Single aluminium foil
15. **The cell suspension formed within**
    A. 24 hrs B. 3-4 days
    C. 2-4 weeks D. 4-6 weeks
16. **In callus culture which type of cells are formed usually**
    A. Parenchyma cells
    B. Sclerenchyma cells
    C. Colenchyma cells
    D. None of the above

17. **Which type of media generally used in callus culture?**
A. Semi solid media B. Liquid media
C. Solid media D. None of the above

18. **When cells from callus able to generate into whole plant, phenomenon is known as**
A. Dedifferrentiation
B. Redifferentiation
C. Organogenesis
D. Cell division

19. **In suspension culture, generally used ....light during incubation**
A. UV light
B. High intensity of light
C. Low intensity light
D. None of the above

20. **Which component is necessary during suspension culture?**
A. High intensity light
B. Continuous agitation
C. Agar
D. Incubation at 45 C

21. **During suspensionculture, continuous agitation can be obtained at ....rpm**
A. 100-200rpm B. 300-400rpm
C. 10-20rpm D. No agitation needed

22. **Which one is type of suspension culture?**
A. Continuous culture
B. Batch culture
C. Both a and b
D. Protoplast culture

23. **Which process occurs during incubation period?**
A. Cell division
B. Cell differentiation
C. Formation of primary metabolite
D. All of above

24. **The growth of cells stops after sometime in primary culture media?**
A. Sufficient ingredient
B. Formation of toxic metabolites
C. Initiation of exponential phase
D. Initiation of lag phase

25. **From primary media the inoculums is transferred to secondary media process is**
A. Primary culture B. Subculture
C. Broth media D. All of the above

26. **Growth phase diagram curve plot between**
A. Cell number v/s time
B. Time v/s size
C. Time v/s cell size
D. Cell colony v/s time

27. **The phase at which the ingredient becomes limited and accumulation of toxic metabolites is**
A. Lag phase B. Exponential phase
C. Stationary D. linear

28. **Prolongation of stationary phase leads to**
A. Lysis of cell B. Formation of toxic
C. Extensive death D. All of the above

29. **Cell doubling time in nicotiana tobacumis........**
A. 48 hrs B. 36 hrs
C. 22 hrs D. 20hrs

30. **Addition of cellulose and pectinase in culture media leads to**
A. Cell dispersion B. Callus formation
C. Cell lysis D. Cell death

31. **Disadvantage of batch cultures**
A. Lage phase short time
B. Exponential growth achieved
C. No period of steady state
D. All of the above

32. **Which culture are used to overcome no period steady state**
A. Batch culture
B. Continuous culture
C. Protoplast culture
D. Zygotic embryo culture

33. **Open and type and close type culture are type of**
A. Batch culture
B. Zygote embryo culture
C. Protoplast
D. Continuous culture

34. **Turbodiostat culture type of**
A. Batchculture
B. Open type continuous culture
C. Closed type continuous culture
D. Protoplast culture

35. Chemostat is which type of culture

A. Open type B. Closed type
C. Protoplast D. Batch type

36. Main disadvantage of continuous culture i.e. not used in large scale up.........

A. Require lot of attraction
B. Equipment not available
C. Both A and B
D. No steady state period

37. After enzymatic degradation protoplast fuse together form homokaryons, this type of protoplast fusion is known as

A. Cybridization B. Spontaneous fusion
C. Totipotency D. Electro fusion

38. Plasmodermatal connection between cells can be reduced by.........

A. Plasmolyticum B. Charophycae
C. Both D. None

39. NaNo3 induced fusion, the solution of NaNo3 used in

A. Isotonic B. Hypertonic
C. Hypotonic D. None of the above

40. The NaNo3 fusion was completely described by

A. Kuster B. Evaus and cocking
C. Pow et al D. Carlson

41. The first somatic hybrid in plant by using fusogen was developed by

A. Keller and Melcher B. Carlson
C. Kuster D. Evaus and cocking

42. Which method is not used in protoplast fusion?

A. PEG treatment
B. Chemical fusion
C. Electro fusion
D. Electroporation

43. Kellers and Melcher used which treatment to produce protoplast fusion in genus nicotiana

A. PEG treatment
B. NaNo3 treatment
C. High pH and high Ca 2+ treatment
D. Mechanism of fusion

44. PH used for protoplast fusion of tobacco

A. Weak acid B. Weak base
C. Neutral D. Highly alkaline

45. The concretion of Ca2+ used for protoplast fusion

A. 50 mm B. 10m
C. 1mm D. 20mm

46. PEG acceptance as fusogen of plant protoplast because

A. Formation of high frequency Hetrokaryons
B. Lowcytotoxicity
C. Both A andB
D. Low heterokaryons formation

47. In which fusion of technique high formation of Binucleat, heterokaryons produced

A. Nano3 treatment
B. High PH and Ca 2+
C. PEG treatment
D. Electro fusion

48. Problem associated in using highly alkaline solution

A. Large clumps of protoplast
B. Aggregation between two or three protoplast
C. Protoplast lysis
D. Low frequency heterokaryons

49. Main advantages over other method of protoplast fusion of PEG treatment

A. Large clumpot protoplast achieved
B. Aggregation between two or three protoplast
C. Toxic method
D. Low frequency heterokaryone

50. For plant protoplast fusion most widely used method is ....

A. High PEG and high Ca2+
B. High Ca and PH
C. Peg treatment
D. NaNo3 treatment

51. PEG perceut used in protoplast fusion are...

A. 15-45% B. 10-15%
C. 60-70 % D. 95%

52. PEG higher than 1000 mw causes

A. Adhesion
B. High frequency fusion of protoplast
C. Both A and B
D. Cohesion

53. Prolongation of incubation in PEG solution leads to

A. Decrease heterokaryon formation
B. Homokaryone formation
C. Cell lysis
D. Increase heterokaryon formation

54. EcrMechanism of fusion Protoplast adhesion is,

A. Temperature dependent
B. Temperature independen
C. PH independent
D. None of the baove

55. Plant protoplast carries which charge

A. Amphiphiles
B. Negative charge
C. Positive charge
D. No charge

56. Net Depending on species the charge on protoplast varyup to

A. -10 to -30 mv B. -40 to - 60mv
C. 0 to -10 mv D. +10 to +40 mv

57. For membrane fusion the membrane must have molecular distance of

A. 20 A0 B. 30 A0
C. 100 A 0 D. 80 A0

58. Disadvantage of using high PH high Ca2+ ion treatment

A. Increase negative charge
B. Neutralic charge
C. Tight adhesion
D. Reduces heterokaryon formation

59. Which concentration solution completely removes the charges from tobacco

A. 10 mm Cacl2.2H2o
B. 30mm cacl2. 2H2o
C. 60mm cacl2 . 2H2o
D. 100mm cacl2 . 2H2o

60. PEG molecules forms ...... binds with protein, bohydrate etc.

A. Hydrogen bond
B. Covalent bond
C. Ionic bond
D. Weak Vander wall force

61. In Ca 2+ and PEG treatment, Ca2+ works via

A. Form bridge between negative protein and PEG
B. Bridge betwen molecules of protoplast
C. Form hydrogen bond
D. Strong covalent bond

62. When PEG used in animal cell to cause

A. Structure alteration
B. Chemical charge
C. Hydrogen bond form
D. None of the above

63. When PEG used, the aggregation of intramembranous protein occurs in

A. Animal cell B. Plant cell
C. Both A and B D. None of the above

64. Chemical fusion have some disadvantages

A. Fusogen are toxic
B. Produces random multiple cell aggregate
C. Fusogen must removed before culture
D. All of the above

65. Whichof the following method of fusion is rapid?

A. Nano3 treatment
B. High PH and high Ca2+
C. Mechanism of fusion
D. Electro fusion

66. Electro fusion is completed with in

A. 15 minutes B. 30minutes
C. 1 hour D. 2 hour

67. Which one fusion is more beneficial for solanum tuberosum

A. Nano3 treatment
B. Electro fusion
C. High PEG
D. All of the above

68. Solenumbrevideus produced more effectively by

A. Nano3 treatment
B. PEG treatment
C. Electro fusion
D. All of the above

69. **Electro fusion of protoplast was fuisty demonstrated by**
A. Senda et al
B. Zimmermann
C. Abkong
D. Kao and wetter

70. **Zimmermann electro fusion system is .... times more effective than other fusion system**
A. 200 times B. 500 times
C. 1000 times D. 10,000 times

71. **Micro droplet method resemble with**
A. Electro fusion
B. Chemical fusion
C. Mechanism of fusion
D. None of the above

72. **Microdroplet method of electrofusion was developed by**
A. Kao and wetter B. Senda et al
C. Ahkongetal D. Koop et al

73. **Electrodes are made up of .... during electrofusion**
A. Copper B. Zinc
C. Platinum D. Silver

74. **By microdroplet method .... one to one fusion could perform in 1 hour**
A. 100 B. 50
C. 10 D.200

75. **Electro fusion is suitable for fusion of**
A. Sclerenchyma cells
B. Mesophyll
C. Root cells
D. All of the above

76. **Electro fusion frequency can be increased by**
A. 1 mM cacl2 B. 10mMcacl2
C. 10 mM mgcl2 D. 40mM cacl2

77. **Sterilization on electro fusion can be achieved by**
A. 70 percent ethanol
B. Volume of sterile water
C. Use of surfactant
D. Use of 70 percent ethanol followed by sterile water

78. **Self replicating extra chromosomal DNA present in cells is**
A. R-DNA B. Plasmid
C. Cosmid D. protein

79. **Agrobacteria tumefacienus is..... catogery of organism**
A. Negative bacteria B.Positive bacteria
C. Virus D. fungi

80. **The common opines found in bacteria**
A. Octopines B. Nopaline
C. Both A and B D. None of the above

81. **Which RE is used as purpose of molecular scissoring**
A. RE type I B. RE type II
C. RE type III D. All of the above

82. **Which of material required for transformation of zactorial genes into host**
A. Cytoplasm B. plasmid
C. Ribosomes D. protein

83. **The Ti – plasmid made up of .... nucleotide**
A. 23000 nucleotide B. 20000 nucleotide
C. 200,000 nucleotide D. 25000 nucleotide

84. **..... nucleotide are introduced into host cell**
A. 20000 nucleotide B. 2,00,000 nucleotide
C. 25000 nucleotide D. 23000 nucleotide

85. **35000 bp region of plasmid outside the T –DNA region turned as**
A. Virulence region
B. Overdrive region
C. Both A and B
D. They are region needed for replication

86. **In octopaline, the plasmid contains .... distict loci**
A. 8 B. 2
C. 1 D. 10

87. **The nopaline plasmid contains lack loci**
A. Vir F B. Vir H
C. Both D. Vir A and B

88. **Which genes are introduced alongside T-DNA intumerfaciens for regeneration and growth**
A. Oncogenes
B. Plasmid conjugation genes
C. Catabolism genes
D. Antibiotic resistance genes

89. **Which of genes are deleted from T-DNA**
A. Oncogenes
B. Catabolism genes
C. Antibiotic resistance genes
D. Plasamid conjugation genes

90. **Which one of following is cis vector**
A. PGV B. SEV
C. Both D. pBin19

91. **Large size of the ti plasmid vector doesn't have**
A. Unique restriction site
B. ORI
C. Resistance genes
D. Bacterial selectable marker

92. **The problem of not having the unique restriction site was overcome by**
A. PBR322
B. Cointegrating vectors
C. Binary vectors
D. All of above

93. **T- DNA of RI- plasmid lacks an gene for..................**
A. Auxin B. Cytokinen
C. Nopalines D. Octapine

94. **Cauliflower mosaiac virus contains ...... as genetic material**
A. RNA
B. Double stranded RNA
C. Single stranded DNA
D. Double stranded DNA

95. **Methotrexate resistant Dihydro folate reductase gene of E. Coli using cauliflower mosaic virus introduced into**
A. Turnip Plant
B. Tulsi plant
C. Both
D. Agrobacterium tumifaciens

96. **Cauliflower mosaic virus have disadvantage of**
A. Larger genes can't incorporated
B. Smaller genes can't incorporated
C. No formation of rDNA
D. All of the above

97. **The main disadvantages ofusing polyamines and dextran for chemical transformation is**
A. Reduce cell viability
B. Call DNA damage
C. No transformation of DNA
D. Cell lysis

98. **PH used when PEG used for chemical transformation**
A. Acidic B. Basic
C. Weak acid D. Strong base

99. **The concentration of PEG used in chemical transformation**
A. 10 percent B. 25-30 percent
C. 50 percent D. 95 percent

100. **Which of the chemical transformation was best suited**
A. Polyamines and dextran
B. PEG treatement
C. Cacl2 precipitation method
D. All of the above

101. **Heat shoch was given in the CaCl2 method for**
A. Open pores of the host
B. PPT CaCl2
C. Sealing of pores
D. For selection of untransformed DNA

102. **CaCl2 solution containing host and vector kept on after heat shock due to**
A. Open pore
B. Sealing of pores
C. For section of untransformed cells
D. For selection of transformed cells

103. **Electrodes used they cause .... to cells**
A. Lysis of cells
B. Temporarily permeable to DNA
C. Protoplast degradation
D. DNA damage

104. **Disadvantage of using electroporation method**
A. Open pores for long time
B. Produce large pores
C. Both A and B
D. High energy require

105. Addition of .... can cause increased transformation frequency of DNA in electroporation

A. PEG
B. Use of carrier DNA
C. Linearizing of plasmid
D. All of the above

106. Sir shimamoto used electroporation method for transfer of DNA into

C. Maize D. Beans
A. Rice B. Wheat

107. Diameter of fine tipped of microinjection used for DNA transfer

A. 0.5-10 micrometer
B. 20-23 micrometer
C. 10-15 micrometer
D. 30-35 micrometer

108. Cell are imbolizied on .... support

A. Solid support B. Agarose
C. Tragacanth D. A and b

109. Micropipette used in microinjection method for

A. Suction of cell B. For transfer of DNA
C. Both D. None

110. Disadvantage of microinjection

A. Slow process
B. Expensive step up
C. High skilled and experienced person
D. All of the above

111. .... technique is modified technique instead of microinjection

A. Lasser microinjection
B. Electroporation
C. Particle bombarded
D. None

112. Frequency of transformation was in which one of organelles

A. Ribosome B. Cytoplasm
C. Nucleus D. Mitrochondria

113. Which one of following is direct genes transfrmation method

A. Electroporation B. Agrobactarium
C. Virus mediated D. All of the above

114. Particle bombardment method also known as

A. Microinjection
B. Electroporation
C. Biolistic
D. Lesser cell processor

115. In particles bombardment method coating of DNA is done on

A. Tungsten B. Gold particle
C. Both D. Zinc

116. By biolistic gun transformation, the DNA can into

A. Soyabean B. Wheat
C. Maice D. All of the above

117. First biolistic gun was designed by

A. Christo B. Santord
C. Gray finer D. None of the above

118. Whichone of following disadvantage can be overcome by biolistic gun transfer

A. Host range specificity
B. Regeneration of complete plant
C. Damage of vector
D. Both A and B

119. BIORAD laboratorie produced .... gun

A. pDS 1000 /He B. pDS 3000/He
C. pDS 1000/Xe D. pDS 3000/Xe

120. Why gold is preferred over tungsten?

A. W is heterogeneous in size
B. Tungsten catalytically degraded DNA
C. Toxic
D. All of the above

121. Microcarrier penetration can be influenced by :-

A. He pressure
B. Distance between rupture disk of different thickness
C. Position of target cell
D. All of the above

122. For plant the pressure of He gas used

A. 1000 psi B. 1100 psi
C. 3000 psi D. 2000 psi

123. Which of following vector contain T –DNA replaced by novel sequence of DNA

A. Co-integrating vector
B. Binary vector
C. P Bin 19
D. Nine of the above

124. Which one of following is binary vector

A. P Bin 19 B. PBR222
C. SEV D. PGV3850

125. Which one of following is physical method

A. Electroporation B. Microinjection
C. Biolistic gun D. All of the above

126. For long term storage of germplasm the temperature required is

A. -1960C B. -100C
C. -500C D. -1000C

127. The temperature requirement wasMaintained by which of the following chemical

A. Liquid nitrogen B. Helim
C. Inert gases D. All of the above

128. Cultured cells shows .... during germplasm conservation

A. Homogeneity
B. Heterogenety
C. Mutation occurs
D. None of the above

129. Shoot apices posses .... features

A. Raising virus free plant
B. High regeneration
C. Rapid clonal multiplication
D. All of the above

130. AlHapliody is highly unstable in

A. Susupension culture
B. Shoot tip culture
C. Axillary bud proliferation
D. All of the above

131. Freeze preservation involves which process

A. Storage B. Thawing
C. Reculture D. All of the above

132. One of the key cause of cell damage during freeze preservation

A. Formation of crystals
B. Cell rupture
C. Increased in concentration of solutes
D. All of the above

133. Thawing process affect.....

A. Viability of cells
B. Damage OF NUCLEUS
C. Crystal form
D. Increased in concentration

134. Which of the following cells are conserved easily

A. Larger cells
B. Highly vacuolated cells
C. Small cells
D. Non meristmatic cells

135. Cell suspension are frozen in .... for storage

A. Early lag phase
B. Late lage phase
C. Stationary phase
D. Late stationary phase

136. Which of the following will better survive during conservation

A. SHOOT APICES
B. Embryo
C. Highly vacuolated cells
D. Young globular embryos

137. To overcome from supercoiling survival which of the following condition is mandatory for solanum Tuberosum

A. Culturing for 48 hour
B. Culturing in light
C. Both Aad B
D. Cooling for 20 hour

138. For high frequency of survival of shoot apices ehile freezing they must be preculture in ....

A. 5 percent DMSO B. 20 percent DMSO
C. 5 Percent DMF D. 20 percent DMF

139. For dessication purpose in germplasm conservation which of the following component used

A. Crystalline freezing cryoprotectant
B. Amorphous freezing cryoprotectant
C. Metastable cryoprotectant
D. None of the above

140. The optimum water content for cryopreservation of tea

A. 13% B. 35%
C. 20% D. 25%

141. The significance of the process vitrification is
A. No need of cryoprotectant
B. Protected from internal damage of ice crystals
C. Prefreezing required
D. None of these

142. Cryoprotectant are substances prevent from
A. From toxic solution effect
B. Prevent from formation of larger ice crystals
C. Bth A and B
D. Dehydration

143. Which of the most commonly and effective cryoprotectant found
A. DMSO B. Glycerol
C. 10% proline D. None of these

144. Which of t5he following is found to natural protecting agent
A. DMF B. DMSO
C. Glycerol D. Proline

145. Dmso should be stored at temperature
A. > 190C B. -100C
C. 100C D. -200C

146. Addition of which agent enhanced cryoprotectant action
A. Glycerol B. DMSO
C. DMF D. cryroseeds

147. In which of the following method the the solution is stored at 0 to -1000C temperature
A. Prefreezing
B. Preculture
C. Slow cooling method
D. Vitrification

148. In which of the following condition cryoprotectant not require
A. Dessicationpreatreatment
B. Vitrification
C. Slow cooling method
D. Rapid cooling method

149. In which of the following procdure the cooling between -10 to-70 0c require
A. Slow cooling method
B. Dessication
C. Rapid cooling method
D. prefreezing

150. For strawberry ultrarapid cooling method the cooling gave ......% surviaval
A. 40-60% B. 20-40%
C. 10% D. Upto100%

151. Which one of the enzyme was immobilized firstly
A. Amino acyclase B. Lipase
C. Dehydrogenase D. Amino reductase

152. Amino acyclase was isolated by
A. Asperigillusoryzea
B. Asperigelisniger
C. Mycobacterium
D. None of the above

153. The first immobilized enzyme was used for
A. Production of alpha amino acids
B. Production of fats
C. Production of carbohydrates
D. None of the above

154. Advantages of enzyme immobilization are
A. Reus of enzyme
B. Continous use
C. Stability of products
D. All od the above

155. Which one of the following are where enzyme immobilization was used
A. Production of jams
B. Diagnosis of gout
C. Manufacturing of liquid orals
D. All of the above

156. Application of enzyme immobilization is
A. In food industry
B. Biomedical application
C. Industrial production
D. All of the above

157. One of the following is the feature of matrix
A. Reaction will be minimum with enzyme and reactant
B. Soluble
C. Permanent hold
D. Ph unstable

158. Which one of the following matrial used for enzyme immobilization
A. Natural B. Synthetic
C. Inorganic D. All of these

159. Which one of the following falls under natural polymer
A. Carrageenan B. Silica
C. Charcoal D. Diatomaceous atom

160. Celite is the trade name of which of the polymer
A. Cellulose
B. Diatomaceous atom
C. Charcoal
D. Activated charcoal

161. Which of the following have good gelling properties
A. Carrageenan B. Pectin
C. Both a and b D. Starch

162. Which of the following are insoluble supports
A. Synthetic B. Inorganic
C. Natural D. None of these

163. Which one of the following used as a synthetic polymer
A. DEAE cellulose B. PVC
C. PEG D. All of the above

164. Based on matrix or immobilization the techniques are classified into
A. Surface immobilization
B. Within support immobilization
C. A both A and B
D. Depth immobilization

165. Which one of the following method is surface immobilization method
A. Complexation B. Copolymerisation
C. Encapsulation D. Entrapment

166. Which one of the following is within support immobilization method
A. Copolymerization B. Adsorption
C. Covalent bond D. Complexation

167. Advantage of covalent bonding are
A. No leakage B. Simple method
C. Wide application D. All of the above

168. Disadvantage of using covalent bonding
A. Loss of fumctional conformation of enzy
B. Inactivation of enzyme
C. Both A and B
D. Desorption

169. Adsorption method was defined by
A. Nelson B. Griffin
C. Nelson and griffin D. Griffith

170. Adsorption method was firstly used on
A. Invertase B. Amino reductase
C. Amino reductase D. Lipase

171. Adsorption method was used in
A. 1920 B. 1916
C. 1924 D. 1930

172. The bond formed during adsorption are
A. Hydrogen
B. Dipole dipole
C. Covalent bond
D. Complexation occurs

173. Method for adsorption for immobilization of enzyme
A. Electrode position process
B. Sedimentation
C. Filteration
D. Complexation

174. Disadvantage of adsorption method
A. Desorption
B. Incactivation of enzyme
C. Chemical modification
D. Permanent bond

175. Advantage of using adsorption method
A. Easy to carry
B. Minimum activation
C. Cheap method
D. All of the above

176. The disadvantage of using entrapment method
A. Leakage of high MW enzyme
B. Leakge of low MW enzyme
C. Permanent method
D. Impermeable to reactants

177. Which of the following method used for entrapment
A. Inclusion of ggels
B. Inclusion of fibres
C. Inclusion of microcapsules
D. All of the above

178. Disadvantage of using entrapment method
A. Pore diffusion limited
B. Deactivation of enzyme
C. Conformation of enzyme change
D. None of above

179. Advantage of entrapment method
A. Fast method
B. Less conformation changes
C. Mild condition required
D. All of the above

180. Colpolymerisation also known as
A. Cross linking B. Interlinking
C. Deformation D. Co- linkimg

181. Commonly used polyfunctional reagents are
A. Glutaraldehyde B. Starch
C. Cellulose D. PVC

182. Diazonium salt is used as in enzyme immobilization
A. Polyfunctional agent
B. Chelating agent
C. Both A and B
D. Monofunctional agent

183. Which of the following techniqus used with pure enzyme
A. Coplymerisation B. Adsorption
C. Entrapment D. Encapsulation

184. Disadvantage of colymerisation techniques
A. Denature of enzyme
B. Loss of catalytic activities
C. Structural changes
D. All of these

185. Which of the following method does not require matrix and support
A. Cross linking B. Adsorption
C. Entrapment D. Encapsulation

186. For encapsulation the capsule should make up of
A. Semipermeable membrane
B. PVC
C. Agar
D. None of these

187. Disadvantage of using encapsulation method
A. Pore size limitation
B. Small substances cross membrane
C. Both A and B
D. Deactivity of enzyme

188. Which of the following method commercial ed for produsuction
A. Coplymerisation B. Adsorption
C. Entrapment D. Encapsulation

189. Dynamic batch process technique is a sub- type
A. Adsorption immobilization
B. Entrapment
C. Encapsulation
D. Copolymerisation

190. Static process is techniques used in
A. Encapsulation B. Entrapment
C. Encapsulation D. Coplymerisation

191. The first somatic hybrids was perfomed between which species
A. Nicotiana glauca and N. langsdorffii
B. Brassica sp. And datura
C. Datura and N. Langsdorffii
D. Nicotiana and brassica sp.

192. The Incubating culturing for the growth of microorganism is
A. 15-200c B. 35 -400c
C. 25-300c D. 45-500c

193. Forceps and needles are sterilized by
A. 70% ethanol followed by flaming
B. 95% ethanol followed by flaming and heating
C. 95% phenol followed by flaming
D. 70% phenol

194. The ttemperaturesfor dry heat sterilization is
A. 160-180 C for 1 hr
B. 160-180 c for 3 hr
C. 190 c for 1 hr
D. 200 c for 3 hr

195. The temperature for moist heat sterilization is
A. 121 C 30 psi B. 121 C 15 psi
C. 130 C 15 psi D. 170 C 15 psi

196. If autocalve is not available which of the following instrument is used as moist heat sterilization

A. Pressure cooker B. Hot air oven

C. Radiation D. Ethylene gas

197. Which of the following is the source of contamination of the medium

A. Explants B. The operator

C. Medium D. All of the above

198. Which one of the following is thermolabile ingredient in tissue culture

A. Pantothenic acid

B. Plant growth regulators

C. ABA

D. All of the above

199. Which one of the plastic can be dry heat sterilised

A. Teflon FEP

B. Polyallomer

C. Polymethylpentene

D. Polypropylene

200. In glass bead steriliser the temperature can raised upto

A. 250 C in 30 mins

B. 250C in 5-7secs

C. 250 C in 15-20 mins

D. 150 C in 10 secs

201. The temperature for infrared steriliser raised upto

A. 250 C B. 150 C

C. 700 C D. 200 C

202. The exposure of content in infrared steriliser is upto

A. 1 min B. 2-5 secs

C. 10 min D. 15-20 min

203. The exposure of content in glass bead steriliser upto

A. 5-7 secs B. 1 min

C. 7 mins D. 2 min

204. The increase in temp will .... of protoplast fusion

A. Increase frequency

B. Constant

C. Decrease

D. Firstly decrease then increase

205. Which of the following condition allows protoplast adhesion

A. 15 C temperature B. Acidic PH

C. 35 C temperature D. Basic PH

206. When there is diluted enzymes are used the protoplast fusion is

A. Poor protoplast fusion

B. Formation of more heterokaryons

C. High membrane adhesion

D. High fusion frequency

207. Limitation of the immobilized cell system are

A. Biomass must be produced in suspension culture

B. Gel matrix introduces an additional diffusion barrier

C. Secretion of products in external medium

D. All of the above

208. The shelves are made up of

A. Glass B. Rigid wire

C. Iron frames D. All of the above

209. The junction of the walls should be

A. Rough B. Angular

C. Rounded D. None of these

210. The location of the laboratory should be

A. Away from cities

B. Towards the cities

C. In high populated area

D. None of the above

211. The chemical conversionofthe exogenously substances by living cells derived from cell cultures is known as

A. Metabolism

B. Biotransformation

C. Formation of primary metabolites

D. Distubution

212. The yield of product will .... as the no. Of step increases

A. Increases

B. Decreases

C. Constant

D. First increase latter decrease

213. Which of the biotransformation will be more efficient

A. Multiple step B. Single step

C. Both A and B D. Conversion by heat

214. Arbutin a secondary metabolite produced by which of the following
A. Arginine B. napthaquinone
C. Arginosuccinate D. Hydroquinone

215. Arbutin a metabolite obtained from hydroquinone is used as
A. Antidiabetic
B. Skin depigmentation agent
C. Anti rheumatic
D. Anticancer

216. Vincristine a metabolite used as
A. Anticancer
B. Anti diabetic
C. Anti parkinsonian agent
D. Anti rheumatic

217. Vincristine and vinblastine are generally
A. Dimeric alkaloids
B. Monomeric alkaloids
C. Tetrameric alkaloids
D. Trimeric alkaloids

218. Vincristine and vinblastine are
A. Hydroquinone alkaloids
B. Quinine alkaloids
C. Indole alkaloids
D. Isoquinone alkaloids

219. Vincristine and vinblastine are produced from
A. C. roseus B. D .lanata
C. B. atropa D. D . purpurea

220. c. rosseus however not able to produce vincristine and viblastine due to
A. Inability to produce vindoline
B. Inability to produce catharanthine
C. Indole
D. All of the above

221. The catharanthinea and vindoline are
A. Dimeric alkaloids
B. Monomeric alkaloids
C. Tatramericalakliods
D. Trimeric alakloids

222. Which of the following is used in heart disease
A. Arbutin B. Hydroquinone
C. Digitalis D. Vincristine

223. Which of the following is the method for isolation of cells
A. Enzymatic method
B. Chemical method
C. Physical method
D. None of the above

224. Advantage of the mechanical method over enzymatic method is
A. Cell damage
B. Eliminates the exposure of cells to harmful effect
C. Cell culture can be increased
D. None of the above

225. The process of starvation is known as
A. Cells arrested in G1 and G2 phase
B. Cell cycle inhibition
C. Arrest of M phase
D. Arrest of s phase

226. Assessment of viability of cultured cell can be done by
A. Reduction of tetrazolium ion
B. Fluorescein diaacetate
C. Phase contrast microscopy
D. All of the above

227. Assessment of growth in suspension culture can be done by
A. Cell counting
B. Phase contrast microscopy
C. Reduction of tetrazolium ion
D. Fluorescien diacetate

228. Which of the following method is growth assessment method except
A. Packed cell volume
B. Cell dry weight
C. Cell fresh weight
D. Evan blue staining

229. eva Which of the following is viability assessment method except
A. Cell dry weight
B. Evans blue staining
C. Fluorescien diacetate
D. Phase contrast microscopy

230. Assessment of growth can be done by
A. 15 ml graduated centrifuges
B. Cell fresh weight
C. Cell counting
D. All of the above

231. For agitation of medium in the suspension culture the rpm is set at

A. 30-150 rpm min-1
B. 150 -200 rpm min-1
C. 200-300 rpm min-1
D. Above 300 rpm

232. For agitation of suspension medium which of the following equipment is used

A. Mechanical stirrer
B. Magnetic stirrer
C. Orbital platform shaker
D. None of these

233. Shychroni culture means

A. Follows cell cycle phase in order
B. Continous media provide
C. Dosent follow cell cycle in order
D. Rapid multiplication of cells

234. Which of the following methodused to achiveshychronization

A. Inhibition B. Starvation
C. Both D. Agitation

235. For counting of cell for assessment of growth which instrument is used

A. Haemocytometer B. Coloni counter
C. Both D. Coulter current

236. Packed cell volume can be expressed as

A. Ml pellet ml-1 B. ml-1 pellet ml-1
C. cm-1 pellet ml-1 D. Ml 2 pellet

237. In which of the following method the cells are dried for 12 hr AT 60 C

A. Cell fresh weight
B. CELL dry weight
C. Packed cell volume
D. Cell counting

238. In which of the following method the growth assement based on the height of the sediment

A. Cell counting
B. Non invasive method
C. Cell fresh weight
D. Packed cell volume

239. Microscopic assessment of cell viability based on

A. Ribosome streaming
B. Mitochondria activaton
C. Both
D. Cytoplasmic streaming

240. Which f the following test gives green fluorescence

A. FDA
B. Evans blue staining
C. Reduction of tetrazolium ion
D. None of these

241. Which of the following compound is non polar

A. Tetrazolium salt B. Fluoscien
C. FDA D. Evans blue

242. Which of the following culture is true about chemostat cultures

A. Maintain steady state
B. Maintain metabolism
C. Determine effect of individual growth limiting nutrients
D. All of the above

243. Strret and co-workers used cell counting method for which cells

A. Sycamore cells
B. Mesophyll
C. Paranchymatous
D. Colenchymatous

244. Street and co-workers used which method for assessment of growth in suspension culture

A. Cell counting
B. Packed cell volume
C. Cell fresh weight
D. Cell dry weight

245. Agitation of medium serves which function

A. Exert mild pressure on cell aggregates
B. Uniform distribution of cells
C. Breaking them into smaller clumps
D. All of these

246. Limitation of germplasm storage is

A. Some plant cannot bear dessication or exposure to low temp
B. Seeds may destroyed by pathogen
C. Not applicable to vegetatively propagated crops
D. All of the above

247. Advantages of germplasm storage
A. Free from virus
B. Plants do not require splitting and pruning
C. Maintained free from pest
D. All of the above

248. Beta vulgaris can be stored at
A. 5 c for 6 months B. 5 c for 12 mnths
C. 15 c for 6 months D. 15 c for 12 months

249. Oxygen lowering can be done by
A. Cover by mineral oil
B. Cover by peppermint oil
C. Cover by rose water
D. None of these

250. The growth reduction techniques was first applied by
A. Ahking B. Caplin
C. Street D. kustur

251. Which of the following factor will not affect somatic embryogenesis
A. Explants B. Growth regulators
C. Hybridisation D. Polyamines

252. Which of the following material used for somatic embryogenesis
A. Immature zygotic embryo
B. Soyabean cotyledons
C. Both
D. Mature zygotic embryo

253. Which of the following process will reduce the quality and quantity of somatic embryogenesis
A. Flowering B. Stress of any kind
C. Both D. Leaves formation

254. Which of the following have high tendency to form embryogenic callus
A. Basal portion of leaves
B. Distance from explants from base
C. Flowering
D. Stress of any kind

255. Genotypic variation could be due to in somatic embryogenesis
A. Levels of hormons
B. Ph
C. Temperature
D. None of these

256. Which of the following is not used as growth regulator for somatic embryogenesis
A. Auxin B. Cytokinen
C. ABA D. Polyamines

257. Which of the following Auxin is most widely used for alfalfa
A. 2,4 D
B. 2(2,4 – dichlorophenoxy) propanoic acid
C. 2- chloro[hosphoric acid
D. None of these

258. Which of the following growth regulators breaks in presence of irradiation
A. Cytokinen B. Auxin
C. ABA D. Giberllenin

259. Which of the following is not used for the induction of somatic embryogenesis
A. Giberllenin B. ABA
C. auxin D. GA3

260. Which of the following compound inhibits somatic embryogenesis
A. Kinetin B. GA3
C. Giberllenin D. All of the above

261. Who is the father of tissue culture
A. Bonner B. Haberlandt
C. LaibachD. Ganthert

262. The production of secondary metabolites require the use of
A. Protoplast B. Cell suspension
C. Meristem D. Auxillary buds

263. Synthetic seeds is produced by encapsulating somatic embryo with
A. NaCl B. Sodium alginate
C. Sodium acetate D. Sodium nitrate

264. Hormone pair required for a callus to differentiate are
A. Auxin and cytokinen
B. Auxin and ethylene
C. Cytokinin and gibberllin
D. Auxin and absiccic acid

265. DMSO (dimethyl sulfoxide) is used as
A. Gelling agent B. Alkylating agent
C. Cryoprotectant D. Chelating agent

266. The most widely used chemical for protoplast fusion, as a fusogen, is

A. Manitol B. Sorbitol
C. Mannil D. Polyethylene glycol

267. Cybrids are produced by

A. Fusion of two different nuclei from two different species
B. Fusion of two same nuclei from same SPECIES
C. Nucleus of one species but cytoplasm from both the parent species
D. None of the above

268. Callus is

A. Tissue that form embryo
B. An insoluble carbohydrate
C. Tissue that grows to form embryoid
D. Unorganised actively dividing mass of cells maintained in cultured

269. Part of plant used for culturing is called

A. Scion B. Explants
C. Stock D. Callus

270. Growth hormone producing apical dominance is

A. Auxin B. Gibberellin
C. Ethylene D. Cytokinen

271. A medium which is composed of chemically defined compound is called as

A. Natural media B. Synthetic media
C. Artificial media D. None of these

272. To obtain haploid plant, we culture

A. Entire anther B. Nucleus
C. Embryo D. Apical bud

273. Somaclonal variations are the ones

A. Caused by mutagens
B. Produced during tissue culture
C. Caused by gamma rays
D. Induced during sexual embryogeny

274. Which of the following plant cell will show totipotency

A. Xylem vessels B. Sieve tubes
C. Meristem D. Cork cells

275. Which vector is mostly used in crop improvement

A. Plasmid B. Cosmid
C. Agrobactarium D. Phasmid

276. Somatic hybridization is achived through

A. Grafting
B. Protoplast fusion
C. Recombinant DNA technology
D. Conjugation

277. The plant brassica napus has been modified to produce

A. Vitamin A B. Hirudin
C. Insulin D. Lysine rich seed

278. Plant tissue culture was redefined method for

A. Hybridization
B. Vegetative propogation
C. Selection
D. Asexual reproduction

279. The enzymsrequired to obtain naked protoplast are

A. Cellulase and proteinase
B. Cellulase and pectinase
C. Cellulase and amylase
D. Cellulase and amylase

280. Agrobactarium based gene transfer is efficient in

A. Only with dicots
B. Only with monocots
C. Majority monocots and few dicots
D. Both dicots and monocots

281. Two or more `adjoining somatic protoplasts are fused without any inducer is called

A. Spontaneous B. Induced
C. Protoplast D. Somatic cell

282. The genetic variability regenerated during tissue culture is termed as

A. Somoclonal variation
B. Organogenesis
C. Micropropagation
D. Adrogenesis

283. The somaclonal variation in a large number of plants is defined by

A. Larkin and sharp B. Evans and sharp
C. Hein and Mee D. Stepar and Bidney

284. The precursors for the synthesis of nopalines in Ti plasmid is
A. Phosphoenolpyruvate + amino acid
B. Pyruvate + amino acid
C. Alpha-ketoglutarate + amino acid
D. Oxalate + amino acid

285. Somatic embryogenesis is
A. Germ line cells developing into embryos
B. Non-germ line cells developing into embryos
C. Embryos developing from zygotes
D. Embryonic tissue becoming somatic

286. The gene transfer techniquw involves the use of a fatty bubbles to carry a gene into a somatic cells is
A. Electrofusion B. Liposome transfer
C. Laser transfer D. Biolistics

287. Which amino acid is a derivative of glyphosate
A. Alanine B. Serine
C. Valine D. Glycine

288. The gene transfer technique involves a tiny needle that used to inject DNA into a cell lacking that DNA sequence is termed is
A. Electroporation
B. Liposome transfer
C. Microinjection
D. Particles bombardment

289. A new variety derived from tissue culture is referred as
A. Somaclones
B. Invitro miroclones
C. Proto muticlones
D. Chloroclones

290. Protoplast fusion and somatic hynridization in plant are based on
A. Protoplast isolation
B. Cell wall gets disrupted
C. Fusion of pronuclei
D. Protoplast fusion

291. Which of the following plant cell will show totipotency?
A. Xylem vessels B. Sieve tube
C. Meristem D. Cork cells

292. Somaclonal variation are the ones
A. Caused by mutagens
B. Produce during tissue culture
C. Caused by gamma rays
D. Induced during sexual embryogene

293. To obatain haploid plant we culture
A. Entire anther B. Nucleus
C. Embryo D. Apical bud

294. A medium which is composed of chemically defined compound is called
A. Natural media B. Synthetic media
C. Artificial media D. None of above

295. Growth hormone producing apical dominance is
A. Auxin B. Gibberellins
C. Ethylene D. Cytokinin

296. Part of plant used for culturing is called
A. Scion B. Explant
C. Stock D. Callus

297. Cybrids are produced by
A. Fusion of two different nuclei from two different species
B. Fusion of two same nuclei from same species
C. Nucleus of one species but cytoplasm from both the parent species
D. None of above

298. Which of the following is considered as the disadvantage of conventional plant tissue culture for clonal propagation
A. Multiplication of sexually derived sterile hybrids
B. Less multiplication of disease free plants
C. Storage and transportation of propagates
D. Both (b) and (c)

299. Protoplasts can be produced from suspension cultures, callus tissues or intact tissues by enzymatic treatment with
A. Cellulotyic enzymes
B. Pectolytic enzymes
C. Both cellulotyic and pectolytic enzymes
D. None of above

300. A(n) is and excised piece of leaf or stem tissue used in micropropagation
A. Microshoot B. Medium
C. Explants D. Scion

301. Protein consists of
A. Carbon containing
B. Oxygen containing
C. Hydrogen containing
D. Nitrogen containing

302. Protein are the polymer of
A. Carbonyl group B. Amino acid
C. Nucleotide D. Carbon

303. What is the average nitrogen content of protein
A. 15 B. 17
C. 18 D. 16

304. The most active site of protein synthesis is the
A. Nucleus B. Ribosome
C. Mitrochondria D. Cell wall

305. In a protein and amino acid are linked by which bonds
A. Hydrogen bond B. Peptide bond
C. Ionic bond D. Metallic bond

306. Firstly discovered protein are
A. Louis pasture B. Marie Curie
C. John moulder D. Darvin

307. ____Is a major elements present in the protein
A. Hydrogen B. Sulphur
C. Carbon D. Nitrogen group

308. Keratin is example of
A. Chrooprotein B. Lipoprotein
C. Phosphoprotein D. Seleroprotein

309. Which protein present in the hair
A. Keratin B. Elastein
C. Myocein D. Tryptophan

310. The protein soluble in
A. Acetone
B. Benzene
C. Alcohol and water
D. Aqueous alcohol

311. Which is the most abundant protein in mammals is
A. Albumin B. Hemoglobin
C. Collegen D. Elastein

312. Which protein present in the cereals
A. Thyronine B. Proline
C. Albumin D. Gluteline

313. Protein content of egg is
A. 10% B. 13%
C. 30% D. 20%

314. Protein content of meat is
A. 10% B. 13%
C. 16% D. 20%

315. Protein content of rice is
A. 10% B. 13%
C. 5% D. 7%

316. Structural protein is
A. Karetein B. Collegen
C. Both A and b D. None of the above

317. What is the pH of albumin
A. 6.8 B. 9.6
C. 4.7 D. 8.3

318. Transport proteins is
A. Hemoglobin B. Albumin
C. Serum D. All of these

319. Hormonal proteins is
A. Serum B. Pepsin
C. Insulin D. Albumin

320. Contractile proteins is
A. Actin B. Myosin
C. Both a & b D. None pf these

321. Storege proteins is
A. Actin B. Albumin
C. Gluteline D. Myosin

322. Genetic proteins is
A. Nucleoprotein B. Nuroprotein
C. Cycloprotein D. Lipoprotein

323. Globular proteins is
A. Albumin B. Lactin
C. Globulin D. All of these

324. Simple proteins are mainly composed of
A. Only nitrogen group
B. Amino acid residues
C. Hydrogen & Corban
D. Sulfateinos

325. Scleroproteins is
A. Keratein B. Elastein
C. Collagen D. All of these

326. Which of the following types of conjugate proteins

A. Glycoproteins B. Nucleoproteins
C. Lipoproteins D. All of these

327. Which types of protein are example of phosphoproteins

A. Avamucoids B. Giladin
C. Ovouitellin D. Elastin

328. Whcih types of protein are example of metalopropteins

A. Mucin B. Silderophilin
C. Both a and b D. None

329. Which types of protein are example of chronoprotein

A. Amalase B. Prolase
C. Analase D. Catalase

330. Which types of protein are example of globulins proteins

A. Glutaline B. Salmine
C. Tuberin D. Liquline

331. Types of derived protein is

A. Proteans B. Proteoses
C. Meta proteins D. All of these

332. Which one of the following isometric pH of alanine is

A. 6.7 B. 8.5
C. 7.4 D. 6.2

333. Which one of the following in most abundant protein present in the bones is

A. Collagen type1 B. Collagen type2
C. Collagen type3 D. None of these

334. Apolipoprotein are

A. C1 B. Al
C. Al1 D. All of these

335. Which types of Plasma proteins are

A. Prothrombin B. Fibrinogen
C. Thrombine D. Calsinogen

336. All enzyme are made up of

A. Carbohydrates B. Lipid
C. Proteins D. Nucleic ACid

337. Histone is

A. Acidic protein B. Neutral protein
C. Basic protein D. Buffer

338. Protein may be separated by

A. Electrophoresis B. Ultracentrifuge
C. Chromatography D. All of these

339. Blood protein included is

A. Fibrinogen B. Glabuline
C. Albumin D. All of these

340. What do you x by elastase

A. Convert to enzyme
B. Breck down of protein
C. Convert to lipid
D. Breck down of lipid

341. Plasma proteins are also called as

A. Lipoprotein B. Phosphoprotein
C. Glycoprotein D. Metaloprotein

342. The secondary structure of protein arestablized by

A. Vonder wall force B. Hydrogen bonding
C. Ionic bonding D. Metallic bonding

343. Which of the following are rare amino acids in a protein

A. Leucine B. Lysine
C. Tryptophan D. Serine

344. One of the amino acid are do not optically active

A. Leucine B. Alanine
C. Glycine D. Valine

345. ___is the branched chain aminoacid are

A. Tyrosine B. Serine
C. Alanine D. Cystine

346. ____is the hydroxyl containing amino acid are

A. Cystine B. Tyrosine
C. Lysine D. Serine

347. ___is the sulfar containing amino acid are

A. Alanine B. Valine
C. Methionine D. Lysine

348. ___is the aromatic amino acid are

A. Tryptophan B. Valine
C. Lysine D. Serin

349. ___is the heterocyclic amino acid ar

A. Arginine B. Guanine
C. Cytocine D. Tryptophan

350. Formation of peptide bonds except
A. Amino acid and Corban
B. Amino acid and carboxyl group
C. Amino acid and hydrogen
D. All of these

351. Dipeptide is
A. 2 amino acid and 2 peptide bond
B. 2 amino acid and 1 peptide bond
C. 2 amino acid and 3 peptide bond
D. None of these

352. Peptide bonds is a
A. Inoic bonds B. Hydrogen bonds
C. Covalent bonds D. Metallic bonds

353. Tripeptide is
A. 3 amino acid and 1 peptide
B. 3 amino acid and 2 peptide
C. 3 amino acid and 3 peptide
D. 2 amino acid and 1 peptide

354. One of the following functions of peptides bonds is
A. Oxidation
B. Dehydration synthesis
C. Complexation
D. Reduction

355. Condensation reaction is used synthesis
A. Polypeptide B. Dipeptide
C. Tripeptide D. All of these

356. Dehydration reaction is used for synthesis
A. Amino acid B. Glutathione
C. Glturate D. Peptide

357. Which of the following glutathione is the example of
A. Polypeptide B. Dipeptide
C. Tripeptide D. Mono peptide

358. One of the following human insulin is a example of
A. Mono peptide B. Dipeptide
C. Tripeptide D. Polypeptide

359. All of the following arginine and cornosine is a example of
A. Mono peptide B. Dipeptide
C. Tripeptide D. Polypeptide

360. Chemical name of dipeptide is
A. Glycine-A-alanine B. Glycine-L-serin
C. Glycine-L-alanin D. Glycine-y-valine

361. Chemical name of tripeptide
A. Glucose B. Glucoxyl
C. Glutathione D. Glycine

362. Polyelectrolyte are the widely used for
A. Water balance B. Impulse response
C. Oil recovery D. All of these

363. Which protein present in the epidermal tissue of the body's
A. Keratin B. Elastin
C. Collagen D. None of these

364. Primary structure of protein represent the sequence of
A Carboxyl group B Amino acid
C Hydrogen bonding D Ionic bonding

365. Which one of the structure gives the 3 dimensional view of protein
A. Primary structure
B. Secondary structure
C. Tertiary structure
D. All of these

366. Which of the protein are responsible for structural and strength of body
A. Keratin B. Collagen
C Elastin D. All of these

367. ___is the essential amino acid are
A. Aspartate B. Methionine
C. Tyrosine D. Serine

368. ____is the non essential amino acid
A. Syrian B. Taurine
C. Azaserine D. Ornithine

369. What do you mean by protein except
A. Holding of the first place
B. Holding of the second place
C. Holding of the cell
D. Holding of the plasma

370. Which method use for nitrogen estimation
A. Mohar's method B. Marr's method
C. Aldol method D. Kjeldohl's method

371. Secondary structure of protein represented are
A. Sequence of Amino acid
B. Three dimensional structure
C. Spatial arrangements of protein
D. None of these

372. Senger's reagents are usefull
A. Holding of protein
B. Protein sequencing
C. Nitrogen estimation
D. Degradation of protein

373. What is the Chemical name of Edman's reagents is
A. Densyl chloride
B. Phenyl iso propayl
C. Phenylalanine
D. Phenyl iso thiocyanate

374. Chemical name of senger's reagents is
A. 1 fluro 2,4 dinitrobromide
B. 2 fluro 3,4 dinitrobromide
C. 1 fluro 2,4 dinitrobenzene
D. 1 fluro,4dinitrobromide

375. Sequnomator machine are
A. Holding machine
B. Stability testing machine
C. Aromatic machine
D. None of these

376. Edman degradation firstly developed by
A. Jhon crick B. Pehr Edman
C. Jhon maxx D. Smith and edman

377. Edman degradation method areusefull
A. Selecting Amino acid
B. Sequencing of Amino gruop
C. Degradation of protein
D. Holding of protein

378. Secondary structure of protein is
A. Beta-helix and Beta-sheet
B. Beta-helix and Alpha-sheet
C. Alpha-helix and Beta-sheet
D. Alpha -helix and Alpha-sheet

379. Which of the following alpha-helix and Beta-sheet structure was firstly proposed by
A. Zwitter and poul
B. Densyl and edman
C. Pouling and Caroy
D. Senger and moldur

380. The term motif is use for described
A. Primary structure of protein
B. Secondary structure of protein
C. Tertiary structure of protein
D. Supersecondary structure of protein

381. The example of oligomeric protein is
A. Tryptophan and lysin
B. Hemoglobin and lectate
C. Serine and luesin
D. Histamine and thyopsinr

382. Which of the following a zwitterion ions is
A. Negative ions B. Positive ions
C. Both a and b D. None of these

383. Hemoglobin has a major quantities preset in which amino acid
A. Histsdine B. Alanine
C. Cystine D. Tyrosine

384. Which one of the do not non covalent bond is
A. Metellic bonds B. Hydrogen bonds
C. Vonder wall D. None of these

385. Protein molecular weight depends on the number of
A. Carboxyl group B. Amino acid
C. Hydrogen group D. Carbon content

386. Which test perform for protein identifications is
A. Sulfar test B. Biuret test
C. Polye's test D. Mineral test

387. Alpha helix is stabilized by
A. Nitrogen bonds B. Ionic bonds
C. Matellic bond D. Hydrogen bonds

388. Primary structure of protein can be determined by the help of
A. Edman's reagents
B. Sanger reagents
C. Ninhydrin
D. None of these

389. Secretine consist of
A. 10 amino acid B. 21 amino acid
C. 27 amino acid D. 35 Amino acids

390. PH of amino acid depends on the
A. Optical rotation
B. Chain length
C. Diffusion coefficient
D. Dissociation constants

391. Protein anabolism is stimulated by
A. Epinephrine B. Testosterone
C. Non epinephrine D. None of these

392. Alpha helix is formed by which bonds
A. Electrostatic bonds
B. Ionic bonds
C. Matellic bonds
D. Hydrogen bonds

393. One of the following has a phenoli group present in amino acid
A. Hydroxyl lysine
B. Histamine
C. Serotonin
D. Histadin

394. Which of the following an amino acid are optically active except
A. Lysine
B. Serine
C. Alanine
D. Glyasine

395. Full form of GABA
A. Glutathione amino butyric acid
B. Glutrate amino boric acid
C. Glutathione amino boric acid
D. Gama amino butyric acid

396. 2-amino-3-oH propanoic acid is also called as
A. Valine
B. Phenyl alanine
C. Serine
D. Phenyl valine

397. Which of the following protein produced polypeptide form protein by
A. Reduction
B. Oxidation
C. Hydrolyzing
D. None of the above

398. Amino acids exist as
A. Zwitterions
B. Cataions
C. Anaion
D. None of the above

399. Which of the following can't undergo transmitted
A. Serine
B. Thyrosine
C. Glutathione
D. Theronine

400. Which types of protein present in the major quantity in the human blood
A. Glucose
B. Urea
C. Amide
D. Hemoglobin

401. One of the following an amino acid produce a vesocantritor an decarboxylation
A. Arginine
B. Tyrosine
C. Theronine
D. Histamine

402. Fibronectin is a
A. Contractile proteins
B. Glycoprotein
C. Tissue protein
D. Lipoprotein

403. Actin is a
A. Contractile proteins
B. Glycoprotein
C. Lipoprotein
D. Muscle protein

404. The Golgi complex are done
A. Protein synthesis
B. Forms glycoprotein
C. Produced ATP
D. All of these

405. What is the main function of plasma albumin
A. Osmosis
B. Transport
C. Immunity
D. Replication

406. Polore amino acid is
A. Alanine
B. Leucine
C. Arginine
D. Valine

407. ____is the ketogenic amino acid is
A. Valine
B. Custine
C. Leusine
D. Theronine

408. One of the amino acid not found in protein is
A. Lysine
B. Beta alanine
C. Proline
D. Histadine

409. Sakaguchi reaction is idenfication for the an amino acid
A. Tyrosine
B. Proline
C. Arginine
D. Cystine

410. Millions nasse's reaction is characterized by
A. Tryptophan
B. Tyrosine
C. Phenylalanine
D. Arginine

411. ___is the example of metalloprotein
A. Casine
B. Ceruloplasmin
C. Gletine
D. Saline

412. Hemoglobin is the example of
A. Phosphoprotein
B. Lipoprotein
C. Chromaprotein
D. Metalloprotein

413. Carrier proteins can be
A. Transport only one substances
B. Exchange one substances to anther
C. Transport more than one substances
D. Perform all of these function

414. Denaturation is except
A. Disorganization of positive protein structure
B. Organization of amino group
C. Organization of nitrogen group
D. All of the above

415. Which of the following denaturation protein cannot be
A. Dehydration B. Oxidation
C. Reduction D. Crystallization

416. Protein deficiency disease is known as
A. Animia B. Kwashiorkor
C. Acutal confusion D. Parkinson disease

417. The following is largest immonoglobin globulin is
A. LgA B. LgD
C. LgG D. LgM

418. one of the following most abundant immunoglobulin is
A. LgA B. LgM
C. LgD D. LgG

419. Transamination process is required
A. ATP B. NDA
C. FDA D. PLP

420. Chemical name of seratonine
A. 5-hydroxy-tryptophan
B. Dopamine
C. Morphine
D. 5-hydroxy-tryptamine

421. transamination metabolism catelysed by a group of enzyme
A. Deaminase B. Dehydrogenase
C. Glutaminase D. Transaminase

422. All transaminase are required
A. PLP B. PPP
C. PAP D. LPL

423. The process of transamination reaction is except
A. Inreversible reaction
B. Reversible reaction
C. Cataylic reaction
D. None of these

424. Transamination metabolism is important for
A. Production of amino acid
B. Product of non protein amino acid
C. Production of lipid
D. Production of carbohydrates

425. Amino acid convrt into keto acid are Reaction occur
A. Deamination
B. Metabolism of urea
C. Metabolism of ammonia
D. Transamination

426. Transamination ping pong Bi Bi mechanism are proposed by
A. Nieman pick B. Sir j Dimer
C. Wotson and crik D. Bravstein

427. Full form of AST are the important diagnostic enzyme
A. Aspartate trandeminase
B. Acidic acid transferase
C. Aspartate transaminase
D. Acut amino transferase

428. Full form of ALT enzyme
A. Alanine deamination
B. Alanine transaminase
C. Alanine transdeamination
D. All of these

429. Serums AST is the mostly used for treatment
A. Ranin disorder B. Hartunp disease
C. Cardiac disorders D. Cancer

430. What do mean by deamination
A. Removal of amine group
B. Removal of acitic acid group
C. Removal of amino group
D. Removal of lipid

431. Which enzyme is catelysed by the deamination reaction
A. Deaminaylase
B. Deaminase
C. Deaminastrasfrease
D. All of these

432. Which does oxidative deamination process take place are
A. Intestine and stomach
B. Lungs and heart
C. Kidney and liver
D. Pancreas and blood vessels

433. Which enzyme is catelysed by the oxidative deamination reaction
A. Glutamatase
B. Glutamates dehydrogenase
C. Glutrate deaminase
D. Glutamine oxidatase

434. Which of the following hormone to inhibit the GDH enzyme
A. TcH B. T2 and T3
C. Striod and thyroid D. Histamine

435. Which of the following zin containing mitrochondrial enzyme
A. Tranamiase
B. Glutrate deaminase
C. Alanine transaminase
D. Glutrate dehydrogenase

436. Which one of the following a collection centre of amino group
A. Keto glutathione B. Aspartate
C. Glutamate D. Fumarate

437. Deamination process is
A. Reversible B. Inreversible
C. Potential D. None of these

438. Deamination process results in
A. Elimination of amino acid
B. Elimination of ammonia
C. Absorption of water
D. Absorption pf nuteriant

439. The end product of protein metabolism
A. Ammonia
B. Urea
C. Ammonium chloride
D. Citric acid

440. Which is key enzyme the convrt trypsinogen to trypsin
A. Secretine B. Elastase
C. Chymotrypsin D. Endoclase

441. Endopeptidase enzyme is
A. Brack down peptide bonds of c-terminal amino acid acid
B. Breck down peptide bonds N- terminal amino acid
C. Both a and b
D. None of these

442. Exopeptide enzyme is
A. The peptide bond C- terminal acitic
B. Breck down peptide bond of N-terminal amino acid
C. Both a and b
D. None of these

443. Proteolytic enzymes are alsp called as
A. Hydrogenase B. Peptidases
C. Pentosase D. Proteases

444. Where does absorption of protein take place
A. Stomach B. Intestine
C. Liver D. Kidney

445. Where does digestion of protein take place
A. Stomach and liver
B. Stomach and intestine
C. Stomach and duodenum
D. Intestine

446. One of the following enzyme are secret in stomach
A. Maltase B. TCH
C. Lipase D. Pepsin

447. One of the following enzyme secret in pancreas
A. Pepsin
B. Trypsin and chymatrypsin
C. Pepsinogen
D. None of these

448. Wjat is th main function of renin enzyme of the body
A. Killing to microorganisms
B. Curdling of milk
C. Control pepsin secretion
D. Rapidly absorption

449. Pancreatic juice are secretion of take place
A. Ductal cells B. Acinar cells
C. Both a and b D. None of these

450. Secretine a Harmone produced by the duadenul cells
A. T cell B. Beta cells
C. Alpha cells D. S cells

451. Cck(chlolecystelakinine) is a hormone released by

A. Alpha cells
B. Beta cells
C. I call
D. S cells

452. One of the following cannot pancreatic protease enzyme

A. Rennie
B. Trypsinogen
C. Trypsin
D. Chymotrypsin

453. Carboxypeptidase enzyme are also called as

A. Na -proteases
B. Zh-protases
C. Arg-protases
D. Cl-protases

454. The combined action of pancreatic protease results in the formation of

A. Free amino acid and trypeptide
B. Free amino acid and poly peptide
C. Free amino acid qnd small peptide
D. None of these

455. Aminopeptidase enzyme are secreted by

A. Small intestine
B. Stomach
C. Large intestine
D. Liver

456. Where is amino acid and dipeptide is absorbed in

A. Crypt and villi
B. Liminal
C. Epithelial cells
D. Cornia

457. Meister cycle is

A. Absorption mechanism
B. Elemination
C. Transport mechanism
D. Degradation

458. What is the pH of gestric juice in humans

A. 1 to 2.5
B. 3.5 to 4
C. 1.5 to 3.5
D. 4.2 to 5

459. What is the pH of small intestine in humans

A. 8.5 to 9
B. 5.4 to 6
C. 6.2 to 7.5
D. 6.0 to 7.4

460. What is the pH of large intestine

A. 6.5 to 8.5
B. 5.5 to 7.0
C. 1o.2 to 10.4
D. 7.5 to 7.8

461. Function of large intestine is

A. Recovery of water
B. Electrolyte formation
C. Indugstible food matters by bacteria
D. All of these

462. Renin enzyme is absent in

A. Babbis
B. Youngest
C. Adult
D. None of these

463. Main function of pancreatic lipase enzyme

A. Emulsification
B. Dissolution
C. Alkaline
D. Absorption

464. Work of human pancreatic lipase enzyme

A. Digestion of monosaccharides
B. Digestion of trisccharide
C. Digestion of fats
D. All of these

465. One of the following glands are secretion of intestinal fluid

A. Adrinal glands
B. Memory glands
C. Sweet glands
D. Berumar and lieberkumn

466. Denaturation of protein results in

A. Destruction of primary structure
B. Produce of peptides bond
C. Distribution of hydrogen bonds
D. None of the above

467. What is the ph of renin enzyme is

A. 2.0
B. 4.0
C. 8.0
D. 6.0

468. What is the ph of chymotrypsin enzyme is

A. 2.0
B. 4.0
C. 6.0
D. 8.0

469. What is the ph of trypsine enzyme is

A. 2.2 to 3
B. 2.0to 4.0
C. 5.2 to 6.2
D. 8.0

470. What is the ph of pepsine enzyme is

A. 1.0 to 2.0
B. 5.8 to 6.3
C. 5.3 to 6.0
D. 4.2 to 5.0

471. Hopkins cole test is specific for the amino acid

A. Glutathione
B. Serine
C. Lysine
D. Tryptophan

472. What is the term use of zymogen

A. intracellular enzyme
B. Inactivated enzyme
C. Serum suppersent
D. None of these

473. What is the coenzyme
A. Enzyme substrate complex
B. Heat stable, non protein, organic molecules
C. Subtract concentration
D. Soluble collaidal protein molecules

474. What is the ph of gestric lipases is
A. 3.0 to 4.0 B. 2.5 to 3.5
C. 3.0to 6.0 D. 4.0

475 What' is the ph of pancreatic lipase
A. 7.5 B. 8.0
C. 6.0 D. 7.0

476 Which of the following is a proteolytic enzymes
A. Trypsin B. Pepsin
C. Chymotrypsin D. All of the above

477 One of the following proenzyme is
A. Pepsin B. Chymotrypsin
C. Elastase D. Renin

478 Which class of pepsine
A. Aminopeptidase B. Endopeptidase
C. Exopeptidase D. Protulase

479 Zymogen is a
A. Hormone B. Receptors
C. Vitamin D. Enzyme

480 After Digestion amino acid results in
A. Converted into glucose in the intestine
B. Are excreted to extent of 50 %
C. Converted into glucose in the glutrate
D. Are absorbed into protein circulation

481 The symptoms of ammonia poisoning include
A. Metal confusion B. Diarrhoea
C. Vomating D. Constipation

482 One of the following protein moiety of an enzyme is know as
A. Co enzyme B. Apoenzyme
C. Pre enzyme D. None of these

483 What is the ammonia formula
A. N2h4 B. Nh3
C. Nh4 D. N2h4

484 Chemical formula of ammonium
A. NH3 B. N2 H2
C. N2 H3 D. NH4

485 Stores house of ammonia is
A. Glutamine B. Fumarate
C. Glutathione D. Glutrate

486 The Haber process is the name of to gives a production of
A. Salt B. Glutamine
C. Minimal D. Ammonia

487 What do you mean by term of ureotalic
A. Convert NH3 to uric acid
B. Convert NH3 to water
C. Convert NH3 to urea
D. None of these

488 Increase in the level of ammonia in the blood is
A. Hypomania B. Hyperamonnemia
C. Uremia D. None of these

489 Urea synthesis in
A. Cytoplasm B. Mitochondria
C. Both a and b D. Liver

490 Urea cycle is
A. Transport mechanism
B. Second metabolism
C. First metabolism
D. None of these

491 In which year urea cyclr is firstly elucidated
A. 1933 B. 1935
C. 1923 D. 1932

492 ____ krebshasInslet cycle is also known as
A. TCA cycle B. Nitrogen cycle
C. Crebs cycle D. Urea cycle

493 The two' nitrogen of urea are derived from
A. Glutrate and ammonia
B. Ornithine and citrulline
C. Furamatesnd ammonia
D. Aspartate and ammonia

494 CPSI carbonyl phosphate synthase enzyme located in
A. Cytoplasm B. Lysosome
C. Mitrochondroa D. Ribosome

495 CPSI-2 enzyme are located in
A. Mitrochondria B. Ribosome
C. Lysosome D. Cytoplasm

496 Which one of the following enzyme involved in pyrimidine synthesis

A. Cpsi-1 B. Rinne
C. Cpsi-2 D. Lysine

497 The Corban atom source while producing urea in the urea cycle

A. Glucose B. Aspartic acid
C. Arginine D. Co2

498 Which enzyme is rate limiting in urea cycle

A. Argunino succinct
B. Corbamoylphasphat synthase
C. Arginase
D. Glutrate

499 The main purpose of urea cycle is

A. Elimination to water
B. Elimination to toxic ammonia
C. Elimination to protein
D. Elimination to minirals

500 Uremia cause by

A. Blood urea level high
B. Blood urea level is low
C. Blood pressure low
D. Blood pressure high

501 Urea cycle is linked by

A. Gluconeogenesis B. Glycolysis
C. HMP shunt D. TCA cycle

502 Urea cycle is also known as

A. Ornithine cycle B. TcA cycle
C. Nitrogen cycle D. Citric acid cycle

503 Arginiase enzyme is mostly found in

A. Kidney B. Intestine
C. Gollbleddr D. Liver

504 Normal blood urea concentration is

A. 40-45 mg /dl B. 10 -40 mg /dl
C. 30-50 mg /dl D. 40-60 mg /dl

505 Metabolic defects in urea cycle

A. Alkloidsis B. Azatemia
C. Hyperaommnia D. All of these

506 BUN test is determined the workingof

A. Kidney B. Heart'
C. Lungs D. Intestine

507 Blood urea increase

A. Acut glomerulonephritis
B. Ureamia
C. Chronic nephritis
D. All of these

508 N acrtylglutamate is required for the activation of the enzyme

A. Arginiase
B. Carbamoyl phosphate synthase
C. Argunino succinct
D. All of these

509 Which in enzyme cataysd by the reaction of glutamate canvrt to glutamine

A. Glutaminetranfrase
B. Glutaminereductase
C. Glutamineoxidase
D. Glutaminase

510 Ammonia ions to the brain vis

A. Beneficial B. Non toxic
C. Toxic D. No effect

511 In water ures is

A. Soluble B. Very soluble
C. In soluble D. Partially soluble

512 Ornithine in the presence of carbomyl phosphate form

A. Furamate B. Arginine
C. Citrulline D. Arginino succinct

513 Daily extraction of urea is ____gm

A. 20 gm B. 30gm
C. 40gm D. 60gm

514 What is the ph of urine

A. 7.5 B. 6.0
C. 8.3 D. 4.5

515. Which of the following enzyme located in the mitrochondria

A. Cytochrome oxidase
B. DihydrolipylDehydrogenase
C. Succinate dehydrogenase
D. All of these

516 Hematourea is also called as

A. HemolyticAnemiaB. Stone in kidney
C. Yellow fever D. Non of these

517 Which amino acid involved in urea cycle

A. Arginiase B. Histadine
C. Ornithine D. Citrulline

518 Which integrator between the urea cycle and TCA cycle
A. Glutamate B. Glutamine
C. Pryuvate D. Fumarate

519 Uremia occur in
A. Cirrhosis of the liver
B. Coronry thrombosis
C. Both a and b
D. None of these

520 Which is inhibitors for succinate dehydrogenase id
A. Citrate B. Oxilatase
C. Maltase D. Arsenite

521 Urease is also called as
A. Lingase B. Hydrolase
C. Lyase D. Isomerase

522 The following number of amino acid involved during the urea cycle
A. 4 B. 3
C. 5 D. 6

523 One of the following ketogenic amino acid is
A. Glutamine B. Leucine
C. Serin D. Tyrosine

524 Example of ligase is
A. Elastase
B. Succinate thiokinase
C. Hydrolase
D. Hydrolase

525. In Which Year DNA Technology experiment Perform ?
A. 1873 B. 1973
C. 1956 D. 1867

526. Who Is Founder Of DNA Technology ?
A. Peter lobban And Dale Kaiser
B. Werner arber And Hamilton Smith
C. Poul Berg And Denial Nathan`s
D. Herbert W.Boyer And Stanly N. Cohen

527. How many Chronological Categories Divided By Biotechnologist ?
A. 2 B. 4
C. 9 D. 5

528. How Many Host Cell Are-
A. 6 B. 4
C. 2 D. 8

529. Which Type Of Host Cell Mostly Used In coloning ?
A. Eukaryotes B. Microorganizm
C. Potozoans D. Protists

530. In Wich Year DNA Recombinat Technology Found ?
A. 1940- 1930 B. 1870-1880
C. 1970-1980 D. 1980-1990

531. why do we use the DNA recombinant tech
A. for making rDNA
B. for coloning host cell
C. for making DNA double halix
D. for amplefyandcopies the same DNA

532. in which position bases and sugar are attached in DNA
A. C-2 B. C-1
C. C-4 D. C-5

533. what is the basic protein of DNA
A. coronin B. histone
C. elastine D. f-spondin

534. in which process chimeric molecule obtained in DNA recombinant
A. purification
B. Replication
C. manipulation and isolation
D. obstruction

535. what is the key tool in DNA recombinant research
A. restriction enzymes
B. protein
C. host cell
D. bacteria

536. who has cut DNA at specific DNA sequence
A. eukaryotic cell B. enzymes
C. nitrogen base D. viruses

537. the pair of site specific DNA methylases and restriction enzymes are present in
A. M.DNA B. bacterium
C. histone D. host DNA

538. is the name of the phage in which restricted enzymes restricted the growth of bacterial viruses
A. isolation B. Bacteriophages
C. enzymatic process
D. amplification

539. what is the type of DNA that inserted in gene of interest into the vacter DNA

A. R DNA
B. self replicating DNA
C. non replicating DNA
D. M DNA

540. give the example of self replicating DNA

A. plasmid B. bacterial DNA
C. pyramidine D. drosophila

541. in which cell vector DNA can be multiply

A. host cell B. bacterium
C. plasmid D. clones

542. why DNA vector called gene coloning vector

A. clone have many identical gene vacter
B. plasmid are replicated
C. non- coding DNA
D. group of enzymes cut DNA

543. a plasmid consist of it's on DNA with a foreign DNA the DNA called-

A. non- coding DNA B. recombinant DNA
C. coding DNA D. vactor DNA

544. what is more replicated DNA vacter

A. large DNA molecule
B. small DNA molecule
C. non combined DNA molecule
D. bactorial DNA

545. what form of DNA vacter used in the preservation of DNA destruction by the receipt vactor

A. large DNA B. circular DNA
C. triangular DNA D. Small DNA

546. where is the another DNA preservation mechanism occurs

A. DNA of viruses inserted into host chromosomes itself
B. bacteriophages
C. DNA of plasmid enter in host cell
D. in coloning vector

547. what is the first protein produce through DNA recombinant

A. insulin B. erythropoitin
C. somatostatin D. nterferon

548. recombinant DNA molecule is produced by

A. joining of two DNA fragments
B. joining of two or more DNA fragments
C. both a and b
D. joining of two or more DNA fragments originating from different organisms

549. Restriction enzymes are also called as

A. biological scissors
B. molecular scalpels
C. molecular knives
D. all of these

550. The first successful transformation of rDNA molecule into a bacterium was carried out by

A. Nathan, Arber and Smith
B. Watson, Crick and Wilkins
C. Boyer and Cohen
D. Paul Berg

551. Who discovered restriction enzymes

A. Nathan, Arber and Smith in 1970
B. Watson, Crick and Wilkins in 1970
C. Boyer and Cohen in 1975
D. Paul Berg in 1975

552. The gene formed by the joining of DNA segments from two different sources are called as

A. recombinant gene B. joined gene
C. both a and b D. chimaeric gene

553. Restriction enzymes are named for A.the person who discovered B.the bacterium they are derived fromC.the viral DNA that attackD.none of the above

A. non-coding sequences
B. satellites
C. palindromes with rotational symmetry
D. tandem repeats

554. Transfer of recombinant plasmid into E. Coli cells needs

A. heat treatment B. UV rays treatment
C. Cacl2 treatment D.

555. An ideal plasmid to be used for recombinant DNA technology must have

A. minimum amount of DNA
B. relaxed replication control
C. one recognition site for one restriction endonuclease
D. all of these

556. Restriction endonucleases have the ability of cutting

A. DNA at random sites
B. DNA at specific sites
C. Both a and b
D. DNA and RNA at random sites

557. Which group of enzymes are popularly called "Molecular stichers"

A. restriction Endonuclease
B. ligases
C. RNA polymerase
D. DNA polymerase

558. Which of the following statement about plasmids is correct?

A. plasmids are present in bacteria only
B. plasmids are present in all organisms
C. plasmids present in bacteria and phages
D. plasmids present in plants and animals

559. E. coli is generally used for gene cloning because

A. it supports the replication of recombinant DNA
B. it is easy to transform
C. it is free from elements that interferes with replication andrecombination of DNA
D. all of these

560. Which of the following involves remarkable capacity of short segment of DNA to move fromone place to another?

A. DNA transposition
B. DNA replication
C. Translation
D. Transcription

561. Which of the following process occurs in regions where no large –scale sequence similarity is apparent?

A. Homologous genetic recombination
B. Site specific recombination
C. Non-homologous recombination
D. Replicative recombination

562. Which of the following occurs between particular short sequences present on otherwisedissimilar parental molecules?

A. Homologous genetic recombination
B. Site specific recombination
C. Non-homologous recombination
D. Replicative recombination

563. The sequences of the recombination sites recognized by site-specific recombinases are

A. Partially asymmetric
B. Partially symmetricg
C. Symmetric
D. Palindromic

564. Which of the following contain only the sequences required for transposition and the genes for proteins that promote the process?

A. Insertion sequences
B. Complex transposons
C. Transposons
D. Chromosomes

565. Gene cloning refers to the

A. production of large number of copies of the gene being cloned
B. production of asexual progeny from a single individual or a cell
C. both a and b
D. none of these

566. The plasmid used by Cohen and Boyer for their transformation experiment was

A. PSC 101 B. PUC 17
C. PBR 322 D. E.coli plasmids

567. Isoschizomers recognize

A. same recognition sequence but different recognition site
B. same recognition site and recognition sequence
C. same recognition site and different recognition sequence
D. differentrecognition site and different recognition sequence

568. DNA Ligase, used in recombinant DNA technology is obtained from

A. E.coli only
B. E.coli and also Ligase encoded by T4 phage
C. Saccharomyces
D. retroviruses

569. The DNA molecule to which the gene of insert is integrated for cloning is called

A. Carrier B. transformer
C. vector D. none of these

570. The mechanism of intake of DNA fragments from the surrounding medium by a cell is called

A. transformation B. transduction
C. both a and b D. conjugation

571. The first successful transformation of rDNA molecule into a bacterium was carried out by a) (transformation) Nathan, Arber and Smith

A. Nathan, Arber and Smith
B. Watson, Crick and Wilkins
C. Boyer and Cohen
D. Paul Berg

572. Main tools required for recombinant DNA technology are

A. vector, desired gene
B. vector, desired gene, mRNA of desired gene, host, restriction enzymes, ligases
C. desired gene, host, vector
D. Vector, desired gene, mRNA of desired gene, host

573. An ideal plasmid to be used for recombinant DNA technology must have

A. Minimum amount of DNA 2. relaxed replication control
B. relaxed replication control
C. one recognition site for one restriction endonuclease
D. all of these

574. Gene therapy, a technique that helps in

A. saving endangered species
B. curing genetic disorders
C. clonal propagation
D. producing monoclonal antibodies

575 defects of increasing serum lipase

A. Acutparatitis B. Achehyderiya
C. Reumatoid D. Uremia

576 DNA denoted by

A. Use of acid B. Use of heat
C. Use of alkline D. All of these

577 Number of nucleotides pairs persent in DNA

A. 1500-300 B. 400-1000
C. 1600-9000 D. All of these

578 Double helix structure model of the DNA was discribed by

A. Aldone B. Pouling and Corry
C. Wotson and Crick D. Zwittermaxx

579 Which one of the following is absent in the sugar moiety of DNA

A. Uracil B. Adinine
C. Thymine D. Deoxyribonucleic

580 One of the following persent in sugar moiety of DNA

A. Lysosome B. Riboulase
C. Deoxyribose D. Ribose

581 Which one of the DNA molecules except

A. Adinin content does not equal thymin content
B. Guanine content equal cystine content
C. Adnine content equal uracil content
D. None of the above

582 The gene which is transcribed during the repression

A. Structural B. Oprator
C. Pronator D. Regulator

583 The enzyme DNA ligaseis require

A. The double helix
B. Synthesis of pyrimadine
C. Contact thr end of two DNA chain
D. Synthesis of RNA

584 DNA three hydrogen bonds are formed between constituent

A. Adinin and guanine
B. Thymin and cystine
C. Adinin and thymine
D. Guanine and cytosine

585 Which is the number of hydrogen bonds between adenine and thymine in DNA molecules is

A. One B. Two
C. Three D. Four

586 The following synthesis of DNA is also known as

A. Transcription B. Translation
C. Replication D. Duplication

587 One of the following DNA fragments are sealed by

A. DNA ligase B. Host DNA
C. DNA polymerase D. None of these

588 Which one of the following present in the restriction endonuclase

A. Eukaryotic B. Host cell
C. Virus D. Alll pf these

589 Restriction endonuclease split

A. Single DNA B. RNA
C. Double DNA D. None of these

590 Restriction endonuclase can recognise

A. Hamopolymer sequence
B. Uvr sequence
C. Polindremic sequence
D. Non of these

591 All of the following may be used expression vector except

A. Plasmid B. Bactriophase
C. E.coli D. None of these

592 A plasmid is except

A. Single strand liners DNA
B. Double standed liner DNA
C. Ring standed circular DNA
D. Double standard cricular DNA

593 Southern blotting techniques can be identified by

A. RNA B. Ribosome
C. DNA D. t RNA

594 A particular RAN in a mixture can be identified by

A. Nothern blotting
B. Sownthren blotting
C. Western blotting
D. Eostren blotting

595 An antibody prabe is use in

A. Sownthren blotting
B. Northern blotting
C. Western blotting
D. Eostern blotting

596 The first protein synthesized by r DNA technology was

A. Insulin B. Glucose
C. Blood D. Glutathione

597 Monoclonal antibodies are are proposed by cloning

A. Mylona cells B. Lymphocyte
C. Eukrytic gene D. Hypridema cell

598 Mylona cells are lacking in the enzyme of

A. DNA transfease B. TMP
C. HGPRT D. All pf theses

599 Which of the following used as a cloning vector

A. Lamda phage B. Cosmid
C. Plasmid D. All of these

600 A cosmid consists of

A. Large bacteria plasmid
B. Small bacteria plasmid
C. Hybrid of plasmid and phage
D. All of these

601 Dose sequence of DNA can be proposed by

A. Sanger didoxy method
B. Glibret method
C. Both a and b
D. None of these

602 Which one of the following gene is except

A. A single protein molecules
B. A bit of DNA molecules
C. A group of protein
D. None of these

603 Restriction enzyme have been found in

A. Humans B. Birds
C. Bacteria D. None of these

604 The Trade name for insulin produced by recombinant DNA technology

A. Intron B B. Humalin
C. Intron A D. Pratropin

605 The first synthesis vaccine development by recombinant DNA technology

A. Humalin B. HB s Ag
C. Intron A D. None of these

606 One oof the following enzyme produced single standard DNA

A. DNA polymerase B. DNA transferase
C. DNA ligase D. None of these

607 The first pharmaceutical products of recombinant DNA technology approval for human use

A. Vaccine B. Insulin
C. Growth hormone D. None of these

608 Western blotting in the technique of the identification of

A. Protein B. DNA
C. RNA D. None of these

609 Safe use of hepatitis B vaccine are trade name is

A. Pratropin B. Recombivone
C. Kagenate D. Humatrape

610 In which year the firstly develop on indigenous hepatitis B vaccine in the world

A. 1988 B. 1997
C. 1987 D. 1933

611 In which year the firstly systhtic vaccine development in india

A. 1997 B. 2000
C. 1988 D. 2002

612 One of the following is not a DNA sequencing techniques

A. Maxan and glibeet
B. Microorganisms
C. Automatic DNA sequence
D. Autoradiography

613 PCR is a

A. Detection of microorganisms
B. Sequence in a DNA molecules
C. Development of nervous system
D. Cell free aplification techniques

614. Which is the first cloned cell strain isolated by capillary cloning from mouse L-cells

A. L929 B. B253
C. C666 D. JM109

615. Which amongst the following is not a animal cell culture media

A. Eagle's Basal Medium
B. DMEM
C. RPMI 1640
D. Soyabean Casein Digest media

616. Most common pH for animal cell growth is

A. 7.4 B. 7.8
C. 6.5 D. 8.2

617. The common sources of serum for serum containing media is

A. Calf serum B. Fatal bovine serum
C. Human serum D. All of the above

618. ___________ is commonly used as pH indicator of animal cell culture media

A. Methyl blue B. Phenyl red
C. Crystal violet D. Safranin

619. Most suitable media for cultivation of HeLa cells is

A. Alpha MEM with FB
B. M199 with FB
C. Eagle's MEM with calf serum
D. None of the above

620. Primary culture is

A. The stage of culture after isolation of the cell but before first sub culture
B. The stage of culture before isolation of the cell but after first sub culture
C. Both
D. None

621. Techniques for the disaggregation of tissue in primary culture is

A. Mechanical disaggregation
B. Enzymatic disaggregation
C. Both
D. None

622. The enzymatic disaggregation of tissue in primary culture is done by

A. Cold trypsinization
B. Warm trypsinization
C. Collagenase method
D. All of the above

623. For warm trypsinization ______ % trypsin is used

A. 1% B. 5%
C. 10% D. 2.5%

624. In case of mechanical disaggregation of tissue for animal cell culture the initial sieve size is

A. 100 μm B. 200 μm
C. 300 μm D. 400 μm

625. The non viable cells are removed from primary disaggregate by centrifuging the cells on a mixture of

A. Poly ethylene glycol
B. Ficoll& sodium metrizoate
C. Methyl parabene
D. Calcium chloride

626. The first human cell line from a cervical carcinoma is

A. FM 3 B. MCF-7
C. HeLa D. IMR-90

627. Animal cell cloning is done by seeding the cell into

A. Agar gel B. Agarose gel
C. Methocel D. All of the above

628. In cold trypsinization _________% crude trypsin in serum free RPMI 1640 is used

A. 0.12% B. 0.39%
C. 0.11% D. 0.25%

629. What is xenotransplantation

A. Transplanting plant parts
B. Transplanting organ parts between the species
C. Transplanting bacterial body
D. Transplanting viral body

630. When an tissue is transferred from one part of body to other in same individual, the condition is called as

A. Autograft B. Xenograft
C. Allograft D. None of the above

631. As per American iron and steel Institute (AISI) which grade of stainless steel is commonly used for the construction of a fermentor

A. 205 B. 610
C. 316 D. 390

632. For 30,000 to 40,000 lit. fermentor the thickness of the construction material for the side vessels is approximately

A. 2mm B. 7mm
C. 5mm D. 10mm

633. For 30,000 to 40,000 lit. fermentor the thickness of the construction material for the top and bottom plate is approximately

A. 10 mm B. 5 mm
C. 7mm D. 15mm

634. 'O' ring in a fermentor is a type of-

A. sparger B. Valve
C. Impeller D. Seal

635. The size of batch fermentor for pilot plant varies from

A. 1-2 litres B. 25-100 gallons
C. 250000-500000 gallons
D. None of the above

636. Microbes in continuous fermentation process constantly adjust to internal and external changes in a steady state through a process called

A. Homoeostasis B. Respiration
C. Osmosis D. Diffusion

637. Largest practical diameter for glass fermentor is

A. 20 cm B. 100 cm
C. 90 cm D. 60 cm

638. Internal coil and external jackets are used for the control of

A. Temperature B. Pressure
C. Time D. Aeration

639. __________ is used for agitation in a fermentor

A. Spargers B. Internal coils
C. Baffles D. impellers

640. __________ is used for aeration in a fermentor

A. Spargers B. External Jackets
C. Baffles D. impellers

641. To prevent the vortex and improve aeration efficiency________ is used in a fermentor

A. pH probe B. Heating jackets
C. Baffles D. None

642. Disc turbine, vaned disc, open turbine are the names of __________

A. Agitator
B. Aerator
C. Stirring gland and bearings
D. Baffles

643. Scaba, ProchemMaxflo T, Lightnin A315 are_________.

A. Modern Agitator
B. Modern Aerator
C. Modern Stirring gland and bearings
D. Modern Baffles

644. The effective sealing of the stirring shaft assembly in a fermentor is achieved by the use of

A. Ring Sparger
B. Stirring gland and bearings
C. Marine propeller
D. All of the above

645. Porous sparger is primarily used __________ fermentor vessel
A. Agitated B. Non agitated
C. Both D. None

646. In orifice sparger the size of sparger hole should be
A. 6mm B. 1mm
C. 2mm D. 3mm

647. Combined sparger-agitator on small scale was developed by
A. Herbert et.al.
B. Walker and Holdsworth
C. Winkler
D. Cameron and Godfrey

648. For the production of single-cell protein ______ fermentor is commonly used
A. Deep jet B. Air lift
C. Cyclone column D. Packed tower

649. The cyclone column fermentor is used for
A. SCP
B. Non filamentous culture
C. Filamentous culture
D. Animal cells

650. _________ type of fermentor is commonly used with the use of immobilized cells.
A. Rotating disc B. Air Lift
C. Cyclone column D. Packed tower

651. _________ type of fermentor is commonly used for the treatment of effluent
A. Rotating disc B. Air Lift
C. Cyclone column D. Packed tower

652. The cells that requires solid support for their replication are called as
A. Anchorage dependent cells
B. Anchorage independent
C. Both
D. None

653. The maximum cell density obtained in stirred and air lift fermentor are often
A. 102 cells cm-3 B. 104 cells cm-3
C. 103 cells cm-3 D. 106 cells cm-3

654. In immobilised animal cell stirred fermentor the shear stress is due to
A. Sparging
B. Break up of bubble on medium surface
C. Both A and B
D. Media component

655. The sensor which is an integral part of the fermentor and the measured value is used directly for process control is called as
A. On-line sensor B. Off-line sensor
C. In-line sensor D. None

656. The sensor which is an integral part of the fermentor and the measured value cannot be used directly for process control is called as
A. On-line sensor B. Off-line sensor
C. In-line sensor D. None

657. The sensor which is not an integral part of the fermentor and the measured value cannot be used directly for process control is called as
A. On-line sensor B. Off-line sensor
C. In-line sensor D. None

658. In a fermentor______ is used for the measurement of temperature
A. Mercury in glass thermometers
B. Electric resistance thermometers
C. Thermistors
D. All of the above

659 The measurement of gas flow in fermentor is done by
A. Rotameter
B. Thermal mass flowmeter
C. Both A and B
D. Thermometer

660. The measurement of liquid flow in fermentor is done by
A. Sterile burette
B. Rotameter
C. Electrical flow transducer
D. All of the above

661. Metering pump and piston pump is used in fermentor for
A. Temperature measurement
B. Flow rate measurement
C. Turbidity measurement
D. Pressure measurement

662. __________ is used for the measurement of pressure in a fermentor

A. Bourdon tube pressure gauge
B. Diaphragm gauge
C. Pressure bellows
D. All of the above

663. During normal operation a positive head pressure of _____ atmosphere absolute is maintained

A. 1.2 B. 2.1
C. 5.0 D. 10

664. The measurement of power consumption of a fermentor is done by

A. Watt meter
B. Torsion dynamometer
C. Rotmeter
D. Both A and B

665. Tachometer is used monitoring ______ in fermentor

A. Rate of drying
B. Rate of gas flow
C. Rate of rotation of stirrer shaft
D. Rate of liquid flow

666. Hollow cones, horizontal rotating shaft, centrifugal separator and jet spraying on deflector plate are the examples of

A. Mechanical antifoam devices
B. Pressure measurement devices
C. pH measurement devices
D. None

667. In a fermentation reaction salts such as ammonium and sodium sulphate are used for the recovery and fractionation of ___________.

A. Lipids B. Carbohydrates
C. Proteins D. None

668. Triazine dyes are ________ binding dyes used for its precipitation

A. Lipids B. Carbohydrates
C. Proteins D. None

669. Kieselghur is the most common material used for the filtration of bacteria in a fermentation process. It has voidage of approx.

A. 0.55 B. 0.85
C. 0.65 D. 0.25

670. In fungal mycelia filtration, the fibrous cake is separated from drum by

A. String discharge
B. Scraper discharge
C. Scraper discharge with pre coating of the drum
D. None

671. The yeast cell can be collected on a filter drum by

A. String discharge
B. Scraper discharge
C. Scraper discharge with pre coating of the drum
D. Both B and C

672. Basket centrifuge are useful for separating

A. Mould
B. Mycelia
C. Crystalline compound
D. All of the above

673. The centrifugation of cell lysate, fermentation broth and coarse material such as sewage sludge is done by

A. Solid bowl scroll centrifuge
B. Multi chamber centrifuge
C. Tubular bowl centrifuge
D. Basket centrifuge

674. Multi chamber centrifuge is used when the particles size is between

A. 0.1 to 100 μm B. 0.1 to 300 μm
C. 0.1 to 200 μm D. 0.1 to 400 μm

675. The physio mechanical method use for cell disruption is

A. Liquid shear B. Solid shear
C. Ultrasonication D. All of the above

676. The chemical method use for cell disruption is

A. Detergent
B. Osmotic shock
C. Enzyme Treatment
D. All of the above

677. Cell disruption by APV-Manton Gaulin-homogenizer is based on

A. Solid shear B. Liquid shear
C. Freeze thawing D. Agitation

678. B-Glucosidase is obtained from S.cervisiae after cell disruption by _______ method

A. Freeze thawing
B. Alkali treatment
C. Solid shear
D. Agitation with abrasives

679. For cell disruption High frequency ultrasonic vibrations of _____ kHz is used

A. ~ 30 kHz B. ~ 10 kHz
C. ~ 20 kHz D. ~ 50 kHz

680. Sodium dodecyl sulphate (SDS), Triton X-100 are used for

A. Cell aggregation B. Cell disruption
C. Cell growth D. All of the above

681. Triton X-100 in combination of guanidine HCl is widely used for the release of

A. Carbohydrate B. Vitamin
C. Lipid D. Protein

682. Luciferase extraction from Photobacterium fischeri is commonly done with the help of ____ method

A. Alkali treatment
B. Osmotic shock
C. Enzyme treatment
D. Ultrasonication

683. Alkali treatment method can be used for the hydrolysis of microbial cell if

A. Enzyme will tolerate a pH of 11.5 to 12.5
B. Enzyme will tolerate a pH of 8 to 9
C. Enzyme will tolerate a pH of 8.5 to 9.5
D. Enzyme will tolerate a pH of 9 to 10

684. Biochemically fermentation is

A. Generation of energy by catabolism of organic compound
B. Production of product by the mass culture of micro-organism
C. Both A and B
D. None

685. The commercially important fermentation process includes-

A. Those that produce microbial metabolite
B. Those that modify compound which are added to the fermentor
C. Those that produce biomass
D. All of the above

686. In Pharmaceutical Industry enzyme amylase and protease is produced by fermentation technology is mainly used as

A. Digestive aid B. Counter irritant
C. Anti allergic D. Anti aging

687. For a biochemical process, which statement is true

A. Involve low concentration of substrate and product
B. Reactions are restricted to aqueous phase
C. Conditions of temperature and pH are mild
D. All of the above

688. Microbiological reactions are

A. Homogenous B. Hetrogenous
C. Both A and B D. None of the above

689. Which enzyme amongst is responsible for alcohol fermentation

A. Protease B. Zymase
C. Lipase D. Pectinase

690. Pasteur's first experiment on fermentation was performed on

A. Yogurt B. Milk
C. Fruit juice D. None

691. Pseudomonas species and E.Coli can be differentiated by

A. Acid fast staining
B. Shape
C. Glucose fermentation Vs respiration
D. All of the above

692. Bacteria used in fermentation of milk in dairy industry is

A. E.Coli
B. Lactobacillus
C. Pseudomonas species
D. S.aureus

693. Sterilization of fermentor is done by

A. Chemical method
B. Application of radiation
C. Heat
D. All of the above

694. Pyruvate decarboxylase reaction with CO2 is observed in

A. Ethanol fermentation
B. Penicilline fermentation
C. Citric acid fermentation
D. None

695. The first successful transgenic mammal was developed by _______ method

A. Gene gun B. Electroporation
C. Micoinjection D. Ultrasonication

696. In 2006 USFDA approve _______ recombinant protein derived from transgenic goat

A. antithrombin B. Insulin
C. Growth hormone D. Globulin

697. In 2011, European Medicines Evaluation Agency approved _______ produced in rabbits for the treatment of hereditary angioedema

A. Recombinant antithrombin
B. C1-esterase inhibitor
C. Recombinant insulin
D. None

698. Nuclear transfer and intranuclear microinjection of DNA are the common methods for

A. Transgenic animal production
B. Mab Production
C. Vaccine production
D. All of the above

699. In animal cell culture: A culture without foreign or undesirable life form is called as

A. Cell culture
B. Axenic culture
C. Chemically defined medium
D. None

700. The viable cell generated from the fusion of cytoplasm is called as

A. Hybrid B. Turbid
C. Cybrid D. None

701. When the nucleus of the cell contains exact multiples of the haploid number of chromosomes, the cell is called as

A. Diploid B. Euploid
C. Hetrokaryon D. Hetroploid

702. The culture that is started directly from cell, tissue, organ taken directly from organism is called

A. Secondary culture B. Primary culture
C. Sub culture D. Organ culture

703. The cell reconstructed by the fusion of karyoplast and cytoplast is called as

A. Recon B. Synkaryon
C. Totipotent cell D. None

704. The transfer of cell from one culture vessel to another is called as

A. Massage B. Discharge
C. Passage D. None

705. The in vitro similarity of the cell in animal cell culture to the tissue in form is called as

A. Histiotypic B. Hetroploid
C. Homoploid D. Euploid

706. The cells that grow only when attached to a surface is called as

A. Anchorage independent cells
B. Autocrine cells
C. Anchorage dependent cells
D. Clone

707. The population of cell obtain from the mitosis of cell in animal cell culture is said to be

A. Recon B. Clone
C. Autocrine cells D. None

708. The first animal cell product produces in-vitro in the year 1954 was

A. Salk polio vaccine
B. Insulin
C. Monoclonal antibodies
D. Hepatitis vaccine

709. The cell line obtain from the late embryonic stage of Drosophila melanogaster is

A. Schneider-2 B. HeLa
C. COS 1 D. Sf9

710. _____ cell line is derived from kidney of normal African green monkey and widely used in the production of polio (sabin) vaccine.

A. Sf9 B. COS 7
C. Vero D. Schneider-2

711. The first cell line was observed in

A. Mouse B. Monkey
C. E.coli D. None

712. The human embryonic lung cell line is

A. HeLa B. MRC-5
C. COS 1 D. COS 7

713. Animal cell culture media does not contain_____

A. Growth factor B. Nitrogen source
C. Starch D. Serum

714. Carbohydrates consist of-

A. Carbon, Nitrogen, Oxygen
B. Oxygen, Hydrogen and Water
C. Carbon, Hydrogen and Oxygen
D. None of the above

715. What is the term represents the entire spectrum of sugars of an organism presents in either or complex form of molecules?

A. Glucagon B. Glycome
C. Glycose D. (A) &(B) Both

716. What hormone regulate carbohydrate metabolism?

A. Insulin B. Oxytocin
C. Enzyme D. Vitamin

717. Which types of carbohydrates stories from in animals?

A. Glycerol B. Glycogen
C. Glucose D. Galactose

718. Which types of carbohydrates storage form in the photosynthesis in plant.

A. Starch B. Lactose
C. Protein D. Fats

719. What is the blood concentration of glucose in a normal healthy individual is-

A. 6.0-6.5 mM B. 3.4-5.0 Mm
C. 5.0-6.5 mM D. 4.5-5.0 mM

720. Which pathway is metabolic pathway that lead to a simpler structure from a Complex structure constitute.

A. Anabolic Pathways
B. Catabolic Pathways
C. Metabolic Pathways
D. None of the above

721. Which process is called the metabolic pathway from glucose to pyruvate occurs in 10 metabolic steps are

A. Glycolysis B. Glycosides
C. Glyconeogenesis
D. Glycogenesis

722. Drug compressibility about 27% by addition of-

A. Glident B. Starch
C. Binder D. Talc

723. Glucose are reabsorbed in the

A. Proximal tubule B. Distal tubule
C. Collecting duct D. Loop of henle

724. Insulin contains how many amino acids?

A. 51 B. 68
C. 5 D. 58

725. Which formula is monosaccharides hexoses-

A. C6H11O6 B. C6H12O6
C. C6H10O12 D. C6H11O5

726. What is pentoses monosaccharides are also known as-

A. Ribose B. Fructose
C. Glucose D. Lactose

727. Which is hexoses monosaccharide are also known as-

A. Glucose and fructose
B. Glucose and ribose
C. Ribose and fructose
D. Fructose and lactose

728. Which saccharide are yield two to ten monosaccharides units on hydrolysis

A. Disaccharides
B. Oligosaccharides
C. Monosaccharides
D. Polysaccharide

729. Carbohydrates glycogen is first discovered by

A. Robert Brown B. Alexander Fleming
C. Claude Bernard D. Louis Pasteur

730. Which are the examples of disaccharides-

A. Maltose B. Trehalose
C. Robinose D. Rassinose

731. Glycogen are example of?

A. Heteropolysaccharides
B. Trisaccharides
C. Homeo polysaccharides
D. Monosaccharides

732. Which are the types of oligosaccharides
A. Tetrasaccharides
B. Hompolysaccharides
C. Hexasaccharides
D. Disaccharides

733. Which are the example of heptoses in monosaccharides-
A. T-glucoheptose B. Glucoheptose
C. Glucohexose D. Polyglucoheptoses

734. Which of the following sugars is a test rose
A. fructose B. Lactose
C. Idose D. Erythrose

735. Which of the following sugars is found in RNA?
A. Ribose B. Sucrose
C. Xylose D. Glucose

736. Which of the following sugars is found in DNA?
A. d-ribulose B. 2-deoxy-d-ribose
C. d- fructose D. d- xylose

737. amongst the following is a sugar alcohol?
A. Mannitol B. Gluconic acid
C. Maltose D. Dextrose

738. Which of the following sugars is a monosaccharides?
A. Starch B. Maltose
C. Sucrose D. Mannose

739. What is cellulose polymer as a-
A. Heteropolymers
B. Homopolymer
C. Nucleotide
D. Nucleoside

740. ________ is the polymer of fructose?
A. Inulin B. Mannitol
C. Dextrose D. Starch

741. What is the ratio of hydrogen and oxygen in water carbohydrates-
A. 2:1 B. 1:1
C. 3:1 D. 1:5

742. Majority of monosaccharides found in human body are of-
A. L- type B. DL- type
C. D- type D. N-type

743. What are the test that are carried out for carbohydrates?
A. Molisch's test B. Fehling's test
C. Anthrone test D. All of the above

744. Amylopectin is composed of chains of units.
A. 20 to 40 D-glucose
B. 22 to 30 D-glucose
C. 24 to 30 D-glucose
D. 30 to 35 D- glucose

745. Relative sweetness of which artificial sugar is highest.
A. Sacchorian B. Nectrain
C. Cyclamate D. Invertase

746. Lactose is also hydrolysed by an enzyme that hydrolyses B-Glycosides.
A. Emulsin B. Lactonic acid
C. D-Galactose D. Insulin

747. Lactose reacts with Phenylhydrazine in presence of acetic acid to produce.
A. Emulsin B. Lactosazone
C. Inulin D. All of the above

748. Sucrose in aqueous solution reacts with hydroxides of calcium, rarium and stronsiun to produce.
A. Sucrosates B. Lactose
C. Fructose D. Galactose

749. The percentage of amylopectin in natural starch is?
A. 70-80% B. 60-90%
C. 80-90% D. 60-80%

750. Lactose reacts with dimethyl sulphate in alkaline solution to form in
A. Octa methyl lactose
B. Tetra methyl Electron
C. Penta methyl lactose
D. Caramel

751. One projection commonly used for representation of D and L glyceraldehyde B known as-
A. Robert projection
B. Fischer projection
C. Enantiomers
D. Paschuer projection

752. The simpler way of drawing Fischer projection is to use

A. Horizontal lines B. Diagonal lines
C. Vertical lines D. All of the above

753. In Aldotroses how many optical isomers are possible

A. 2 to 6 B. 2 to 8
C. 2 to 4 D. Only 4

754. What is cellulose polymer as a

A. Hetero polymers B. Homo polymers
C. Keto polymers D. Nucleoside

755. _________ Is the polymer of fructose?

A. Inulin B. Mannitol
C. Dextrose D. Starch

756. What is colour of starch-i2 complex?

A. Grey colour B. Blue colour
C. Red colour D. Pink colour

757. What is the plant cell walls composed of

A. Polysaccharide B. Oligosaccharides
C. Monosaccharides D. Disaccharides

758. What is the bonds that links monosaccharides in polysaccharides?

A. Nuclear Bond B. Metallic Bond
C. Glycosidic Bond D. Ionic bond

759. The D and Let erythrose an mirror images so also be called

A. Mesoisomers B. Enantiomers
C. Superimpossble D. None of the above

760. How many optical ispmers are possible in epimers?

A. 2 to 16 B. 4 to 16
C. 8 to 16 D. 6 to 16

761. What is a Deoxy sugar-

A. Hydrogen atom is replaced by hydroxyl group
B. Hydroxyl group is replaced by carbon atom
C. Hydroxyl group is replaced by hydrogen atom
D. None of the above

762. Aldohexoses contain how many numbers of asymmetric carbon atom.

A. 2 B. 3
C. 4 D. 5

763. The process of conversion of Aldose into higher Aldose it is first reacted with

A. HCN B. H2SO4
C. HCL D. HNO3

764. Glucose may be occured from.

A. Starch B. Sucrose
C. Cellulose D. All of the above

765. The process of epimerization is related to

A. Conversion ofan aldose into lower aldose
B. Conversion of ketose into aldose
C. Conversion on aldose into epimers aldose
D. Conversion of aldose into higher ketose

766. Glucose reacts with acetic anhydride in the presence of pyridine to form

A. Tetra acetate B. Penta acetate
C. Hexa acetates D. Tri acetate

767. Oxidation of Gluconic acid with nitro acid gives

A. Gluconic acid B. Glyconic acid
C. Both (A) & (B) D. Beta- gluconic acid

768. Action of strong alkali on D- glucose leads to

A. Crystal green products
B. Brow resiners products
C. Reddish brown products
D. Orange blue products

769. D- Glucose reacts with thiols to form

A. Dimethyl mercarptal
B. Mercarptals
C. Dithioacetals
D. Both (A) & (B)

770. The structure of glucon is-

A. Penta hydroxy hexonal
B. Penta hydroxy heptonal
C. Penta hydroxy octanal
D. Penta hydroxy pentanal

771. Uses of glucose include-

A. All of the below
B. Production of food conds
C. As a preserves
D. Silvering of mirror

772. D- Glucose enolate amino after stabilized with resonance to form an

A. Enetriol B. Enediol
C. Enepentol D. Eneoctol

773. Calcium is removed by filtration and converted to fructose by passing
A. Alfa-D Glucose B. H2SO4
C. CO 2 D. NH3

774. D- fructose undergoes aeondenstion reaction with semicarbazide
A. D- fructose B. Cyanomannitol
C. Semicarbazone D. None of the above

775. Dextran is used as a __________?
A. Plasma substitute B. Haemoglobin
C. Sugar substitute D. Fat substitute

776. Maltose on hydrolysis yields
A. Glucose + fructose
B. Fructose
C. Glucose + Glucose
D. Fructose + Fructose

777. Fructose is a
A. Reducing aldo hexose
B. Reducing keto hexose
C. Increasing keto hexose
D. Increasing aldo hexose

778. Lactose on hydrolysis yields
A. Glucose and Maltose
B. Glucose and lactose
C. Galactose and fructose
D. Glucose and Galactose

779. Saliva, A mixed secretion of several glands, has a pH of -
A. 6.4-6.9 B. 6.4-6.5
C. 6.1-6.9 D. 6.0-7.0

780. Saliva contains a carbohydrates which is known as-
A. Lipase B. Salivary amylse
C. Salivary maltose D. Billirubin

781. pH of stomach is ________?
A. 0.5 to 2.5 B. 3.5 to 6.2
C. 1.5 to 3.5 D. 4.0 to 7.5

782. D- fructose reacts with acetic anhydride in pyridine solution to form
A. Anomeric pentaacetate
B. Anomeric Hexaacetates
C. Cationic pentaacetate
D. All of the above

783. Glucose is converted to Glucose -6-phosphate by the action of the enzyme.
A. Pentakinase B. Hexakinase
C. Heptakinase D. Octakinase

784. The pancreatic secreatio mainly contains maltose, which converts to
A. Maltose to Glucose
C. Maltose to Galactose
B. Fructose to Glucose
D. None

785. Glucose-1-Phosphate is converted to Glucose-6-phosphate by the action of enzyme
A. Phosphoenol Pyruvate
B. Phosphoglucomutase
C. Phosphofructokinase
D. Glycerol

786. Formation of Galactose-1-Phosphate to galactose and ATP molecules are catalysed by:
A. Hexokinase
B. Glucokinase
C. Galactokinase
D. Glucose-1-P transferase

787. Formation of Glucose-1-P and Galactose to convert Galactose-1-P + UDP- Glucose is catalysed by:
A. Octakinase
B. Galactose-2-P
C. Glucokinase
D. Galactose-1-P uridyl transferase

788. Glycogenolysis is a process and the glucogen in muscle is finally break down to produce:
A. Glucose-1-phosphate
B. Glucose-6-Phosphate
C. Acetic acid
D. Pyruvate acid

789. Glycogenesis is a process by which glucagon in synthesized from?
A. Pyruvate acid B. ATP
C. Lactose D. Glucose

790. Glycolysis is a process by which glycogen on glucose is broken down to produce :
A. Lipids B. Amino acids
C. Pyruvate acid D. Glucose

791. The most prominent site of glycolysis is-
A. Muscles B. Liver
C. Kidney D. Pancreas

792. Main site of gluconeogenesis are:
A. Splean B. Kidney
C. Liver D. Brain

793. TCA cycle in enzymes are found in the
A. Nucleolus B. Stomach
C. Golgibodies D. Mitochondria

794. How many molecules of ATP are produced when one molecule of glucose gets completely oxidised?
A. 32 B. 36
C. 24 D. 38

795. Range of renal thresold value for glucose is form:
A. 120 to160mg% B. 100 to 120mg%
C. 160 to180mg% D. 180 to 200mg%

796. The first stage is the 'direct' oxidation of glucose -6-p to-in the HMP shunt.
A. 6-phosphogluconate
B. Guanosine thriphosphate
C. 4-phosphogluconate
D. None of the above

797. Ribulose -5-P is isomerized to a mixture of the ketopentoses which are in the HMP shunt.
A. Xylulose-5-p & glucose-6-p
B. Glucose-6-p & fructose-1-p
C. Xylulose-5-p & ribose-5-p
D. Xylulose-4-p & Glucose-2-p

798. There enists in an aererobic cells a group of respiratory pigments which is known as-,
A. Cytochromes
B. Cytoplasmic reticlulumn
C. Mitochondria
D. Ribosomes

799. Full form of ETF is -
A. Electrone technique factor
B. Electrone transferring factor
C. Electrone technical factore
D. None of the above

800. Electrone transferring factore is probably-
A. Emylax B. Nucleoside
C. Flavoprotein D. NADPH

801. In diabetes mellitus rate of carbohydrates oxidation is -
A. Decreased B. Increased
C. Normal D. None of the above

802. The rate of Glucose production by gluconeogenesis can vary form to above g/24 hours in the adult human subjects -
A. Zero above 100 B. Zero above 500
C. Zero above 300 D. Zero above 700

803. Full form of EMP pathway is -
A. Embden meyerhofparnas pathway
B. Electrone magnetic pathway
C. Aembdenmachenical pathway
D. None of the above

804. Which disease is a rare type of glycogenesis and is characterized by the formation of a polysaccharide in liver that resembles amylopectin in its structure-
A. Amylopectinogenesis
B. Amylopectinosis
C. Flavoproteins
D. Ubiquinone

805. Drug (s) affecting oxidative phosphorylation is/are
A. Uncouplers like 2,4-di nitrophenol
B. Hypocholinergic drug
C. Cholinergic drug
D. Antidiabetic drugs

806. In erythrocytes ,the most abundantly found phosphate ester is:
A. glucose -1-P
B. glucose-6-P
C. fructose-6-P
D. 2,3-di phosphoglycerate

807. Good qualitative test for the detection of urinary sugar is
A. Benedict's test B. Ramedict'stdest
C. alkaline test D. urinary's test

808. fructose-6-P is converted into F-1, 6-di P .with the help of the enzyme-
A. phospho fructokinase
B. phospho glucokinase
C. phospholactokinase
D. Xylulose-5-P

809. pyruvic acid is converted into F-1,6-diP with the help of the enzyme-

A. 6-phospho gluconate
B. lactic dehydrogenase
C. Ribose-5-P
D. Glucose oxidase

810. which is responsible for converting F-1,6-diP into dihydrocy acetone phosphate and glyceraldehyde phosphate-

A. galactolase B. Ribulose
C. Aldolase D. None of the above

811. which is catalyses the reaction of glucose -1-P to glucose -6-P?

A. phosphoglucomutase
B. phosphoglycerate
C. phosphomutase
D. phosphoglucose

812. fumarase is responsible for the conversion of into?

A. Fumaric acid into malic acid
B. Fumaric acid into tartaric acid
C. lactic acid into malic acid
D. flavoprotein

813. isocitric acid is converted into alpha-keto glucose acid woth help of the enzyme

A. Isocitrate hydroenase
B. Isocitrate oxygenase
C. Isocitrate dehydrogenase
D. None of the above

814. coenzymes required for the conversion of pyruvic acid into acetyl coA are-

A. NAD, triar. phosphate
B. lipoic acid
C. coA-sh
D. all of the above

815. compelete oxidation of glucose requires six molecules of oxygen for each molecules of glucose, the equation may be shows as-

A. $C6H12O6+6O2=6CO2+6H2O$
B. $C6H12O6+4O2=6CO2+4H2O$
C. $C2H5OH+2O2=CH3-CHO+2H2O$
D. None of the above

816. The respiratory quotient for glucose catabolism is -

A. 2.0 B. 3.5
C. 1.0 D. 1.5

817. which is enzyme is widely used for the qualitative detection and quantitative analysis by glucose in biological specimens?

A. Lactose
B. glucose hydroxidase
C. Maltose
D. glucose oxidase

818. pentosusia is quite common in people who eat a great deal of?

A. Fruits B. Glucose
C. Dry fruits D. None of the above

819. Liver and.muscle glycogen are very in controlled senere diabetes mellitus?

A. High B. Low
C. Medium D. Very low

820. Liver glycogen is very ....in glycogenosis

A. High B. very high
C. low D. reduce

821. Liver glycogen is very............in von gierkels disease-

A. low B. medium
C. high D. None of the above

822. ....may be considered the universal coenzymes of sugar metabolism-

A. uridine nucleotide B. pyridine nucleotide
C. starch D. galactose

823. ptyalin acts on starch and glycogen produncing limited quantities of -

A. lactose B. maltose
C. fructose D. galactose

824. The intestinal mucosal cells secrete a mixture succes entericus which contains-

A. All of the above
B. maltose
C. invertase (sucrose)
D. lactose

825. The sugar mainly in the milk is

A. Lactose B. Maltose
C. Fructose D. Glucose

826. Carbohydrates are not digested in the

A. Small intestine B. Mouth
C. Stomach D. None of the above

827. Which of the invert sugar is
A. Galactose
B. Maltose
C. Fructose
D. Hydrolytic products of sucrose

828. Which is animal starch in a polysaccharide is
A. Dextrin B. Glycogenesis
C. Inulin D. Galactose

829. Inulin is the unit of
A. Fructose B. Glycogen
C. Mannnose D. Galactose

830. Heteroglycan is a
A. Amaylase B. Dextron
C. Agar D. Chitin

831. The amylopectin are mainly number of branches is
A. 30 B. 80
C. 50 D. 40

832. Reduction in glucose with sodium amalgum forms
A. Sorbitol B. Cubitol
C. Mannitol D. Amphytol

833. Glucose on oxidation does not give
A. Galactose B. Glycosaccharic acid
C. Glycoside D. Pyruvate acid

834. Number of stereoisomers of glucose is
A. 8 B. 14
C. 12 D. 16

835. Ribulose is a
A. Ketopentoses B. Oxytetrases
C. Ketotetrose D. None

836. Which found in hyaluronic acid is
A. Muscles B. Intestines
C. Joints D. Brain

837. Epimeric pairs which of the following is
A. Glucose and Galactose
B. Galactose
C. Glucose and maltose
D. All of these

838. Glycogen branching in approximately after
A. Four Glucose units
B. Ten Glucose units
C. Eight Glucose units
D. Twenty Glucose units

839. Iodine gives a red color called as
A. Glycogen B. Octin
C. Starch D. Starch

840. Gluconeogenesis is decreased by the
A. Inulin B. Glycogen
C. Insulin D. Pyruvate acid

841. Not present is a Glucose-6-P in
A. Liver and kidney
B. Muscles and adipose tissue
C. Kidney and adipose tissue
D. Both (A) &(B)

842. Glucose uptake in liver cells is
A. Insulin independent
B. Energy consumption
C. Insulin dependent
D. None

843. McArdle's disease is due to the deficiency of
A. Glucose-1-P
B. Glucose -6-P
C. Muscles phosphorylase
D. All of these

844. Action of salivary amylase on starch leads to the formation are
A. Maltotriose B. Galactose
C. Maltose D. Both (A) & (C)

845. Uridine phosphate Glucose UDPG is a
A. Required for synthesis of glucoronic acid
B. Required for metabolism of galactose
C. Both (A) &(B)
D. None

846. Catalytic activity is required in salivary amylase presence of
A. Bromide ions B. Chloride ions
C. Tri peptide ionsD. Fluride ions

847. Gluconeogenesis is ethanol decreased by
A. ConvertingNAD+into NADH and decreasing
B. Inhibiting Glucose -1-P
C. Inhibiting phosphorylase
D. Decreased in pyridine

848. Mucopolysaccharide are the
A. Vitamins
B. Hamopolysaccharides
C. Amino acids
D. Lipids

849. The heptoses ketose sugar formed as a result of chemical reaction in HMP shunt:
A. Glycoheptulose B. Galactohexose
C. Sedoheptulose D. Mannoheptose

850. Honey contains the hydrolytic products of
A. Inulin B. Maltose
C. Glucose D. All of these

851. Glycosides are found in many
A. Minerals B. Vitamins
C. Drugs D. Protein

852. What is dietary carbohydrates are polysaccharide sources in
A. Fructose, Glucose
B. Starch, Glycogen
C. lactose, sucrose
D. All of the above

853. What is dietary carbohydrates are disaccharides in
A. lactose, Sucrose
B. Lactose, Maltose
C. Glucose
D. Starch

854. HMP shunt (Hexose monophosphate shunt) Is also known as
A. PPP (pentoses phosphate pathway)
B. EMP (embdenmeyerhofparnas pathway)
C. Krebs cycle
D. Glycogenesis

855. The enzymes of HMP shunt are located in
A. Cytoplasmic reticulum
B. Cytosol
C. Adrenal cortex
D. Liver

856. The digestion of carbohydrates largely in
A. Stomach B. Pancreas
C. Intestine D. Gall bladder

857. One of the following are general formula of monosaccharides
A. CnH2On B. CnH2nOn
C. CnH2nOn D. CnH2O2n

858. The triose sugar is called as a
A. Glucose B. Ribulose
C. Glycerol D. Fructose

859. which are the most important epimers of Glucose is a
A. Galactose B. Ribose
C. Xylose D. Ribulose

860. Digestion of food starts in a
A. Stomach B. Mouth
C. Jejunum D. Intestine

861. Erythromycin contains are
A. Glycerol and sugar
B. Tetra methyl amino sugar
C. Dimethyl amino sugar
D. Ribulose &Fructose

862. The amount of saliva secrets by an adult about is a
A. 300-500ml B. 700-1000ml
C. 800 - 950ml D. 1100 -1500ml

863. The pH range of pancreatic juice in
A. 1.5 to 2.3 B. 7.3 to 8.2
C. 8.5 to 9.8 D. 10 to 11.5

864. The pH value of bile lies in the maximum range of a
A. 5 - 6.5 B. 7 - 8.5
C. 8.5 - 9.6 D. 9.6 - 9.9

865. The carbohydrates is most easily absorbed in
A. Maltose B. Glucose
C. Fructose D. Galactose

866. The test for generally detection of carbohydrates is
A. Molisch's test B. Iodine test
C. Sulfor test D. Glucose tete

867. The depressed activity in glycogen synthetase is
A. Glycogen B. Cyclic AMP
C. Inulin D. Glycogenesis

868. The reaction succinyl COA to succinate requires to a
A. ADP B. GDC
C. ATP D. NADPH

869. UDPG is oxidized to UDP glucoronic acid by UDP dehydrogenase in presence of a

A. NADP B. ATP
C. NAD+ D. ADP

870. The converted in alanine to Glucose is called as

A. Glycogenesis B. Glycogen
C. Gluconeogenesis D. Glycolysis

871. Glucose will be converted to fatty acids in the diet has excess of

A. Glycogen B. Carbohydrates
C. Protein D. Lipids

872. In EMP pathway-2-phosphoglycerate is converted to

A. Pyridine
B. Pyruvate acids
C. Phosphate enol pyruvate
D. 1,3 biphosphoglycerate

873. Which are the mainly two important byproduct of HMP shunt are

A. NADPH and pentose sugars
B. Tetra hydroxy sugar
C. NADH and hexose sugars
D. Pentose sugar

874. The HMP shunt pathway are the four membered aldose sugar phosphate formed is a

A. Maltose P B. Xylose P
C. Ribulose P D. Erythrose P

875. Increased in the production of pentose is

A. EMP pathway B. ENT shunt
C. HMP shunt D. None

876. The following is an enzymes required for glycolysis pathway

A. Pyruvate B. Pyruvate kinase
C. Hexokinase D. Glucose -1-P

877. which are the pathway can gets the our body from in pentoses

A. Glycogenesis
B. EMP pathway
C. Glycolysis pathway
D. Glycolytic pathway

878. Glucose tolerance is decreased in

A. Acromegaly B. Thyroid disease
C. Diabetes mellitus D. Thyrotoxicosis

879. Glycolysis, fructose 1,6diphosphate is decomposed by the enzyme are

A. Aldolase B. Ketolase
C. Maltolase D. Enolase

880. The following dehydrogenase enzymes of the hexose monophosphate shunt are

A. NADPH specific B. FAD+ non specific
C. FAD specific D. NADP+ specific

881. Which of the following is a not envolved an enzymes in glycolysis

A. Glucose oxidase B. Maltose
C. Fructose oxidase D. Aldolose

882. This phenomenon is termed as a tissue from lactic acid from Glucose

A. Reduction
B. Oxidation
C. Anaerobic glycolysis
D. None

883. Glucose should be converted to a glycogenesis pathway

A. UDP Glucose B. Pyruvic acid
C. Pyridine D. All of these

884. Glucose enters the cells by

A. Insulin dependent transport
B. Inulin independent transport
C. Insulin independent transport
D. Enzymatic transport

885. Which one of the following is a rate limiting enzymes of gluconeogenesis is?

A. Monokinase
B. Pyruvate carboxylase
C. Phosphorylase
D. Pyruvate

886. Succinate dehydrogenase steps in the produced in numbers of ATP is

A. 2 B. 4
C. 6 D. 8

887. The totally contened in Glucose in the body is

A. 10 - 30 gms B. 20 - 60 gms
C. 20 - 30 gms D. 80 - 90 gms

888. What termed in a synthesis of Glucose from amino acids is a

A. Gluconeogenesis B. Lipogenesis
C. Glycolysis D. None

889. UDp Glucose is converted to UDP - glucoronic acid is generated by

A. ATP B. ADP
C. GTP D. NAD

890. Glycogen synthesis is a regulator of the enzyme

A. Pyruvate B. Hexokinase
C. Pyruvic acid D. Citric acid

891. A disaccharides linked by alfa-1-4 Glycosideic linkages is a

A. Maltose B. Lactose
C. Galactose D. Inulin

892. Carbohydrates is a reducing ability to a

A. Methyl group B. Acetyl group
C. Carboxyl group D. Hydroxyl group

893. Not reduced by the Barfoed's solution is

A. Sucrose B. Fructose
C. Maltose D. Mannose

894. Important constituents in a glucosamine

A. Hompolysaccharides
B. Mucopolysaccharide
C. Monosaccharides
D. Oligosaccharides

895. Precursor of the phenylalanine is

A. Hydrogen B. Pectins
C. Resins D. Tyrosine

896. Pyruvate to acetyl CoA and CO2 for the conversation of

A. Involves the participation of lipoic acid
B. Acetic acid
C. Lactate pyruvate
D. Requires oxidation

897. Gluconeogenesis is the unique reaction to following

A. Pyruvic acid
B. Oxaloacetate phosphoenol pyruvate
C. Glucose-6- phosphate
D. None of these

898. Phosphofructokinase is the reaction catalysed by

A. Is the rate limiting reaction of the glycolytic pathway
B. Is inhibited by the Glucose 2, 6 di phosphate
C. Rate limiting reaction of the glycogen pathway
D. Aceteldehyde

899. High energy required in the form in conversion of oxaloacetate to phosphoenol pyruvate

A. O2 and ATP
B. CO2 and ATP
C. ATP, protein and CO2
D. Vitamins

900. How many ATP molecules will be required for the conversation of 2- molecules of lactic acid to Glucose

A. 6 B. 10
C. 8 D. 12

901. Which of the following is glycolysis is regulated by

A. All of the below
B. Pyruvate kinase
C. Hexokinase
D. Phosphofructokinase

902. Which hormones is not involved in carbohydrates metabolism?

A. Glucogan B. ACTH
C. Vasopressin D. Cortisol

903. Liver in converting Glucose to glycogen is

A. UTP B. UDC
C. UDP D. GTP

904. Succinate dehydrogenase for the inhibitor is

A. Citrate B. Pyruvate
C. Melouate D. None

905. Clearing factor is a

A. Starch B. Lipoprotein lypase
C. Glycosides D. Hydroxy lypase

906. Maltose are attacks only is

A. Beta glucosides B. Glycosides
C. Alfa glucosides D. All of these

907. Pantothenic acid is acts on the

A. NADPH B. NADP+
C. NAD+ D. ADP+

908. Boisynthesis of UDP glucoronic acid is required for the

A. Chondroitin sulphates
B. Glucose C. Maltose
D. Galactose

909. The coenzyme of transketolase is
A. phosphoenol pyruvate
B. TPP
C. NAD
D. ADP

910. Diabetes mellitus and starvartin two conditions for the increased pathway
A. Glycolysis B. Gluconeolysis
C. EMP pathway D. Gluconeogenesis

911. Which of the following compounds cannot give to the net synthesis of glucose
A. Glycerol B. Acetate
C. Acetyl CoA D. Pyruvate

912. After digestion in aminoacids
A. Absorbed into Glucose phosphate
B. Alanine
C. Are absorbed into portal circulation
D. Galactose

913. Consist for the blood group substance is
A. Fructose B. Glycose
C. Lactose D. Glycogen

914. Oxidation of galactose with concentrate HNO3 yields
A. Acetic acid B. Mucic acid
C. Lactic acid D. All of these

915. The glysamino glycan which doest not contains uronic acid is a
A. Acetic acetate B. Lactic acid
C. Pyruvate D. Keratan sulphate

916. The major sugar of insect of insects hemolymph is
A. Trehalose B. Betahelose
C. Octahelose D. Mannitol

917. Keratan sulphate is found in abundance in a
A. Cortex B. Mitochondria
C. Cornea D. Cytoplasm

918. Pyruvate carboxylase is regulated by
A. All of the below B. Induction
C. Repression D. Allosteric regulation

919. Glucose is inhibited in active uptake
A. Digoxin B. Insulinoma
C. Phlorrizin D. All of these

920. Which of the following actively absorbed in the intestine
A. Galactose B. Ribulose
C. Maltose D. Mannose

921. In place of glucoronic acid chondroitin sulphate B contains
A. Acetic acid B. Induronic acid
C. Phenyl acetate D. Galactose

922. Hexokinase hasin a high affinity for Glucose than the
A. Glucokinase B. Glucokinase
C. Fructokinase D. None

923. The citric acid cycle is carrier of the
A. Oxaloacetate B. Hexokinase
C. Malate D. D-fructose

924. Galactose is phosphorylated by galactokinase to form in
A. Galactose-6-phosphate
B. Galactose-1-Phosphate
C. Glucose -6-phosphate
D. All of these

925. Tricarboxylic acid cycle to be continuous requires the regeneration of
A. Oxaloacetic acid B. Beta oxaloacetic acid
C. Alfa oxaloacetate D. Malic acid

926. Rothera test is not given by
A. Keto hydroxy acetate
B. Glycose
C. Beta hydroxy butyrate
D. Glucagon

927. The physiological glycosuria is met with in the
A. Alimentary Glycosuria
B. NAD+
C. Renal gylcosuria
D. None of these

928. Amylo 1,6 glucosidase is called as
A. With branching enzymes
B. Phosphorylase
C. Both (A) &(B)
D.De branching enzymes

929. A inhibitor for succinate dehydrogenase is a
A. Meloute B. Citrate
C. Acetate D. None

930. Which is the substrate for aldolose activity in aglycolytic

A. Fructose 6-Biphosphate
B. Glucose 1- phosphate
C. Fructose 1- biphosphate
D. Glyceraldehyde

931. What is dietary carbohydrates are monosaccharides in

A. Maltose & galactose
B. Lactose
C. Glucose & fructose
D. None of the above

932. HMP shunt is a process by which are synthesized

A. All of the below
B. Ribose -5-phosphate
C. NADPH
D. Xylulose-5-phosphate

933. The phenomenon of inhibitor of glycolysis by O2 is termed as a

A. Fischer effect B. Ionic effect
C. Pasteur effect D. None

934. One molecules of Glucose gives the __ molecules of CO2 I EM TCA cycle

A. 3 B. 6
C. 4 D. 8

935. Fluoride inhibits_____ and glycolysis is

A. Enolose B. Acetic acid
C. Actonose D. None

936. Decreased in the Glucose tolerance is

A. Thyrotoxicosis B. Diabetes mellitus
C. Adrenalectomy D. All of these

937. Hexokinase has high affinity for Glucose than a

A. Glucokinase B. Fruktokinase
C. Glycokinase D. Maltose

938. The conversion of alanine to Glucose is termed

A. Glycolysis
B. Oxidative carboxylation
C. Gluconeogenesis
D. Decarboxylase

939. Which are the following metabolite Glucose and fatty acid metabolism

A. Sucrose B. Glucose
C. Maltose D. Mannose

940. Sugar is cerebrosides consist of mostly the

A. Galactose B. Fats
C. Manninose D. Protein

941. Iodine solution produces no color with

A. Starch B. Vitamins
C. Cellulose D. All of these

942. Active transport of sugar is a depressed by the agent

A. Malonate B. Ribulose
C. Maltose D. Fructose

943. Reduction of glucose with Ca++ in water produces

A. Mannitol B. Sorbitol
C. Acetic acid D. Fructose

944. Related in alfa D- Glucose and Beta D-Glucose is

A. Anomers B. Ketomers
C. Epimers D. None

945. Main constituent of a galactose is

A. Dairy milk B. sucrose
C. Milk sugar D. Fructose

946. D- mannnose is present in some plant products as a

A. Mannitol B. Gums
C. Agar D. Resins

947. Reduced glutathione function in RBCs to a

A. Reduce oxidized agent such as H2O2
B. Produce NAD+
C. Produce ATP
D. Reduce hemoglobin

948. For conversion of oxaloacetate to phosphoenol pyruvate, required high energy molecules in the form of

A. CO2 and ADP B. ATP
C. Both D. GTP Or ITP

949. The following co-enzyme is needed for the oxidative decarboxylation of ketoacids is a

A. TPP B. UDP
C. ADP D. All of the these

950. Required ions for maximum activity in pyruvate kinase

A. K++ B. Na+
C. K+ D. Ca2+

951. The formation of citrate from oxaloacetate and acetyl CoA is a

A. Condensation B. Reduction
C. Oxidation D. Phosphorylation

952. Tricarboxylic acid cycle to be continuous required the regeneration of

A. Glucoronic acid B. Oxaloacetic acid
C. Lactic acid D. Pyruvic acid

953. Physiological glycosuria is met with in the

A. Respiration
B. Stomach glycosuria
C. Alimentary glycosuria
D. Renal glycosuria

954. Oxidative decarboxylation of pyruvate required is

A. COASH B. NAD+
C. NADPH D. None

955. Mainly test for ketohexoses is

A. Molisch test B. Glucose test
C. Seliwanoff's test D. Diabetes test

956. The smallest monosaccharides having furanose ring structure is a

A. Mannose B. Erythrose
C. Galactose D. Ribose

957. who is the father of microbiological

A. A.V.Leeuwenhock
B. Sr.J.J.Thmson
C. Alexander flaming
D. Robert

958. Salt and sugar presence food behave they are called as-

A. reduce a hypertonic environment
B. produce a hypertonic environment
C. produce a hypotonic environment
D. None of the above

959. citrus canker is mainly caused by

A. stepto bacillus B. lactobacillus
C. phytomonas D. phytomonty

960. mainly responsible for fermentation of dairy milk in bacteria-

A. Lactobacillus B. Octobacillus
C. Salmonella D. None of the above

961. The body in fungal disease that affect the internal organs and spread are through

A. Non -systemic mycoses
B. mycoses
C. tuberculaهresis
D. systemic mycoses

962. Which are the mainly contain in bacterial pili?

A. protein B. vitamins
C. carbohydrates D. yeast

963. Culture medium used in fungus is

A. Agar B. Moulds
C. Nutrient agar D. None of the above

964. The industrial production of citric acid is fungus used in-

A. Aspergillus migricans
B. Encephalitis
C. Lysogen
D. None of the above

965. The alcoholic production are mailnyused microorganisms-

A. panicillin G
B. I.coli
C. Saccharomyces serviceaed
D. A.nigar

966. Industrial alcohol will be produced by used in starter culture are

A. T.p yeast B. lower yeast
C. feeder yeast D. bottom yeast

967. Which of the mainly food poisoning is caused by-

A. clostridumwelchi B. ulcer
C. urinary infection D. clostridium

968. Candidiasis is caused by

A. Candida coli
B. Yeast
C. Candidates albicans
D. Floccum

969. A alcoholic fermentation, CO, evolved duriny

A. formation of acetaldehyde
B. Both (a)&(b)
C. Decarboxylation of pyruvic acid
D. None of the above

970. which is process in the following conditions food material are preserved at a temperature just above freezing temperatures?

A. Chilling B. freezing
C. milling D. phosphorylation

971. In E.coh at the site on between-

A. curing
B. bio and galgenes
C. gal and biogenes
D. gal and tgenes

972. Acetone butanol fermentation process is a by product include

A. Isoketonal B. Riboflavin
C. pyruvic acid D. acetic acid

973. Fungus used in industrial production of citric acid is:

A. catalyse B. Aspergillus oryzac,
C. Aspergillus D. Bacillus subtilis

974. The alcohol fermentation mainly used microorganisms is -

A. Bacillus cervisiae
B. E.coli
C. lactobacillus subtilis
D. A.spergilus.niger

975. closed System is also called as

A. Batch fermentation
B. continuous fermentation
C. middle fermentation
D. Both(A)&(C)

976. The medium used in. differntiateNon-lactose and lactose fermentors are

A. starch medium
B. glucose medium
C. mac conkeys medium
D. acetic medium

977. which are the following organism used for fermentation are

A. yeast B. bacteria
C. lurva D. fungi

978. mainly depends on the industrial microbiology as-

A. Nucleotids B. aseptic condition
C. fermentation D. None of the above

979. The part of inoculum fermentor and mixing of midium useful is.

A. Roller B. Impeller
C. Shaft D. All of the above

980. The top portion is fermentation are left without broth is called

A. Head space B. stearm
C. Shaft D. sparger

981. which controlled by the fermentation over heating of fermentation is-

A. steam bath B. cooling Jacket
C. hot air D. cool air

982. Basically for the principal in industrial microbiology is-

A. mainly aseptic condition
B. fungi
C. Fermentation
D. bacteria

983. The laboratory fermentation is capacity of-

A. 15-20 lit. B. 12-15 lit.
C. 200 lit. D. 400 lit.

984. The Raw material used in the production of ethanol is.

A. sulphite waste liquor
B. Hellulose
C. maltose
D. cellulose

985. Vaccines against viruses are usually

A. Given at birth
B. Either live-attenuated or killed
C. Expensive
D. Mainly polysaccharide

986. A. Fumigates can produce

A. Exotoxins B. Fumigates
C. Endotoxins D. All of these

987. which is the fermentation are submerged :

A. Batch fermentation
B. Topically fermentation
C. continuous fermentation
D. Both (a) and (c)

988. which types of fermentation are more than one microorganisms is used to ontain the required product as-

A. Dual fermentation
B. Batch fermentation
C. continuous fermentation
D. None of the above

989. The fermentor are mainly production of desirable prduction is

A. higherstream process
B. Batch fermentation
C. Downstream process
D. upstream process

990. The production od alcohol is used for Raw -material as-

A. starch
B. sulphite waste water
C. Both
D. None

991. The most infection foof borne disease is called as-

A. Botulim B. lytic
C. lysogen D. All of thes

992. who is bacterial transformation was discovered by?

A. Ederberg and beadle
B. Alsons and beadle
C. Ederberg and tatum
D. None

993. The alcohol fermentation in most commonly used microorganisms is-

A. Steptomyces B. A spergillusniger
C. E.Coli D. Bacillus myses

994. algae are rich in..

A. carbohydrates B. protein
C. Both (A) & (B) D. None

995. The fermentation experiment.firstpasteur conducted is.

A. milk B. fruit juices
C. Both (a)&(b) D. glucose

996. E.coli was firstly islolated by.

A. Robert brown B. Ercherich
C. Louis Pasteur D. Sr.J.J.Thomson

997. ffungi producing mucelium are called as.

A. Yeast B. oryzae
C. Moulds D. filament fungus

998. fungus in the culture medium used for.

A. Nutricient agar
B decrease Nutrition agar
C. Minimum agar
D. None

999. Sun ray fungus are the

A. Actimomyces e. Coli
B. Streptococcus
C. Actimomycesirraeli
D. Bacteriostatic

1000. Which Of The Following Type Of MatarialFormationProcess

A. Batch Formation
B. Continous Process
C. Both A&B
D. Cultural Condition

1001. What Are The Products Of Formation

A. Alcohol
B. Organic Solvents
C. Lectic &AciticAcid
D. All Of There

1002. Normally Principle In Industrial Microbiology Is-

A. Fermentation
B. Producing Volatile
C. Growth Condition
D. Arobic&Anarobic Condition

1003. Who The Discovered Formentation By

A. Louis Posteur B. J.J Thomson
C. ErmestRutherford D. Artoine Lavoisier

1004. What Is The Meaning Or Formations Prosses

A. Conversion Of Sugar Into Fat
B. Coversion Of Yeast Into Food
C. Converted Of Sugar into Alcohol
D. None Of Above

1005. All of The Following Are Major Commeridly Important Fermantaion Exepts As The Produce

A. Those That produce Microbial Cell (Or Biomars)
B. Those That produce microbial Anzymes

C. These That Produce Envourment Products

D. These That Produce production or Organic Solvent

1006. Which Type Of Yeast industrial Alcohol Wilol be Produced By Using Starter Culture

A. Plant Yeast B. Bottem Yeast

C. Middile Yeast D. None

1007. Which CreationIsSpeacially Observed In Ethanol Fermentor Are

A. Ethylene DecrbolaseAcidaldehyde + H_2O

B. Pyruvate DecarrbolaseAcidaldehyde $+CO_2$

C. Pyruvate DecrbolaseAcidaldehyde $+O_2$

D. Metal Decrbolase Acidaldehyde+Co2

1008. The Pyruvate Dehydrogese Multi enzyme Complex present in The Occur In

A. Aerobic Bacteria

B. Macrophilic Bacteria

C. Facultative Anaerobic Bacteria

D. Both A & C

1009. Which Are The Main Example of Traditional microbial Formation

A. Vinager B. Yeast

C. Penicilin D. Oxytetracycline

1010. In Alcohol Fermentation CO2 Is Produced In

A. Oxidation of Acetaldehyde

B. Formation Of Acetaldehyde

C. Oxidation of Acetic Acid

D. Both A&B

1011. Which Of The Following Condition In VinegerFermantation Involved is

A. Yeast With Hydroxy Acid Bacteria

B. Yeast With Acetic acid Bactiria

C. Yeast With Ammonium Acetate Bacteria

D. All of Above

1012. Which Type Fermantation Processes in tobacco and tea leaves are fermented to give flavour and taste.

A. Curing

B. Alcoholic fermentation

C. Penicillin

D. Canning

1013. Technique which are used in to enable better visualisation of cells and cell parts under the microscope

A. Coloring B. Painting

C. Staining D. Sketching

1014. Which stain is also used as redox indicator in analytical industry

A. Crystal violet B. Iodine

C. Safranin D. All of the above

1015. Which stain is useful in plant cell staining

A. Crystal violet B. Glycogen red

C. Safranin D. None of the above

1016. The method of staining in which bacteria are stained by using a simple stain

A. Gram Staining

B. Acid fast staining

C. Differential staining

D. Simple Staining

1017. The method of staining that colours the background and leaves the cell uncoloured

A. Simple Staining B. Gram Staining

C. Relief staining D. None

1018. Which dye is used in preparing a temporary mount of stomata in a leaf peal

A. Iodine B. Crystal violet

C. Safranin D. All of the above

1019. What is the main importance of staining

A. Improve visuality

B. Morphological study

C. Structural study

D. All of the above

1020. On the basis of chemical nature, staining is classified into

A. 3 types B. 5 types

C. 10 types D. 8 types

1021. In staining, the acidic stain carries

A. Positive charge B. Negative charge

C. Both a and b D. Neutral

1022. In staining, the basic stain carries

A. Positive charge B. Negative charge

C. Both A and B D. Neutral

1023. The example of acidic stain is

A. Crystal violet B. Leishman stain
C. Methylene blue D. Nigrosin

1024. The example of basic stain is

A. Malachite green B. Safranin
C. Carol fuschin D. All of the above

1025. The example of neutral stain is

A. Geimsa stain B. Wright stain
C. Leishman stain D. All of the above

1026. The main objective of Staining is

A. See organisms
B. Differentiate organisms
C. Identify structure
D. All of the above

1027. The stain generally consist of

A. Chromogen B. Auxochrome
C. Both a and b D. None of the above

1028. When benzene ring reacts with the chromophore group then the compound which formed is called

A. Chromogen B. Auxochrome
C. Auxogen D. None of the above

1029. Which staining requires the simple use of stain only

A. Simple Staining B. Acid fast staining
C. Gram Staining D. All of the above

1030. Staining procedure that make visible the difference between bacterial cell or parts of a bacterial cell are termed as

A. Gram Staining B. Differential staining
C. Direct staining D. Simple Staining

1031. Which staining types are comes under the special staining

A. Capsule staining
B. Endospores staining
C. Flagella staining
D. All of the above

1032. Basic dyes easily release_______ and accept_______ ion

A. Release OH ion and accept H ion
B. Release H and accept OH
C. Both a and b
D. None of the above

1033. Acidic dyes easily release _______ and accept_______ ion

A. Release H ion and accept OH
B. Release OH and accept H ion
C. Both a and b
D. None of the above

1034. Exposure time of safranin to stain the bacteria

A. 30-60 second B. 15-30 second
C. 1-2 minutes D. 5-10 second

1035. Exposure time of crystal violet is

A. 20-60 second B. 1-2 minutes
C. 30-60 second D. 15-40 second

1036. The main drawback of simple staining is

A. Examine shape
B. Rapid method
C. Cannot classify organisms type
D. Morphological study

1037. In which staining, the positive charged colour portion of the basic dye combine with the negatively charged bacterium and the organisms become directly stained

A. Gram Staining B. Acid fast staining
C. Direct staining D. All of the above

1038. In which staining, acidic dye which does not combine with the negative cell of the bacteria

A. Indirect staining B. Direct staining
C. Capsule staining D. All of the above

1039. Which purpose of made to fix the bacteria onto the slide and to prevent the sample from being lost during a Staining procedure

A. Immobilization B. Smear
C. Spread D. Cover

1040. The process by which integral and external structure of cells and microorganisms are preserved and fixed in position with the help of heat called

A. Heat fixation
B. Hang up
C. Thermal addiction
D. All of the above

1041. The method of Staining used to distinguish and classify bacterial species into two large group

A. Gram Staining
B. Acid fast staining
C. Capsule staining
D. All of the above

1042. Who introduced the technique of gram Staining

A. E.van Gram B. Wilkinson Gram
C. Christian Gram D. Richard Gram

1043. Which stain are used as counter stain

A. Carol fuschin B. Crystal violet
C. Safranin D. All of the above

1044. Which dye are act as mordant in gram Staining

A. Crystal violet B. Iodine
C. Safranin D. None of the above

1045. Which bacteria cell wall consist thick layer of peptidoglycan

A. Proteus B. Yersinia
C. Neisseria D. Mycobacterium

1046. Which bateria consist thin layer of peptidoglycan and high lipid content

A. Staraptocoocus B. Staphylococcus
C. Clostridium D. Traponema

1047. In gram Staining,the gram positive bateria appear

A. Deep violet B. Pink
C. Orange D. None of the above

1048. In gram Staining, the gram negative bacteria appear

A. Red B. Deep voilet
C. Blue D. None of the above

1049. Which bacteria/organisms cannot be detected/visualised using gram Staining method

A. Chlamydia B. Vibrio
C. Clostridium D. Nocardia

1050. Acid fast staining is also called as

A. Ziehl- Neelson B. Louis - maria
C. Pasturization D. None of the above

1051. Acid -fast staining are very useful to identify which type of organisms

A. Clostridium B. Staphyllocoocus
C. Staraptocoocus D. Mycobacterium

1052. In acid fast staining,the acid fast positive cell appear

A. Pink colour B. Blue
C. Orange D. All of the above

1053. In acid fast staining,the acid fast negative cell appear light blue colour because of

A. Carol fuschin B. Iodine
C. Methylene blue D. None of the above

1054. Which staining helps to distinguish gram positive bacteria with waxy mycolic acids in their cell wall

A. Gram Staining
B. Ziehlneelson staining
C. Endospore staining
D. Flagella staining

1055. Which bacteria are acid fast bacteria

A. Mycobacterium tuberculosis
B. Nocardia
C. Both a and b
D. None of the above

1056. A substance used to set dyes on fabrics by forming a coordination complex with the dye,which then attached to the fabrics

A. Counterstain B. Mordant
C. Decolonisation D. None of the above

1057. Technique which are used to demonstrate presence of capsule surrounding cells

A. Capsule staining
B. Cytoplasmic inclusion stain
C. Giemsa staining
D. None of the above

1058. Technique which are used to identify intracellular deposits of starch,glycon, phosphate,hydroxybutyrate and other substances

A. Cytoplasmic inclusion staining
B. Protoplasmic inclusion staining
C. Mitochondrial inclusion staining
D. None of the above

1059. Technique which are used to demonstrate spore structure in bacteria as well as free spores

A. Endospore staining
B. Exospore staining
C. Intraspore staining
D. Extraspore staining

1060. Technique which are particularly applicable for staining rickettsias and some protozoa

A. Giemsa staining
B. Rickett staining
C. Protozoal staining
D. Acid fast staining

1061. Technique which are used to demonstrate presence and arrangement of flagella

A. Flagella staining
B. Endospore staining
C. Hair staining
D. All of the above

1062. Sometime gram positive organisms fail to retain the primary crystal violet stain,so they may show variations in this respect.This reaction known

A. Gram variable reaction
B. Gram alteration reaction
C. Gram changes reaction
D. All of the above

1063. Which instrument are used to identify and visualise some tricky samples including bacteria, algae, and fungi in microbiology laboratory

A. Hand glass B. Hand lens
C. Microscope D. Eye glass

1064. A instrument that uses visible light and magnifying lenses to examine small objects which is not visible to the naked eye

A. Microscope
B. Light microscope
C. Floroscent microscope
D. None of the above

1065. Enlargement of the image is called

A. Glorification B. Amplification
C. Magnification D. All of the above

1066. The ability to distinguish two very small and closely spaced objects as seperate entities is known as

A. Resolution B. Magnification
C. Both a and b D. None of the above

1067. The science of investigating small object using such as instrument is called

A. Microscopy B. Macroscopy
C. Nanoscopy D. Micoscopy

1068. Help in measurement of the size of microscopic object is

A. Micometery B. Micrometery
C. Nanometery D. Macrometery

1069. In which microscopy,the microscopic field is brightly lighted and the organisms appear dark

A. Dark field microscopy
B. Bright field microscopy
C. Phase contrast microscopy
D. Floroscent microscopy

1070. The technique used to observe unstained samples causing them to appear brightly light against a dark almost purely black background is called

A. Phase contrast microscopy
B. Bright field microscopy
C. Dark field microscopy
D. All of the above

1071. Who invented dark field microscopy

A. Anton van Leeuwenhoek
B. Anwasksman C. Girolamo fraeastoro
D. None of the above

1072. Which light having maximum resolution

A. Green B. Yellow
C. Orange D. Blue

1073. Which microscope are used to magnify and visualised live cells

A. Floroscent microscope
B. Dark field microscope
C. Phase contrast microscope
D. Light microscope

1074. In a microscope,which device are used to draw clear magnified sketches of objects

A. Light microscope
B. Dark field microscope
C. Bright field microscope
D. Camera lucida

1075. Objects can be magnified under electron microscope is

A. 3,00,000 times B. 3,50,000 times
C. 2,00,000times D. 5,00,000 times

1076. For gross morphological feature of bacteria, yeast, mood, algae, and protozoa, which Microscopy technique is used

A. Bright field microscopy
B. Floroscent microscopy
C. Phase contrast microscopy
D. Dark field microscopy

1077. The secondary electrons radiated back in scanning microscope is collected by

A. Anode B. Cathode
C. Specimen D. All of the above

1078. Which microscope are used to study internal structure of cell

A. SEM B. TEM
C. Compound microscope
D. Light microscope

1079. The maximum magnification of light microscope is usually

A. 1000 times B. 1500 times
C. 2000 times D. 2500 times

1080. The object can be magnified under bright field microscopy is

A. 2000-3000 B. 1000-2000
C. 4000-5000 D. 3000-4000

1081. An optical microscope that uses flouroscene and phosophorescenes instead of, or in addition to scattering, reflection and absorption to study the properties of organic and inorganic substance

A. Floroscent microscope
B. Light microscope
C. Scanning electron microscope
D. Transmission electron microscope

1082. Which microscope uses electron to create an image of the target and has higher magnification or resolving power

A. Light microscope
B. Election microscope
C. Compound microscope
D. None of the above

1083. A Microscopy technique in which a beam of electrons is transmitted through a specimen to form a image

A. TEM
B. SEM
C. Light microscope
D. Compound microscope

1084. Electron microscope that produces image of a sample by scanning the surface with a focused beam of electrons

A. TEM
B. SEM
C. Florescent microscope
D. Dark field microscope

1085. Examination of viruses and ultra structure of microbial cells can be done by the help of

A. Electron microscope
B. Light microscope
C. Florescent microscope
D. Phase contrast microscope

1086. We can gather information on crystalline structure, stress, internal fracture with the help of which microscope

A. Transmission electron microscope
B. Scanning electron microscope
C. Compound microscope
D. Phase contrast microscope

1087. In which microscope, electron create an object by detecting reflector knocked-off electron

A. Transmission electron microscope
B. Florescent microscope
C. Light microscope
D. Scanning electron microscope

1088. Which microscopy is used very effectively in microanalysis and failure analysis of solid inorganic materials

A. SEM B. TEM
C. both a and b D. None of the above

1089. In fluorescence microscopy, which of the following perform the function of remove all light except blue light

A. Exciter filter B. Barrier filter
C. Both A and B D. None of the above

1090. In fluorescence microscopy, which blocks out blue light and allows any other light emitted by the fluorescing specimen to pass through a reach the eye

A. Exciter filter B. Barrier filter
C. Both A and B D. None of the above

1091. Minimum distance for the eye to focus any object

A. 10 cm. B. 20cm.
C. 25 cm. D. 15 cm.

1092. An optical microscopy techniques that convert phase shifts in light passing through a transparent specimen to brightness change in the image

A. Phase contrast microscopy
B. Dark field microscopy
C. Bright field microscopy
D. Florescent microscopy

1093. Which kingdom have Archaebacteria and Eubacteria sub kingdom

A. Monera B. Protista
C. Plantae D. Animalia

1094. Which kingdom includes prokaryotic cells lacking organised nucleus and membrane bound cell organelles

A. Plantae B. Animalia
C. Monera D. None of the above

1095. Which kingdom include mushrooms, rhizomes and mucor

A. Fungi B. Animalia
C. Protista D. All of the above

1096. Humans are comes under which kingdom

A. Animals B. Plants
C. Monera D. Both A and B

1097. In which year Whittaker proposed 5 kingdom

A. 1968 B. 1963
C. 1969 D. 1962

1098. The production of new living organisms or organelles called

A. Abiogenesis B. Biogenesis
C. Micro-biogenesis D. All of the above

1099. Who proposed biogenesis theory

A. Louis Pasteur B. Warner Lambert
C. Roger bacon D. None of the above

1100. The original evaluation of life or living organisms from inorganic or inanimate substance

A. Abiogenesis B. Biogenesis
C. Both a and b D. None of the above

1101. Which has proved by experiment that bacteria are the cause of same diseases

A. Louis Pasteur B. Aristotle
C. John Needham D. Francesco Redi

1102. Who is the father of microbiology

A. Robert Koch B. Louis Pasteur
C. Aristotle D. None of the above

1103. Who is the father of bacteriology

A. Leeuwenhoek B. Louis Pasteur
C. John Tyndall D. Schwann

1104. The process in which an organisms convert a carbohydrate into alcohol or acid

A. Breakdown B. Fermentation
C. Evaporation D. None of the above

1105. Who investigate the anthrax disease cycle in 1876

A. Robert Koch B. Fred Koch
C. Charles Koch D. David Koch

1106. The example of prokaryotic cell

A. Yeast B. Fungi
C. Protozoa D. Bacteria

1107. Example of eukaryotic cell

A. Yeast B. Algae
C. Both a and b D. None

1108. The size range of protozoa is

A. 2.0 - 200 mm B. 5 -100mm
C. 4.0-600 mm D. None of the

1109. Which scientist firstly observe and accurately record and report microorganisms

A. Antony van Leeuwenhoek
B. John Phillip
C. John Tyndall
D. Fanny hesse

1110. Who proposed fractional sterilization to kill spores

A. John Tyndall B. Howard T.Ricketts
C. Franz schultze D. None of the above

1111. Fermentation which is carried out by bacteria is called

A. Acetic acid fermentation

B. Butyric acid fermentation

C. Formic acid fermentation

D. Lactic acid fermentation

1112. Who established principles for germ theory of disease

A. Jacob henle B. Louis Pasteur

C. Robert Koch D. None of the above

1113. ___ is a type of genetic modification in plants.

A. Spontaneous fusion

B. Induced fusion C. Protoplast fusion

D. None of above

Answer Key

Chapter 1: Pharmaceutics

1. (D)
2. (C)
3. (A)
4. (A)
5. (D)
6. (C)
7. (A)
8. (A)
9. (A)
10. (A)
11. (D)
12. (C)
13. (C)
14. (B)
15. (C)
16. (C)
17. (A)
18. (A)
19. (B)
20. (C)
21. (C)
22. (D)
23. (D)
24. (A)
25. (A)
26. (A)
27. (C)
28. (A)
29. (A)
30. (D)
31. (D)
32. (A)
33. (B)
34. (C)
35. (A)
36. (A)
37. (A)
38. (A)
39. (D)
40. (A)
41. (A)
42. (A)
43. (D)
44. (A)
45. (C)
46. (D)
47. (B)
48. (B)
49. (A)
50. (A)
51. (A)
52. (A)
53. (D)
54. (C)
55. (C)
56. (D)
57. (D)
58. (C)
59. (A)
60. (A)
61. (D)
62. (C)
63. (A)
64. (D)
65. (D)
66. (C)
67. (A)
68. (D)
69. (D)
70. (C)
71. (A)
72. (D)
73. (C)
74. (A)
75. (D)
76. (A)
77. (C)
78. (A)
79. (B)
80. (D)
81. (A)
82. (A)
83. (C)
84. (B)
85. (D)
86. (A)
87. (C)
88. (A)
89. (A)
90. (A)
91. (C)
92. (A)
93. (D)
94. (D)
95. (A)
96. (B)
97. (C)
98. (B)
99. (C)
100. (B)
101. (B)
102. (C)
103. (C)
104. (A)
105. (A)
106. (A)
107. (B)
108. (C)
109. (A)
110. (A)
111. (C)
112. (A)
113. (C)
114. (B)
115. (B)
116. (C)
117. (C)
118. (A)
119. (A)
120. (A)
121. (B)
122. (C)
123. (D)
124. (A)
125. (C)
126. (A)
127. (C)
128. (A)
129. (D)
130. (D)
131. (A)
132. (C)
133. (B)
134. (A)
135. (B)
136. (B)
137. (C)
138. (D)
139. (A)
140. (B)
141. (A)
142. (A)
143. (C)
144. (D)
145. (A)
146. (B)
147. (D)
148. (B)
149. (C)
150. (A)
151. (A)
152. (D)
153. (A)
154. (B)
155. (A)
156. (B)
157. (A)
158. (D)
159. (C)
160. (A)
161. (D)
162. (C)
163. (B)
164. (C)
165. (B)
166. (C)
167. (A)
168. (D)
169. (D)
170. (B)
171. (D)
172. (C)
173. (A)
174. (B)
175. (B)
176. (C)
177. (D)
178. (A)
179. (B)
180. (B)
181. (A)
182. (A)
183. (A)
184. (B)
185. (A)
186. (B)
187. (B)
188. (C)
189. (D)
190. (A)
191. (B)
192. (B)
193. (C)
194. (B)
195. (A)
196. (A)
197. (C)
198. (B)
199. (A)
200. (D)
201. (B)
202. (C)
203. (A)
204. (B)

205. (B)
206. (B)
207. (B)
208. (A)
209. (C)
210. (C)
211. (D)
212. (A)
213. (B)
214. (B)
215. (D)
216. (C)
217. (D)
218. (C)
219. (D)
220. (D)
221. (D)
222. (A)
223. (C)
224. (C)
225. (D)
226. (C)
227. (D)
228. (C)
229. (D)
230. (D)
231. (D)
232. (A)
233. (B)
234. (C)
235. (D)
236. (C)
237. (B)
238. (C)
239. (C)
240. (C)
241. (D)
242. (D)
243. (B)
244. (A)
245. (A)
246. (D)
247. (A)
248. (B)
249. (D)
250. (C)
251. (D)
252. (A)
253. (C)
254. (D)
255. (D)
256. (C)
257. (A)
258. (B)
259. (B)
260. (A)
261. (C)
262. (A & B)
263. (A)
264. (A)
265. (A)
266. (B)
267. (A)
268. (D)
269. (A)
270. (D)
271. (A)
272. (A)
273. (A)
274. (C)
275. (B)
276. (D)
277. (B)
278. (B)
279. (A)
280. (C)
281. (A)
282. (B)
283. (D)
284. (A)
285. (D)
286. (B)
287. (A)
288. (C)
289. (D)
290. (C)
291. (C)
292. (D)
293. (A)
294. (C)
295. (C)
296. (A)
297. (B)
298. (C)
299. (D)
300. (D)
301. (A)
302. (B)
303. (A)
304. (C)
305. (A)
306. (B)
307. (B)
308. (A)
309. (C)
310. (D)
311. (D)
312. (A)
313. (B)
314. (D)
315. (A)
316. (B)
317. (B)
318. (B)
319. (A)
320. (C)
321. (B)
322. (D)
323. (A)
324. (C)
325. (C)
326. (C)
327. (A)
328. (D)
329. (C)
330. (A)
331. (A)
332. (D)
333. (A)
334. (B)
335. (B)
336. (C)
337. (B)
338. (A)
339. (A)
340. (C)
341. (A)
342. (A)
343. (B)
344. (C)
345. (D)
346. (A)
347. (C)
348. (A)
349. (B)
350. (A)
351. (D)
352. (D)
353. (C)
354. (B)
355. (A)
356. (A)
357. (A)
358. (B)
359. (C)
360. (B)
361. (A)
362. (C)
363. (D)
364. (D)
365. (D)
366. (B)
367. (A)
368. (B)
369. (A)
370. (B)
371. (D)
372. (A)
373. (C)
374. (A)
375. (C)
376. (D)
377. (C)
378. (B)
379. (D)
380. (A)
381. (A)
382. (D)
383. (A)
384. (B)
385. (C)
386. (C)
387. (C)
388. (D)
389. (B)
390. (D)
391. (A)
392. (A)
393. (C)
394. (B)
395. (D)
396. (A)
397. (B)
398. (A)
399. (B)
400. (C)
401. (A)
402. (C)
403. (B)
404. (B)
405. (D)
406. (C)
407. (A)
408. (D)
409. (A)
410. (D)
411. (D)
412. (D)
413. (D)
414. (A)
415. (A)
416. (B)
417. (A)
418. (A)
419. (B)
420. (A)
421. (A)
422. (A)
423. (D)
424. (B)
425. (C)
426. (A)

427.	(D)	464.	(C)	501.	(B)	538.	(C)	575.	(A)	612.	(D)
428.	(A)	465.	(A)	502.	(A)	539.	(D)	576.	(D)	613.	(A)
429.	(A)	466.	(B)	503.	(A)	540.	(B)	577.	(B)	614.	(B)
430.	(D)	467.	(C)	504.	(A)	541.	(D)	578.	(C)	615.	(A)
431.	(B)	468.	(A)	505.	(D)	542.	(A)	579.	(D)	616.	(B)
432.	(B)	469.	(B)	506.	(C)	543.	(A)	580.	(D)	617.	(A)
433.	(C)	470.	(C)	507.	(B)	544.	(D)	581.	(A)	618.	(B)
434.	(A)	471.	(D)	508.	(C)	545.	(C)	582.	(B)	619.	(C)
435.	(B)	472.	(A)	509.	(A)	546.	(D)	583.	(A)	620.	(B)
436.	(D)	473.	(A)	510.	(B)	547.	(B)	584.	(C)	621.	(C)
437.	(C)	474.	(C)	511.	(A)	548.	(A)	585.	(C)	622.	(D)
438.	(B)	475.	(A)	512.	(C)	549.	(A)	586.	(C)	623.	(C)
439.	(D)	476.	(A)	513.	(B)	550.	(C)	587.	(B)	624.	(B)
440.	(D)	477.	(B)	514.	(A)	551.	(B)	588.	(A)	625.	(A)
441.	(D)	478.	(C)	515.	(D)	552.	(D)	589.	(C)	626.	(B)
442.	(A)	479.	(B)	516.	(B)	553.	(C)	590.	(A)	627.	(A)
443.	(C)	480.	(B)	517.	(D)	554.	(C)	591.	(B)	628.	(D)
444.	(B)	481.	(C)	518.	(A)	555.	(A)	592.	(C)	629.	(A)
445.	(D)	482.	(B)	519.	(D)	556.	(B)	593.	(A)	630.	(B)
446.	(B)	483.	(B)	520.	(B)	557.	(C)	594.	(C)	631.	(C)
447.	(D)	484.	(A)	521.	(B)	558.	(C)	595.	(A)	632.	(C)
448.	(A)	485.	(C)	522.	(B)	559.	(A)	596.	(A)	633.	(A)
449.	(D)	486.	(A)	523.	(C)	560.	(B)	597.	(B)	634.	(B)
450.	(D)	487.	(B)	524.	(B)	561.	(A)	598.	(C)	635.	(D)
451.	(D)	488.	(A)	525.	(D)	562.	(A)	599.	(B)	636.	(A)
452.	(A)	489.	(C)	526.	(C)	563.	(A)	600.	(D)	637.	(C)
453.	(C)	490.	(C)	527.	(A)	564.	(C)	601.	(B)	638.	(C)
454.	(A)	491.	(A)	528.	(D)	565.	(D)	602.	(A)	639.	(B)
455.	(C)	492.	(D)	529.	(B)	566.	(B)	603.	(B)	640.	(A)
456.	(B)	493.	(B)	530.	(A)	567.	(B)	604.	(A)	641.	(C)
457.	(C)	494.	(C)	531.	(D)	568.	(C)	605.	(D)	642.	(D)
458.	(A)	495.	(A)	532.	(C)	569.	(C)	606.	(C)	643.	(A)
459.	(C)	496.	(D)	533.	(A)	570.	(A)	607.	(C)	644.	(B)
460.	(A)	497.	(B)	534.	(D)	571.	(D)	608.	(A)	645.	(A)
461.	(C)	498.	(D)	535.	(C)	572.	(B)	609.	(A)	646.	(D)
462.	(B)	499.	(D)	536.	(A)	573.	(D)	610.	(C)	647.	(C)
463.	(B)	500.	(C)	537.	(A)	574.	(A)	611.	(A)	648.	(D)

649. (C)
650. (D)
651. (B)
652. (C)
653. (C)
654. (A)
655. (D)
656. (C)
657. (A)
658. (D)
659. (B)
660. (C)
661. (A)
662. (B)
663. (D)
664. (A)
665. (B)
666. (C)
667. (A)
668. (B)
669. (D)
670. (C)
671. (B)
672. (D)
673. (C)
674. (B)
675. (C)
676. (A)
677. (C)
678. (B)
679. (D)
680. (B)
681. (D)
682. (C)
683. (A)
684. (A)
685. (D)
686. (B)
687. (A)
688. (D)
689. (C)
690. (A)
691. (D)
692. (C)
693. (B)
694. (D)
695. (B)
696. (A)
697. (C)
698. (C)
699. (D)
700. (A)
701. (C)
702. (B)
703. (D)
704. (B)
705. (A)
706. (B)
707. (C)
708. (D)
709. (A)
710. (A)
711. (B)
712. (B)
713. (A)
714. (C)
715. (D)
716. (B)
717. (D)
718. (A)
719. (B)
720. (A)
721. (B)
722. (A)
723. (A)
724. (C)
725. (D)
726. (B)
727. (C)
728. (B)
729. (C)
730. (C)
731. (A)
732. (A)
733. (C)
734. (D)
735. (C)
736. (A)
737. (C)
738. (C)
739. (A)
740. (B)
741. (A)
742. (C)
743. (D)
744. (B)
745. (D)
746. (A)
747. (C)
748. (A)
749. (A)
750. (A)
751. (C)
752. (D)
753. (C)
754. (D)
755. (B)
756. (C)
757. (D)
758. (A)
759. (C)
760. (A)
761. (C)
762. (B)
763. (A)
764. (A)
765. (C)
766. (B)
767. (C)
768. (D)
769. (D)
770. (A)
771. (B)
772. (A)
773. (C)
774. (D)
775. (A)
776. (B)
777. (C)
778. (B)
779. (C)
780. (A)
781. (A)
782. (B)
783. (C)
784. (A)
785. (D)
786. (A)
787. (C)
788. (D)
789. (D)
790. (B)
791. (A)
792. (A)
793. (B)
794. (B)
795. (D)
796. (C)
797. (D)
798. (A)
799. (C)
800. (C)
801. (D)
802. (D)
803. (A)
804. (D)
805. (D)
806. (A)
807. (D)
808. (C)
809. (D)
810. (C)
811. (B)
812. (C)
813. (C)
814. (C)
815. (C)
816. (B)
817. (A)
818. (D)
819. (D)
820. (B)
821. (C)
822. (A)
823. (B)
824. (A)
825. (D)
826. (A)
827. (D)
828. (A)
829. (B)
830. (C)
831. (D)
832. (B)
833. (C)
834. (D)
835. (A)
836. (C)
837. (B)
838. (A)
839. (B)
840. (C)
841. (B)
842. (A)
843. (A)
844. (D)
845. (B)
846. (C)
847. (A)
848. (B)
849. (D)
850. (B)
851. (C)
852. (D)
853. (A)
854. (C)
855. (B)
856. (A)
857. (D)
858. (A)
859. (D)
860. (D)
861. (D)
862. (D)
863. (D)
864. (B)
865. (D)
866. (A)
867. (C)
868. (D)
869. (B)
870. (A)

871. (B)
872. (C)
873. (D)
874. (A)
875. (C)
876. (B)
877. (B)
878. (D)
879. (C)
880. (B)
881. (C)
882. (C)
883. (B)
884. (A)
885. (C)
886. (B)
887. (A)
888. (C)
889. (B)
890. (B)
891. (C)
892. (A)
893. (B)
894. (B)
895. (A)
896. (D)
897. (C)
898. (B)
899. (A)
900. (A)
901. (B)
902. (A)
903. (C)
904. (D)
905. (A)
906. (A)
907. (B)
908. (C)
909. (B)
910. (A)
911. (A)
912. (D)
913. (C)
914. (B)
915. (D)
916. (D)
917. (A)
918. (A)
919. (A)
920. (A)
921. (A)
922. (B)
923. (C)
924. (C)
925. (A)
926. (C)
927. (D)
928. (D)
929. (B)
930. (D)
931. (A)
932. (D)
933. (A)
934. (D)
935. (A)
936. (A)
937. (A)
938. (B)
939. (B)
940. (B)
941. (A)
942. (D)
943. (D)
944. (B)
945. (A)
946. (C)
947. (D)
948. (A)
949. (B)
950. (B)
951. (D)
952. (D)
953. (A)
954. (D)
955. (D)
956. (C)
957. (D)
958. (B)
959. (D)
960. (D)
961. (A)
962. (C)
963. (B)
964. (A)
965. (B)
966. (D)
967. (C)
968. (D)
969. (A)
970. (D)
971. (B)
972. (B)
973. (C)
974. (D)
975. (B)
976. (A)
977. (B)
978. (D)
979. (D)
980. (D)
981. (C)
982. (D)
983. (B)
984. (A)
985. (D)
986. (D)
987. (A)
988. (C)
989. (B)
990. (B)
991. (A)
992. (A)
993. (A)
994. (B)
995. (B)
996. (C)
997. (D)
998. (D)
999. (A)
1000. (B)
1001. (C)
1002. (A)
1003. (B)
1004. (C)
1005. (C)
1006. (B)
1007. (C)
1008. (D)
1009. (B)
1010. (A)
1011. (D)
1012. (D)
1013. (A)
1014. (B)
1015. (D)
1016. (B)
1017. (C)
1018. (D)
1019. (B)
1020. (D)
1021. (C)
1022. (B)
1023. (C)
1024. (D)
1025. (D)
1026. (C)
1027. (A)
1028. (A)
1029. (B)
1030. (C)
1031. (A)
1032. (C)
1033. (A)
1034. (A)
1035. (A)
1036. (D)
1037. (A)
1038. (C)
1039. (A)
1040. (A)
1041. (A)
1042. (A)
1043. (D)
1044. (A)
1045. (B)
1046. (A)
1047. (A)
1048. (A)
1049. (B)
1050. (D)
1051. (C)
1052. (D)
1053. (A)
1054. (B)
1055. (A)
1056. (A)
1057. (D)
1058. (D)
1059. (D)
1060. (A)
1061. (A)
1062. (D)
1063. (A)
1064. (A)
1065. (D)
1066. (A)
1067. (A)
1068. (D)
1069. (A)
1070. (D)
1071. (C)
1072. (A)
1073. (A)
1074. (A)
1075. (A)
1076. (C)
1077. (D)
1078. (D)
1079. (A)
1080. (D)
1081. (C)
1082. (A)
1083. (D)
1084. (A)
1085. (A)
1086. (B)
1087. (D)
1088. (B)
1089. (C)
1090. (D)
1091. (D)
1092. (B)

1093.	(B)	1130.	(D)	1167.	(D)	1204.	(D)	1241.	(A)	1278.	(A)
1094.	(C)	1131.	(A)	1168.	(A)	1205.	(D)	1242.	(C)	1279.	(D)
1095.	(B)	1132.	(C)	1169.	(C)	1206.	(A)	1243.	(A)	1280.	(A)
1096.	(C)	1133.	(B)	1170.	(B)	1207.	(C)	1244.	(B)	1281.	(A)
1097.	(B)	1134.	(A)	1171.	(D)	1208.	(A)	1245.	(A)	1282.	(D)
1098.	(B)	1135.	(C)	1172.	(D)	1209.	(D)	1246.	(B)	1283.	(B)
1099.	(C)	1136.	(D)	1173.	(A)	1210.	(A)	1247.	(B)	1284.	(C)
1100.	(A)	1137.	(A)	1174.	(B)	1211.	(B)	1248.	(D)	1285.	(D)
1101.	(D)	1138.	(D)	1175.	(A)	1212.	(D)	1249.	(B)	1286.	(A)
1102.	(C)	1139.	(C)	1176.	(B)	1213.	(A)	1250.	(C)	1287.	(A)
1103.	(B)	1140.	(A)	1177.	(D)	1214.	(D)	1251.	(A)	1288.	(B)
1104.	(B)	1141.	(C)	1178.	(C)	1215.	(D)	1252.	(C)	1289.	(B)
1105.	(A)	1142.	(D)	1179.	(A)	1216.	(B)	1253.	(B)	1290.	(D)
1106.	(B)	1143.	(D)	1180.	(C)	1217.	(A)	1254.	(D)	1291.	(A)
1107.	(C)	1144.	(B)	1181.	(A)	1218.	(D)	1255.	(A)	1292.	(D)
1108.	(D)	1145.	(C)	1182.	(A)	1219.	(D)	1256.	(B)	1293.	(D)
1109.	(C)	1146.	(C)	1183.	(C)	1220.	(D)	1257.	(C)	1294.	(D)
1110.	(B)	1147.	(A)	1184.	(A)	1221.	(B)	1258.	(D)	1295.	(D)
1111.	(C)	1148.	(A)	1185.	(B)	1222.	(D)	1259.	(A)	1296.	(A)
1112.	(B)	1149.	(B)	1186.	(C)	1223.	(B)	1260.	(B)	1297.	(A)
1113.	(C)	1150.	(A)	1187.	(A)	1224.	(A)	1261.	(C)	1298.	(D)
1114.	(B)	1151.	(B)	1188.	(D)	1225.	(C)	1262.	(B)	1299.	(C)
1115.	(A)	1152.	(C)	1189.	(C)	1226.	(A)	1263.	(A)	1300.	(B)
1116.	(C)	1153.	(D)	1190.	(B)	1227.	(A)	1264.	(B)	1301.	(B)
1117.	(B)	1154.	(D)	1191.	(A)	1228.	(C)	1265.	(D)	1302.	(C)
1118.	(D)	1155.	(B)	1192.	(C)	1229.	(A)	1266.	(A)	1303.	(B)
1119.	(A)	1156.	(D)	1193.	(C)	1230.	(D)	1267.	(B)	1304.	(C)
1120.	(C)	1157.	(D)	1194.	(B)	1231.	(D)	1268.	(D)	1305.	(D)
1121.	(A)	1158.	(A)	1195.	(D)	1232.	(B)	1269.	(C)	1306.	(C)
1122.	(C)	1159.	(C)	1196.	(A)	1233.	(C)	1270.	(B)	1307.	(D)
1123.	(A)	1160.	(D)	1197.	(A)	1234.	(B)	1271.	(A)	1308.	(C)
1124.	(D)	1161.	(A)	1198.	(D)	1235.	(D)	1272.	(A)	1309.	(D)
1125.	(C)	1162.	(D)	1199.	(C)	1236.	(C)	1273.	(B)	1310.	(D)
1126.	(B)	1163.	(A)	1200.	(C)	1237.	(B)	1274.	(A)	1311.	(A)
1127.	(A)	1164.	(D)	1201.	(C)	1238.	(D)	1275.	(D)	1312.	(B)
1128.	(A)	1165.	(C)	1202.	(C)	1239.	(A)	1276.	(D)	1313.	(D)
1129.	(D)	1166.	(B)	1203.	(D)	1240.	(A)	1277.	(C)	1314.	(B)

1315. (C)
1316. (D)
1317. (B)
1318. (D)
1319. (A)
1320. (B)
1321. (C)
1322. (B)
1323. (C)
1324. (C)
1325. (D)
1326. (B)
1327. (C)
1328. (C)
1329. (D)
1330. (A)
1331. (C)
1332. (D)
1333. (C)
1334. (B)
1335. (D)
1336. (A)
1337. (B)
1338. (D)
1339. (A)
1340. (C)
1341. (A)
1342. (A)
1343. (B)
1344. (C)
1345. (D)
1346. (B)
1347. (A)
1348. (C)
1349. (D)
1350. (D)
1351. (D)
1352. (A)
1353. (A)
1354. (B)
1355. (D)
1356. (D)
1357. (A)
1358. (C)
1359. (D)
1360. (C)
1361. (D)
1362. (D)
1363. (D)
1364. (C)
1365. (D)
1366. (A)
1367. (D)
1368. (B)
1369. (D)
1370. (C)
1371. (D)
1372. (A)
1373. (B)
1374. (A)
1375. (D)
1376. (D)
1377. (D)
1378. (D)
1379. (C)
1380. (B)
1381. (C)
1382. (C)
1383. (C)
1384. (B)
1385. (B)
1386. (C)
1387. (A)
1388. (A)
1389. (A)
1390. (B)
1391. (B)
1392. (A)
1393. (B)
1394. (D)
1395. (C)
1396. (D)
1397. (A)
1398. (C)
1399. (D)
1400. (D)
1401. (D)
1402. (B)
1403. (C)
1404. (B)
1405. (D)
1406. (D)
1407. (A)
1408. (D)
1409. (A)
1410. (B)
1411. (C)
1412. (C)
1413. (D)
1414. (A)
1415. (B)
1416. (D)
1417. (B)
1418. (A)
1419. (C)
1420. (A)
1421. (D)
1422. (A)
1423. (C)
1424. (A)
1425. (B)
1426. (C)
1427. (D)
1428. (D)
1429. (D)
1430. (C)
1431. (D)
1432. (B)
1433. (A)
1434. (A)
1435. (D)
1436. (B)
1437. (A)
1438. (B)
1439. (C)
1440. (D)
1441. (B)
1442. (A)
1443. (C)
1444. (C)
1445. (A)
1446. (B)
1447. (B)
1448. (B)
1449. (B)
1450. (D)
1451. (D)
1452. (D)
1453. (C)
1454. (C)
1455. (B)
1456. (C)
1457. (C)
1458. (D)
1459. (C)
1460. (D)
1461. (B)
1462. (D)
1463. (A)
1464. (A)
1465. (C)
1466. (A)
1467. (B)
1468. (B)
1469. (C)
1470. (A)
1471. (D)
1472. (B)
1473. (B)
1474. (B)
1475. (B)
1476. (B)
1477. (A)
1478. (B)
1479. (B)
1480. (C)
1481. (B)
1482. (C)
1483. (D)
1484. (C)
1485. (B)
1486. (A)
1487. (C)
1488. (B)
1489. (B)
1490. (C)
1491. (D)
1492. (A)
1493. (D)
1494. (A)
1495. (B)
1496. (A)
1497. (B)
1498. (B)
1499. (D)
1500. (A)
1501. (C)
1502. (B)
1503. (D)
1504. (D)
1505. (C)
1506. (D)
1507. (A)
1508. (A)
1509. (C)
1510. (D)
1511. (A)
1512. (B)
1513. (A)
1514. (C)
1515. (B)
1516. (C)
1517. (C)
1518. (C)
1519. (A)
1520. (A)
1521. (D)
1522. (D)
1523. (B)
1524. (A)
1525. (B)
1526. (A)
1527. (B)
1528. (A)
1529. (A)
1530. (A)
1531. (A)
1532. (A)
1533. (B)
1534. (C)
1535. (A)
1536. (C)

1537. (B)
1538. (A)
1539. (A)
1540. (C)
1541. (A)
1542. (B)
1543. (B)
1544. (A)
1545. (B)
1546. (A)
1547. (C)
1548. (A)
1549. (A)
1550. (C)
1551. (A)
1552. (A)
1553. (C)
1554. (D)
1555. (B)
1556. (D)
1557. (D)
1558. (A)
1559. (D)
1560. (B)
1561. (D)
1562. (B)
1563. (D)
1564. (C)
1565. (C)
1566. (D)
1567. (A)
1568. (B)
1569. (D)
1570. (B)
1571. (C)
1572. (D)
1573. (A)
1574. (D)
1575. (B)
1576. (A)
1577. (D)
1578. (A)
1579. (B)
1580. (A)
1581. (D)
1582. (D)
1583. (B)
1584. (D)
1585. (D)
1586. (B)
1587. (D)
1588. (D)
1589. (D)
1590. (D)
1591. (A)
1592. (B)
1593. (A)
1594. (B)
1595. (C)
1596. (D)
1597. (D)
1598. (B)
1599. (D)
1600. (A)
1601. (A)
1602. (B)
1603. (A)
1604. (B)
1605. (D)
1606. (D)
1607. (D)
1608. (D)
1609. (C)
1610. (A)
1611. (A)
1612. (C)
1613. (A)
1614. (A)
1615. (B)
1616. (A)
1617. (A)
1618. (C)
1619. (D)
1620. (C)
1621. (A)
1622. (B)
1623. (B)
1624. (C)
1625. (B)
1626. (A)
1627. (D)
1628. (B)
1629. (A)
1630. (D)
1631. (B)
1632. (D)
1633. (D)
1634. (C)
1635. (C)
1636. (D)
1637. (A)
1638. (D)
1639. (D)
1640. (C)
1641. (C)
1642. (C)
1643. (C)
1644. (D)
1645. (D)
1646. (D)
1647. (D)
1648. (D)
1649. (B)
1650. (B)
1651. (D)
1652. (A)
1653. (D)
1654. (A)
1655. (C)
1656. (C)
1657. (C)
1658. (A)
1659. (B)
1660. (C)
1661. (C)
1662. (B)
1663. (D)
1664. (C)
1665. (C)
1666. (C)
1667. (B)
1668. (C)
1669. (C)
1670. (C)
1671. (D)
1672. (B)
1673. (B)
1674. (B)
1675. (C)
1676. (A)
1677. (D)
1678. (A)
1679. (D)
1680. (D)
1681. (B)
1682. (C)
1683. (B)
1684. (D)
1685. (D)
1686. (A)
1687. (A)
1688. (B)
1689. (D)
1690. (B)
1691. (D)
1692. (C)
1693. (B)
1694. (C)
1695. (B)
1696. (A)
1697. (D)
1698. (C)
1699. (B)
1700. (C)
1701. (B)
1702. (A)
1703. (A)
1704. (C)
1705. (A)
1706. (C)
1707. (A)
1708. (C)
1709. (B)
1710. (A)
1711. (B)
1712. (A)
1713. (C)
1714. (D)
1715. (A)
1716. (B)
1717. (B)
1718. (C)
1719. (B)
1720. (C)
1721. (A)
1722. (C)
1723. (A)
1724. (B)
1725. (B)
1726. (B)
1727. (B)
1728. (B)
1729. (B)
1730. (C)
1731. (C)
1732. (C)
1733. (D)
1734. (A)
1735. (C)
1736. (A)
1737. (B)
1738. (A)
1739. (C)
1740. (A)
1741. (A)
1742. (B)
1743. (A)
1744. (B)
1745. (D)
1746. (C)
1747. (A)
1748. (C)
1749. (D)
1750. (A)
1751. (B)
1752. (D)
1753. (C)
1754. (A)
1755. (C)
1756. (B)
1757. (A)
1758. (B)

1759. (A)
1760. (D)
1761. (B)
1762. (A)
1763. (B)
1764. (C)
1765. (B)
1766. (C)
1767. (C)
1768. (B)
1769. (B)
1770. (C)
1771. (C)
1772. (A)
1773. (B)
1774. (C)
1775. (D)
1776. (D)
1777. (A)
1778. (D)
1779. (D)
1780. (C)
1781. (A)
1782. (C)
1783. (A)
1784. (A)
1785. (B)
1786. (D)
1787. (A)
1788. (C)
1789. (B)
1790. (A)
1791. (B)
1792. (C)
1793. (A)
1794. (C)
1795. (A)
1796. (C)
1797. (A)
1798. (C)
1799. (A)
1800. (C)
1801. (A)
1802. (C)
1803. (D)
1804. (B)
1805. (A)
1806. (D)
1807. (A)
1808. (B)
1809. (A)
1810. (A)
1811. (D)
1812. (A)
1813. (C)
1814. (B)
1815. (D)
1816. (A)
1817. (A)
1818. (B)
1819. (D)
1820. (A)
1821. (D)
1822. (C)
1823. (D)
1824. (D)
1825. (A)
1826. (C)
1827. (B)
1828. (C)
1829. (A)
1830. (B)
1831. (D)
1832. (D)
1833. (A)
1834. (C)
1835. (A)
1836. (C)
1837. (D)
1838. (A)
1839. (C)
1840. (D)
1841. (A)
1842. (C)
1843. (B)
1844. (C)
1845. (A)
1846. (A)
1847. (C)
1848. (A)
1849. (C)
1850. (A)
1851. (D)
1852. (A)
1853. (C)
1854. (A)
1855. (A)
1856. (C)
1857. (A)
1858. (C)
1859. (A)
1860. (C)
1861. (A)
1862. (C)
1863. (A)
1864. (C)
1865. (A)
1866. (A)
1867. (C)
1868. (A)
1869. (A)
1870. (B)
1871. (A)
1872. (C)
1873. (B)
1874. (A)
1875. (B)
1876. (A)
1877. (C)
1878. (A)
1879. (B)
1880. (A)
1881. (C)
1882. (B)
1883. (A)
1884. (B)
1885. (C)
1886. (B)
1887. (C)
1888. (B)
1889. (C)
1890. (B)
1891. (D)
1892. (B)
1893. (C)
1894. (C)
1895. (A)
1896. (A)
1897. (C)
1898. (C)
1899. (D)
1900. (C)
1901. (A)
1902. (B)
1903. (D)
1904. (C)
1905. (A)
1906. (C)
1907. (A)
1908. (D)
1909. (D)
1910. (A)
1911. (C)
1912. (A)
1913. (D)
1914. (A)
1915. (B)
1916. (A)
1917. (D)
1918. (C)
1919. (B)
1920. (C)
1921. (A)
1922. (C)
1923. (A)
1924. (B)
1925. (A)
1926. (B)
1927. (A)
1928. (D)
1929. (C)
1930. (B)
1931. (A)
1932. (A)
1933. (C)
1934. (D)
1935. (A)
1936. (D)
1937. (A)
1938. (D)
1939. (B)
1940. (B)
1941. (A)
1942. (C)
1943. (B)
1944. (D)
1945. (A)
1946. (D)
1947. (A)
1948. (B)
1949. (D)
1950. (C)
1951. (A)
1952. (B)
1953. (A)
1954. (D)
1955. (A)
1956. (C)
1957. (C)
1958. (A)
1959. (B)
1960. (C)
1961. (A)
1962. (D)
1963. (A)
1964. (B)
1965. (C)
1966. (C)
1967. (B)
1968. (A)
1969. (B)
1970. (A)
1971. (B)
1972. (D)
1973. (A)
1974. (C)
1975. (C)
1976. (A)
1977. (A)
1978. (C)
1979. (D)
1980. (A)

1981. (C)
1982. (B)
1983. (A)
1984. (C)
1985. (B)
1986. (A)
1987. (A)
1988. (C)
1989. (D)
1990. (C)
1991. (A)
1992. (B)
1993. (A)
1994. (C)
1995. (C)
1996. (B)
1997. (B)
1998. (B)
1999. (A)
2000. (D)
2001. (A)
2002. (D)
2003. (B)
2004. (A)
2005. (C)
2006. (B)
2007. (A)
2008. (C)
2009. (A)
2010. (A)
2011. (C)
2012. (A)
2013. (C)
2014. (B)
2015. (D)
2016. (A)
2017. (A)
2018. (A)
2019. (A)
2020. (A)
2021. (A)
2022. (A)
2023. (C)
2024. (B)
2025. (B)
2026. (B)
2027. (B)
2028. (C)
2029. (A)
2030. (A)
2031. (A)
2032. (C)
2033. (C)
2034. (A)
2035. (B)
2036. (C)
2037. (C)
2038. (A)
2039. (A)
2040. (A)
2041. (C)
2042. (A)
2043. (D)
2044. (A)
2045. (C)
2046. (C)
2047. (A)
2048. (A)
2049. (A)
2050. (C)
2051. (C)
2052. (A)
2053. (A)
2054. (A)
2055. (A)
2056. (A)
2057. (C)
2058. (A)
2059. (A)
2060. (C)
2061. (A)
2062. (A)
2063. (A)
2064. (B)
2065. (A)
2066. (A)
2067. (A)
2068. (A)
2069. (A)
2070. (C)
2071. (A)
2072. (A)
2073. (A)
2074. (D)
2075. (A)
2076. (B)
2077. (A)
2078. (D)
2079. (A)
2080. (A)
2081. (C)
2082. (A)
2083. (A)
2084. (A)
2085. (B)
2086. (A)
2087. (A)
2088. (C)
2089. (B)
2090. (B)
2091. (A)
2092. (A)
2093. (B)
2094. (A)
2095. (A)
2096. (A)
2097. (A)
2098. (A)
2099. (C)
2100. (B)
2101. (B)
2102. (B)
2103. (B)
2104. (C)
2105. (A)
2106. (A)
2107. (A)
2108. (A)
2109. (C)
2110. (A)
2111. (A)
2112. (B)
2113. (A)
2114. (A)
2115. (A)
2116. (A)
2117. (A)
2118. (B)
2119. (A)
2120. (B)
2121. (B)
2122. (C)
2123. (A)
2124. (B)
2125. (C)
2126. (A)
2127. (D)
2128. (A)
2129. (B)
2130. (C)
2131. (D)
2132. (A)
2133. (B)
2134. (C)
2135. (D)
2136. (A)
2137. (B)
2138. (C)
2139. (D)
2140. (A)
2141. (C)
2142. (A)
2143. (A)
2144. (A)
2145. (A)
2146. (A)
2147. (B)
2148. (A)
2149. (A)
2150. (A)
2151. (A)
2152. (A)
2153. (A)
2154. (A)
2155. (A)
2156. (A)
2157. (A)
2158. (A)
2159. (A)
2160. (A)
2161. (B)
2162. (C)
2163. (D)
2164. (A)
2165. (A)
2166. (B)
2167. (A)
2168. (A)
2169. (A)
2170. (B)
2171. (C)
2172. (D)
2173. (A)
2174. (B)
2175. (C)
2176. (D)
2177. (B)
2178. (A)
2179. (C)
2180. (B)
2181. (A)
2182. (A)
2183. (D)
2184. (A)
2185. (A)
2186. (D)
2187. (A)
2188. (D)
2189. (C)
2190. (C)
2191. (A)
2192. (A)
2193. (A)
2194. (A)
2195. (A)
2196. (A)
2197. (B)
2198. (B)
2199. (D)
2200. (A)
2201. (B)
2202. (C)

2203. (A)
2204. (D)
2205. (C)
2206. (B)
2207. (A)
2208. (A)
2209. (B)
2210. (A)
2211. (A)
2212. (A)
2213. (A)
2214. (A)
2215. (A)
2216. (A)
2217. (A)
2218. (B)
2219. (A)
2220. (A)
2221. (A)
2222. (A)
2223. (A)
2224. (B)
2225. (C)
2226. (A)
2227. (C)
2228. (D)
2229. (C)
2230. (A)
2231. (A)
2232. (A)
2233. (A)
2234. (A)
2235. (A)
2236. (A)
2237. (D)
2238. (A)
2239. (C)
2240. (B)
2241. (D)
2242. (B)
2243. (C)
2244. (A)
2245. (C)
2246. (B)
2247. (D)
2248. (B)
2249. (C)
2250. (A)
2251. (C)
2252. (C)
2253. (B)
2254. (A)
2255. (D)
2256. (C)
2257. (B)
2258. (A)
2259. (C)
2260. (B)
2261. (C)
2262. (A)
2263. (C)
2264. (B)
2265. (B)
2266. (A)
2267. (D)
2268. (C)
2269. (A)
2270. (B)
2271. (B)
2272. (A)
2273. (D)
2274. (A)
2275. (A)
2276. (A)
2277. (A)
2278. (B)
2279. (B)
2280. (B)
2281. (D)
2282. (B)
2283. (A)
2284. (A)
2285. (C)
2286. (A)
2287. (A)
2288. (A)
2289. (A)
2290. (A)
2291. (A)
2292. (C)
2293. (B)
2294. (A)
2295. (D)
2296. (A)
2297. (D)
2298. (C)
2299. (A)
2300. (B)
2301. (A)
2302. (A)
2303. (C)
2304. (C)
2305. (C)
2306. (D)
2307. (D)
2308. (D)
2309. (A)
2310. (B)
2311. (D)
2312. (B)
2313. (A)
2314. (B)
2315. (D)
2316. (C)
2317. (C)
2318. (A)
2319. (C)
2320. (A)
2321. (D)
2322. (A)
2323. (D)
2324. (A)
2325. (B)
2326. (B)
2327. (A)
2328. (A)
2329. (B)
2330. (D)
2331. (C)
2332. (D)
2333. (C)
2334. (B)
2335. (A)
2336. (C)
2337. (C)
2338. (A)
2339. (C)
2340. (C)
2341. (A)
2342. (A)
2343. (B)
2344. (C)
2345. (A)
2346. (D)
2347. (C)
2348. (D)
2349. (D)
2350. (D)
2351. (A)
2352. (D)
2353. (A)
2354. (C)
2355. (B)
2356. (B)
2357. (B)
2358. (A)
2359. (B)
2360. (A)
2361. (A)
2362. (B)
2363. (A)
2364. (D)
2365. (B)
2366. (C)
2367. (A)
2368. (B)
2369. (A)
2370. (A)
2371. (A)
2372. (B)
2373. (D)
2374. (B)
2375. (A)
2376. (B)
2377. (D)
2378. (A)
2379. (B)
2380. (D)
2381. (C)
2382. (C)
2383. (D)
2384. (A)
2385. (A)
2386. (C)
2387. (D)
2388. (A)
2389. (A)
2390. (B)
2391. (A)
2392. (C)
2393. (D)
2394. (B)
2395. (A)
2396. (C)
2397. (C)
2398. (D)
2399. (A)
2400. (B)
2401. (C)
2402. (B)
2403. (A)
2404. (B)
2405. (D)
2406. (A)
2407. (C)
2408. (C)
2409. (D)
2410. (A)
2411. (B)
2412. (C)
2413. (A)
2414. (D)
2415. (A)
2416. (B)
2417. (A)
2418. (B)
2419. (A)
2420. (C)
2421. (B)
2422. (B)
2423. (A)
2424. (A)

2425. (C)
2426. (D)
2427. (A)
2428. (B)
2429. (D)
2430. (C)
2431. (B)
2432. (C)
2433. (B)
2434. (A)
2435. (B)
2436. (B)
2437. (C)
2438. (A)
2439. (C)
2440. (A)
2441. (D)
2442. (B)
2443. (C)
2444. (B)
2445. (C)
2446. (D)
2447. (C)
2448. (B)
2449. (C)
2450. (B)
2451. (A)
2452. (B)
2453. (B)
2454. (B)
2455. (A)
2456. (C)
2457. (C)
2458. (B)
2459. (B)
2460. (B)
2461. (A)
2462. (A)
2463. (B)
2464. (A)
2465. (C)
2466. (C)
2467. (D)
2468. (B)
2469. (A)
2470. (A)
2471. (C)
2472. (B)
2473. (C)
2474. (A)
2475. (B)
2476. (B)
2477. (C)
2478. (C)
2479. (B)
2480. (A)
2481. (B)
2482. (C)
2483. (B)
2484. (A)
2485. (C)
2486. (B)
2487. (C)
2488. (A)
2489. (B)
2490. (B)
2491. (B)
2492. (C)
2493. (A)
2494. (C)
2495. (B)
2496. (B)
2497. (C)
2498. (C)
2499. (C)
2500. (B)
2501. (B)
2502. (C)
2503. (B)
2504. (A)
2505. (B)
2506. (A)
2507. (D)
2508. (D)
2509. (B)
2510. (B)
2511. (B)
2512. (A)
2513. (C)
2514. (A)
2515. (C)
2516. (C)
2517. (B)
2518. (C)
2519. (B)
2520. (A)
2521. (B)
2522. (B)
2523. (A)
2524. (B)
2525. (A)
2526. (C)
2527. (A)
2528. (D)
2529. (D)
2530. (B)
2531. (D)
2532. (D)
2533. (C)
2534. (B)
2535. (A)
2536. (A)
2537. (D)
2538. (B)
2539. (C)
2540. (B)
2541. (B)
2542. (A)
2543. (A)
2544. (D)
2545. (A)
2546. (C)
2547. (A)
2548. (B)
2549. (A)
2550. (A)
2551. (B)
2552. (C)
2553. (A)
2554. (B)
2555. (A)
2556. (D)
2557. (C)
2558. (D)
2559. (B)
2560. (B)
2561. (D)
2562. (A)
2563. (C)
2564. (A)
2565. (A)
2566. (A)
2567. (C)
2568. (D)
2569. (C)
2570. (C)
2571. (B)
2572. (C)
2573. (C)
2574. (A)
2575. (A)
2576. (B)
2577. (C)
2578. (C)
2579. (C)
2580. (A)
2581. (A)
2582. (D)
2583. (A)
2584. (D)
2585. (D)
2586. (A)
2587. (D)
2588. (B)
2589. (D)
2590. (C)
2591. (B)
2592. (C)
2593. (C)
2594. (D)
2595. (D)
2596. (B)
2597. (A)
2598. (D)
2599. (C)
2600. (D)
2601. (D)
2602. (D)
2603. (B)
2604. (A)
2605. (D)
2606. (B)
2607. (C)
2608. (C)
2609. (B)
2610. (D)
2611. (B)
2612. (C)
2613. (B)
2614. (B)
2615. (B)
2616. (A)
2617. (C)
2618. (B)
2619. (B)
2620. (A)
2621. (B)
2622. (C)
2623. (A)
2624. (C)
2625. (A)
2626. (C)
2627. (C)
2628. (D)
2629. (B)
2630. (B)
2631. (C)
2632. (D)
2633. (D)
2634. (B)
2635. (A)
2636. (C)
2637. (D)
2638. (B)
2639. (A)
2640. (C)
2641. (D)
2642. (A)
2643. (C)
2644. (A)
2645. (C)
2646. (D)

2647. (B)
2648. (A)
2649. (D)
2650. (D)
2651. (C)
2652. (D)
2653. (C)
2654. (A)
2655. (D)
2656. (C)
2657. (D)
2658. (A)
2659. (B)
2660. (A)
2661. (C)
2662. (C)
2663. (D)
2664. (C)
2665. (D)
2666. (D)
2667. (A)
2668. (B)
2669. (A)
2670. (D)
2671. (C)
2672. (A)
2673. (C)
2674. (D)
2675. (A)
2676. (B)
2677. (B)
2678. (C)
2679. (A)
2680. (A)
2681. (B)
2682. (D)
2683. (D)
2684. (C)
2685. (A)
2686. (B)
2687. (D)
2688. (A)
2689. (A)
2690. (A)
2691. (B)
2692. (D)
2693. (A)
2694. (D)
2695. (C)
2696. (D)
2697. (D)
2698. (B)
2699. (D)
2700. (A)
2701. (C)
2702. (A)
2703. (B)
2704. (D)
2705. (B)
2706. (A)
2707. (C)
2708. (C)
2709. (C)
2710. (B)
2711. (C)
2712. (A)
2713. (A)
2714. (D)
2715. (B)
2716. (D)
2717. (B)
2718. (B)
2719. (B)
2720. (A)
2721. (D)
2722. (B)
2723. (A)
2724. (D)
2725. (C)
2726. (C)
2727. (A)
2728. (C)
2729. (A)
2730. (D)
2731. (D)
2732. (D)
2733. (B)
2734. (B)
2735. (A)
2736. (D)
2737. (C)
2738. (C)
2739. (C)
2740. (D)
2741. (D)
2742. (B)
2743. (C)
2744. (A)
2745. (D)
2746. (B)
2747. (C)
2748. (A)
2749. (C)
2750. (D)
2751. (B)
2752. (D)
2753. (A)
2754. (B)
2755. (A)
2756. (B)
2757. (C)
2758. (C)
2759. (B)
2760. (B)
2761. (D)
2762. (D)
2763. (C)
2764. (D)
2765. (C)
2766. (B)
2767. (C)
2768. (C)
2769. (B)
2770. (A)
2771. (C)
2772. (C)
2773. (A)
2774. (B)
2775. (A)
2776. (B)
2777. (C)
2778. (A)
2779. (A)
2780. (A)
2781. (C)
2782. (C)
2783. (B)
2784. (A)
2785. (C)
2786. (D)
2787. (D)
2788. (A)
2789. (D)
2790. (B)
2791. (C)
2792. (A)
2793. (D)
2794. (D)
2795. (B)
2796. (C)
2797. (A)
2798. (D)
2799. (C)
2800. (D)
2801. (A)
2802. (D)
2803. (D)
2804. (D)
2805. (A)
2806. (B)
2807. (B)
2808. (C)
2809. (B)
2810. (B)
2811. (C)
2812. (C)
2813. (A)
2814. (B)
2815. (B)
2816. (D)
2817. (C)
2818. (A)
2819. (C)
2820. (C)
2821. (A)
2822. (A)
2823. (B)
2824. (D)
2825. (B)
2826. (A)
2827. (A)
2828. (D)
2829. (B)
2830. (B)
2831. (A)
2832. (D)
2833. (B)
2834. (D)
2835. (B)
2836. (B)
2837. (A)
2838. (D)
2839. (C)
2840. (A)
2841. (A)
2842. (C)
2843. (D)
2844. (C)
2845. (B)
2846. (D)
2847. (A)
2848. (A)
2849. (C)
2850. (B)
2851. (D)
2852. (A)
2853. (C)
2854. (B)
2855. (C)
2856. (A)
2857. (D)
2858. (B)
2859. (D)
2860. (A)
2861. (B)
2862. (C)
2863. (A)
2864. (B)
2865. (C)
2866. (A)
2867. (C)
2868. (B)

2869.	(A)	2906.	(C)	2943.	(B)	2980.	(D)	3017.	(A)	3054.	(B)
2870.	(B)	2907.	(A)	2944.	(C)	2981.	(B)	3018.	(D)	3055.	(A)
2871.	(C)	2908.	(B)	2945.	(A)	2982.	(C)	3019.	(A)	3056.	(C)
2872.	(A)	2909.	(A)	2946.	(B)	2983.	(B)	3020.	(D)	3057.	(B)
2873.	(B)	2910.	(B)	2947.	(C)	2984.	(D)	3021.	(D)	3058.	(A)
2874.	(D)	2911.	(D)	2948.	(D)	2985.	(D)	3022.	(B)	3059.	(C)
2875.	(A)	2912.	(B)	2949.	(B)	2986.	(D)	3023.	(A)	3060.	(D)
2876.	(A)	2913.	(A)	2950.	(A)	2987.	(C)	3024.	(B)	3061.	(B)
2877.	(C)	2914.	(C)	2951.	(B)	2988.	(D)	3025.	(D)	3062.	(C)
2878.	(A)	2915.	(A)	2952.	(D)	2989.	(C)	3026.	(D)	3063.	(C)
2879.	(B)	2916.	(A)	2953.	(B)	2990.	(A)	3027.	(A)	3064.	(B)
2880.	(A)	2917.	(A)	2954.	(C)	2991.	(D)	3028.	(D)	3065.	(C)
2881.	(A)	2918.	(B)	2955.	(B)	2992.	(D)	3029.	(A)	3066.	(D)
2882.	(B)	2919.	(C)	2956.	(A)	2993.	(D)	3030.	(A)	3067.	(B)
2883.	(C)	2920.	(A)	2957.	(C)	2994.	(A)	3031.	(B)	3068.	(D)
2884.	(B)	2921.	(C)	2958.	(B)	2995.	(A)	3032.	(B)	3069.	(B)
2885.	(D)	2922.	(D)	2959.	(B)	2996.	(C)	3033.	(C)	3070.	(A)
2886.	(A)	2923.	(B)	2960.	(C)	2997.	(C)	3034.	(C)	3071.	(C)
2887.	(A)	2924.	(A)	2961.	(A)	2998.	(A)	3035.	(C)	3072.	(C)
2888.	(B)	2925.	(C)	2962.	(D)	2999.	(A)	3036.	(C)	3073.	(D)
2889.	(A)	2926.	(C)	2963.	(B)	3000.	(D)	3037.	(C)	3074.	(B)
2890.	(A)	2927.	(B)	2964.	(B)	3001.	(C)	3038.	(B)	3075.	(A)
2891.	(A)	2928.	(D)	2965.	(A)	3002.	(A)	3039.	(A)	3076.	(B)
2892.	(B)	2929.	(C)	2966.	(C)	3003.	(A)	3040.	(B)	3077.	(D)
2893.	(C)	2930.	(B)	2967.	(C)	3004.	(A)	3041.	(B)	3078.	(A)
2894.	(A)	2931.	(D)	2968.	(B)	3005.	(B)	3042.	(B)	3079.	(A)
2895.	(D)	2932.	(A)	2969.	(D)	3006.	(D)	3043.	(B)	3080.	(C)
2896.	(A)	2933.	(C)	2970.	(A)	3007.	(A)	3044.	(A)	3081.	(C)
2897.	(A)	2934.	(D)	2971.	(B)	3008.	(C)	3045.	(A)	3082.	(B)
2898.	(A)	2935.	(A)	2972.	(B)	3009.	(C)	3046.	(D)	3083.	(D)
2899.	(A)	2936.	(A)	2973.	(D)	3010.	(D)	3047.	(A)	3084.	(C)
2900.	(A)	2937.	(A)	2974.	(C)	3011.	(A)	3048.	(B)	3085.	(D)
2901.	(B)	2938.	(D)	2975.	(B)	3012.	(D)	3049.	(D)	3086.	(B)
2902.	(A)	2939.	(A)	2976.	(A)	3013.	(A)	3050.	(C)	3087.	(A)
2903.	(B)	2940.	(A)	2977.	(B)	3014.	(D)	3051.	(D)	3088.	(A)
2904.	(A)	2941.	(C)	2978.	(C)	3015.	(A)	3052.	(C)	3089.	(D)
2905.	(A)	2942.	(A)	2979.	(A)	3016.	(B)	3053.	(A)	3090.	(C)

3091. (D)
3092. (A)
3093. (A)
3094. (D)
3095. (A)
3096. (A)
3097. (D)
3098. (A)
3099. (A)
3100. (A)
3101. (B)
3102. (A)
3103. (A)
3104. (D)
3105. (C)
3106. (C)
3107. (D)
3108. (A)
3109. (B)
3110. (A)
3111. (D)
3112. (B)
3113. (A)
3114. (B)
3115. (A)
3116. (C)
3117. (C)
3118. (D)
3119. (B)
3120. (B)
3121. (A)
3122. (B)
3123. (A)
3124. (A)
3125. (A)
3126. (A)
3127. (A)
3128. (A)
3129. (A)
3130. (A)
3131. (A)
3132. (C)
3133. (C)
3134. (A)
3135. (C)
3136. (A)
3137. (A)
3138. (A)
3139. (D)
3140. (A)
3141. (D)
3142. (D)
3143. (A)
3144. (A)
3145. (A)
3146. (D)
3147. (A)
3148. (A)
3149. (B)
3150. (A)
3151. (B)
3152. (A)
3153. (D)
3154. (A)
3155. (C)
3156. (C)
3157. (D)
3158. (C)
3159. (C)
3160. (A)
3161. (A)
3162. (D)
3163. (A)
3164. (A)
3165. (C)
3166. (D)
3167. (A)
3168. (D)
3169. (C)
3170. (D)
3171. (B)
3172. (C)
3173. (D)
3174. (B)
3175. (A)
3176. (B)
3177. (C)
3178. (C)
3179. (D)
3180. (B)
3181. (C)
3182. (D)
3183. (A)
3184. (B)
3185. (C)
3186. (B)
3187. (B)
3188. (C)
3189. (D)
3190. (C)
3191. (C)
3192. (C)
3193. (D)
3194. (A)
3195. (B)
3196. (A)
3197. (D)
3198. (C)
3199. (A)
3200. (C)
3201. (B)
3202. (B)
3203. (C)
3204. (B)
3205. (C)
3206. (D)
3207. (D)
3208. (C)
3209. (D)
3210. (A)
3211. (B)
3212. (B)
3213. (C)
3214. (C)
3215. (B)
3216. (C)
3217. (B)
3218. (A)
3219. (B)
3220. (B)
3221. (A)
3222. (A)
3223. (D)
3224. (C)
3225. (B)
3226. (B)
3227. (C)
3228. (B)
3229. (B)
3230. (A)
3231. (B)
3232. (C)
3233. (C)
3234. (C)
3235. (B)
3236. (A)
3237. (B)
3238. (D)
3239. (C)
3240. (B)
3241. (B)
3242. (B)
3243. (A)
3244. (C)
3245. (D)
3246. (A)
3247. (C)
3248. (B)
3249. (D)
3250. (B)
3251. (D)
3252. (B)
3253. (A)
3254. (B)
3255. (C)
3256. (A)
3257. (D)
3258. (B)
3259. (D)
3260. (A)
3261. (B)
3262. (A)
3263. (C)
3264. (B)
3265. (B)
3266. (C)
3267. (A)
3268. (C)
3269. (A)
3270. (C)
3271. (D)
3272. (C)
3273. (C)
3274. (C)
3275. (C)
3276. (B)
3277. (D)
3278. (B)
3279. (C)
3280. (D)
3281. (A)
3282. (B)
3283. (A)
3284. (A)
3285. (D)
3286. (D)
3287. (A)
3288. (A)
3289. (D)
3290. (B)
3291. (A)
3292. (B)
3293. (B)
3294. (A)
3295. (A)
3296. (A)
3297. (A)
3298. (B)
3299. (C)
3300. (B)
3301. (A)
3302. (A)
3303. (B)
3304. (B)
3305. (A)
3306. (A)
3307. (B)
3308. (A)
3309. (C)
3310. (B)
3311. (A)
3312. (A)

3313.	(B)	3350.	(B)	3387.	(D)	3424.	(C)	3461.	(A)	3498.	(D)
3314.	(D)	3351.	(A)	3388.	(D)	3425.	(A)	3462.	(B)	3499.	(A)
3315.	(A)	3352.	(A)	3389.	(C)	3426.	(B)	3463.	(A)	3500.	(A)
3316.	(A)	3353.	(D)	3390.	(A)	3427.	(C)	3464.	(C)	3501.	(C)
3317.	(A)	3354.	(A)	3391.	(B)	3428.	(B)	3465.	(A)	3502.	(C)
3318.	(A)	3355.	(B)	3392.	(C)	3429.	(B)	3466.	(A)	3503.	(A)
3319.	(A)	3356.	(A)	3393.	(B)	3430.	(B)	3467.	(C)	3504.	(C)
3320.	(A)	3357.	(B)	3394.	(C)	3431.	(A)	3468.	(B)	3505.	(A)
3321.	(C)	3358.	(A)	3395.	(B)	3432.	(A)	3469.	(A)	3506.	(A)
3322.	(C)	3359.	(A)	3396.	(C)	3433.	(B)	3470.	(B)	3507.	(C)
3323.	(A)	3360.	(B)	3397.	(B)	3434.	(B)	3471.	(A)	3508.	(A)
3324.	(C)	3361.	(C)	3398.	(C)	3435.	(B)	3472.	(B)	3509.	(A)
3325.	(A)	3362.	(D)	3399.	(B)	3436.	(B)	3473.	(B)	3510.	(B)
3326.	(D)	3363.	(C)	3400.	(C)	3437.	(A)	3474.	(C)	3511.	(D)
3327.	(A)	3364.	(A)	3401.	(D)	3438.	(C)	3475.	(B)	3512.	(B)
3328.	(B)	3365.	(D)	3402.	(B)	3439.	(B)	3476.	(C)	3513.	(D)
3329.	(A)	3366.	(A)	3403.	(A)	3440.	(B)	3477.	(D)	3514.	(B)
3330.	(A)	3367.	(D)	3404.	(C)	3441.	(A)	3478.	(A)	3515.	(C)
3331.	(D)	3368.	(A)	3405.	(C)	3442.	(B)	3479.	(B)	3516.	(B)
3332.	(B)	3369.	(C)	3406.	(A)	3443.	(B)	3480.	(A)	3517.	(A)
3333.	(A)	3370.	(A)	3407.	(B)	3444.	(C)	3481.	(A)	3518.	(D)
3334.	(D)	3371.	(A)	3408.	(B)	3445.	(B)	3482.	(A)	3519.	(C)
3335.	(D)	3372.	(A)	3409.	(A)	3446.	(D)	3483.	(B)	3520.	(C)
3336.	(A)	3373.	(A)	3410.	(B)	3447.	(C)	3484.	(A)	3521.	(B)
3337.	(A)	3374.	(B)	3411.	(C)	3448.	(A)	3485.	(D)	3522.	(C)
3338.	(A)	3375.	(D)	3412.	(B)	3449.	(B)	3486.	(B)	3523.	(A)
3339.	(B)	3376.	(D)	3413.	(A)	3450.	(B)	3487.	(D)	3524.	(C)
3340.	(D)	3377.	(A)	3414.	(A)	3451.	(A)	3488.	(B)	3525.	(B)
3341.	(C)	3378.	(B)	3415.	(A)	3452.	(B)	3489.	(C)	3526.	(C)
3342.	(A)	3379.	(A)	3416.	(A)	3453.	(B)	3490.	(A)	3527.	(D)
3343.	(A)	3380.	(C)	3417.	(A)	3454.	(C)	3491.	(B)	3528.	(A)
3344.	(D)	3381.	(B)	3418.	(B)	3455.	(B)	3492.	(D)	3529.	(D)
3345.	(A)	3382.	(C)	3419.	(A)	3456.	(A)	3493.	(B)	3530.	(C)
3346.	(B)	3383.	(A)	3420.	(A)	3457.	(D)	3494.	(A)	3531.	(D)
3347.	(A)	3384.	(C)	3421.	(C)	3458.	(C)	3495.	(A)	3532.	(A)
3348.	(B)	3385.	(D)	3422.	(D)	3459.	(A)	3496.	(D)	3533.	(A)
3349.	(D)	3386.	(B)	3423.	(D)	3460.	(A)	3497.	(C)	3534.	(C)

3535. (C)
3536. (B)
3537. (B)
3538. (C)
3539. (A)
3540. (B)
3541. (C)
3542. (B)
3543. (A)
3544. (B)
3545. (B)
3546. (D)
3547. (D)
3548. (A)
3549. (A)
3550. (A)
3551. (C)
3552. (B)
3553. (B)
3554. (D)
3555. (A)
3556. (D)
3557. (D)
3558. (D)
3559. (B)
3560. (C)
3561. (D)
3562. (D)
3563. (A)
3564. (B)
3565. (D)
3566. (A)
3567. (D)
3568. (B)
3569. (A)
3570. (D)
3571. (D)
3572. (C)
3573. (B)
3574. (D)
3575. (D)
3576. (A)
3577. (C)
3578. (C)
3579. (B)
3580. (A)
3581. (D)
3582. (A)
3583. (C)
3584. (C)
3585. (A)
3586. (B)
3587. (D)
3588. (D)
3589. (A)
3590. (C)
3591. (D)
3592. (D)
3593. (C)
3594. (C)
3595. (D)
3596. (D)
3597. (B)
3598. (A)
3599. (C)
3600. (D)
3601. (A)
3602. (B)
3603. (C)
3604. (C)
3605. (A)
3606. (C)
3607. (A)
3608. (A)
3609. (D)
3610. (D)
3611. (A)
3612. (C)
3613. (D)
3614. (C)
3615. (A)
3616. (C)
3617. (B)
3618. (D)
3619. (D)
3620. (A)
3621. (C)
3622. (D)
3623. (A)
3624. (B)
3625. (B)
3626. (C)
3627. (A)
3628. (C)
3629. (A)
3630. (B)
3631. (D)
3632. (B)
3633. (A)
3634. (C)
3635. (B)
3636. (D)
3637. (C)
3638. (A)
3639. (A)
3640. (B)
3641. (D)
3642. (C)
3643. (A)
3644. (C)
3645. (D)
3646. (D)
3647. (C)
3648. (A)
3649. (B)
3650. (C)
3651. (C)
3652. (D)
3653. (C)
3654. (A)
3655. (A)
3656. (C)
3657. (A)
3658. (A)
3659. (C)
3660. (B)
3661. (D)
3662. (A)
3663. (D)
3664. (B)
3665. (D)
3666. (B)
3667. (A)
3668. (A)
3669. (D)
3670. (A)
3671. (D)
3672. (D)
3673. (A)
3674. (A)
3675. (B)
3676. (B)
3677. (A)
3678. (A)
3679. (B)
3680. (A)
3681. (B)
3682. (A)
3683. (C)
3684. (A)
3685. (A)
3686. (B)
3687. (D)
3688. (A)
3689. (A)
3690. (C)
3691. (C)
3692. (D)
3693. (A)
3694. (A)
3695. (C)
3696. (A)
3697. (B)
3698. (A)
3699. (A)
3700. (B)
3701. (A)
3702. (C)
3703. (A)
3704. (B)
3705. (A)
3706. (B)
3707. (A)
3708. (A)
3709. (A)
3710. (D)
3711. (B)
3712. (C)
3713. (D)
3714. (C)
3715. (A)
3716. (A)
3717. (C)
3718. (B)
3719. (D)
3720. (A)
3721. (A)
3722. (B)
3723. (B)
3724. (C)
3725. (C)
3726. (C)
3727. (D)
3728. (D)
3729. (B)
3730. (C)
3731. (C)
3732. (C)
3733. (D)
3734. (D)
3735. (C)
3736. (A)
3737. (C)
3738. (B)
3739. (D)
3740. (D)
3741. (D)
3742. (D)
3743. (B)
3744. (C)
3745. (B)
3746. (C)
3747. (D)
3748. (A)
3749. (B)
3750. (A)
3751. (B)
3752. (D)
3753. (A)
3754. (D)
3755. (A)
3756. (B)

3757.	(C)	3794.	(C)	3831.	(D)	3868.	(C)	3905.	(A)	3942.	(D)
3758.	(D)	3795.	(D)	3832.	(D)	3869.	(C)	3906.	(C)	3943.	(A)
3759.	(A)	3796.	(D)	3833.	(A)	3870.	(A)	3907.	(A)	3944.	(C)
3760.	(D)	3797.	(A)	3834.	(C)	3871.	(B)	3908.	(B)	3945.	(C)
3761.	(D)	3798.	(C)	3835.	(C)	3872.	(C)	3909.	(D)	3946.	(A)
3762.	(A)	3799.	(C)	3836.	(D)	3873.	(A)	3910.	(C)	3947.	(A)
3763.	(A)	3800.	(D)	3837.	(D)	3874.	(C)	3911.	(D)	3948.	(C)
3764.	(D)	3801.	(D)	3838.	(A)	3875.	(A)	3912.	(A)	3949.	(A)
3765.	(A)	3802.	(A)	3839.	(C)	3876.	(C)	3913.	(D)	3950.	(D)
3766.	(D)	3803.	(C)	3840.	(D)	3877.	(A)	3914.	(A)	3951.	(B)
3767.	(D)	3804.	(D)	3841.	(A)	3878.	(A)	3915.	(B)	3952.	(D)
3768.	(A)	3805.	(A)	3842.	(C)	3879.	(B)	3916.	(B)	3953.	(A)
3769.	(D)	3806.	(C)	3843.	(C)	3880.	(D)	3917.	(C)	3954.	(C)
3770.	(A)	3807.	(C)	3844.	(A)	3881.	(A)	3918.	(A)	3955.	(A)
3771.	(B)	3808.	(A)	3845.	(A)	3882.	(A)	3919.	(A)	3956.	(C)
3772.	(A)	3809.	(A)	3846.	(A)	3883.	(B)	3920.	(D)	3957.	(C)
3773.	(D)	3810.	(A)	3847.	(D)	3884.	(D)	3921.	(A)	3958.	(B)
3774.	(B)	3811.	(D)	3848.	(D)	3885.	(D)	3922.	(A)	3959.	(D)
3775.	(A)	3812.	(D)	3849.	(C)	3886.	(D)	3923.	(A)	3960.	(A)
3776.	(B)	3813.	(C)	3850.	(A)	3887.	(C)	3924.	(A)	3961.	(C)
3777.	(D)	3814.	(A)	3851.	(B)	3888.	(A)	3925.	(A)	3962.	(A)
3778.	(A)	3815.	(A)	3852.	(A)	3889.	(A)	3926.	(C)	3963.	(B)
3779.	(A)	3816.	(D)	3853.	(A)	3890.	(C)	3927.	(A)	3964.	(A)
3780.	(D)	3817.	(C)	3854.	(C)	3891.	(D)	3928.	(A)	3965.	(C)
3781.	(C)	3818.	(A)	3855.	(B)	3892.	(C)	3929.	(B)	3966.	(C)
3782.	(A)	3819.	(A)	3856.	(A)	3893.	(D)	3930.	(A)	3967.	(A)
3783.	(A)	3820.	(A)	3857.	(A)	3894.	(A)	3931.	(A)	3968.	(A)
3784.	(A)	3821.	(B)	3858.	(A)	3895.	(A)	3932.	(A)	3969.	(A)
3785.	(B)	3822.	(B)	3859.	(D)	3896.	(C)	3933.	(A)	3970.	(A)
3786.	(B)	3823.	(D)	3860.	(A)	3897.	(A)	3934.	(A)	3971.	(D)
3787.	(D)	3824.	(A)	3861.	(A)	3898.	(C)	3935.	(B)	3972.	(D)
3788.	(A)	3825.	(D)	3862.	(D)	3899.	(C)	3936.	(D)	3973.	(D)
3789.	(D)	3826.	(C)	3863.	(A)	3900.	(C)	3937.	(A)	3974.	(C)
3790.	(C)	3827.	(A)	3864.	(C)	3901.	(D)	3938.	(C)	3975.	(A)
3791.	(A)	3828.	(C)	3865.	(A)	3902.	(A)	3939.	(C)	3976.	(A)
3792.	(C)	3829.	(D)	3866.	(C)	3903.	(A)	3940.	(C)	3977.	(C)
3793.	(D)	3830.	(C)	3867.	(D)	3904.	(A)	3941.	(C)	3978.	(A)

3979. (C)
3980. (D)
3981. (D)
3982. (A)
3983. (C)
3984. (A)
3985. (A)
3986. (A)
3987. (A)
3988. (B)
3989. (A)
3990. (C)
3991. (D)
3992. (A)
3993. (C)
3994. (C)
3995. (D)
3996. (C)
3997. (A)
3998. (A)
3999. (D)
4000. (A)
4001. (D)
4002. (A)
4003. (B)
4004. (C)
4005. (C)
4006. (C)
4007. (A)
4008. (A)
4009. (D)
4010. (A)
4011. (D)
4012. (D)
4013. (C)
4014. (D)
4015. (C)
4016. (A)
4017. (D)
4018. (D)
4019. (A)
4020. (A)
4021. (A)
4022. (D)
4023. (D)
4024. (C)
4025. (A)
4026. (B)
4027. (D)
4028. (B)

Chapter 2: Pharmaceutical Chemistry and Pharmacology

1.	(C)	37.	(A)	73.	(B)	109.	(D)	145.	(B)
2.	(A)	38.	(C)	74.	(A)	110.	(B)	146.	(B)
3.	(C)	39.	(C)	75.	(C)	111.	(A)	147.	(D)
4.	(B)	40.	(C)	76.	(C)	112.	(C)	148.	(D)
5.	(B)	41.	(A)	77.	(B)	113.	(B)	149.	(B)
6.	(D)	42.	(A)	78.	(B)	114.	(C)	150.	(C)
7.	(B)	43.	(B)	79.	(A)	115.	(D)	151.	(C)
8.	(C)	44.	(B)	80.	(B)	116.	(C)	152.	(D)
9.	(A)	45.	(C)	81.	(A)	117.	(D)	153.	(A)
10.	(A)	46.	(A)	82.	(D)	118.	(D)	154.	(C)
11.	(A)	47.	(B)	83.	(B)	119.	(D)	155.	(A)
12.	(A)	48.	(B)	84.	(A)	120.	(A)	156.	(C)
13.	(C)	49.	(D)	85.	(A)	121.	(B)	157.	(A)
14.	(B)	50.	(A)	86.	(D)	122.	(C)	158.	(B)
15.	(C)	51.	(C)	87.	(D)	123.	(C)	159.	(C)
16.	(D)	52.	(A)	88.	(A)	124.	(B)	160.	(B)
17.	(D)	53.	(C)	89.	(A)	125.	(C)	161.	(C)
18.	(A)	54.	(D)	90.	(B)	126.	(A)	162.	(B)
19.	(C)	55.	(B)	91.	(A)	127.	(C)	163.	(B)
20.	(C)	56.	(C)	92.	(C)	128.	(D)	164.	(B)
21.	(D)	57.	(A)	93.	(C)	129.	(D)	165.	(B)
22.	(B)	58.	(B)	94.	(A)	130.	(C)	166.	(B)
23.	(D)	59.	(D)	95.	(A)	131.	(C)	167.	(D)
24.	(C)	60.	(A)	96.	(D)	132.	(D)	168.	(B)
25.	(D)	61.	(B)	97.	(A)	133.	(C)	169.	(A)
26.	(D)	62.	(D)	98.	(D)	134.	(D)	170.	(B)
27.	(A)	63.	(D)	99.	(C)	135.	(A)	171.	(B)
28.	(B)	64.	(D)	100.	(A)	136.	(C)	172.	(D)
29.	(D)	65.	(A)	101.	(C)	137.	(D)	173.	(C)
30.	(D)	66.	(B)	102.	(C)	138.	(C)	174.	(B)
31.	(A)	67.	(A)	103.	(B)	139.	(B)	175.	(C)
32.	(B)	68.	(C)	104.	(A)	140.	(A)	176.	(C)
33.	(B)	69.	(D)	105.	(D)	141.	(B)	177.	(C)
34.	(C)	70.	(A)	106.	(B)	142.	(D)	178.	(C)
35.	(B)	71.	(A)	107.	(B)	143.	(B)	179.	(D)
36.	(A)	72.	(A)	108.	(C)	144.	(A)	180.	(A)

181. (D)
182. (C)
183. (D)
184. (C)
185. (B)
186. (C)
187. (C)
188. (A)
189. (B)
190. (C)
191. (B)
192. (D)
193. (D)
194. (C)
195. (B)
196. (B)
197. (D)
198. (C)
199. (A)
200. (C)
201. (A)
202. (B)
203. (A)
204. (B)
205. (B)
206. (B)
207. (D)
208. (B)
209. (A)
210. (D)
211. (B)
212. (C)
213. (A)
214. (A)
215. (A)
216. (C)
217. (D)
218. (B)
219. (C)
220. (B)
221. (B)
222. (C)
223. (C)
224. (D)
225. (B)
226. (B)
227. (B)
228. (C)
229. (B)
230. (C)
231. (B)
232. (D)
233. (A)
234. (C)
235. (B)
236. (B)
237. (D)
238. (A)
239. (A)
240. (D)
241. (D)
242. (D)
243. (D)
244. (C)
245. (D)
246. (B)
247. (D)
248. (C)
249. (B)
250. (B)
251. (B)
252. (B)
253. (C)
254. (B)
255. (C)
256. (C)
257. (B)
258. (A)
259. (D)
260. (B)
261. (D)
262. (D)
263. (B)
264. (D)
265. (B)
266. (A)
267. (B)
268. (B)
269. (A)
270. (B)
271. (A)
272. (C)
273. (C)
274. (B)
275. (D)
276. (C)
277. (C)
278. (A)
279. (B)
280. (C)
281. (B)
282. (C)
283. (B)
284. (B)
285. (B)
286. (A)
287. (C)
288. (A)
289. (B)
290. (C)
291. (A)
292. (C)
293. (A)
294. (B)
295. (B)
296. (A)
297. (C)
298. (B)
299. (D)
300. (C)
301. (D)
302. (A)
303. (B)
304. (A)
305. (B)
306. (B)
307. (A)
308. (A)
309. (A)
310. (D)
311. (A)
312. (C)
313. (C)
314. (C)
315. (D)
316. (C)
317. (D)
318. (A)
319. (A)
320. (A)
321. (B)
322. (B)
323. (D)
324. (C)
325. (A)
326. (A)
327. (A)
328. (B)
329. (C)
330. (A)
331. (A)
332. (A)
333. (C)
334. (B)
335. (A)
336. (A)
337. (C)
338. (B)
339. (A)
340. (A)
341. (B)
342. (D)
343. (C)
344. (B)
345. (B)
346. (B)
347. (D)
348. (D)
349. (A)
350. (A)
351. (A)
352. (A)
353. (C)
354. (A)
355. (A)
356. (A)
357. (A)
358. (A)
359. (C)
360. (D)
361. (A)
362. (A)
363. (C)
364. (A)
365. (D)

366. (C)
367. (A)
368. (D)
369. (D)
370. (A)
371. (C)
372. (C)
373. (C)
374. (A)
375. (C)
376. (C)
377. (A)
378. (A)
379. (D)
380. (C)
381. (A)
382. (A)
383. (A)
384. (D)
385. (A)
386. (D)
387. (A)
388. (A)
389. (A)
390. (A)
391. (C)
392. (A)
393. (A)
394. (A)
395. (A)
396. (A)
397. (A)
398. (A)
399. (A)
400. (A)
401. (A)
402. (C)
403. (a)
404. (a)
405. (a)
406. (a)
407. (a)
408. (c)
409. (a)
410. (a)
411. (A)
412. (A)
413. (C)
414. (A)
415. (A)
416. (A)
417. (A)
418. (A)
419. (A)
420. (A)
421. (A)
422. (A)
423. (C)
424. (A)
425. (A)
426. (A)
427. (A)
428. (A)
429. (C)
430. (A)
431. (A)
432. (A)
433. (B)
434. (C)
435. (A)
436. (B)
437. (B)
438. (B)
439. (B)
440. (C)
441. (B)
442. (A)
443. (B)
444. (B)
445. (B)
446. (D)
447. (B)
448. (B)
449. (D)
450. (D)
451. (D)
452. (D)
453. (D)
454. (D)
455. (B)
456. (A)
457. (C)
458. (D)
459. (A)
460. (B)
461. (B)
462. (A)
463. (A)
464. (B)
465. (A)
466. (B)
467. (C)
468. (C)
469. (A)
470. (C)
471. (A)
472. (C)
473. (B)
474. (D)
475. (B)
476. (A)
477. (D)
478. (B)
479. (A)
480. (A)
481. (B)
482. (B)
483. (B)
484. (A)
485. (A)
486. (B)
487. (D)
488. (C)
489. (B)
490. (C)
491. (B)
492. (C)
493. (C)
494. (A)
495. (D)
496. (C)
497. (A)
498. (B)
499. (A)
500. (A)
501. (A)
502. (C)
503. (B)
504. (B)
505. (B)
506. (B)
507. (B)
508. (C)
509. (B)
510. (B)
511. (B)
512. (B)
513. (C)
514. (B)
515. (B)
516. (B)
517. (B)
518. (A)
519. (A)
520. (B)
521. (A)
522. (C)
523. (B)
524. (A)
525. (B)
526. (A)
527. (B)
528. (C)
529. (C)
530. (D)
531. (A)
532. (A)
533. (A)
534. (A)
535. (A)
536. (A)
537. (A)
538. (A)
539. (A)
540. (A)
541. (A)
542. (A)
543. (B)
544. (B)
545. (B)
546. (B)
547. (A)
548. (B)
549. (B)
550. (C)

551.	(B)	588.	(B)	625.	(B)	662.	(C)	699.	(B)
552.	(B)	589.	(B)	626.	(D)	663.	(D)	700.	(D)
553.	(B)	590.	(C)	627.	(A)	664.	(B)	701.	(A)
554.	(C)	591.	(D)	628.	(C)	665.	(A)	702.	(D)
555.	(A)	592.	(A)	629.	(D)	666.	(C)	703.	(A)
556.	(C)	593.	(B)	630.	(A)	667.	(C)	704.	(C)
557.	(A)	594.	(A)	631.	(A)	668.	(C)	705.	(A)
558.	(C)	595.	(A)	632.	(C)	669.	(A)	706.	(C)
559.	(B)	596.	(C)	633.	(B)	670.	(C)	707.	(D)
560.	(A)	597.	(A)	634.	(C)	671.	(C)	708.	(B)
561.	(A)	598.	(B)	635.	(B)	672.	(D)	709.	(D)
562.	(C)	599.	(A)	636.	(C)	673.	(B AND D)	710.	(D)
563.	(C)	600.	(A)	637.	(A)	674.	(A)	711.	(C)
564.	(A)	601.	(B)	638.	(D)	675.	(C)	712.	(D)
565.	(C)	602.	(C)	639.	(A)	676.	(C)	713.	(B)
566.	(A)	603.	(D)	640.	(B)	677.	(C)	714.	(A)
567.	(A)	604.	(C)	641.	(D)	678.	(C)	715.	(C)
568.	(C)	605.	(B)	642.	(D)	679.	(B)	716.	(B)
569.	(A)	606.	(A)	643.	(C)	680.	(D)	717.	(D)
570.	(C)	607.	(C)	644.	(A)	681.	(D)	718.	(A)
571.	(A)	608.	(D)	645.	(A)	682.	(D)	719.	(A)
572.	(A)	609.	(B)	646.	(B)	683.	(C)	720.	(B)
573.	(D)	610.	(C)	647.	(B)	684.	(C)	721.	(D)
574.	(A)	611.	(A)	648.	(D)	685.	(D)	722.	(C)
575.	(C)	612.	(A)	649.	(C)	686.	(A)	723.	(C)
576.	(B)	613.	(C)	650.	(C)	687.	(C)	724.	(D)
577.	(A)	614.	(D)	651.	(C)	688.	(B)	725.	(C)
578.	(C)	615.	(B)	652.	(C)	689.	(D)	726.	(D)
579.	(B)	616.	(C)	653.	(D)	690.	(A)	727.	(C)
580.	(A)	617.	(A)	654.	(D)	691.	(D)	728.	(A)
581.	(A)	618.	(B)	655.	(A)	692.	(B)	729.	(D)
582.	(B)	619.	(A)	656.	(D)	693.	(C)	730.	(C)
583.	(A)	620.	(D)	657.	(D)	694.	(B)	731.	(A)
584.	(D)	621.	(A)	658.	(C)	695.	(D)	732.	(A)
585.	(A)	622.	(B)	659.	(A)	696.	(A)	733.	(A)
586.	(B)	623.	(D)	660.	(C)	697.	(A)	734.	(D)
587.	(A)	624.	(C)	661.	(B)	698.	(B)	735.	(A)

736.	(C)	773.	(c)	810.	(D)	847.	(D)	884.	(C)
737.	(B)	774.	(A)	811.	(D)	848.	(C)	885.	(B)
738.	(B)	775.	(B)	812.	(D)	849.	(B)	886.	(C)
739.	(B)	776.	(D)	813.	(B)	850.	(C)	887.	(B)
740.	(D)	777.	(B)	814.	(D)	851.	(A)	888.	(B)
741.	(D)	778.	(A)	815.	(A)	852.	(C)	889.	(A)
742.	(B)	779.	(D)	816.	(D)	853.	(B)	890.	(D)
743.	(C)	780.	(D)	817.	(A)	854.	(A)	891.	(B)
744.	(B)	781.	(D)	818.	(D)	855.	(B)	892.	(C)
745.	(C)	782.	(D)	819.	(C)	856.	(A)	893.	(D)
746.	(C)	783.	(B)	820.	(B)	857.	(C)	894.	(B)
747.	(C)	784.	(D)	821.	(D)	858.	(B)	895.	(C)
748.	(C)	785.	(A)	822.	(C)	859.	(C)	896.	(A)
749.	(A)	786.	(B)	823.	(A)	860.	(D)	897.	(A)
750.	(B)	787.	(A)	824.	(B)	861.	(D)	898.	(B)
751.	(C)	788.	(A)	825.	(D)	862.	(B)	899.	(D)
752.	(C)	789.	(B)	826.	(B)	863.	(C)	900.	(D)
753.	(B)	790.	(A)	827.	(D)	864.	(A)	901.	(D)
754.	(A)	791.	(A)	828.	(B)	865.	(A)	902.	(D)
755.	(C)	792.	(C)	829.	(A)	866.	(D)	903.	(D)
756.	(C)	793.	(D)	830.	(B)	867.	(B)	904.	(D)
757.	(B)	794.	(C)	831.	(B)	868.	(D)	905.	(A)
758.	(C)	795.	(B)	832.	(D)	869.	(C)	906.	(C)
759.	(B)	796.	(D)	833.	(B)	870.	(B)	907.	(A)
760.	(B)	797.	(D)	834.	(A)	871.	(C)	908.	(C)
761.	(C)	798.	(B)	835.	(A)	872.	(D)	909.	(C)
762.	(A)	799.	(D)	836.	(A)	873.	(B)	910.	(C)
763.	(A)	800.	(A)	837.	(D)	874.	(D)	911.	(A)
764.	(A)	801.	(B)	838.	(B)	875.	(C)	912.	(A)
765.	(C)	802.	(C)	839.	(D)	876.	(D)	913.	(B)
766.	(A)	803.	(B)	840.	(A)	877.	(C)	914.	(D)
767.	(B)	804.	(B)	841.	(D)	878.	(C)	915.	(C)
768.	(B)	805.	(D)	842.	(D)	879.	(C)	916.	(C)
769.	(B)	806.	(B)	843.	(B)	880.	(B)	917.	(C)
770.	(D)	807.	(D)	844.	(C)	881.	(C)	918.	(B)
771.	(A)	808.	(C)	845.	(D)	882.	(A)	919.	(C)
772.	(B)	809.	(B)	846.	(D)	883.	(C)	920.	(D)

921.	(A)	958.	(A)	995.	(A)	1032.	(A)	1069.	(A)
922.	(C)	959.	(A)	996.	(B)	1033.	(A)	1070.	(A)
923.	(D)	960.	(A)	997.	(A)	1034.	(A)	1071.	(A)
924.	(B)	961.	(A)	998.	(A)	1035.	(A)	1072.	(C)
925.	(D)	962.	(D)	999.	(B)	1036.	(A)	1073.	(A)
926.	(D)	963.	(D)	1000.	(B)	1037.	(A)	1074.	(A)
927.	(D)	964.	(A)	1001.	(A)	1038.	(A)	1075.	(C)
928.	(C)	965.	(B)	1002.	(A)	1039.	(A)	1076.	(A)
929.	(C)	966.	(A)	1003.	(A)	1040.	(A)	1077.	(A)
930.	(A)	967.	(A)	1004.	(A)	1041.	(A)	1078.	(D)
931.	(C)	968.	(A)	1005.	(A)	1042.	(A)	1079.	(A)
932.	(B)	969.	(A)	1006.	(D)	1043.	(A)	1080.	(A)
933.	(D)	970.	(A)	1007.	(A)	1044.	(A)	1081.	(A)
934.	(A)	971.	(A)	1008.	(A)	1045.	(A)	1082.	(A)
935.	(A)	972.	(A)	1009.	(A)	1046.	(A)	1083.	(A)
936.	(B)	973.	(A)	1010.	(A)	1047.	(A)	1084.	(B)
937.	(A)	974.	(A)	1011.	(A)	1048.	(A)	1085.	(A)
938.	(A)	975.	(A)	1012.	(A)	1049.	(A)	1086.	(A)
939.	(A)	976.	(A)	1013.	(A)	1050.	(A)	1087.	(D)
940.	(A)	977.	(A)	1014.	(D)	1051.	(A)	1088.	(A)
941.	(A)	978.	(A)	1015.	(A)	1052.	(A)	1089.	(A)
942.	(A)	979.	(A)	1016.	(B)	1053.	(A)	1090.	(A)
943.	(A)	980.	(A)	1017.	(A)	1054.	(A)	1091.	(A)
944.	(B)	981.	(A)	1018.	(A)	1055.	(A)	1092.	(A)
945.	(A)	982.	(B)	1019.	(D)	1056.	(B)	1093.	(A)
946.	(A)	983.	(A)	1020.	(B)	1057.	(A)	1094.	(A)
947.	(B)	984.	(A)	1021.	(C)	1058.	(A)	1095.	(A)
948.	(A)	985.	(C)	1022.	(B)	1059.	(A)	1096.	(A)
949.	(A)	986.	(A)	1023.	(A)	1060.	(B)	1097.	(A)
950.	(A)	987.	(B)	1024.	(D)	1061.	(C)	1098.	(A)
951.	(C)	988.	(A)	1025.	(A)	1062.	(B)	1099.	(A)
952.	(A)	989.	(A)	1026.	(A)	1063.	(A)	1100.	(A)
953.	(D)	990.	(A)	1027.	(A)	1064.	(B)	1101.	(A)
954.	(A)	991.	(A)	1028.	(A)	1065.	(C)	1102.	(A)
955.	(D)	992.	(A)	1029.	(A)	1066.	(C)	1103.	(A)
956.	(A)	993.	(A)	1030.	(A)	1067.	(A)	1104.	(A)
957.	(A)	994.	(A)	1031.	(A)	1068.	(A)	1105.	(D)

1106.	(A)	1143.	(A)	1180.	(D)	1217.	(A)	1254.	(A)
1107.	(A)	1144.	(A)	1181.	(D)	1218.	(A)	1255.	(D)
1108.	(A)	1145.	(B)	1182.	(D)	1219.	(A)	1256.	(B)
1109.	(A)	1146.	(D)	1183.	(D)	1220.	(B)	1257.	(C)
1110.	(A)	1147.	(A)	1184.	(C)	1221.	(C)	1258.	(A)
1111.	(A)	1148.	(A)	1185.	(A)	1222.	(C)	1259.	(C)
1112.	(A)	1149.	(D)	1186.	(D)	1223.	(A)	1260.	(D)
1113.	(A)	1150.	(C)	1187.	(D)	1224.	(D)	1261.	(C)
1114.	(D)	1151.	(A)	1188.	(A)	1225.	(D)	1262.	(B)
1115.	(D)	1152.	(A)	1189.	(A)	1226.	(C)	1263.	(A)
1116.	(A)	1153.	(A)	1190.	(D)	1227.	(D)	1264.	(B)
1117.	(D)	1154.	(A)	1191.	(A)	1228.	(C)	1265.	(B)
1118.	(A)	1155.	(D)	1192.	(A)	1229.	(A)	1266.	(A)
1119.	(A)	1156.	(C)	1193.	(D)	1230.	(C)	1267.	(A)
1120.	(A)	1157.	(A)	1194.	(A)	1231.	(B)	1268.	(C)
1121.	(A)	1158.	(D)	1195.	(D)	1232.	(D)	1269.	(D)
1122.	(A)	1159.	(A)	1196.	(D)	1233.	(D)	1270.	(D)
1123.	(D)	1160.	(D)	1197.	(D)	1234.	(A)	1271.	(D)
1124.	(A)	1161.	(A)	1198.	(D)	1235.	(C)	1272.	(A)
1125.	(A)	1162.	(A)	1199.	(A)	1236.	(D)	1273.	(B)
1126.	(D)	1163.	(B)	1200.	(D)	1237.	(C)	1274.	(C)
1127.	(D)	1164.	(D)	1201.	(D)	1238.	(A)	1275.	(D)
1128.	(A)	1165.	(A)	1202.	(A)	1239.	(B)	1276.	(C)
1129.	(D)	1166.	(B)	1203.	(B)	1240.	(A)	1277.	(C)
1130.	(D)	1167.	(C)	1204.	(A)	1241.	(B)	1278.	(A)
1131.	(A)	1168.	(C)	1205.	(D)	1242.	(B)	1279.	(C)
1132.	(A)	1169.	(D)	1206.	(B)	1243.	(C)	1280.	(A)
1133.	(D)	1170.	(D)	1207.	(B)	1244.	(A)	1281.	(C)
1134.	(A)	1171.	(C)	1208.	(C)	1245.	(A)	1282.	(C)
1135.	(A)	1172.	(B)	1209.	(B)	1246.	(D)	1283.	(A)
1136.	(D)	1173.	(D)	1210.	(A)	1247.	(A)	1284.	(D)
1137.	(A)	1174.	(D)	1211.	(A)	1248.	(B)	1285.	(D)
1138.	(A)	1175.	(A)	1212.	(C)	1249.	(A)	1286.	(D)
1139.	(A)	1176.	(D)	1213.	(C)	1250.	(A)	1287.	(D)
1140.	(A)	1177.	(D)	1214.	(D)	1251.	(D)	1288.	(B)
1141.	(A)	1178.	(A)	1215.	(A)	1252.	(A)	1289.	(B)
1142.	(C)	1179.	(C)	1216.	(C)	1253.	(C)	1290.	(C)

1291. (D)
1292. (B)
1293. (A)
1294. (A)
1295. (A)
1296. (D)
1297. (A)
1298. (D)
1299. (C)
1300. (A)
1301. (D)
1302. (A)
1303. (C)
1304. (A)
1305. (D)
1306. (A)
1307. (B)
1308. (D)
1309. (A)
1310. (A)
1311. (C)
1312. (A)
1313. (A)
1314. (C)
1315. (A)
1316. (B)
1317. (A)
1318. (C)
1319. (A)
1320. (C)
1321. (D)
1322. (D)
1323. (D)
1324. (A)
1325. (D)
1326. (A)
1327. (C)
1328. (D)
1329. (A)
1330. (C)
1331. (D)
1332. (B)
1333. (C)
1334. (A)
1335. (D)
1336. (B)
1337. (B)
1338. (D)
1339. (B)
1340. (A)
1341. (C)
1342. (B)
1343. (D)
1344. (B)
1345. (C)
1346. (A)
1347. (C)
1348. (A)
1349. (D)
1350. (D)
1351. (A)
1352. (C)
1353. (B)
1354. (D)
1355. (A)
1356. (C)
1357. (A)
1358. (A)
1359. (D)
1360. (D)
1361. (B)
1362. (D)
1363. (B)
1364. (A)
1365. (D)
1366. (A)
1367. (B)
1368. (D)
1369. (D)
1370. (D)
1371. (A)
1372. (D)
1373. (A)
1374. (A)
1375. (D)
1376. (B)
1377. (A)
1378. (B)
1379. (D)
1380. (D)
1381. (A)
1382. (A)
1383. (C)
1384. (D)
1385. (C)
1386. (A)
1387. (B)
1388. (A)
1389. (C)
1390. (C)
1391. (A)
1392. (D)
1393. (B)
1394. (A)
1395. (C)
1396. (B)
1397. (C)
1398. (A)
1399. (B)
1400. (C)
1401. (B)
1402. (D)
1403. (A)
1404. (D)
1405. (C)
1406. (A)
1407. (B)
1408. (C)
1409. (D)
1410. (A)
1411. (D)
1412. (D)
1413. (B)
1414. (D)
1415. (B)
1416. (C)
1417. (B)
1418. (B)
1419. (C)
1420. (D)
1421. (A)
1422. (B)
1423. (D)
1424. (D)
1425. (A)
1426. (B)
1427. (A)
1428. (B)
1429. (D)
1430. (A)
1431. (C)
1432. (A)
1433. (B)
1434. (A)
1435. (A)
1436. (C)
1437. (C)
1438. (D)
1439. (B)
1440. (D)
1441. (A)
1442. (B)
1443. (C)
1444. (B)
1445. (A)
1446. (D)
1447. (D)
1448. (B)
1449. (C)
1450. (B)
1451. (D)
1452. (C)
1453. (B)
1454. (B)
1455. (C)
1456. (B)
1457. (A)
1458. (B)
1459. (A)
1460. (C)
1461. (B)
1462. (B)
1463. (A)
1464. (A)
1465. (C)
1466. (D)
1467. (B)
1468. (B)
1469. (C)
1470. (C)
1471. (B)
1472. (A)
1473. (D)
1474. (C)
1475. (A)

1476. (D)
1477. (A)
1478. (C)
1479. (B)
1480. (D)
1481. (A)
1482. (A)
1483. (D)
1484. (D)
1485. (C)
1486. (B)
1487. (B)
1488. (A)
1489. (C)
1490. (A)
1491. (C)
1492. (A)
1493. (B)
1494. (D)
1495. (B)
1496. (D)
1497. (A)
1498. (B)
1499. (A)
1500. (D)
1501. (C)
1502. (D)
1503. (A)
1504. (A)
1505. (D)
1506. (A)
1507. (A)
1508. (C)
1509. (C)
1510. (C)
1511. (A)
1512. (A)
1513. (A)
1514. (D)
1515. (A)
1516. (D)
1517. (C)
1518. (A)
1519. (A)
1520. (A)
1521. (C)
1522. (A)
1523. (D)
1524. (D)
1525. (C)
1526. (D)
1527. (D)
1528. (A)
1529. (A)
1530. (A)
1531. (A)
1532. (A)
1533. (B)
1534. (C)
1535. (D)
1536. (A)
1537. (A)
1538. (B)
1539. (C)
1540. (C)
1541. (A)
1542. (D)
1543. (C)
1544. (D)
1545. (B)
1546. (B)
1547. (A)
1548. (A)
1549. (B)
1550. (C)
1551. (A)
1552. (C)
1553. (C)
1554. (A)
1555. (A)
1556. (A)
1557. (B)
1558. (A)
1559. (B)
1560. (C)
1561. (A)
1562. (A)
1563. (A)
1564. (C)
1565. (D)
1566. (A)
1567. (B)
1568. (D)
1569. (C)
1570. (A)
1571. (C)
1572. (C)
1573. (D)
1574. (A)
1575. (A)
1576. (A)
1577. (D)
1578. (A)
1579. (C)
1580. (D)
1581. (D)
1582. (C)
1583. (A)
1584. (C)
1585. (A)
1586. (A)
1587. (A)
1588. (D)
1589. (C)
1590. (A)
1591. (C)
1592. (B)
1593. (A)
1594. (B)
1595. (A)
1596. (B)
1597. (B)
1598. (A)
1599. (C)
1600. (A)
1601. (A)
1602. (D)
1603. (C)
1604. (A)
1605. (A)
1606. (B)
1607. (A)
1608. (C)
1609. (A)
1610. (A)
1611. (C)
1612. (A)
1613. (A)
1614. (A)
1615. (D)
1616. (B)
1617. (B)
1618. (D)
1619. (A)
1620. (C)
1621. (B)
1622. (B)
1623. (D)
1624. (B)
1625. (D)
1626. (C)
1627. (A)
1628. (D)
1629. (C)
1630. (B)
1631. (A)
1632. (C)
1633. (A)
1634. (C)
1635. (D)
1636. (A)
1637. (C)
1638. (A)
1639. (B)
1640. (B)
1641. (D)
1642. (D)
1643. (C)
1644. (A)
1645. (A)
1646. (A)
1647. (C)
1648. (A)
1649. (C)
1650. (A)
1651. (C)
1652. (A)
1653. (D)
1654. (A)
1655. (A)
1656. (A)
1657. (D)
1658. (A)
1659. (C)
1660. (B)

1661. (A)
1662. (A)
1663. (A)
1664. (A)
1665. (B)
1666. (D)
1667. (C)
1668. (A)
1669. (D)
1670. (C)
1671. (B)
1672. (A)
1673. (D)
1674. (C)
1675. (D)
1676. (A)
1677. (D)
1678. (C)
1679. (A)
1680. (A)
1681. (A)
1682. (A)
1683. (C)
1684. (C)
1685. (B)
1686. (B)
1687. (C)
1688. (D)
1689. (C)
1690. (C)
1691. (D)
1692. (A)
1693. (B)
1694. (C)
1695. (D)
1696. (C)
1697. (C)
1698. (A)
1699. (A)
1700. (C)
1701. (A)
1702. (D)
1703. (B)
1704. (A)
1705. (A)
1706. (D)
1707. (A)
1708. (A)
1709. (B)
1710. (A)
1711. (D)
1712. (D)
1713. (A)
1714. (A)
1715. (C)
1716. (C)
1717. (C)
1718. (B)
1719. (A)
1720. (C)
1721. (B)
1722. (A)
1723. (C)
1724. (D)
1725. (C)
1726. (A)
1727. (B)
1728. (B)
1729. (C)
1730. (C)
1731. (A)
1732. (A)
1733. (D)
1734. (A)
1735. (A)
1736. (B)
1737. (C)
1738. (C)
1739. (D)
1740. (B)
1741. (C)
1742. (C)
1743. (A)
1744. (B)
1745. (C)
1746. (C)
1747. (D)
1748. (A)
1749. (C)
1750. (C)
1751. (D)
1752. (B)
1753. (B)
1754. (A)
1755. (C)
1756. (D)
1757. (D)
1758. (A)
1759. (C)
1760. (C)
1761. (D)
1762. (A)
1763. (D)
1764. (A)
1765. (A)
1766. (D)
1767. (D)
1768. (D)
1769. (A)
1770. (A)
1771. (C)
1772. (D)
1773. (D)
1774. (A)
1775. (B)
1776. (A)
1777. (D)
1778. (C)
1779. (B)
1780. (A)
1781. (B)
1782. (A)
1783. (A)
1784. (C)
1785. (A)
1786. (A)
1787. (C)
1788. (A)
1789. (C)
1790. (A)
1791. (A)
1792. (D)
1793. (A)
1794. (C)
1795. (A)
1796. (D)
1797. (A)
1798. (A)
1799. (C)
1800. (C)
1801. (D)
1802. (A)
1803. (A)
1804. (A)
1805. (A)
1806. (A)
1807. (D)
1808. (A)
1809. (B)
1810. (C)
1811. (C)
1812. (C)
1813. (A)
1814. (A)
1815. (D)
1816. (C)
1817. (A)
1818. (D)
1819. (A)
1820. (A)
1821. (A)
1822. (C)
1823. (A)
1824. (D)
1825. (D)
1826. (B)
1827. (A)
1828. (D)
1829. (A)
1830. (A)
1831. (A)
1832. (B)
1833. (C)
1834. (A)
1835. (A)
1836. (C)
1837. (D)
1838. (A)
1839. (C)
1840. (D)
1841. (A)
1842. (D)
1843. (B)
1844. (A)
1845. (C)

1846. (C)
1847. (D)
1848. (A)
1849. (A)
1850. (C)
1851. (C)
1852. (A)
1853. (A)
1854. (A)
1855. (D)
1856. (A)
1857. (A)
1858. (D)
1859. (D)
1860. (B)
1861. (A)
1862. (C)
1863. (A)
1864. (C)
1865. (A)
1866. (A)
1867. (A)
1868. (C)
1869. (A)
1870. (A)
1871. (A)
1872. (B)
1873. (D)
1874. (C)
1875. (A)
1876. (A)
1877. (A)
1878. (D)
1879. (C)
1880. (A)
1881. (A)
1882. (A)
1883. (A)
1884. (C)
1885. (C)
1886. (A)
1887. (A)
1888. (C)
1889. (A)
1890. (A)
1891. (B)
1892. (A)
1893. (C)
1894. (B)
1895. (C)
1896. (A)
1897. (C)
1898. (B)
1899. (A)
1900. (C)
1901. (A)
1902. (C)
1903. (B)
1904. (A)
1905. (C)
1906. (A)
1907. (A)
1908. (A)
1909. (C)
1910. (D)
1911. (A)
1912. (A)
1913. (A)
1914. (A)
1915. (D)
1916. (A)
1917. (A)
1918. (C)
1919. (A)
1920. (D)
1921. (C)
1922. (B)
1923. (C)
1924. (A)
1925. (C)
1926. (A)
1927. (C)
1928. (A)
1929. (A)
1930. (A)
1931. (B)
1932. (C)
1933. (B)
1934. (C)
1935. (A)
1936. (A)
1937. (C)
1938. (D)
1939. (B)
1940. (D)
1941. (A)
1942. (C)
1943. (A)
1944. (A)
1945. (C)
1946. (A)
1947. (B)
1948. (A)
1949. (D)
1950. (A)
1951. (A)
1952. (A)
1953. (C)
1954. (B)
1955. (D)
1956. (D)
1957. (C)
1958. (A)
1959. (A)
1960. (C)
1961. (B)
1962. (A)
1963. (A)
1964. (A)
1965. (C)
1966. (B)
1967. (C)
1968. (A)
1969. (A)
1970. (D)
1971. (C)
1972. (B)
1973. (C)
1974. (D)
1975. (B)
1976. (A)
1977. (A)
1978. (D)
1979. (B)
1980. (A)
1981. (A)
1982. (D)
1983. (D)
1984. (A)
1985. (A)
1986. (D)
1987. (C)
1988. (B)
1989. (D)
1990. (A)
1991. (D)
1992. (D)
1993. (C)
1994. (D)
1995. (C)
1996. (D)
1997. (B)
1998. (D)
1999. (C)
2000. (D)
2001. (D)
2002. (C)
2003. (D)
2004. (D)
2005. (A)
2006. (C)
2007. (C)
2008. (D)
2009. (C)
2010. (B)
2011. (A)
2012. (A)
2013. (A)
2014. (A)
2015. (C)
2016. (A)
2017. (D)
2018. (A)
2019. (A)
2020. (B)
2021. (B)
2022. (A)
2023. (B)
2024. (A)
2025. (A)
2026. (C)
2027. (D)
2028. (D)
2029. (C)
2030. (B)

2031. (A)
2032. (C)
2033. (D)
2034. (B)
2035. (A)
2036. (A)
2037. (C)
2038. (B)
2039. (A)
2040. (C)
2041. (A)
2042. (B)
2043. (C)
2044. (A)
2045. (D)
2046. (C)
2047. (A)
2048. (A)
2049. (C)
2050. (B)
2051. (A)
2052. (C)
2053. (A)
2054. (B)
2055. (C)
2056. (A)
2057. (C)
2058. (D)
2059. (A)
2060. (A)
2061. (C)
2062. (A)
2063. (A)
2064. (D)
2065. (A)
2066. (C)
2067. (A)
2068. (A)
2069. (A)
2070. (B)
2071. (A)
2072. (D)
2073. (D)
2074. (A)
2075. (D)
2076. (D)
2077. (C)
2078. (A)
2079. (D)
2080. (B)
2081. (C)
2082. (B)
2083. (A)
2084. (A)
2085. (C)
2086. (D)
2087. (B)
2088. (B)
2089. (C)
2090. (A)
2091. (A)
2092. (A)
2093. (A)
2094. (C)
2095. (D)
2096. (A)
2097. (C)
2098. (A)
2099. (A)
2100. (B)
2101. (D)
2102. (C)
2103. (A)
2104. (B)
2105. (B)
2106. (A)
2107. (C)
2108. (B)
2109. (A)
2110. (C)
2111. (D)
2112. (C)
2113. (B)
2114. (D)
2115. (C)
2116. (D)
2117. (D)
2118. (B)
2119. (D)
2120. (D)
2121. (B)
2122. (C)
2123. (A)
2124. (B)
2125. (C)
2126. (C)
2127. (B)
2128. (A)
2129. (B)
2130. (A)
2131. (B)
2132. (C)
2133. (C)
2134. (A)
2135. (A)
2136. (B)
2137. (A)
2138. (C)
2139. (A)
2140. (B)
2141. (D)
2142. (A)
2143. (A)
2144. (C)
2145. (A)
2146. (C)
2147. (A)
2148. (B)
2149. (C)
2150. (B)
2151. (B)
2152. (B)
2153. (A)
2154. (A)
2155. (A)
2156. (A)
2157. (C)
2158. (A)
2159. (C)
2160. (B)
2161. (A)
2162. (A)
2163. (B)
2164. (C)
2165. (C)
2166. (B)
2167. (D)
2168. (B)
2169. (C)
2170. (A)
2171. (A)
2172. (C)
2173. (A)
2174. (A)
2175. (A)
2176. (B)
2177. (A)
2178. (C)
2179. (A)
2180. (D)
2181. (A)
2182. (D)
2183. (A)
2184. (B)
2185. (D)
2186. (B)
2187. (C)
2188. (D)
2189. (C)
2190. (A)
2191. (C)
2192. (D)
2193. (C)
2194. (D)
2195. (C)
2196. (A)
2197. (A)
2198. (C)
2199. (A)
2200. (D)
2201. (D)
2202. (D)
2203. (B)
2204. (A)
2205. (D)
2206. (C)
2207. (C)
2208. (D)
2209. (B)
2210. (A)
2211. (A)
2212. (B)
2213. (D)
2214. (C)
2215. (A)

2216. (A)
2217. (A)
2218. (D)
2219. (C)
2220. (B)
2221. (B)
2222. (C)
2223. (A)
2224. (A)
2225. (A)
2226. (B)
2227. (D)
2228. (C)
2229. (B)
2230. (C)
2231. (C)
2232. (C)
2233. (A)
2234. (A)
2235. (A)
2236. (D)
2237. (B)
2238. (C)
2239. (C)
2240. (A)
2241. (D)
2242. (B)
2243. (A)
2244. (D)
2245. (C)
2246. (B)
2247. (A)
2248. (D)
2249. (A)
2250. (D)
2251. (A)
2252. (D)
2253. (A)
2254. (B)
2255. (A)
2256. (A)
2257. (A)
2258. (D)
2259. (A)
2260. (D)
2261. (A)
2262. (C)
2263. (D)
2264. (A)
2265. (B)
2266. (A)
2267. (C)
2268. (D)
2269. (A)
2270. (B)
2271. (B)
2272. (C)
2273. (A)
2274. (B)
2275. (D)
2276. (B)
2277. (A)
2278. (C)
2279. (D)
2280. (C)
2281. (B)
2282. (C)
2283. (B)
2284. (A)
2285. (D)
2286. (D)
2287. (D)
2288. (A)
2289. (B)
2290. (D)
2291. (D)
2292. (A)
2293. (A)
2294. (D)
2295. (D)
2296. (A)
2297. (B)
2298. (D)
2299. (A)
2300. (A)
2301. (A)
2302. (D)
2303. (A)
2304. (D)
2305. (D)
2306. (B)
2307. (B)
2308. (A)
2309. (A)
2310. (C)
2311. (A)
2312. (C)
2313. (A)
2314. (B)
2315. (C)
2316. (A)
2317. (A)
2318. (C)
2319. (C)
2320. (C)
2321. (B)
2322. (B)
2323. (D)
2324. (A)
2325. (D)
2326. (A)
2327. (D)
2328. (B)
2329. (B)
2330. (D)
2331. (A)
2332. (A)
2333. (A)
2334. (C)
2335. (A)
2336. (C)
2337. (A)
2338. (A)
2339. (D)
2340. (A)
2341. (B)
2342. (D)
2343. (B)
2344. (B)
2345. (B)
2346. (C)
2347. (D)
2348. (B)
2349. (D)
2350. (A)
2351. (D)
2352. (D)
2353. (A)
2354. (B)
2355. (A)
2356. (A)
2357. (A)
2358. (B)
2359. (D)
2360. (D)
2361. (A)
2362. (B)
2363. (A)
2364. (A)
2365. (D)
2366. (A)
2367. (A)
2368. (C)
2369. (A)
2370. (B)
2371. (D)
2372. (C)
2373. (C)
2374. (B)
2375. (A)
2376. (C)
2377. (A)
2378. (C)
2379. (A)
2380. (D)
2381. (B)
2382. (C)
2383. (D)
2384. (A)
2385. (A)
2386. (A)
2387. (A)
2388. (A)
2389. (B)
2390. (C)
2391. (B)
2392. (B)
2393. (C)
2394. (C)
2395. (A)
2396. (A)
2397. (A)
2398. (D)
2399. (A)
2400. (B)

2401. (B)
2402. (B)
2403. (A)
2404. (C)
2405. (B)
2406. (A)
2407. (B)
2408. (A)
2409. (C)
2410. (B)
2411. (B)
2412. (A)
2413. (C)
2414. (B)
2415. (A)
2416. (B)
2417. (B)
2418. (D)
2419. (B)
2420. (B)
2421. (B)
2422. (B)
2423. (D)
2424. (B)
2425. (C)
2426. (A)
2427. (D)
2428. (B)
2429. (D)
2430. (D)
2431. (A)
2432. (B)
2433. (D)
2434. (B)
2435. (B)
2436. (C)
2437. (B)
2438. (D)
2439. (B)
2440. (D)
2441. (C)
2442. (B)
2443. (D)
2444. (D)
2445. (C)
2446. (A)
2447. (B)
2448. (C)
2449. (A)
2450. (C)
2451. (A)
2452. (A)
2453. (B)
2454. (D)
2455. (C)
2456. (C)
2457. (B)
2458. (D)
2459. (B)
2460. (B)
2461. (D)
2462. (B)
2463. (B)
2464. (C)
2465. (C)
2466. (A)
2467. (B)
2468. (B)
2469. (D)
2470. (A)
2471. (C)
2472. (D)
2473. (C)
2474. (D)
2475. (B)
2476. (B)
2477. (B)
2478. (A)
2479. (D)
2480. (A)
2481. (A)
2482. (C)
2483. (A)
2484. (C)
2485. (A)
2486. (A)
2487. (D)
2488. (A)
2489. (B)
2490. (A)
2491. (B)
2492. (D)
2493. (A)
2494. (C)
2495. (B)
2496. (A)
2497. (A)
2498. (A)
2499. (D)
2500. (C)
2501. (C)
2502. (B)
2503. (A)
2504. (C)
2505. (B)
2506. (A)
2507. (A)
2508. (B)
2509. (C)
2510. (A)
2511. (A)
2512. (A)
2513. (C)
2514. (B)
2515. (C)
2516. (C)
2517. (A)
2518. (D)
2519. (A)
2520. (A)
2521. (A)
2522. (B)
2523. (B)
2524. (A)
2525. (A)
2526. (C)
2527. (C)
2528. (A)
2529. (D)
2530. (B)
2531. (C)
2532. (B)
2533. (D)
2534. (C)
2535. (A)
2536. (D)
2537. (C)
2538. (D)
2539. (D)
2540. (D)
2541. (B)
2542. (B)
2543. (A)
2544. (D)
2545. (B)
2546. (C)
2547. (B)
2548. (C)
2549. (C)
2550. (C)
2551. (D)
2552. (C)
2553. (C)
2554. (D)
2555. (C)
2556. (A)
2557. (C)
2558. (B)
2559. (D)
2560. (C)
2561. (D)
2562. (A)
2563. (C)
2564. (B)
2565. (A)
2566. (B)
2567. (B)
2568. (A)
2569. (B)
2570. (B)
2571. (B)
2572. (B)
2573. (B)
2574. (B)
2575. (D)
2576. (A)
2577. (A)
2578. (A)
2579. (B)
2580. (A)
2581. (C)
2582. (A)
2583. (A)
2584. (A)
2585. (A)

2586. (A)
2587. (A)
2588. (A)
2589. (B)
2590. (D)
2591. (C)
2592. (A)
2593. (D)
2594. (A)
2595. (A)
2596. (B)
2597. (D)
2598. (A)
2599. (D)
2600. (D)
2601. (C)
2602. (B)
2603. (C)
2604. (B)
2605. (C)
2606. (A)
2607. (C)
2608. (B)
2609. (A)
2610. (A)
2611. (B)
2612. (C)
2613. (A)
2614. (B)
2615. (A)
2616. (B)
2617. (A)
2618. (D)
2619. (A)
2620. (C)
2621. (A)
2622. (B)
2623. (A)
2624. (D)
2625. (C)
2626. (A)
2627. (B)
2628. (B)
2629. (C)
2630. (B)
2631. (C)
2632. (A)
2633. (B)
2634. (D)
2635. (A)
2636. (B)
2637. (D)
2638. (B)
2639. (A)
2640. (B)
2641. (B)
2642. (D)
2643. (A)
2644. (A)
2645. (A)
2646. (C)
2647. (B)
2648. (A)
2649. (D)
2650. (C)
2651. (D)
2652. (B)
2653. (C)
2654. (C)
2655. (D)
2656. (D)
2657. (A)
2658. (B)
2659. (C)
2660. (B)
2661. (D)
2662. (A)
2663. (B)
2664. (A)
2665. (B)
2666. (C)
2667. (A)
2668. (D)
2669. (C)
2670. (B)
2671. (D)
2672. (C)
2673. (D)
2674. (C)
2675. (D)
2676. (D)
2677. (B)
2678. (A)
2679. (B)
2680. (C)
2681. (B)
2682. (C)
2683. (A)
2684. (C)
2685. (D)
2686. (B)
2687. (D)
2688. (B)
2689. (B)
2690. (A)
2691. (A)
2692. (A)
2693. (C)
2694. (B)
2695. (C)
2696. (B)
2697. (D)
2698. (D)
2699. (B)
2700. (B)
2701. (A)
2702. (C)
2703. (A)
2704. (A)
2705. (C)
2706. (C)
2707. (D)
2708. (B)
2709. (D)
2710. (B)
2711. (D)
2712. (A)
2713. (B)
2714. (D)
2715. (A)
2716. (B)
2717. (A)
2718. (A)
2719. (A)
2720. (C)
2721. (B)
2722. (A)
2723. (C)
2724. (A)
2725. (C)
2726. (A)
2727. (A)
2728. (A)
2729. (A)
2730. (A)
2731. (A)
2732. (C)
2733. (D)
2734. (D)
2735. (B)
2736. (C)
2737. (A)
2738. (A)
2739. (B)
2740. (C)
2741. (B)
2742. (A)
2743. (C)
2744. (B)
2745. (D)
2746. (A)
2747. (A)
2748. (D)
2749. (C)
2750. (A)
2751. (C)
2752. (D)
2753. (A)
2754. (C)
2755. (B)
2756. (C)
2757. (D)
2758. (C)
2759. (A)
2760. (A)
2761. (B)
2762. (B)
2763. (C)
2764. (C)
2765. (D)
2766. (D)
2767. (A)
2768. (C)
2769. (D)
2770. (A)

2771. (C)
2772. (A)
2773. (C)
2774. (A)
2775. (C)
2776. (B)
2777. (A)
2778. (D)
2779. (A)
2780. (A)
2781. (C)
2782. (C)
2783. (D)
2784. (B)
2785. (A)
2786. (B)
2787. (B)
2788. (A)
2789. (C)
2790. (B)
2791. (A)
2792. (A)
2793. (A)
2794. (A)
2795. (C)
2796. (A)
2797. (A)
2798. (A)
2799. (C)
2800. (B)
2801. (A)
2802. (D)
2803. (A)
2804. (B)
2805. (A)
2806. (D)
2807. (B)
2808. (C)
2809. (C)
2810. (A)
2811. (D)
2812. (C)
2813. (C)
2814. (A)
2815. (B)
2816. (A)
2817. (C)
2818. (C)
2819. (A)
2820. (B)
2821. (D)
2822. (C)
2823. (B)
2824. (C)
2825. (C)
2826. (C)
2827. (B)
2828. (A)
2829. (A)
2830. (C)
2831. (D)
2832. (D)
2833. (A)
2834. (C)
2835. (B)
2836. (C)
2837. (D)
2838. (C)
2839. (D)
2840. (C)
2841. (A)
2842. (B)
2843. (B)
2844. (B)
2845. (A)
2846. (C)
2847. (D)
2848. (A)
2849. (B)
2850. (D)
2851. (D)
2852. (B)
2853. (B)
2854. (D)
2855. (C)
2856. (B)
2857. (C)
2858. (A)
2859. (C)
2860. (C)
2861. (B)
2862. (A)
2863. (C)
2864. (C)
2865. (D)
2866. (A)
2867. (A)
2868. (C)
2869. (C)
2870. (B)
2871. (A)
2872. (C)
2873. (A)
2874. (C)
2875. (A)
2876. (B)
2877. (B)
2878. (A)
2879. (A)
2880. (D)
2881. (A)
2882. (D)
2883. (C)
2884. (B)
2885. (D)
2886. (B)
2887. (C)
2888. (B)
2889. (B)
2890. (A)
2891. (B)
2892. (A)
2893. (C)
2894. (B)
2895. (A)
2896. (A)
2897. (A)
2898. (C)
2899. (C)
2900. (A)
2901. (D)
2902. (C)
2903. (A)
2904. (B)
2905. (C)
2906. (B)
2907. (A)
2908. (C)
2909. (D)
2910. (A)
2911. (D)
2912. (D)
2913. (B)
2914. (B)
2915. (D)
2916. (B)
2917. (A)
2918. (C)
2919. (B)
2920. (C)
2921. (A)
2922. (D)
2923. (C)
2924. (A)
2925. (B)
2926. (B)
2927. (A)
2928. (C)
2929. (C)
2930. (C)
2931. (A)
2932. (B)
2933. (B)
2934. (C)
2935. (D)
2936. (A)
2937. (C)
2938. (B)
2939. (A)
2940. (D)
2941. (B)
2942. (B)
2943. (A)
2944. (C)
2945. (A)
2946. (A)
2947. (C)
2948. (C)
2949. (D)
2950. (B)
2951. (D)
2952. (B)
2953. (D)
2954. (A)
2955. (B)

2956. (D)
2957. (A)
2958. (B)
2959. (A)
2960. (A)
2961. (A)
2962. (C)
2963. (B)
2964. (A)
2965. (C)
2966. (A)
2967. (C)
2968. (A)
2969. (A)
2970. (A)
2971. (A)
2972. (A)
2973. (A)
2974. (C)
2975. (D)
2976. (D)
2977. (B)
2978. (C)
2979. (A)
2980. (A)
2981. (B)
2982. (C)
2983. (B)
2984. (A)
2985. (C)
2986. (B)
2987. (D)
2988. (A)
2989. (A)
2990. (D)
2991. (C)
2992. (A)
2993. (C)
2994. (D)
2995. (A)
2996. (C)
2997. (B)
2998. (C)
2999. (D)
3000. (C)
3001. (A)
3002. (A)
3003. (B)
3004. (B)
3005. (C)
3006. (C)
3007. (D)
3008. (D)
3009. (A)
3010. (C)
3011. (D)
3012. (A)
3013. (A)
3014. (C)
3015. (A)
3016. (A)
3017. (C)
3018. (A)
3019. (D)
3020. (A)
3021. (A)
3022. (C)
3023. (C)
3024. (D)
3025. (B)
3026. (A)
3027. (B)
3028. (B)
3029. (A)
3030. (C)
3031. (B)
3032. (A)
3033. (A)
3034. (A)
3035. (A)
3036. (C)
3037. (A)
3038. (A)
3039. (A)
3040. (C)
3041. (B)
3042. (A)
3043. (D)
3044. (A)
3045. (B)
3046. (A)
3047. (D)
3048. (B)
3049. (C)
3050. (C)
3051. (A)
3052. (D)
3053. (C)
3054. (C)
3055. (A)
3056. (B)
3057. (A)
3058. (C)
3059. (C)
3060. (A)
3061. (B)
3062. (D)
3063. (C)
3064. (B)
3065. (C)
3066. (C)
3067. (C)
3068. (B)
3069. (A)
3070. (A)
3071. (C)
3072. (D)
3073. (D)
3074. (A)
3075. (C)
3076. (B)
3077. (C)
3078. (D)
3079. (C)
3080. (D)
3081. (C)
3082. (A)
3083. (B)
3084. (B)
3085. (B)
3086. (A)
3087. (C)
3088. (D)
3089. (A)
3090. (A)
3091. (D)
3092. (D)
3093. (B)
3094. (B)
3095. (D)
3096. (C)
3097. (B)
3098. (C)
3099. (A)
3100. (C)
3101. (C)
3102. (B)
3103. (A)
3104. (C)
3105. (B)
3106. (A)
3107. (B)
3108. (A)
3109. (A)
3110. (B)
3111. (D)
3112. (B)
3113. (C)
3114. (D)
3115. (A)
3116. (A)
3117. (C)
3118. (C)
3119. (B)
3120. (A)
3121. (C)
3122. (A)
3123. (C)
3124. (A)
3125. (B)
3126. (B)
3127. (A)
3128. (A)
3129. (D)
3130. (A)
3131. (D)
3132. (C)
3133. (B)
3134. (D)
3135. (B)
3136. (C)
3137. (B)
3138. (B)
3139. (A)
3140. (B)

3141. (A)
3142. (C)
3143. (B)
3144. (A)
3145. (A)
3146. (A)
3147. (C)
3148. (C)
3149. (A)
3150. (D)
3151. (C)
3152. (A)
3153. (B)
3154. (C)
3155. (B)
3156. (A)
3157. (C)
3158. (D)
3159. (A)
3160. (D)
3161. (D)
3162. (B)
3163. (B)
3164. (D)
3165. (B)
3166. (A)
3167. (C)
3168. (B)
3169. (C)
3170. (A)
3171. (C)
3172. (A)
3173. (D)
3174. (C)
3175. (A)
3176. (C)
3177. (A)
3178. (B)
3179. (A)
3180. (C)
3181. (D)
3182. (D)
3183. (A)
3184. (B)
3185. (A)
3186. (D)
3187. (A)
3188. (A)
3189. (B)
3190. (C)
3191. (B)
3192. (D)
3193. (B)
3194. (A)
3195. (B)
3196. (D)
3197. (A)
3198. (D)
3199. (A)
3200. (B)
3201. (C)
3202. (C)
3203. (C)
3204. (B)
3205. (A)
3206. (B)
3207. (B)
3208. (D)
3209. (C)
3210. (D)
3211. (C)
3212. (C)
3213. (B)
3214. (A)
3215. (B)
3216. (B)
3217. (D)
3218. (D)
3219. (A)
3220. (C)
3221. (B)
3222. (D)
3223. (B)
3224. (D)
3225. (A)
3226. (A)
3227. (A)
3228. (A)
3229. (C)
3230. (D)
3231. (B)
3232. (A)
3233. (A)
3234. (B)
3235. (D)
3236. (C)
3237. (B)
3238. (A)
3239. (C)
3240. (D)
3241. (B)
3242. (A)
3243. (C)
3244. (A)
3245. (A)
3246. (B)
3247. (D)
3248. (A)
3249. (D)
3250. (B)
3251. (C)
3252. (C)
3253. (B)
3254. (A)
3255. (C)
3256. (A)
3257. (C)
3258. (D)
3259. (B)
3260. (C)
3261. (A)
3262. (C)
3263. (B)
3264. (B)
3265. (D)
3266. (A)
3267. (D)
3268. (A)
3269. (C)
3270. (D)
3271. (A)
3272. (B)
3273. (C)
3274. (A)
3275. (D)
3276. (B)
3277. (A)
3278. (B)
3279. (C)
3280. (A)
3281. (D)
3282. (B)
3283. (C)
3284. (D)
3285. (A)
3286. (C)
3287. (B)
3288. (C)
3289. (C)
3290. (D)
3291. (A)
3292. (C)
3293. (B)
3294. (D)
3295. (A)
3296. (C)
3297. (D)
3298. (B)
3299. (D)
3300. (B)
3301. (A)
3302. (C)
3303. (D)
3304. (B)
3305. (A)
3306. (C)
3307. (D)
3308. (C)
3309. (B)
3310. (A)
3311. (C)
3312. (B)
3313. (D)
3314. (A)
3315. (D)
3316. (B)
3317. (C)
3318. (D)
3319. (B)
3320. (C)
3321. (C)
3322. (A)
3323. (B)
3324. (D)
3325. (A)

3326. (C)
3327. (B)
3328. (D)
3329. (C)
3330. (A)
3331. (B)
3332. (A)
3333. (A)
3334. (C)
3335. (B)
3336. (A)
3337. (C)
3338. (B)
3339. (D)
3340. (B)
3341. (C)
3342. (B)
3343. (B)
3344. (A)
3345. (B)
3346. (D)
3347. (C)
3348. (B)
3349. (A)
3350. (A)
3351. (D)
3352. (B)
3353. (C)
3354. (A)
3355. (D)
3356. (B)
3357. (C)
3358. (D)
3359. (A)
3360. (C)
3361. (B)
3362. (A)
3363. (A)
3364. (C)
3365. (B)
3366. (B)
3367. (D)
3368. (C)
3369. (A)
3370. (D)
3371. (B)
3372. (C)
3373. (A)
3374. (D)
3375. (B)
3376. (C)
3377. (A)
3378. (B)
3379. (A)
3380. (D)
3381. (A)
3382. (C)
3383. (C)
3384. (D)
3385. (B)
3386. (A)
3387. (C)
3388. (C)
3389. (D)
3390. (A)
3391. (C)
3392. (C)
3393. (B)
3394. (D)
3395. (A)
3396. (D)
3397. (C)
3398. (A)
3399. (B)
3400. (C)
3401. (C)
3402. (B)
3403. (C)
3404. (C)
3405. (D)
3406. (A)
3407. (B)
3408. (B)
3409. (A)
3410. (B)
3411. (C)
3412. (B)
3413. (C)
3414. (C)
3415. (B)
3416. (C)
3417. (A)
3418. (A)
3419. (B)
3420. (C)
3421. (B)
3422. (C)
3423. (D)
3424. (C)
3425. (A)
3426. (B)
3427. (D)
3428. (C)
3429. (C)
3430. (B)
3431. (D)
3432. (A)
3433. (B)
3434. (C)
3435. (A)
3436. (B)
3437. (C)
3438. (D)
3439. (B)
3440. (A)
3441. (D)
3442. (B)
3443. (C)
3444. (D)
3445. (A)
3446. (D)
3447. (A)
3448. (D)
3449. (C)
3450. (C)
3451. (C)
3452. (A)
3453. (D)
3454. (B)
3455. (A)
3456. (D)
3457. (B)
3458. (D)
3459. (A)
3460. (B)
3461. (C)
3462. (B)
3463. (C)
3464. (A)
3465. (D)
3466. (B)
3467. (A)
3468. (C)
3469. (A)
3470. (D)
3471. (B)
3472. (B)
3473. (D)
3474. (C)
3475. (B)
3476. (C)
3477. (B)
3478. (C)
3479. (A)
3480. (C)
3481. (B)
3482. (B)
3483. (B)
3484. (B)
3485. (C)
3486. (D)
3487. (A)
3488. (A)
3489. (D)
3490. (B)
3491. (D)
3492. (B)
3493. (C)
3494. (A)
3495. (C)
3496. (A)
3497. (D)
3498. (A)
3499. (B)
3500. (D)
3501. (D)
3502. (A)
3503. (D)
3504. (C)
3505. (C)
3506. (D)
3507. (B)
3508. (A)
3509. (C)
3510. (A)

3511. (A)
3512. (D)
3513. (C)
3514. (A)
3515. (A)
3516. (B)
3517. (A)
3518. (A)
3519. (A)
3520. (A)
3521. (C)
3522. (B)
3523. (A)
3524. (A)
3525. (D)
3526. (A)
3527. (B)
3528. (B)
3529. (A)
3530. (D)
3531. (D)
3532. (B)
3533. (D)
3534. (B)
3535. (B)
3536. (C)
3537. (C)
3538. (D)
3539. (B)
3540. (A)
3541. (C)
3542. (C)
3543. (D)
3544. (C)
3545. (C)
3546. (C)
3547. (B)
3548. (D)
3549. (D)
3550. (C)
3551. (A)
3552. (C)
3553. (C)
3554. (A)
3555. (A)
3556. (B)
3557. (D)
3558. (C)
3559. (C)
3560. (A)
3561. (C)
3562. (B)
3563. (A)
3564. (C)
3565. (C)
3566. (B)
3567. (B)
3568. (A)
3569. (D)
3570. (A)
3571. (C)
3572. (D)
3573. (B)
3574. (C)
3575. (A)
3576. (B)
3577. (C)
3578. (C)
3579. (A)
3580. (A)
3581. (B)
3582. (A)
3583. (B)
3584. (C)
3585. (D)
3586. (C)
3587. (A)
3588. (A)
3589. (C)
3590. (D)
3591. (A)
3592. (B)
3593. (A)
3594. (C)
3595. (A)
3596. (C)
3597. (B)
3598. (B)
3599. (D)
3600. (A)
3601. (C)
3602. (D)
3603. (A)
3604. (B)
3605. (C)
3606. (B)
3607. (A)
3608. (B)
3609. (C)
3610. (C)
3611. (A)
3612. (A)
3613. (A)
3614. (A)
3615. (D)
3616. (A)
3617. (B)
3618. (C)
3619. (A)
3620. (C)
3621. (D)
3622. (A)
3623. (A)
3624. (B)
3625. (D)
3626. (A)
3627. (C)
3628. (D)
3629. (A)
3630. (A)
3631. (C)
3632. (B)
3633. (D)
3634. (A)
3635. (B)
3636. (C)
3637. (A)
3638. (B)
3639. (D)
3640. (A)
3641. (C)
3642. (B)
3643. (D)
3644. (A)
3645. (B)
3646. (D)
3647. (D)
3648. (B)
3649. (D)
3650. (D)
3651. (A)
3652. (D)
3653. (A)
3654. (A)
3655. (C)
3656. (D)
3657. (A)
3658. (B)
3659. (D)
3660. (C)
3661. (B)
3662. (D)
3663. (B)
3664. (C)
3665. (A)
3666. (B)
3667. (C)
3668. (A)
3669. (B)
3670. (A)
3671. (A)
3672. (C)
3673. (A)
3674. (A)
3675. (D)
3676. (C)
3677. (A)
3678. (C)
3679. (D)
3680. (A)
3681. (C)
3682. (B)
3683. (C)
3684. (C)
3685. (A)
3686. (D)
3687. (B)
3688. (A)
3689. (B)
3690. (B)
3691. (C)
3692. (D)
3693. (C)
3694. (A)
3695. (B)

3696. (C)
3697. (A)
3698. (D)
3699. (A)
3700. (B)
3701. (A)
3702. (B)
3703. (B)
3704. (A)
3705. (C)
3706. (A)
3707. (B)
3708. (D)
3709. (A)
3710. (B)
3711. (C)
3712. (C)
3713. (A)
3714. (B)
3715. (A)
3716. (C)
3717. (C)
3718. (A)
3719. (C)
3720. (C)
3721. (A)
3722. (A)
3723. (D)
3724. (D)
3725. (C)
3726. (C)
3727. (D)
3728. (C)
3729. (A)
3730. (C)
3731. (B)
3732. (D)
3733. (A)
3734. (C)
3735. (A)
3736. (B)
3737. (A)
3738. (C)
3739. (A)
3740. (A)
3741. (A)
3742. (B)
3743. (A)
3744. (C)
3745. (D)
3746. (A)
3747. (B)
3748. (A)
3749. (D)
3750. (A)
3751. (B)
3752. (C)
3753. (A)
3754. (B)
3755. (B)
3756. (D)
3757. (D)
3758. (A)
3759. (D)
3760. (C)
3761. (D)
3762. (C)
3763. (A)
3764. (A)
3765. (B)
3766. (D)
3767. (A)
3768. (B)
3769. (C)
3770. (A)
3771. (A)
3772. (A)
3773. (B)
3774. (C)
3775. (C)
3776. (D)
3777. (B)
3778. (B)
3779. (A)
3780. (B)
3781. (C)
3782. (D)
3783. (A)
3784. (A)
3785. (C)
3786. (C)
3787. (B)
3788. (D)
3789. (C)
3790. (D)
3791. (A)
3792. (A)
3793. (D)
3794. (D)
3795. (C)
3796. (B)
3797. (B)
3798. (A)
3799. (C)
3800. (D)
3801. (D)
3802. (C)
3803. (A)
3804. (C)
3805. (B)
3806. (D)
3807. (A)
3808. (D)
3809. (A)
3810. (B)
3811. (D)
3812. (B)
3813. (C)
3814. (A)
3815. (C)
3816. (D)
3817. (C)
3818. (B)
3819. (A)
3820. (D)
3821. (A)
3822. (A)
3823. (B)
3824. (A)
3825. (D)
3826. (A)
3827. (C)
3828. (C)
3829. (D)
3830. (A)
3831. (B)
3832. (A)
3833. (A)
3834. (B)
3835. (A)
3836. (D)
3837. (C)
3838. (B)
3839. (B)
3840. (B)
3841. (A)
3842. (B)
3843. (C)
3844. (B)
3845. (A)
3846. (C)
3847. (A)
3848. (A)
3849. (B)
3850. (C)
3851. (A)
3852. (C)
3853. (C)
3854. (D)
3855. (A)
3856. (C)
3857. (B)
3858. (B)
3859. (C)
3860. (D)
3861. (D)
3862. (A)
3863. (C)
3864. (B)
3865. (A)
3866. (D)
3867. (B)
3868. (A)
3869. (C)
3870. (A)
3871. (D)
3872. (B)
3873. (B)
3874. (A)
3875. (C)
3876. (D)
3877. (D)
3878. (C)
3879. (A)
3880. (D)

3881.	(C)	3918.	(C)	3955.	(D)	3992.	(B)	4029.	(A)
3882.	(D)	3919.	(D)	3956.	(B)	3993.	(A)	4030.	(C)
3883.	(A)	3920.	(A)	3957.	(C)	3994.	(D)	4031.	(A)
3884.	(C)	3921.	(A)	3958.	(A)	3995.	(D)	4032.	(C)
3885.	(D)	3922.	(C)	3959.	(C)	3996.	(D)	4033.	(D)
3886.	(C)	3923.	(D)	3960.	(B)	3997.	(D)	4034.	(B)
3887.	(B)	3924.	(D)	3961.	(C)	3998.	(A)	4035.	(A)
3888.	(D)	3925.	(A)	3962.	(B)	3999.	(C)	4036.	(C)
3889.	(D)	3926.	(B)	3963.	(B)	4000.	(A)	4037.	(D)
3890.	(B)	3927.	(C)	3964.	(B)	4001.	(C)	4038.	(B)
3891.	(A)	3928.	(A)	3965.	(D)	4002.	(A)	4039.	(C)
3892.	(C)	3929.	(B)	3966.	(A)	4003.	(C)	4040.	(B)
3893.	(A)	3930.	(C)	3967.	(C)	4004.	(C)	4041.	(B)
3894.	(A)	3931.	(A)	3968.	(A)	4005.	(A)	4042.	(C)
3895.	(A)	3932.	(D)	3969.	(C)	4006.	(D)	4043.	(A)
3896.	(B)	3933.	(C)	3970.	(D)	4007.	(A)	4044.	(C)
3897.	(C)	3934.	(B)	3971.	(A)	4008.	(A)	4045.	(C)
3898.	(A)	3935.	(D)	3972.	(A)	4009.	(C)	4046.	(D)
3899.	(B)	3936.	(A)	3973.	(C)	4010.	(B)	4047.	(D)
3900.	(C)	3937.	(D)	3974.	(B)	4011.	(B)	4048.	(B)
3901.	(B)	3938.	(D)	3975.	(C)	4012.	(C)	4049.	(D)
3902.	(A)	3939.	(B)	3976.	(C)	4013.	(C)	4050.	(B)
3903.	(B)	3940.	(C)	3977.	(B)	4014.	(B)	4051.	(C)
3904.	(B)	3941.	(A)	3978.	(A)	4015.	(A)	4052.	(D)
3905.	(A)	3942.	(C)	3979.	(C)	4016.	(D)	4053.	(A)
3906.	(D)	3943.	(B)	3980.	(B)	4017.	(B)	4054	(B)
3907.	(A)	3944.	(D)	3981.	(A)	4018.	(C)	4055.	(C)
3908.	(D)	3945.	(C)	3982.	(C)	4019.	(D)	4056.	(D)
3909.	(C)	3946.	(C)	3983.	(D)	4020.	(A)	4057.	(A)
3910.	(A)	3947.	(C)	3984.	(B)	4021.	(B)	4058.	(D)
3911.	(B)	3948.	(A)	3985.	(A)	4022.	(D)	4059.	(A)
3912.	(A)	3949.	(B)	3986.	(C)	4023.	(B)	4060.	(B)
3913.	(B)	3950.	(C)	3987.	(B)	4024.	(C)	4061.	(A)
3914.	(C)	3951.	(B)	3988.	(A)	4025.	(D)	4062.	(B)
3915.	(A)	3952.	(A)	3989.	(B)	4026.	(B)	4063.	(D)
3916.	(D)	3953.	(C)	3990.	(?)	4027.	(A)	4064.	(C)
3917.	(A)	3954.	(A)	3991.	(C)	4028.	(A)	4065.	(C)

4066. (D)
4067. (D)
4068. (A)
4069. (C)
4070. (D)
4071. (A)
4072. (C)
4073. (C)
4074. (A)
4075. (B)
4076. (A)
4077. (D)
4078. (A)
4079. (A)
4080. (D)
4081. (A)
4082. (B)
4083. (C)
4084. (D)
4085. (A)
4086. (D)
4087. (C)
4088. (B)
4089. (B)
4090. (B)
4091. (C)
4092. (D)
4093. (B)
4094. (A)
4095. (B)
4096. (A)
4097. (B)
4098. (A)
4099. (B)
4100. (D)
4101. (B)
4102. (C)
4103. (D)
4104. (D)
4105. (A)
4106. (D)
4107. (B)
4108. (A)
4109. (A)
4110. (A)
4111. (C)
4112. (C)
4113. (A)
4114. (A)
4115. (D)
4116. (A)
4117. (A)
4118. (C)
4119. (D)
4120. (B)
4121. (D)
4122. (D)
4123. (A)
4124. (A)
4125. (D)
4126. (A)
4127. (A)
4128. (A)
4129. (C)
4130. (D)
4131. (D)
4132. (A)
4133. (C)
4134. (D)
4135. (A)
4136. (D)
4137. (A)
4138. (A)
4139. (A)
4140. (A)
4141. (A)
4142. (A)
4143. (C)
4144. (A)
4145. (A)
4146. (A)
4147. (A)
4148. (A)
4149. (A)
4150. (A)
4151. (A)
4152. (A)
4153. (A)
4154. (A)
4155. (D)
4156. (A)
4157. (C)
4158. (A)
4159. (D)
4160. (D)
4161. (D)
4162. (A)
4163. (A)
4164. (A)
4165. (A)
4166. (A)
4167. (C)
4168. (A)
4169. (C)
4170. (A)
4171. (D)
4172. (D)
4173. (D)
4174. (C)
4175. (C)
4176. (C)
4177. (B)
4178. (C)
4179. (B)
4180. (C)
4181. (C)
4182. (D)
4183. (A)
4184. (B)
4185. (A)
4186. (B)
4187. (C)
4188. (C)
4189. (C)
4190. (D)
4191. (C)
4192. (B)
4193. (A)
4194. (D)
4195. (B)
4196. (A)
4197. (D)
4198. (A)
4199. (D)
4200. (B)
4201. (C)
4202. (D)
4203. (C)
4204. (D)
4205. (A)
4206. (D)
4207. (A)
4208. (A)
4209. (D)
4210. (A)
4211. (A)
4212. (A)
4213. (A)
4214. (A)
4215. (A)
4216. (A)
4217. (A)
4218. (A)
4219. (A)
4220. (A)
4221. (A)
4222. (C)
4223. (A)
4224. (A)
4225. (A)
4226. (A)
4227. (A)
4228. (A)
4229. (C)
4230. (A)
4231. (A)
4232. (A)
4233. (A)
4234. (A)
4235. (A)
4236. (B)
4237. (A)
4238. (A)
4239. (A)
4240. (A)
4241. (A)
4242. (A)
4243. (A)
4244. (A)
4245. (A)
4246. (A)
4247. (C)
4248. (A)
4249. (A)
4250. (A)

4251.	(A)	4276.	(C)	4301.	(B)	4326.	(B)	4351.	(A)
4252.	(A)	4277.	(A)	4302.	(A)	4327.	(C)	4352.	(A)
4253.	(B)	4278.	(A)	4303.	(A)	4328.	(C)	4353.	(A)
4254.	(C)	4279.	(B)	4304.	(D)	4329.	(C)	4354.	(A)
4255.	(C)	4280.	(C)	4305.	(C)	4330.	(B)	4355.	(B)
4256.	(C)	4281.	(A)	4306.	(A)	4331.	(C)	4356.	(D)
4257.	(A)	4282.	(B)	4307.	(C)	4332.	(B)	4357.	(A)
4258.	(C)	4283.	(C)	4308.	(C)	4333.	(A)	4358.	(A)
4259.	(B)	4284.	(A)	4309.	(A)	4334.	(B)	4359.	(A)
4260.	(D)	4285.	(B)	4310.	(A)	4335.	(A)	4360.	(D)
4261.	(B)	4286.	(A)	4311.	(A)	4336.	(D)	4361.	(A)
4262.	(A)	4287.	(C)	4312.	(D)	4337.	(A)	4362.	(D)
4263.	(C)	4288.	(D)	4313.	(A)	4338.	(D)	4363.	(C)
4264.	(C)	4289.	(A)	4314.	(D)	4339.	(A)	4364.	(D)
4265.	(A)	4290.	(B)	4315.	(A)	4340.	(C)	4365.	(D)
4266.	(D)	4291.	(A)	4316.	(B)	4341.	(B)	4366.	(B)
4267.	(D)	4292.	(D)	4317.	(D)	4342.	(D)	4367.	(D)
4268.	(C)	4293.	(A)	4318.	(D)	4343.	(B)	4368.	(D)
4269.	(A)	4294.	(D)	4319.	(A)	4344.	(B)	4369.	(B)
4270.	(D)	4295.	(A)	4320.	(C)	4345.	(B)	4370.	(D)
4271.	(B)	4296.	(D)	4321.	(A)	4346.	(A)	4371.	(C)
4272.	(C)	4297.	(D)	4322.	(C)	4347.	(D)		
4273.	(D)	4298.	(D)	4323.	(D)	4348.	(A)		
4274.	(A)	4299.	(A)	4324.	(A)	4349.	(A)		
4275.	(D)	4300.	(C)	4325.	(D)	4350.	(C)		

Chapter 3A: Pharmacognosy and Phytochemistry

1.	(B)	38.	(C)	75.	(C)	112.	(C)	149.	(A)	186.	(D)
2.	(B)	39.	(A)	76.	(D)	113.	(C)	150.	(A)	187.	(C)
3.	(C)	40.	(A)	77.	(C)	114.	(C)	151.	(B)	188.	(A)
4.	(A)	41.	(A)	78.	(C)	115.	(C)	152.	(D)	189.	(A)
5.	(B)	42.	(B)	79.	(B)	116.	(B)	153.	(A)	190.	(A)
6.	(C)	43.	(D)	80.	(C)	117.	(A)	154.	(C)	191.	(A)
7.	(D)	44.	(A)	81.	(D)	118.	(C)	155.	(A)	192.	(A)
8.	(B)	45.	(B)	82.	(D)	119.	(A)	156.	(A)	193.	(D)
9.	(C)	46.	(C)	83.	(B)	120.	(C)	157.	(A)	194.	(B)
10.	(D)	47.	(C)	84.	(D)	121.	(B)	158.	(A)	195.	(C)
11.	(C)	48.	(A)	85.	(B)	122.	(B)	159.	(A)	196.	(B)
12.	(C)	49.	(C)	86.	(A)	123.	(C)	160.	(C)	197.	(C)
13.	(C)	50.	(D)	87.	(D)	124.	(B)	161.	(A)	198.	(A)
14.	(C)	51.	(B)	88.	(A)	125.	(B)	162.	(A)	199.	(A)
15.	(C)	52.	(A)	89.	(D)	126.	(A)	163.	(A)	200.	(A)
16.	(A)	53.	(C)	90.	(D)	127.	(B)	164.	(A)	201.	(D)
17.	(C)	54.	(A)	91.	(A)	128.	(A)	165.	(A)	202.	(C)
18.	(A)	55.	(C)	92.	(B)	129.	(D)	166.	(D)	203.	(C)
19.	(C)	56.	(B)	93.	(B)	130.	(B)	167.	(A)	204.	(A)
20.	(C)	57.	(D)	94.	(C)	131.	(A)	168.	(C)	205.	(C)
21.	(C)	58.	(B)	95.	(D)	132.	(A)	169.	(C)	206.	(B)
22.	(B)	59.	(C)	96.	(C)	133.	(B)	170.	(C)	207.	(D)
23.	(D)	60.	(C)	97.	(C)	134.	(C)	171.	(A)	208.	(D)
24.	(B)	61.	(A)	98.	(D)	135.	(C)	172.	(D)	209.	(C)
25.	(A)	62.	(B)	99.	(C)	136.	(D)	173.	(C)	210.	(C)
26.	(A)	63.	(A)	100.	(C)	137.	(C)	174.	(A)	211.	(A)
27.	(B)	64.	(C)	101.	(D)	138.	(C)	175.	(A)	212.	(B)
28.	(A)	65.	(B)	102.	(C)	139.	(C)	176.	(A)	213.	(A)
29.	(B)	66.	(A)	103.	(A)	140.	(C)	177.	(A)	214.	(A)
30.	(B)	67.	(C)	104.	(D)	141.	(C)	178.	(A)	215.	(B)
31.	(D)	68.	(A)	105.	(A)	142.	(C)	179.	(D)	216.	(B)
32.	(C)	69.	(D)	106.	(A)	143.	(B)	180.	(A)	217.	(B)
33.	(C)	70.	(C)	107.	(D)	144.	(D)	181.	(B)	218.	(B)
34.	(C)	71.	(C)	108.	(C)	145.	(D)	182.	(A)	219.	(D)
35.	(B)	72.	(D)	109.	(B)	146.	(D)	183.	(A)	220.	(D)
36.	(B)	73.	(C)	110.	(B)	147.	(D)	184.	(A)	221.	(D)
37.	(B)	74.	(A)	111.	(A)	148.	(A)	185.	(A)	222.	(A)

223. (A)
224. (A)
225. (C)
226. (C)
227. (B)
228. (A)
229. (D)
230. (B)
231. (C)
232. (A)
233. (C)
234. (A)
235. (B)
236. (D)
237. (A)
238. (D)
239. (C)
240. (C)
241. (B)
242. (C)
243. (C)
244. (A)
245. (B)
246. (C)
247. (C)
248. (A)
249. (C)
250. (A)
251. (D)
252. (B)
253. (C)
254. (C)
255. (A)
256. (A)
257. (A)
258. (D)
259. (D)
260. (D)
261. (C)
262. (B)
263. (A)
264. (C)
265. (C)
266. (B)
267. (D)
268. (A)
269. (A)
270. (A)
271. (D)
272. (B)
273. (D)
274. (A)
275. (A)
276. (B)
277. (D)
278. (B)
279. (D)
280. (B)
281. (B)
282. (A)
283. (D)
284. (B)
285. (D)
286. (C)
287. (B)
288. (B)
289. (A)
290. (C)
291. (A)
292. (D)
293. (D)
294. (A)
295. (A)
296. (A)
297. (A)
298. (D)
299. (D)
300. (D)
301. (A)
302. (C)
303. (C)
304. (B)
305. (A)
306. (C)
307. (A)
308. (C)
309. (C)
310. (D)
311. (C)
312. (A)
313. (A)
314. (B)
315. (A)
316. (A)
317. (C)
318. (D)
319. (B)
320. (D)
321. (B)
322. (A)
323. (C)
324. (D)
325. (D)
326. (A)
327. (D)
328. (A)
329. (D)
330. (A)
331. (D)
332. (B)
333. (A)
334. (C)
335. (D)
336. (A)
337. (B)
338. (A)
339. (B)
340. (B)
341. (A)
342. (B)
343. (B)
344. (B)
345. (D)
346. (B)
347. (A)
348. (A)
349. (A)
350. (C)
351. (C)
352. (D)
353. (D)
354. (D)
355. (B)
356. (A)
357. (D)
358. (D)
359. (D)
360. (B)
361. (D)
362. (A)
363. (D)
364. (A)
365. (C)
366. (A)
367. (C)
368. (D)
369. (A)
370. (A)
371. (C)
372. (A)
373. (D)
374. (A)
375. (B)
376. (A)
377. (D)
378. (A)
379. (C)
380. (D)
381. (A)
382. (A)
383. (A)
384. (A)
385. (A)
386. (A)
387. (C)
388. (A)
389. (C)
390. (A)
391. (A)
392. (D)
393. (A)
394. (D)
395. (D)
396. (A)
397. (D)
398. (A)
399. (D)
400. (A)
401. (A)
402. (D)
403. (A)
404. (A)
405. (D)
406. (D)
407. (A)
408. (A)
409. (A)
410. (D)
411. (A)
412. (B)
413. (B)
414. (C)
415. (A)
416. (A)
417. (B)
418. (D)
419. (D)
420. (A)
421. (A)
422. (A)
423. (B)
424. (A)
425. (D)
426. (A)
427. (A)
428. (D)
429. (D)
430. (B)
431. (D)
432. (A)
433. (A)
434. (D)
435. (A)
436. (C)
437. (D)
438. (D)
439. (A)
440. (A)
441. (D)
442. (A)
443. (D)
444. (A)
445. (D)
446. (D)
447. (C)
448. (A)
449. (D)
450. (C)

451.	(A)	489.	(D)	527.	(D)	565.	(A)	603.	(D)	641.	(A)
452.	(A)	490.	(C)	528.	(A)	566.	(A)	604.	(D)	642.	(C)
453.	(C)	491.	(D)	529.	(C)	567.	(A)	605.	(D)	643.	(C)
454.	(C)	492.	(B)	530.	(B)	568.	(A)	606.	(D)	644.	(D)
455.	(A)	493.	(D)	531.	(A)	569.	(D)	607.	(A)	645.	(A)
456.	(D)	494.	(A)	532.	(A)	570.	(B)	608.	(D)	646.	(D)
457.	(C)	495.	(B)	533.	(A)	571.	(A)	609.	(B)	647.	(C)
458.	(A)	496.	(A)	534.	(D)	572.	(A)	610.	(D)	648.	(A)
459.	(D)	497.	(D)	535.	(A)	573.	(B)	611.	(A)	649.	(A)
460.	(C)	498.	(A)	536.	(D)	574.	(D)	612.	(A)	650.	(B)
461.	(C)	499.	(C)	537.	(D)	575.	(A)	613.	(A)	651.	(B)
462.	(A)	500.	(A)	538.	(B)	576.	(B)	614.	(B)	652.	(B)
463.	(D)	501.	(B)	539.	(D)	577.	(A)	615.	(D)	653.	(C)
464.	(D)	502.	(D)	540.	(D)	578.	(A)	616.	(A)	654.	(A)
465.	(D)	503.	(D)	541.	(D)	579.	(A)	617.	(D)	655.	(A)
466.	(A)	504.	(A)	542.	(A)	580.	(C)	618.	(C)	656.	(A)
467.	(D)	505.	(A)	543.	(D)	581.	(A)	619.	(A)	657.	(B)
468.	(A)	506.	(A)	544.	(A)	582.	(C)	620.	(B)	658.	(C)
469.	(A)	507.	(B)	545.	(C)	583.	(A)	621.	(D)	659.	(C)
470.	(A)	508.	(A)	546.	(B)	584.	(C)	622.	(A)	660.	(A)
471.	(C)	509.	(A)	547.	(A)	585.	(D)	623.	(B)	661.	(B)
472.	(C)	510.	(A)	548.	(C)	586.	(D)	624.	(A)	662.	(B)
473.	(A)	511.	(D)	549.	(D)	587.	(A)	625.	(B)	663.	(A)
474.	(A)	512.	(A)	550.	(C)	588.	(D)	626.	(B)	664.	(B)
475.	(D)	513.	(C)	551.	(C)	589.	(A)	627.	(C)	665.	(C)
476.	(D)	514.	(B)	552.	(B)	590.	(A)	628.	(A)	666.	(A)
477.	(D)	515.	(D)	553.	(A)	591.	(A)	629.	(C)	667.	(B)
478.	(A)	516.	(D)	554.	(C)	592.	(D)	630.	(B)	668.	(A)
479.	(A)	517.	(B)	555.	(C)	593.	(A)	631.	(A)	669.	(A)
480.	(C)	518.	(A)	556.	(D)	594.	(D)	632.	(B)	670.	(B)
481.	(A)	519.	(A)	557.	(A)	595.	(D)	633.	(A)	671.	(A)
482.	(A)	520.	(A)	558.	(B)	596.	(D)	634.	(C)	672.	(B)
483.	(C)	521.	(C)	559.	(A)	597.	(D)	635.	(A)	673.	(A)
484.	(D)	522.	(A)	560.	(D)	598.	(C)	636.	(A)	674.	(A)
485.	(C)	523.	(A)	561.	(C)	599.	(D)	637.	(D)	675.	(B)
486.	(D)	524.	(B)	562.	(D)	600.	(D)	638.	(D)	676.	(C)
487.	(C)	525.	(C)	563.	(B)	601.	(B)	639.	(B)	677.	(A)
488.	(C)	526.	(A)	564.	(A)	602.	(D)	640.	(B)	678.	(A)

679.	(D)	717.	(A)	755.	(A)	793.	(C)	831.	(A)	869.	(A)
680.	(B)	718.	(A)	756.	(B)	794.	(A)	832.	(A)	870.	(C)
681.	(D)	719.	(A)	757.	(A)	795.	(C)	833.	(B)	871.	(A)
682.	(A)	720.	(B)	758.	(A)	796.	(A)	834.	(A)	872.	(C)
683.	(C)	721.	(A)	759.	(B)	797.	(A)	835.	(B)	873.	(C)
684.	(C)	722.	(C)	760.	(A)	798.	(D)	836.	(A)	874.	(A)
685.	(A)	723.	(D)	761.	(A)	799.	(A)	837.	(C)	875.	(C)
686.	(D)	724.	(A)	762.	(A)	800.	(B)	838.	(A)	876.	(C)
687.	(A)	725.	(C)	763.	(A)	801.	(A)	839.	(D)	877.	(B)
688.	(A)	726.	(A)	764.	(C)	802.	(C)	840.	(A)	878.	(A)
689.	(C)	727.	(A)	765.	(B)	803.	(D)	841.	(A)	879.	(A)
690.	(A)	728.	(A)	766.	(A)	804.	(B)	842.	(A)	880.	(C)
691.	(C)	729.	(A)	767.	(A)	805.	(A)	843.	(C)	881.	(C)
692.	(A)	730.	(A)	768.	(A)	806.	(D)	844.	(A)	882.	(B)
693.	(A)	731.	(A)	769.	(A)	807.	(B)	845.	(A)	883.	(A)
694.	(B)	732.	(A)	770.	(B)	808.	(A)	846.	(A)	884.	(A)
695.	(B)	733.	(B)	771.	(B)	809.	(A)	847.	(A)	885.	(D)
696.	(C)	734.	(B)	772.	(A)	810.	(B)	848.	(C)	886.	(B)
697.	(A)	735.	(B)	773.	(B)	811.	(C)	849.	(B)	887.	(A)
698.	(A)	736.	(A)	774.	(B)	812.	(D)	850.	(D)	888.	(C)
699.	(B)	737.	(A)	775.	(B)	813.	(A)	851.	(C)	889.	(D)
700.	(C)	738.	(A)	776.	(A)	814.	(B)	852.	(A)	890.	(C)
701.	(A)	739.	(A)	777.	(A)	815.	(A)	853.	(C)	891.	(D)
702.	(C)	740.	(A)	778.	(A)	816.	(C)	854.	(A)	892.	(A)
703.	(A)	741.	(C)	779.	(A)	817.	(A)	855.	(A)	893.	(C)
704.	(A)	742.	(A)	780.	(B)	818.	(A)	856.	(A)	894.	(B)
705.	(A)	743.	(A)	781.	(B)	819.	(C)	857.	(C)	895.	(C)
706.	(B)	744.	(D)	782.	(A)	820.	(A)	858.	(A)	896.	(A)
707.	(A)	745.	(A)	783.	(A)	821.	(C)	859.	(B)	897.	(C)
708.	(A)	746.	(A)	784.	(B)	822.	(A)	860.	(B)	898.	(D)
709.	(B)	747.	(A)	785.	(A)	823.	(A)	861.	(A)	899.	(A)
710.	(A)	748.	(D)	786.	(A)	824.	(A)	862.	(B)	900.	(C)
711.	(B)	749.	(A)	787.	(A)	825.	(D)	863.	(A)	901.	(A)
712.	(A)	750.	(C)	788.	(B)	826.	(A)	864.	(A)	902.	(C)
713.	(B)	751.	(A)	789.	(B)	827.	(A)	865.	(A)	903.	(A)
714.	(D)	752.	(A)	790.	(A)	828.	(B)	866.	(A)	904.	(D)
715.	(A)	753.	(A)	791.	(A)	829.	(B)	867.	(B)	905.	(A)
716.	(A)	754.	(B)	792.	(A)	830.	(A)	868.	(B)	906.	(D)

907. (A)
908. (C)
909. (D)
910. (A)
911. (B)
912. (A)
913. (D)
914. (D)
915. (C)
916. (A)
917. (B)
918. (A)
919. (C)
920. (C)
921. (D)
922. (D)
923. (B)
924. (D)
925. (A)
926. (A)
927. (C)
928. (C)
929. (D)
930. (A)
931. (C)
932. (A)
933. (C)
934. (A)
935. (B)
936. (D)
937. (C)
938. (D)
939. (C)
940. (A)
941. (B)
942. (C)
943. (A)
944. (B)
945. (D)
946. (A)
947. (C)
948. (D)
949. (C)
950. (D)
951. (B)
952. (D)
953. (B)
954. (B)
955. (A)
956. (A)
957. (C)
958. (C)
959. (D)
960. (B)
961. (B)
962. (C)
963. (D)
964. (C)
965. (A)
966. (D)
967. (A)
968. (C)
969. (A)
970. (A)
971. (B)
972. (A)
973. (B)
974. (D)
975. (D)
976. (A)
977. (D)
978. (A)
979. (D)
980. (A)
981. (B)
982. (A)
983. (B)
984. (D)
985. (D)
986. (B)
987. (B)
988. (D)
989. (A)
990. (A)
991. (C)
992. (D)
993. (D)
994. (A)
995. (B)
996. (D)
997. (A)
998. (D)
999. (A)
1000. (D)
1001. (A)
1002. (D)
1003. (A)
1004. (C)
1005. (A)
1006. (A)
1007. (D)
1008. (A)
1009. (C)
1010. (A)
1011. (B)
1012. (C)
1013. (B)
1014. (A)
1015. (D)
1016. (C)
1017. (D)
1018. (B)
1019. (A)
1020. (C)
1021. (B)
1022. (C)
1023. (A)
1024. (B)
1025. (C)
1026. (B)
1027. (A)
1028. (C)
1029. (D)
1030. (B)
1031. (C)
1032. (C)
1033. (B)
1034. (D)
1035. (A)
1036. (C)
1037. (A)
1038. (B)
1039. (D)
1040. (C)
1041. (D)
1042. (B)
1043. (C)
1044. (B)
1045. (C)
1046. (B)
1047. (C)
1048. (B)
1049. (C)
1050. (A)
1051. (B)
1052. (A)
1053. (B)
1054. (A)
1055. (C)
1056. (B)
1057. (D)
1058. (A)
1059. (C)
1060. (A)
1061. (B)
1062. (B)
1063. (A)
1064. (C)
1065. (C)
1066. (B)
1067. (A)
1068. (A)
1069. (B)
1070. (D)
1071. (B)
1072. (D)
1073. (A)
1074. (C)
1075. (B)
1076. (D)
1077. (C)
1078. (A)
1079. (B)
1080. (C)
1081. (A)
1082. (D)
1083. (A)
1084. (D)
1085. (C)
1086. (B)
1087. (A)
1088. (D)
1089. (A)
1090. (B)
1091. (A)
1092. (B)
1093. (C)
1094. (B)
1095. (A)
1096. (D)
1097. (A)
1098. (D)
1099. (B)
1100. (A)
1101. (C)
1102. (A)
1103. (C)
1104. (A)
1105. (C)
1106. (A)
1107. (D)
1108. (D)
1109. (A)
1110. (A)
1111. (B)
1112. (B)
1113. (A)
1114. (C)
1115. (A)
1116. (C)
1117. (A)
1118. (D)
1119. (A)
1120. (D)
1121. (D)
1122. (A)
1123. (D)
1124. (D)
1125. (D)
1126. (C)
1127. (D)
1128. (D)
1129. (A)
1130. (A)
1131. (A)
1132. (D)
1133. (D)
1134. (A)

1135.	(A)	1173.	(C)	1211.	(A)	1249.	(C)	1287.	(A)	1325.	(B)
1136.	(B)	1174.	(A)	1212.	(B)	1250.	(B)	1288.	(C)	1326.	(C)
1137.	(A)	1175.	(D)	1213.	(B)	1251.	(B)	1289.	(B)	1327.	(B)
1138.	(D)	1176.	(C)	1214.	(B)	1252.	(B)	1290.	(D)	1328.	(A)
1139.	(D)	1177.	(B)	1215.	(D)	1253.	(C)	1291.	(A)	1329.	(D)
1140.	(A)	1178.	(C)	1216.	(A)	1254.	(D)	1292.	(C)	1330.	(A)
1141.	(B)	1179.	(D)	1217.	(B)	1255.	(C)	1293.	(A)	1331.	(D)
1142.	(B)	1180.	(C)	1218.	(C)	1256.	(A)	1294.	(B)	1332.	(B)
1143.	(A)	1181.	(D)	1219.	(B)	1257.	(D)	1295.	(B)	1333.	(A)
1144.	(D)	1182.	(A)	1220.	(C)	1258.	(A)	1296.	(A)	1334.	(C)
1145.	(A)	1183.	(C)	1221.	(A)	1259.	(C)	1297.	(C)	1335.	(A)
1146.	(C)	1184.	(B)	1222.	(A)	1260.	(A)	1298.	(C)	1336.	(C)
1147.	(A)	1185.	(D)	1223.	(C)	1261.	(A)	1299.	(B)	1337.	(A)
1148.	(D)	1186.	(B)	1224.	(D)	1262.	(B)	1300.	(A)	1338.	(C)
1149.	(D)	1187.	(B)	1225.	(A)	1263.	(A)	1301.	(A)	1339.	(A)
1150.	(A)	1188.	(D)	1226.	(B)	1264.	(B)	1302.	(B)	1340.	(D)
1151.	(B)	1189.	(B)	1227.	(D)	1265.	(D)	1303.	(?)	1341.	(D)
1152.	(C)	1190.	(C)	1228.	(B)	1266.	(D)	1304.	(B)	1342.	(A)
1153.	(D)	1191.	(A)	1229.	(B)	1267.	(A)	1305.	(D)	1343.	(A)
1154.	(D)	1192.	(C)	1230.	(A)	1268.	(D)	1306.	(A)	1344.	(B)
1155.	(A)	1193.	(D)	1231.	(C)	1269.	(A)	1307.	(C)	1345.	(B)
1156.	(A)	1194.	(B)	1232.	(B)	1270.	(D)	1308.	(B)	1346.	(A)
1157.	(D)	1195.	(A)	1233.	(B)	1271.	(A)	1309.	(D)	1347.	(C)
1158.	(A)	1196.	(D)	1234.	(B)	1272.	(B)	1310.	(C)	1348.	(A)
1159.	(A)	1197.	(D)	1235.	(A)	1273.	(A)	1311.	(A)	1349.	(C)
1160.	(D)	1198.	(D)	1236.	(A)	1274.	(B)	1312.	(D)	1350.	(A)
1161.	(A)	1199.	(B)	1237.	(D)	1275.	(D)	1313.	(C)	1351.	(D)
1162.	(D)	1200.	(C)	1238.	(C)	1276.	(D)	1314.	(A)	1352.	(A)
1163.	(C)	1201.	(B)	1239.	(C)	1277.	(B)	1315.	(D)	1353.	(D)
1164.	(B)	1202.	(A)	1240.	(B)	1278.	(B)	1316.	(A)	1354.	(D)
1165.	(B)	1203.	(D)	1241.	(C)	1279.	(D)	1317.	(D)	1355.	(A)
1166.	(D)	1204.	(B)	1242.	(A)	1280.	(A)	1318.	(C)	1356.	(D)
1167.	(C)	1205.	(A)	1243.	(D)	1281.	(A)	1319.	(B)	1357.	(D)
1168.	(D)	1206.	(B)	1244.	(B)	1282.	(C)	1320.	(A)	1358.	(D)
1169.	(D)	1207.	(C)	1245.	(A)	1283.	(D)	1321.	(D)	1359.	(C)
1170.	(B)	1208.	(B)	1246.	(B)	1284.	(D)	1322.	(A)	1360.	(D)
1171.	(A)	1209.	(D)	1247.	(A)	1285.	(A)	1323.	(D)	1361.	(D)
1172.	(C)	1210.	(C)	1248.	(A)	1286.	(B)	1324.	(A)	1362.	(A)

1363. (A)
1364. (A)
1365. (D)
1366. (D)
1367. (A)
1368. (A)
1369. (B)
1370. (A)
1371. (D)
1372. (D)
1373. (A)
1374. (B)
1375. (B)
1376. (A)
1377. (D)
1378. (B)
1379. (D)
1380. (C)
1381. (B)
1382. (C)
1383. (D)
1384. (C)
1385. (D)
1386. (A)
1387. (C)
1388. (B)
1389. (D)
1390. (D)
1391. (B)
1392. (B)
1393. (D)
1394. (B)
1395. (C)
1396. (D)
1397. (B)
1398. (A)
1399. (B)
1400. (C)
1401. (B)
1402. (D)
1403. (C)
1404. (A)
1405. (B)
1406. (B)
1407. (B)
1408. (D)
1409. (A)
1410. (B)
1411. (C)
1412. (B)
1413. (C)
1414. (A)
1415. (A)
1416. (C)
1417. (D)
1418. (A)
1419. (B)
1420. (D)
1421. (B)
1422. (B)
1423. (A)
1424. (C)
1425. (B)
1426. (B)
1427. (B)
1428. (A)
1429. (A)
1430. (D)
1431. (C)
1432. (C)
1433. (B)
1434. (C)
1435. (A)
1436. (D)
1437. (B)
1438. (A)
1439. (B)
1440. (A)
1441. (D)
1442. (D)
1443. (A)
1444. (C)
1445. (C)
1446. (C)
1447. (D)
1448. (C)
1449. (C)
1450. (A)
1451. (D)
1452. (B)
1453. (?)
1454. (D)
1455. (C)
1456. (C)
1457. (A)
1458. (A)
1459. (C)
1460. (C)
1461. (B)
1462. (D)
1463. (C)
1464. (A)
1465. (D)
1466. (C)
1467. (D)
1468. (C)
1469. (A)
1470. (C)
1471. (D)
1472. (B)
1473. (A)
1474. (A)
1475. (A)
1476. (C)
1477. (D)
1478. (B)
1479. (A)
1480. (D)
1481. (D)
1482. (B)
1483. (A)
1484. (C)
1485. (A)
1486. (B)
1487. (D)
1488. (A)
1489. (A)
1490. (B)
1491. (B)
1492. (B)
1493. (A)
1494. (D)
1495. (C)
1496. (A)
1497. (D)
1498. (B)
1499. (D)
1500. (A)
1501. (D)
1502. (B)
1503. (C)
1504. (D)
1505. (A)
1506. (A)
1507. (B)
1508. (D)
1509. (C)
1510. (B)
1511. (D)
1512. (B)
1513. (A)
1514. (A)
1515. (C)
1516. (A)
1517. (C)
1518. (C)
1519. (A)
1520. (B)
1521. (D)
1522. (B)
1523. (D)
1524. (A)
1525. (B)
1526. (A)
1527. (D)
1528. (C)
1529. (C)
1530. (A)
1531. (C)
1532. (A)
1533. (B)
1534. (A)
1535. (B)
1536. (A)
1537. (D)
1538. (A)
1539. (D)
1540. (B)
1541. (C)
1542. (C)
1543. (C)
1544. (A)
1545. (A)
1546. (B)
1547. (B)
1548. (C)
1549. (A)
1550. (D)
1551. (C)
1552. (A)
1553. (A)
1554. (C)
1555. (D)
1556. (?)
1557. (B)
1558. (C)
1559. (C)
1560. (D)
1561. (B)
1562. (D)
1563. (B)
1564. (A)
1565. (C)
1566. (A)
1567. (A)
1568. (A)
1569. (D)
1570. (C)
1571. (B)
1572. (D)
1573. (A)
1574. (B)
1575. (B)
1576. (D)
1577. (D)
1578. (C)
1579. (A)
1580. (D)
1581. (B)
1582. (A)
1583. (D)
1584. (D)
1585. (D)
1586. (A)
1587. (C)
1588. (B)
1589. (D)
1590. (A)
1591. (A)

1592. (B)
1593. (A)
1594. (C)
1595. (B)
1596. (D)
1597. (D)
1598. (A)
1599. (A)
1600. (B)
1601. (C)
1602. (A)
1603. (A)
1604. (D)
1605. (A)
1606. (A)
1607. (C)
1608. (B)
1609. (B)
1610. (A)
1611. (B)
1612. (A)
1613. (C)
1614. (A)
1615. (D)
1616. (A)
1617. (C)
1618. (C)
1619. (A)
1620. (C)
1621. (D)
1622. (B)
1623. (A)
1624. (C)
1625. (A)
1626. (D)
1627. (B)
1628. (C)
1629. (A)
1630. (A)
1631. (C)
1632. (B)
1633. (A)
1634. (B)
1635. (A)
1636. (D)
1637. (C)
1638. (B)
1639. (A)
1640. (C)
1641. (A)
1642. (A)
1643. (D)
1644. (B)
1645. (C)
1646. (D)
1647. (B)
1648. (A)
1649. (B)
1650. (B)
1651. (C)
1652. (A)
1653. (D)
1654. (B)
1655. (A)
1656. (D)
1657. (B)
1658. (C)
1659. (B)
1660. (D)
1661. (C)
1662. (A)
1663. (A)
1664. (D)
1665. (D)
1666. (C)
1667. (B)
1668. (A)
1669. (C)
1670. (D)
1671. (B)
1672. (D)
1673. (D)
1674. (D)
1675. (A)
1676. (A)
1677. (B)
1678. (A)
1679. (C)
1680. (D)
1681. (D)
1682. (C)
1683. (B)
1684. (A)
1685. (A)
1686. (V)
1687. (A)
1688. (A)
1689. (B)
1690. (C)
1691. (A)
1692. (B)
1693. (D)
1694. (B)
1695. (A)
1696. (D)
1697. (A)
1698. (D)
1699. (C)
1700. (C)
1701. (A)
1702. (C)
1703. (A)
1704. (D)
1705. (D)
1706. (B)
1707. (C)
1708. (A)
1709. (B)
1710. (A)
1711. (A)
1712. (D)
1713. (D)
1714. (D)
1715. (A)
1716. (B)
1717. (D)
1718. (A)
1719. (C)
1720. (D)
1721. (B)
1722. (C)
1723. (A)
1724. (D)
1725. (C)
1726. (B)
1727. (A)
1728. (A)
1729. (C)
1730. (D)
1731. (C)
1732. (A)
1733. (C)
1734. (D)
1735. (B)
1736. (C)
1737. (A)
1738. (C)
1739. (A)
1740. (D)
1741. (C)
1742. (D)
1743. (C)
1744. (D)
1745. (C)
1746. (D)
1747. (A)
1748. (A)
1749. (B)
1750. (A)
1751. (C)
1752. (B)
1753. (D)
1754. (D)
1755. (A)
1756. (A)
1757. (B)
1758. (C)
1759. (A)
1760. (A)
1761. (D)
1762. (A)
1763. (A)
1764. (C)
1765. (B)
1766. (B)
1767. (A)
1768. (B)
1769. (A)
1770. (C)
1771. (A)
1772. (D)
1773. (A)
1774. (C)
1775. (C)
1776. (A)
1777. (C)
1778. (D)
1779. (B)
1780. (A)
1781. (C)
1782. (A)
1783. (D)
1784. (B)
1785. (C)
1786. (A)
1787. (A)
1788. (C)
1789. (B)
1790. (A)
1791. (B)
1792. (A)
1793. (D)
1794. (C)
1795. (B)
1796. (A)
1797. (C)
1798. (A)
1799. (A)
1800. (D)
1801. (B)
1802. (C)
1803. (D)
1804. (B)
1805. (A)
1806. (B)
1807. (B)
1808. (C)
1809. (A)
1810. (D)
1811. (B)
1812. (A)
1813. (D)
1814. (B)
1815. (C)

Chapter 3B: Biotechnology and Microbiology

1. (B)
2. (B)
3. (C)
4. (A)
5. (B)
6. (C)
7. (D)
8. (B)
9. (C)
10. (D)
11. (C)
12. (C)
13. (C)
14. (C)
15. (C)
16. (A)
17. (C)
18. (A)
19. (C)
20. (C)
21. (C)
22. (B)
23. (D)
24. (B)
25. (A)
26. (A)
27. (B)
28. (A)
29. (B)
30. (B)
31. (D)
32. (C)
33. (C)
34. (C)
35. (B)
36. (B)
37. (B)
38. (C)
39. (A)
40. (A)
41. (A)
42. (B)
43. (D)
44. (A)
45. (B)
46. (C)
47. (C)
48. (A)
49. (C)
50. (D)
51. (B)
52. (A)
53. (C)
54. (A)
55. (C)
56. (B)
57. (D)
58. (B)
59. (C)
60. (C)
61. (A)
62. (B)
63. (A)
64. (C)
65. (B)
66. (A)
67. (C)
68. (A)
69. (D)
70. (C)
71. (C)
72. (D)
73. (C)
74. (A)
75. (C)
76. (D)
77. (C)
78. (C)
79. (B)
80. (C)
81. (D)
82. (D)
83. (B)
84. (D)
85. (B)
86. (C)
87. (D)
88. (A)
89. (D)
90. (D)
91. (A)
92. (B)
93. (B)
94. (C)
95. (D)
96. (C)
97. (C)
98. (D)
99. (C)
100. (C)
101. (D)
102. (C)
103. (A)
104. (D)
105. (A)
106. (A)
107. (D)
108. (C)
109. (B)
110. (B)
111. (A)
112. (C)
113. (C)
114. (C)
115. (C)
116. (B)
117. (A)
118. (C)
119. (A)
120. (C)
121. (B)
122. (B)
123. (C)
124. (B)
125. (B)
126. (A)
127. (B)
128. (A)
129. (D)
130. (B)
131. (A)
132. (A)
133. (B)
134. (C)
135. (C)
136. (D)
137. (C)
138. (C)
139. (C)
140. (A)
141. (C)
142. (C)
143. (D)
144. (D)
145. (D)
146. (D)
147. (D)
148. (A)
149. (A)
150. (A)
151. (B)
152. (D)
153. (A)
154. (C)
155. (A)
156. (A)
157. (A)
158. (A)
159. (A)
160. (C)
161. (A)
162. (A)
163. (A)
164. (A)
165. (A)
166. (D)
167. (A)
168. (C)
169. (C)
170. (C)
171. (A)
172. (D)
173. (C)
174. (A)
175. (A)
176. (A)
177. (A)
178. (A)
179. (D)
180. (A)
181. (B)
182. (A)
183. (A)
184. (A)
185. (A)
186. (D)
187. (C)
188. (A)
189. (A)
190. (A)
191. (A)
192. (A)
193. (D)
194. (B)
195. (C)
196. (B)
197. (C)
198. (A)
199. (A)
200. (A)
201. (D)
202. (C)
203. (C)
204. (A)
205. (C)
206. (B)
207. (D)
208. (D)
209. (C)
210. (C)
211. (A)
212. (B)
213. (A)
214. (A)
215. (B)
216. (B)

217. (B)
218. (B)
219. (D)
220. (D)
221. (D)
222. (A)
223. (A)
224. (A)
225. (C)
226. (B)
227. (B)
228. (A)
229. (D)
230. (B)
231. (C)
232. (A)
233. (C)
234. (A)
235. (B)
236. (D)
237. (A)
238. (D)
239. (C)
240. (C)
241. (B)
242. (C)
243. (C)
244. (A)
245. (B)
246. (C)
247. (C)
248. (A)
249. (C)
250. (A)
251. (D)
252. (C)
253. (B)
254. (C)
255. (C)
256. (A)
257. (A)
258. (A)
259. (D)
260. (D)
261. (C)
262. (B)
263. (A)
264. (C)
265. (C)
266. (B)
267. (D)
268. (A)
269. (A)
270. (A)
271. (D)
272. (B)
273. (D)
274. (A)
275. (A)
276. (B)
277. (D)
278. (B)
279. (D)
280. (B)
281. (B)
282. (A)
283. (D)
284. (B)
285. (D)
286. (C)
287. (B)
288. (D)
289. (A)
290. (C)
291. (A)
292. (D)
293. (D)
294. (A)
295. (A)
296. (A)
297. (A)
298. (D)
299. (D)
300. (D)
301. (A)
302. (C)
303. (C)
304. (B)
305. (A)
306. (C)
307. (A)
308. (C)
309. (C)
310. (D)
311. (C)
312. (A)
313. (A)
314. (B)
315. (A)
316. (A)
317. (C)
318. (A)
319. (C)
320. (C)
321. (C)
322. (A)
323. (D)
324. (B)
325. (D)
326. (D)
327. (C)
328. (C)
329. (D)
330. (C)
331. (D)
332. (D)
333. (A)
334. (D)
335. (B)
336. (C)
337. (C)
338. (D)
339. (D)
340. (B)
341. (C)
342. (B)
343. (C)
344. (C)
345. (C)
346. (B)
347. (C)
348. (D)
349. (D)
350. (B)
351. (B)
352. (C)
353. (B)
354. (B)
355. (B)
356. (D)
357. (C)
358. (D)
359. (B)
360. (C)
361. (C)
362. (C)
363. (A)
364. (B)
365. (C)
366. (D)
367. (B)
368. (B)
369. (A)
370. (D)
371. (C)
372. (B)
373. (D)
374. (C)
375. (C)
376. (B)
377. (B)
378. (C)
379. (C)
380. (D)
381. (B)
382. (C)
383. (A)
384. (A)
385. (B)
386. (B)
387. (D)
388. (B)
389. (C)
390. (D)
391. (B)
392. (D)
393. (C)
394. (D)
395. (D)
396. (B)
397. (C)
398. (A)
399. (D)
400. (D)
401. (B)
402. (B)
403. (D)
404. (B)
405. (A)
406. (C)
407. (C)
408. (B)
409. (C)
410. (B)
411. (B)
412. (C)
413. (D)
414. (A)
415. (D)
416. (B)
417. (D)
418. (D)
419. (D)
420. (D)
421. (D)
422. (A)
423. (B)
424. (B)
425. (D)
426. (D)
427. (C)
428. (B)
429. (C)
430. (C)
431. (B)
432. (C)
433. (B)
434. (C)
435. (D)
436. (C)
437. (B)
438. (B)
439. (B)
440. (C)
441. (B)
442. (B)
443. (D)
444. (B)

445. (C)
446. (D)
447. (B)
448. (B)
449. (C)
450. (D)
451. (C)
452. (A)
453. (B)
454. (C)
455. (A)
456. (C)
457. (C)
458. (C)
459. (D)
460. (B)
461. (D)
462. (C)
463. (A)
464. (D)
465. (D)
466. (B)
467. (B)
468. (D)
469. (C)
470. (A)
471. (D)
472. (B)
473. (B)
474. (C)
475. (C)
476. (D)
477. (A)
478. (B)
479. (D)
480. (D)
481. (A)
482. (B)
483. (B)
484. (D)
485. (A)
486. (D)
487. (C)
488. (B)
489. (C)
490. (C)
491. (D)
492. (D)
493. (D)
494. (C)
495. (D)
496. (C)
497. (B)
498. (B)
499. (B)
500. (A)
501. (D)
502. (A)
503. (D)
504. (B)
505. (C)
506. (A)
507. (D)
508. (B)
509. (D)
510. (C)
511. (B)
512. (C)
513. (B)
514. (B)
515. (D)
516. (B)
517. (B)
518. (D)
519. (A)
520. (D)
521. (B)
522. (D)
523. (B)
524. (B)
525. (B)
526. (D)
527. (A)
528. (D)
529. (B)
530. (C)
531. (D)
532. (B)
533. (B)
534. (C)
535. (A)
536. (B)
537. (D)
538. (B)
539. (B)
540. (A)
541. (B)
542. (A)
543. (B)
544. (B)
545. (D)
546. (A)
547. (C)
548. (D)
549. (A)
550. (C)
551. (A)
552. (D)
553. (A)
554. (B)
555. (C)
556. (B)
557. (D)
558. (B)
559. (D)
560. (D)
561. (C)
562. (B)
563. (A)
564. (A)
565. (B)
566. (A)
567. (B)
568. (B)
569. (C)
570. (A)
571. (C)
572. (B)
573. (C)
574. (A)
575. (A)
576. (D)
577. (C)
578. (C)
579. (A)
580. (C)
581. (B)
582. (D)
583. (C)
584. (D)
585. (B)
586. (C)
587. (A)
588. (B)
589. (C)
590. (C)
591. (C)
592. (D)
593. (C)
594. (A)
595. (C)
596. (C)
597. (D)
598. (C)
599. (D)
600. (C)
601. (C)
602. (D)
603. (C)
604. (B)
605. (D)
606. (C)
607. (B)
608. (C)
609. (B)
610. (B)
611. (A)
612. (D)
613. (D)
614. (A)
615. (D)
616. (A)
617. (D)
618. (B)
619. (C)
620. (A)
621. (C)
622. (D)
623. (D)
624. (A)
625. (B)
626. (C)
627. (D)
628. (D)
629. (B)
630. (A)
631. (C)
632. (B)
633. (A)
634. (D)
635. (B)
636. (A)
637. (D)
638. (A)
639. (D)
640. (A)
641. (C)
642. (A)
643. (A)
644. (B)
645. (B)
646. (A)
647. (A)
648. (B)
649. (C)
650. (D)
651. (A)
652. (A)
653. (D)
654. (C)
655. (C)
656. (A)
657. (B)
658. (D)
659. (C)
660. (D)
661. (B)
662. (D)
663. (A)
664. (D)
665. (C)
666. (A)
667. (C)
668. (C)
669. (B)
670. (A)
671. (D)
672. (D)

673. (A)
674. (C)
675. (D)
676. (D)
677. (B)
678. (A)
679. (C)
680. (B)
681. (D)
682. (B)
683. (A)
684. (C)
685. (D)
686. (A)
687. (D)
688. (C)
689. (B)
690. (C)
691. (C)
692. (B)
693. (D)
694. (A)
695. (C)
696. (A)
697. (B)
698. (A)
699. (B)
700. (C)
701. (B)
702. (B)
703. (A)
704. (C)
705. (A)
706. (C)
707. (B)
708. (A)
709. (A)
710. (C)
711. (A)
712. (B)
713. (C)
714. (C)
715. (B)
716. (A)
717. (B)
718. (A)
719. (D)
720. (B)
721. (A)
722. (B)
723. (D)
724. (C)
725. (B)
726. (A)
727. (A)
728. (B)
729. (C)
730. (A)
731. (C)
732. (A)
733. (B)
734. (D)
735. (A)
736. (B)
737. (A)
738. (D)
739. (B)
740. (A)
741. (A)
742. (C)
743. (D)
744. (C)
745. (B)
746. (A)
747. (B)
748. (A)
749. (C)
750. (A)
751. (B)
752. (A)
753. (C)
754. (B)
755. (A)
756. (B)
757. (A)
758. (C)
759. (B)
760. (A)
761. (C)
762. (C)
763. (A)
764. (D)
765. (C)
766. (B)
767. (A)
768. (B)
769. (D)
770. (A)
771. (A)
772. (B)
773. (C)
774. (C)
775. (A)
776. (C)
777. (B)
778. (D)
779. (A)
780. (B)
781. (C)
782. (A)
783. (B)
784. (A)
785. (B)
786. (C)
787. (D)
788. (B)
789. (D)
790. (C)
791. (A)
792. (C)
793. (D)
794. (D)
795. (C)
796. (A)
797. (C)
798. (A)
799. (B)
800. (C)
801. (A)
802. (C)
803. (A)
804. (B)
805. (A)
806. (D)
807. (A)
808. (A)
809. (B)
810. (C)
811. (A)
812. (A)
813. (C)
814. (D)
815. (A)
816. (C)
817. (D)
818. (A)
819. (B)
820. (A)
821. (C)
822. (A)
823. (B)
824. (A)
825. (A)
826. (C)
827. (D)
828. (A)
829. (A)
830. (C)
831. (B)
832. (B)
833. (C)
834. (D)
835. (A)
836. (C)
837. (A)
838. (B)
839. (A)
840. (C)
841. (B)
842. (A)
843. (C)
844. (D)
845. (C)
846. (D)
847. (A)
848. (B)
849. (C)
850. (A)
851. (C)
852. (B)
853. (A)
854. (A)
855. (B)
856. (C)
857. (B)
858. (C)
859. (A)
860. (B)
861. (C)
862. (D)
863. (C)
864. (B)
865. (D)
866. (A)
867. (B)
868. (A)
869. (C)
870. (C)
871. (B)
872. (C)
873. (A)
874. (D)
875. (C)
876. (B)
877. (D)
878. (C)
879. (A)
880. (D)
881. (A)
882. (C)
883. (A)
884. (A)
885. (B)
886. (A)
887. (B)
888. (A)
889. (C)
890. (A)
891. (A)
892. (C)
893. (A)
894. (B)
895. (D)
896. (A)
897. (B)
898. (A)
899. (C)
900. (A)

901. (A)
902. (C)
903. (A)
904. (C)
905. (B)
906. (A)
907. (A)
908. (A)
909. (B)
910. (D)
911. (A)
912. (C)
913. (A)
914. (B)
915. (D)
916. (A)
917. (C)
918. (A)
919. (C)
920. (A)
921. (B)
922. (C)
923. (A)
924. (B)
925. (A)
926. (C)
927. (A)
928. (D)
929. (A)
930. (C)
931. (C)
932. (A)
933. (C)
934. (B)
935. (A)
936. (B)
937. (A)
938. (C)
939. (B)
940. (A)
941. (C)
942. (A)
943. (B)
944. (A)
945. (C)
946. (B)
947. (A)
948. (D)
949. (A)
950. (C)
951. (A)
952. (B)
953. (A)
954. (C)
955. (D)
956. (D)
957. (A)
958. (B)
959. (C)
960. (A)
961. (D)
962. (A)
963. (C)
964. (A)
965. (C)
966. (C)
967. (A)
968. (C)
969. (C)
970. (A)
971. (C)
972. (B)
973. (C)
974. (D)
975. (A)
976. (C)
977. (D)
978. (C)
979. (B)
980. (A)
981. (B)
982. (C)
983. (B)
984. (A)
985. (B)
986. (C)
987. (D)
988. (A)
989. (C)
990. (C)
991. (A)
992. (C)
993. (B)
994. (C)
995. (B)
996. (B)
997. (C)
998. (A)
999. (C)
1000. (C)
1001. (D)
1002. (A)
1003. (A)
1004. (C)
1005. (D)
1006. (A)
1007. (B)
1008. (D)
1009. (B)
1010. (D)
1011. (B)
1012. (A)
1013. (C)
1014. (C)
1015. (B)
1016. (D)
1017. (C)
1018. (C)
1019. (D)
1020. (A)
1021. (B)
1022. (A)
1023. (D)
1024. (B)
1025. (D)
1026. (D)
1027. (C)
1028. (A)
1029. (A)
1030. (B)
1031. (D)
1032. (A)
1033. (A)
1034. (A)
1035. (A)
1036. (C)
1037. (C)
1038. (A)
1039. (B)
1040. (A)
1041. (A)
1042. (C)
1043. (C)
1044. (B)
1045. (D)
1046. (D)
1047. (A)
1048. (A)
1049. (A)
1050. (A)
1051. (D)
1052. (A)
1053. (C)
1054. (B)
1055. (C)
1056. (B)
1057. (A)
1058. (A)
1059. (A)
1060. (A)
1061. (A)
1062. (A)
1063. (C)
1064. (B)
1065. (C)
1066. (A)
1067. (A)
1068. (B)
1069. (B)
1070. (C)
1071. (A)
1072. (D)
1073. (C)
1074. (D)
1075. (A)
1076. (A)
1077. (A)
1078. (B)
1079. (B)
1080. (B)
1081. (A)
1082. (B)
1083. (A)
1084. (B)
1085. (A)
1086. (A)
1087. (D)
1088. (A)
1089. (A)
1090. (B)
1091. (C)
1092. (A)
1093. (A)
1094. (C)
1095. (A)
1096. (A)
1097. (C)
1098. (B)
1099. (A)
1100. (A)
1101. (A)
1102. (A)
1103. (B)
1104. (B)
1105. (A)
1106. (D)
1107. (C)
1108. (A)
1109. (A)
1110. (A)
1111. (D)
1112. (A)
1113. (C)

www.ingramcontent.com/pod-product-compliance
Ingram Content Group UK Ltd.
Pitfield, Milton Keynes, MK11 3LW, UK
UKHW061536190726
13845UKWH00005B/120